# Health Informatics

For further volumes:
http://www.springer.com/series/1114

This series is directed to healthcare professionals leading the transformation of healthcare by using information and knowledge. For over 20 years, Health Informatics has offered a broad range of titles: some address specific professions such as nursing, medicine, and health administration; others cover special areas of practice such as trauma and radiology; still other books in the series focus on interdisciplinary issues, such as the computer based patient record, electronic health records, and networked healthcare systems. Editors and authors, eminent experts in their fields, offer their accounts of innovations in health informatics. Increasingly, these accounts go beyond hardware and software to address the role of information in influencing the transformation of healthcare delivery systems around the world. The series also increasingly focuses on the users of the information and systems: the organizational, behavioral, and societal changes that accompany the diffusion of information technology in health services environments.

Developments in healthcare delivery are constant; in recent years, bioinformatics has emerged as a new field in health informatics to support emerging and ongoing developments in molecular biology. At the same time, further evolution of the field of health informatics is reflected in the introduction of concepts at the macro or health systems delivery level with major national initiatives related to electronic health records (EHR), data standards, and public health informatics.

These changes will continue to shape health services in the twenty-first century. By making full and creative use of the technology to tame data and to transform information, Health Informatics will foster the development and use of new knowledge in healthcare.

Charlotte A. Weaver • Marion J. Ball
George R. Kim • Joan M. Kiel

Editors

# Healthcare Information Management Systems

## Cases, Strategies, and Solutions

Fourth Edition

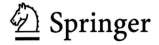 Springer

Charlotte A. Weaver
Gentiva Health Services
Atlanta, Georgia
USA

George R. Kim
Division of Health Sciences Informatics
The Johns Hopkins University
Baltimore, Maryland
USA

Marion J. Ball
Healthcare Informatics
IBM Research
Baltimore, Maryland
USA

Joan M. Kiel
Duquesne University
Pittsburgh, Pennsylvania
USA

ISSN 1431-1917                     ISSN 2197-3741    (electronic)
Health Informatics
ISBN 978-3-319-20764-3       ISBN 978-3-319-20765-0    (eBook)
DOI 10.1007/978-3-319-20765-0

Library of Congress Control Number: 2015950749

Springer Cham Heidelberg New York Dordrecht London

Springer International Publishing AG Switzerland is part of Springer Science+Business Media
(www.springer.com)

*To John and Trish, dear colleagues and cherished friends throughout it all; and as always – to my much treasured son, Kevin.*
Charlotte A. Weaver

*To Dr. Joseph Jasinski who has been my guiding light, advisor, and supporter for the past several years.*
Marion J. Ball

*To my co-editors and co-authors in this effort, in gratitude for the honor of participation, with special acknowledgment to Marion and John Ball, dear friends and mentors.*
George R. Kim

*To Thomas D. Kiel, M.D.*
Joan M. Kiel

# Foreword to the Fourth Edition

In the previous edition of *Healthcare Information Management Systems* (2004), the late Morris F. Collen, MD, FACMI (1914–2014), Director Emeritus of Kaiser Permanente Medical Care's Division of Research and pioneer/historian of healthcare informatics, noted that "the hospital and its associated information system is the most complex organizational structure created by people." He concluded it should be no surprise that healthcare information management systems lagged those used in non-healthcare industries and cited the continual advances in care and technology, the "vicissitudes of healthcare legislation," and the need for intensive training and re-training of healthcare professionals who use information systems as contributors to that lag. Still, he firmly believed that efficient information management systems are essential for high-quality, cost-efficient patient care.

A decade later, the US healthcare industry finds itself redesigning healthcare to achieve the Institute for Healthcare Improvement's Triple Aim of:

- Improving the patient experience of care (including quality and satisfaction)
- Improving the health of populations
- Reducing the per capita cost of healthcare

These, and the goal of building a continuously learning healthcare system, reinforce Dr. Collen's belief that efficient and effective information management systems are necessary to implement effective and efficient care.

Convergent with this vision is the growing, diffusing ecosystem of pervasive data, analytics and Big Data techniques, and personal/social technologies for capturing and managing electronic health data:

- Increasing adoption of electronic health records and health information exchange
- Common use of wearable and mobile technologies and infrastructures that generate, collect, store, and share many forms of personal and exogenous data
- Active research, development, and deployment of platforms, analytics and cognitive computing for processing and visualizing population data for prediction and planning

- Focus of standards development organizations and regulatory agencies on improving interoperability to connect systems and measure outcomes

The turbulent confluence of healthcare redesign and IT innovation is forming the foundation for achieving the Triple Aim. The chapters of this book provide current snapshots of active work in this process from many facets: technical, organizational, workflow, and policy.

To quote computer scientist Alan Kay, "The best way to predict the future is to invent it."

Shahram Ebadollahi, PhD
Vice President
Innovation & Chief Science Officer
IBM Watson Health
New York, USA

# Preface

This is the 4th edition of *Healthcare Information Management Systems*, a book that started in 1991 as a practical guide to preparing clinicians and healthcare organizations for electronic health record adoption. With each edition, the scope has evolved and broadened to include other health information technologies, with shared experiences of healthcare redesign and the role of IT from multiple perspectives. The 3rd edition (2004) included descriptions of comparative experiences from Sweden, Malaysia, Australia, and France. The 4th edition refocuses its scope to the United States, with the aim of capturing a bold and honest description of the current state of electronic health record (EHR) technologies in acute and primary care settings. In the decade since the 3rd edition, EHRs have achieved widespread US adoption in response to legislation and regulatory policy that linked meaningful health IT use to payment incentives and reimbursement penalties. As the country has reached a "tipping point" in EHR adoption under Meaningful Use, agencies, healthcare organizations, and clinicians have not found anticipated gains in efficiency, quality, and costs. Rather, there has been frustration, dissatisfaction, and growing concerns regarding the impact of IT use on patient safety and health outcomes and a not-so-quiet rebellion in the ranks of frontline clinicians. Many informaticists and clinicians suggest that a technology sea change is needed with a second generation of EHRs developed on twenty-first century architectures that more closely match the flexibility and power of mobile and web-based applications available in the general marketplace. And a number of these new technologies and solutions are included here.

Interoperability and data sharing has become another hot topic that has spilled over into the political and public arenas. Starting in 2014, it became not unusual to find stories in the New York Times or Wall Street Journal on the limitations of data sharing of EHR systems, as the lay public have also become engaged users of these medical record systems. This increasing involvement of consumers and other key stakeholders in healthcare is a major theme threaded throughout this 4th edition. Payers, clinicians, the quality and safety, community, the federal government, and consumers are all mobilizing the healthcare industry to achieve the Institute of Healthcare Improvement's Triple Aim: to improve the experience of care, to improve the health of populations, and to reduce the per capita costs of care. The impact of this active engagement has been the steady growth of health IT development/adoption to standardize and connect care and to capture data on healthcare performance, quality, and safety.

Given the growing turmoil over these EHR usability issues, the editors of this book saw an imperative to focus on this current state of health IT as a starting point for renewed dialogue and discourse on health IT as a vital component to enabling healthcare redesign in the United States. Accordingly, as we planned this 4th edition, we made the decision not to keep any of the chapters from the 3rd edition, but rather to build an entirely new book; and thus, in comparing the 3rd and 4th editions, the reader will not find any chapter topics or authors the same. This decision is a testament to the profound changes that have occurred over the past decade in technology and its use and place in every citizen's daily life throughout the world, the economic imperatives for reduction in healthcare costs, and the impact that these two forces have had on healthcare systems. And specifically for the United States, as the sole industrial country that has a "fee-for-service" (FFS) reimbursement structure for its core healthcare commerce, there are unique and singular challenges. At the heart of this structure is the misalignment of incentives, paying on the basis of the more that you do, the more you are paid. However, as many of these chapters detail, this payment structure is on the threshold of changing. As the payer of over 50 % of medical bills in the United States, the Centers for Medicare and Medicaid Services (CMS) is driving fundamental change by linking payment to quality measures, termed "value-based payment" models. Under these new models, health outcomes, preventative care, and population health are financially rewarded. Many project that these payment changes will be in place as early as 2018. And in fact, the partnerships that are happening today under the banner of Accountable Care Organizations are all pilots for this new world of risk-based, value-based, bundled payment models that shift care to wellness and prevention, and away from costly acute care and out into community and home.

The 4th edition is organized into four parts. Part I focuses on the current state of health information technology with respect to its historical evolution. In Chap. 1, McCallie looks at clinical decision support; In Chap. 6, Koppel traces the journey and consequences of Meaningful Use implementation; and in Chaps. 7 and 8 Edmunds, Peddicord and Frisse provide masterful expositions on why interoperability and data sharing are difficult and on the history of key health IT policies. Sittig and colleagues map out the functionality that clinicians have the right to expect from EHR systems in Chap. 2, while Ingram presents the vendor developer's perspective in Chap. 3. Payne provides a view of the CMIO's role in an academic, multiple-site setting that uses multiple EHR systems; Kim, Hudson, and Miller outline a multidisciplinary, clinical team perspective on EHR system functionality needed for patient care and its coordination.

Part II, "the evolving state of health IT: reinventing care, roles and connections," builds on this current state with solutions and strategies emerging from new care delivery models of care, new leadership roles, and IT infrastructure needed to support these care delivery changes. Unertl, Holden, and Lorenzi (Chap. 9) map out their approach to building in usability throughout systems lifecycle; Danis references human factor engineering science in usability for wellness system design (Chap. 10). New care delivery models are addressed in Chaps. 11, 12, 15, 16, and 17 drawing from examples from Kaiser-Permanente (O'Brien and Mattison); Grundy and Hodach on the patient centered medical home (PCMH) initiative; Care Partners Plus (Minniti and colleagues); and Johns Hopkins (Gibbons and Shaikh). We are indebted to Reynolds and Jones for taking on the thorny issue of how healthcare gets paid for (Chap. 14); Andrew Watson for giving his perspective as a practicing surgeon on how technology has digitized every aspect of his work.

The go-forward perspective is introduced in Part III with chapters that explore new areas in the science of patient safety (Rosen et al., Chap. 18); new virtual training environments for healthcare professionals and students (Parvati, Chap. 19); standards, architecture, and infrastructure needed to support a viable and usable Personal Health Record (Yasnoff, Chap. 20); and the new emerging technologies and care delivery models that support person-centric care (Hsueh, Chang and Ramakrishnan, Chap. 21; Zhu and Cahan, Chap. 22); and consumers' choice in care utilization (Yuen-Reed and Mojsilović, Chap. 23). Part III's chapters report on current innovative initiatives in the early conceptual stages of development and testing that are directed at key areas of transformative change.

In Part IV, we look to the future of health information management systems. We are honored to have Dr. Lawrence Weed (and son) (Chap. 26), longtime pioneer and innovator in medical records, provide a guidepost for transforming medical education and the patient record through the use of information technology to couple knowledge to assessment and treatment decision making.

In Chap. 28, McCallie presents the new and emerging technologies for clinical decision support (CDS) with case study examples that offer hope that we will soon have trustworthy and helpful support tools at the fingertips for clinicians. Fackler (Chap. 29) brings his experiences as a pediatric intensivist and vendor developer to present examples of new application programming interface (API) technologies and applications that are just entering today's marketplace. Silva and Ball describe a CAS (Complex Adaptive System) architecture that holds promise for health IT in Chap. 27. And in Chaps. 30, 31, and, 32, a powerhouse of IBM scientists and clinician researchers look at uses of new technologies that are being tested within the IBM laboratories that include wearable sensors for patient-generated health data, data-driven analytics, and cognitive computing to create an active patient-centered learning healthcare system. The book closes (Chap. 33) with a look ahead by Robert Greenes, a leader in the field of informatics, detailing how new architectures for health information technology, management and disruptive technologies, can and will help to overcome current constraints to transform healthcare.

The authors contributing to this book have all done so in the spirit of wanting to help improve upon the current state challenges. The informatics field is made up of committed and dedicated souls that have made this their life's work with the goal of improving the patient's experience, helping the helpers, and taking waste and error out of our healthcare system. We offer this 4th edition of Health Information Management with that same commitment and hope that it will contribute to taking us into a healthcare system that delivers value, is a pleasure to work within, and relieves the taxpayers' burden.

Atlanta, GA, USA                                              Charlotte A. Weaver
Baltimore, MD, USA                                                 Marion J. Ball
Baltimore, MD, USA                                                George R. Kim
Pittsburgh, PA, USA                                                 Joan M. Kiel

# Acknowledgments

This 4th edition emerged from conversations with numerous clinical and informatics colleagues throughout 2014, but most notably from the opportunity to participate in the SHARP-C Project Advisory Board and engage in the many critical discussions that ensued over 2012–2014. So a big thank you to Ted Shortliffe for ensuring broad disciplinary representation in the SHARP-C Advisory Board, and for the excellent leadership and open-mindedness of Jaijie Zhang as SHARP-C's project leader (www.sharpc.org). Across these past four years, the general themes in these discussions focused on the failed promise of electronic health record systems as adoption levels by healthcare organizations reached ubiquitous levels throughout acute and ambulatory care providers. Many of the participants in these conversations are contributing authors in this book. We owe a special thank you to Dr. Andrew Watson, Director of the Center for Connect Medicine at the University of Pittsburgh Medical Center, who hosted a 2-day think tank session for the planning of this book.

We owe a particular debt to Gentiva Health Services, and specifically, Rod Windley and Tony Strange as its executive leaders, who fully supported Charlotte Weaver in her undertaking of this book. Many colleagues behind the scenes also contributed their time, mentoring and critical ideas. We are indebted to, Dr. Shahram Ebadollahi whose inspiration and challenge helped bring about this volume, Dean Linda McCauley for her insightful critiques, and Dr. Robert Herrera who gave us an insider's view of the primary care physician's average day. We also greatly appreciate Jane Snowdon for her professional coaching, advice, and guidance; to Krysia Hudson and Teresa Hancock, who were always standing by to help in any way!!

Most importantly, we thank the authors and co-authors of the chapters that make up this 4th edition book for their hard work, critical thinking, and commitment to capturing the realities of our current state and the promise of the new emerging technologies and policy changes that are erupting on the present-day scene. Their collective voices bring optimism that we will yet see the promise of information technology more fully realized in our healthcare system.

We cannot close these acknowledgments without a warm salute to Grant Weston our editor from Springer-Verlag for his unflinching support of this 4th edition of the Health Information Management series. And to Tracy Marton, our developmental editor, we thank you for your unflagging help in managing all the details, permissions, authors' forms, and for being a partner with this editor team every step of the way!

Charlotte A. Weaver
Marion J. Ball
George R. Kim
Joan M. Kiel

# Contents

# Contributors

**Marion J. Ball, Ed.D** Healthcare and Life Sciences Institute, IBM Research, Johns Hopkins University, Baltimore, MD, USA

**Sasha Ballen, MS** Advanced Comprehensive Care Organization, LLC, Yardley, PA, USA

**Thomas R. Blue, BS, PhD** Research, CarePartners Plus, LLC, Horsham, PA, USA

**Amos Cahan, MD** IBM T.J. Watson Research Center, Yorktown Heights, NY, USA

**Howard Carolan, MPH, MBA** Armstrong Institute of Patient Safety and Quality, Johns Hopkins University School of Medicine, Baltimore, MD, USA

**Henry Chang, PhD** Healthcare Informatics Group, IBM T.J. Watson Research Center, Yorktown Heights, NY, USA

**Frances A. Ciamacco, BS, MS, RHIA** Office of Ethics and Compliance, UPMC, Pittsburgh, PA, USA

**Catalina M. Danis, PhD** Health Informatics Research, IBM T.J. Watson Research Center, Yorktown Heights, NY, USA

**Parvati Dev, PhD** Innovation in Learning, Inc., Los Altos Hills, CA, USA

**Murthy V. Devarakonda, PhD** IBM T.J. Watson Research Center, Yorktown Heights, NY, USA

**Aaron S. Dietz, PhD** Armstrong Institute for Patient Safety and Quality, Johns Hopkins University School of Medicine, Baltimore, MD, USA

**Cynthia Dwyer, BSN** Armstrong Institute for Patient Safety and Quality, Johns Hopkins University School of Medicine, Baltimore, MD, USA

Surgical Intensive Care Unit/Intermediate Care Unit, The Johns Hopkins Hospital, Baltimore, MD, USA

**Shahram Ebadollahi, PhD** IBM Watson Health, Yorktown Heights, NY, USA

**Margo Edmunds, PhD** Department of Evidence Generation and Translation, AcademyHealth, Washington, DC, USA

**James Fackler, MD** Pediatric Anesthesiology and Critical Care Medicine, Johns Hopkins University School of Medicine, Baltimore, MD, USA

**Diane Freed, RN, MSN** Department of Quality, CarePartners Plus, LLC, Horsham, PA, USA

**Mark E. Frisse, MD, MS, MBA** Department of Biomedical Informatics, Vanderbilt University Medical Center, Nashville, TN, USA

**Michael Christopher Gibbons, MD, MPH** Medicine, Public Health and Health Informatics, Urban Health Institute, Johns Hopkins University, Baltimore, MA, USA

**Robert A. Greenes, MD, PhD** Department of Biomedical Informatics, Arizona State University and Mayo Clinic, Scottsdale, AZ, USA

**Paul H. Grundy, MD, MPH, IBM** IBM Industry Academy, IBM Corporation, Armonk, NY, USA

Department of Family and Preventive Medicine, University of Utah, Salt Lake City, UT, USA

**Mark Hagland, MS Journalism** Healthcare Informatics Magazine, Chicago, IL, USA

**Richard J. Hodach, MD, MPH, PhD, FACMQ** American Board of Medical Quality, Tacoma Park, MD, USA

**Richard J. Holden, PhD** Department of BioHealth Informatics, Indiana University School of Informatics and Computing, Indianapolis, IN, USA

**Pei-Yun Sabrina Hsueh, PhD** Healthcare Informatics Group, IBM T.J. Watson Research Center, Yorktown Heights, NY, USA

**Jianying Hu, PhD** Healthcare Analytics Research Group, IBM T.J. Watson Research Center, Yorktown Heights, NY, USA

**Krysia Warren Hudson, DNP, MSN, RN, BC** Department of Acute and Chronic Care, Johns Hopkins University School of Nursing, Baltimore, MD, USA

**James T. Ingram, MD, FACS** Greenway Health, Inc., Carrollton, GA, USA

**Christopher A. Jones, MHA** Quality and Informatics, Wake Forest Baptist Hospital, Area Health Education Center, Winston-Salem, NC, USA

**Joan M. Kiel, PhD, CHPS, MPhil, MPA** HIPAA & HMS Departments, University HIPAA Compliance, Health Management Systems, Duquesne University, Pittsburgh, PA, USA

**George R. Kim, MD** Division of Health Sciences Informatics and Armstrong Institute for Patient Safety and Quality, Johns Hopkins University School of Medicine, Baltimore, MD, USA

**Ross Koppel, PhD, FACMI** LDI Wharton School, University of Pennsylvania, Philadelphia, PA, USA

Department of Sociology, and Center for Clinical Epidemiology and Biostatistics, University of Pennsylvania, Philadelphia, PA, USA

**Christopher A. Longhurst, MD, MS** Division of Systems Medicine, Department of Pediatrics, Stanford University School of Medicine, Stanford, CA, USA

Information Services, Stanford Children's Hospital, Menlo Park, CA, USA

**Nancy M. Lorenzi, PhD, MA, MS** Department of Biomedical Informatics, Schools of Medicine and Nursing, Vanderbilt University, Nashville, TN, USA

**John E. Mattison, MD** Kaiser Permanente Southern California Region, Pasadena, CA, USA

**David P. McCallie Jr., MD** Medical Informatics, Cerner Corp, Kansas City, MO, USA

**Neil Mehta, MBBS, MS** Department of Education and Department of Medicine, Cleveland Clinic, Cleveland Clinic Lerner College of Medicine of Case Western Reserve University, Cleveland, OH, USA

**David L. Meyers, MD, FACEP** Department of Emergency Medicine, Sinai Hospital of Baltimore, Baltimore, MD, USA

**Colette Ann Miller, MSN, RNC-Nic** Baccalaureate Program, Johns Hopkins University School of Nursing, Baltimore, MD, USA

**Martha Jean Minniti, RN** Department of Product Development, CarePartners Plus, Horsham, PA, USA

**Aleksandra Mojsilović, PhD, EE** Data Science, IBM T.J. Watson Research Center, Yorktown Heights, NY, USA

**Ann O'Brien, RN, MSN, CPHIMS** Information Technology and National Patient Care Services, Kaiser Permanente, Oakland, CA, USA

**Thomas H. Payne, MD** Information Technology Services and Department of Medicine, University of Washington, Seattle, WA, USA

**Douglas Peddicord, PhD**  Washington Health Strategies Group, Washington, DC, USA

**Adam Perer, PhD**  Healthcare Analytics Research Group, IBM T.J. Watson Research Center, Yorktown Heights, NY, USA

**Peter J. Pronovost, MD, PhD**  Armstrong Institute for Patient Safety and Quality, Johns Hopkins University School of Medicine, Baltimore, MD, USA

Department of Anesthesiology and Critical Care Medicine, Johns Hopkins University School of Medicine, Joint Appointment in the School of Nursing, School of Medicine, Baltimore, MD, USA

Johns Hopkins Medicine, Baltimore, MD, USA

**Sreeram Ramakrishnan, PhD (Industrial Engineering)**  Wellness Ecosystems and Analytics, Taiwan Colloboratory, IBM T.J. Watson Research, Hawthorne, NY, USA

**Alan Ravitz, MS**  Healthcare, Research and Exploratory Development and Human Factors/Systems Integration, Applied Physics Laboratory, Johns Hopkins University, Laurel, MD, USA

**Harry L. Reynolds Jr.,**  Health Industry Transformation, IBM Global Healthcare and Life Sciences Industry, Durham, NC, USA

**Mark Romig, MD**  Armstrong Institute for Patient Safety and Quality, Johns Hopkins University School of Medicine, Baltimore, MD, USA

**Michael A. Rosen, PhD**  Armstrong Institute for Patient Safety and Quality, Johns Hopkins University School of Medicine, Baltimore, MD, USA

Bloomberg School of Public Health, Johns Hopkins University, Baltimore, MD, USA

**Elise Russo, MPH**  The Section of Health Services Research, Department of Medicine, Houston Veterans Affairs Center for Innovations in Quality, Effectiveness and Safety, Michael E. DeBakey VA Medical Center, Houston, TX, USA

**Adam Sapirstein, MD**  Division of Adult Critical Care Medicine, Johns Hopkins University School of Medicine, Baltimore, MD, USA

Armstrong Institute for Patient Safety and Quality, Johns Hopkins University School of Medicine, Baltimore, MD, USA

**Yahya Shaikh, MD, MPH**  Department of General Preventive Medicine, Johns Hopkins University School of Medicine, Baltimore, MD, USA

**John S. Silva, MD, FACMI**  Silva Consulting Services, Eldersburg, MD, USA

**Hardeep Singh, MD, MPH**  The Section of Health Services Research, Department of Medicine, Houston Veterans Affairs Center for Innovations in Quality, Effectiveness and Safety, Michael E. DeBakey VA Medical Center, Houston, TX, USA

**Dean F. Sittig, PhD**  University of Texas Health Science Center at Houston's School of Biomedical Informatics and the UT-Memorial Hermann Center for Healthcare Quality & Safety, Houston, TX, USA

**Daby M. Sow, PhD**  Exploratory Clinical Analytics and Systems, IBM T.J. Watson Research Center, Yorktown, NY, USA

**Bradley T. Steines, JD**  Corporate Services Division, Office of Ethics and Compliance/Office of Patient and Consumer Privacy, UPMC, Pittsburgh, PA, USA

**Grace Tran, MS**  Applied Physics Laboratory, Human Factors/Systems Integration, Johns Hopkins University, Laurel, MD, USA

**Kim M. Unertl, PhD, MS**  Department of Biomedical Informatics, Vanderbilt University School of Medicine, Nashville, TN, USA

**Fei Wang, PhD**  Computer Science and Engineering, University of Connecticut, Storrs, CT, USA

**Andrew R. Watson, MD, MLitt, FACS**  Department of Surgery, Division of Colorectal Surgery, University of Pittsburgh Medical Center, Pittsburgh, PA, USA

**Charlotte A. Weaver, RN, PhD, FAAN**  Atlanta, GA, USA

**Lawrence L. Weed, MD**  Department of Medicine, University of Vermont, Underhill, VT, USA

**Lincoln Weed, MD, JD**  Axiom Resource Management Inc., Oakton, VA, USA

**William A. Yasnoff, MD, PhD, FACMI**  NHII Advisors, Arlington, VA, USA

**Gigi Yuen-Reed, PhD**  Data Science, IBM T.J. Watson Research, Yorktown Heights, NY, USA

**Xinxin Zhu, MD, PhD**  Department of Healthcare Informatics, IBM T.J. Watson Research Center, Yorktown Heights, NY, USA

# Part I
# The Current State
# of Health Information Management
# in the United States

## Introduction

The first section of the book presents perspectives on the current landscape of information management systems in United States' healthcare. The authors provide historical and contemporary views of the technical, adaptive, organizational and political aspects of "where we are and how we got here" with respect to health IT. In doing so, they lay a foundation for articulating and describing some of the persistent and recurring barriers and problems in implementing and deploying sustainable information systems to improve care and health of individuals and populations.

An inevitable result of the increased uptake of electronic health records and other health IT has been the discovery and identification of new problems, in addition to a better understanding of why progress in health IT can be difficult. Thus, the current landscape is part of a long journey that started before the first edition of this book (1991) and will continue into the future.

- Chapter 1 by David McCallie, (Cerner Corp) presents a historical and environmental scan of clinical decision support tools and systems developed over the past 35+ years, and provides an clear picture of the limitations of those embedded in the EHR systems in use in today's marketplace
- Chapter 2 by Dean Sittig, (Univ Texas) and colleagues provide an grounded view of the EHR functionality that every clinician has a right to expect as they use these systems in the care of adults and children; and list as well the obligations that providers carry in their use of these EHR systems.
- Chapter 3 by James Ingram MD (Greenway Health) discusses the challenges of meeting the fast pace of regulatory and reimbursement changes, balanced with usability of health IT development from the dual perspectives of a vendor developer for ambulatory systems and as a clinician.
- Chapters 4 by Thomas Payne (Univ Washington) provides a CMIO's view of electronic health record (EHR) evolution in a multiple-site setting that uses different EHR systems across facilities; while Chapter 5 by Kim, Hudson and Miller, (Johns Hopkins) gives clinicians' perspectives on EHR functionality development for direct care and care coordination
- Chapter 6 by Ross Koppel (Univ Pennsylvania) provides a medical sociologist's view of the shortcomings of current health IT policy, impact and consequences of Meaningful Use implementation, with recommendations for go-forward efforts.
- In Chapter 7, Edmunds, Peddicord and Frisse (AcademyHealth, Washington Health Strategy Group, and Vanderbilt Univ respectively) take on the perplexing and convoluted reasons why we do not have interoperability in today's EHR systems; and follow this expose in Chapter 8 with a timeline review of critical health IT legislation, policy and (Office of the National Coordinator) ONC Directors as the factual context needed to understand the current state and political landscape.

# Chapter 1
# Clinical Decision Support: History and Basic Concepts

David P. McCallie Jr.

**Abstract** From the earliest implementations of electronic health records (EHR,) clinical decision support (CDS) has been seen as a key benefit of the move to computerization. This chapter will review many of the advances in EHR-based CDS, but will also note where CDS has not yet fully lived up to its promise. Included in this chapter's overview are: the various types of CDS (patient safety, clinical reminders, guidance towards best practice, etc.); the main approaches used for encoding of the clinical knowledge that drives CDS (scripts, rules, guidelines, algorithms, etc.); the different technologies currently used to manage and deliver CDS advice (Arden MLM, expert systems, etc.); as well as aspects of clinicians' user experience of the clinicians who interact with the CDS (alert fatigue, etc.). Understanding where we have come from can help set the stage for the innovations that will be needed to deliver on CDS's full potential, which will be the focus of Chapter 28.

**Keywords** Clinical decision support • Diagnostic decision support • Standardizing CDS knowledge • GELLO • Arden syntax • Medical logic modules • Expert rules systems • vMR • Rules scripting languages • Arden's curly brace • CDS rules maintenance • Alert fatigue • Health eDecisions • Guideline execution engines

## 1.1 The Early Promise of Clinical Decision Support

Early implementers of computer-based medical record systems recognized the value of embedding clinical decision support (CDS) into their designs. The rational was simple – computers, unlike busy or tired clinicians, are good at remembering things, and don't lose concentration. Including CDS for important items such as patient safety alerts and health maintenance reminders was a key goal of early computer patient record systems.

D.P. McCallie Jr., MD
Medical Informatics, Cerner Corp., Kansas City, MO, USA
e-mail: dmccallie@cerner.com

© Springer International Publishing Switzerland 2016                                     3
C.A. Weaver et al. (eds.), *Healthcare Information Management Systems:*
*Cases, Strategies, and Solutions*, Health Informatics,
DOI 10.1007/978-3-319-20765-0_1

Howard Bleich's acid-base interpretation system [4] represents one of the first uses of a computer to help clinicians with decision making. His hard-coded algorithm did the complex math necessary to properly interpret blood-gas and blood chemistry results. By instantly performing the classification of the patient's results, the clinician was relieved of the need to get out a calculator and spend precious time re-keying data.

Influenced by the then burgeoning artificial intelligence (AI) movement, the healthcare application, MYCIN [48], emerged as another pioneering attempt to let the computer augment human decision-making. MYCIN was based as an "inference engine" (expert system) and consisted of approximately 600 rules that were used to make antibiotic treatment recommendations, based on input of facts about the patient and culture results. Each MYCIN rule captured a specific fact about common diseases, the likely causative organisms, as well as knowledge about how to treat specific types of infectious organisms. By combining these facts under the control of the inference engine, MYCIN was able to match human experts in selected test cases [56].

Clem McDonald's work on the Regenstrief Medical Record System, developed for the Wishard Memorial Hospital in Indianapolis (now Eskenazi Health,) typifies another key phase in the use of computerized CDS. In the mid-1970s, McDonald implemented an extensive series of computer-based clinical reminders and alerts. He recognized that the number of necessary clinical reminders and alerts would quickly grow. So instead of hand-crafting each alert deep into computer code, McDonald created one of the first CDS Rule Languages, which he called CARE [32]. The CARE language allowed non-programmer, clinical experts to structure the if-then-else logic of the alert using a simple but flexible scripting language that was then interpreted by the underlying patient record system. The use of a scripting language to capture the clinical logic increased the number of rules that could be authored by experts without requiring programmers. CARE rules grew to be quite sophisticated, and included drug-drug interactions, drug-dose safety alerts, best practice care suggestions, aids for problem list management, as well as preventative reminders. McDonald also performed one of the first randomized trials of the effectiveness of computer decision support, demonstrating that the computer-delivered reminders led to improved care [33].

As computer patient records systems began to spread in other academic centers and as commercial electronic health record (EHR) markets emerged, it became clear that a standard way to replicate the decision logic of alerts and expert systems would help disseminate this new type of clinical knowledge to other medical centers. For a number of reasons, the CARE style of "if-then-else" scripting language approach saw more uptake than the more complicated expert system approach of MYCIN. In the late 1980s, a group of informaticists at Columbia led an important attempt to standardize CDS scripting languages that resulted in the creation of the Arden Syntax [24]. The goal of the Arden Syntax was to encode if-then-else rules in such a way that the rules could run on different EHR systems, regardless of the vendor or the location of the EHR.

Arden Syntax logic modules, often called "Medical Logic Modules" (MLM), consist of several standard sections, known as Categories. Each category contained several "slots" that captured the rule logic. One important slot in the Knowledge Category is the "evoke" slot that determines the triggering event that initially causes the rule to be evaluated. The "logic" slot contains the actual clinical logic, and the "action" slot defines the message that the rule sends to the clinician when triggered. Most modern EHR implementations of rule-based alerting systems follow these general design principles, even if the full Arden Syntax is not followed. Vendors generally apply numerous optimizations to ensure that CDS systems running large numbers of rules do not get bogged down by constantly evaluating potential rules. For example, the number of synchronous "evoke" trigger points is usually limited to specific actions in the clinical workflow, so that rules get evaluated during important clinician actions. Trigger points typically include events such as: open and close of the electronic chart; add diagnosis or problem; add or sign order; or, administer medication, etc. When the clinician's workflow reaches a trigger point, the rule system is invoked and quickly evaluates all of the rules that have been attached to that trigger point. Full evaluation of the deep clinical logic is only performed on the rules that pass an efficient evoke-logic "screening test," in order to minimize needless computation. If the screening test is passed, the rule's full "logic" slot is then evaluated. Such evaluation may involve multiple accesses to the clinical database, a potentially time-consuming event if the rule's logic is complicated. Some rule systems cache data from the database to speed future evaluations, but many systems fetch the data freshly each time the rule is evaluated.

## 1.2 Some Problems Emerge

In the mid-1990s, CDS rules encoded using the Arden Syntax model began to spread to numerous academic centers and to some commercial systems, but early dissemination was limited by difficulty in getting rules written in one facility to run at a different facility. The "logic" slot component of an Arden rule contained machine executable if-then-else code that could be made to run against any system. However, the "curly brace" part of the syntax only contained a textual description of the database action that was necessary for the rule to be able to access EHR data. The text inside the curly braces was not executable code, since there was no standard data model or database language to base it on. This meant that all Arden-based rules had to be hand-coded to the local database system before the rule could be applied. This barrier to implementation was so significant that it came to be called the "*curly brace problem*". The challenge to achieve complete rule portability across environments persists in many rule languages to the current day, as will be discussed below.

Several other core CDS challenges emerged as experience was gained with Arden and other alerting systems. In addition to this *rule portability* problem, early implementations of alert-based CDS began to generate complaints of "*alert fatigue*" due to the growing number of pop-up messages that would interrupt the clinician's workflow. *Accuracy and relevance* of alerts became as issue, as it became clear that much more patient data was necessary than originally realized to ensure that alerts were both sensitive and specific to the clinical situation. For example, a very sick patient in an Intensive Care Unit (ICU) setting should not generate the same alerts that might be expected from a patient in a non-ICU setting, even though the exact same lab results or medications were present in the two patients. In addition, early experience with alerts that had hard-coded if-then-else logic with specific thresholds lead to the realization that selection of the threshold value had a dramatic effect on whether or not a particular alert would fire – this characteristic is referred to as *brittleness*. The result was inconsistent with the gradual variation of human biology that clinicians experienced in clinical settings. For example, a serious alert that would fire with a potassium level of 2.5 mmol/L might remain silent with a level of 2.6. This didn't match clinician's expectations. As more sites tried to use script-based (Arden-like) alerting systems, it was realized that simple if-then-else rules were unable to capture the logic of more complex clinical decisions, leading to the need for advances in techniques of *knowledge modeling and representation*. In addition, as the speed of knowledge advances in medicine grew, the *maintenance* of deployed CDS systems became an issue if CDS rules were allowed to get out of synch with new science knowledge. We will address these core issues in the remainder of this chapter.

## 1.3 Alert Fatigue and Workflow Interruption

The earliest CDS systems followed a simple paradigm of interrupting the clinician's workflow with a pop-up alert. These alerts were typically triggered in response to some action the clinician had taken, such as prescribing a medication, adding a problem to the problem list, or ordering a procedure. These *synchronous alerts* were attention-grabbing but led to clinician irritation as the number of alerts grew, especially if the alert forced the clinician to choose some action to dismiss the alert. The irritation was especially severe if the accuracy or relevancy of the alert was inadequate. Alert fatigue has been well documented [12, 31, 41, 43, 53] to frustrate providers and to cause providers to sometimes dismiss an alert without adequate consideration, or to even disable the entire alerting system.

## 1.4 Efforts to Improve Arden-Like Rules

A number of approaches have emerged to reduce alert fatigue. A key consideration is to *improve the accuracy and relevance* of the alerts, reducing the number of false-positive interruptions, while hopefully not increasing the false-negatives. To achieve improved accuracy, the alert's logic model will often need to be more sophisticated to ensure that the alert only fires when absolutely necessary [14]. For example, a simple drug-lab alert that makes good sense in an ambulatory setting would fire far too frequently in an ICU setting. Typically alerts are tailored to the patient, but a more robust logic model might allow the alerting system to take into account the provider as well, adjusting the alert to reflect the provider's expertise and preferences. A cardiologist may not need to see the same alerts as a general practitioner. Some studies suggest that even with these additional factors, it is difficult to avoid generating too many alerts [8].

Another way to address alert fatigue is to use *smart alert routing* to deliver the alert to a different clinician who may be in a better position to deal with the alert's message than the bedside clinician. For example, a medication-dose alert could be routed to the pharmacologist assigned to the care team instead of to the ordering physician [42]. Additionally, smart routing can be supplemented by *alert prioritization* systems that use the clinical data to refine alerts into categories of urgency. These urgency categories might range from high-priority "stop now" alerts that would be allowed break into the immediate workflow, down to the lowest category of "FYI" alerts that might be queued to the provider's message center for reading at a later time. Recent work at Regenstrief allows for a provider to use a simple configuration tool to customize both the alerts and their personal alert delivery preferences [15].

Synchronous alerts cause many of the alert fatigue problems, but not all alerts need to be triggered in tight synchronization with clinician activity. A major class of alerts, known as *asynchronous alerts*, can be triggered by background system activity that is unrelated to the clinician's workflow. Asynchronous alerting systems are sometimes known as *clinical event monitors*, [28] because they monitor clinical activity such as the availability of a new lab result, the activation of an order, or an unexpected change in vital signs in the background, as data flows in or out of the EHR. Since asynchronous alerts can be triggered outside any particular clinician's workflow, the resulting message needs to be routed to an appropriate recipient. This requires that EHR systems understand provider's roles, and how care teams are structured. Ideally, the alerting system knows provider call schedules to avoid surprising a clinician who has just left his shift. However, even with this knowledge of personnel, roles, and schedules, it may be challenging to ensure delivery of the alert to someone empowered to react appropriately. *Notification escalation* techniques [26, 50, 55] should be employed to ensure that any critical alerts are responded to in a timely fashion. If no response occurs in a specified time, the alert can be escalated to a fallback target. The process repeats until someone eventually responds. In some systems, workflow engines have been used to manage the complexities of alert delivery and escalation [26].

Asynchronous alerts can also be triggered by elapsed time. These *expectation-tracking* alerts will fire unless something satisfies or cancels the alert. Expectation-tracking alerts can be used to ensure that certain types of follow-up occur. A generic form of expectation tracking can be used to implement a *health maintenance reminder* system [17], which keeps track of long-term health maintenance issues such as advising colonoscopy in patients over age 50, etc. Due to the long-term nature of health maintenance issues, specialized systems that are optimized to track the state of the expectations over long periods of time are often used rather than traditional Arden-like medical logic modules.

### 1.4.1   Ambient Alerts: A Better Approach to Delivering Alerts?

A relatively new approach to the alert fatigue problem is the deployment of *ambient alerts* [44, 47] to the healthcare setting. An ambient alert is delivered to the clinician's attention, but in an less intrusive and non-interruptive way, typically off in a sidebar or down at the bottom of the screen. The provider's attention is not immediately distracted from his current activity, but the alert's message is still visible. Ambient alerts can come from synchronous or asynchronous triggers. Ambient alerts can be context-aware, and may even be triggered by specific details of what the provider is doing, at a level of granularity that can be more precise than traditional MLM triggers [15]. For example, if the provider is authoring a history and physical exam, an ambient monitoring system could have access to the actual note being entered, with the ability to use real-time natural language parsing (NLP) to extract specific symptoms and findings to support an ambient differential diagnosis display, without requiring that findings be double-entered into the differential diagnosis engine.

Cerner is one of the commercial EHR vendors planning to use ambient alerting. Information such as non-urgent traditional alerts, risk scores from real-time predictive analytics, real-time differential diagnosis, cumulative radiation doses, and narcotic risk alerts from a local PDMP program (Prescription Drug Monitoring Program) will be displayed in the "smart zone" of the screen. Initial response to the use of ambient alerting has been positive, but it is too early to know what effect these ambient alerts will have on the care process. Some have suggested that utilization of the ambient approach could lead to overlooking of critical messages (Personal communication, Lisa Harris MD, February, 2015).

## 1.5   Expert Systems as Alternative to Arden-Like Rules

Many CDS systems in use today rely on fairly simple Arden-like "if-then-else" Medical Logic Modules (MLMs) to encapsulate the clinical knowledge necessary to drive the decision support. From the developers' perspective the appeal of simple if-then-else MLMs is clear – such rules are easy to create, easy to understand, and easy to implement. However, as the need for greater clinical sophistication increased and the MLMs became more complicated, informaticists have explored alternate ways to represent the clinical knowledge and logic. One such important alternative is the use of *rule-based expert systems*, the approach first pioneered by the MYCIN project, described above.

Rule-based expert systems work as follows: The rules engine ("inference engine") manages a set of independent rules, consisting of simple if-then declarative statements that capture components of the clinical knowledge. The rules engine also manages a "working memory" that contains "facts" which have been asserted by one or more of the rules that have been evaluated as true. Every time new data is made available to the engine, the full set of rules is re-evaluated to find any rule whose "if" condition now matches the newly arrived data. If there is a match, the rules' "then" clause can assert a new fact into the rule engine's working memory. At that point, the process repeats – the new fact is checked against all the other rules to see if any rule matches the new fact, and if so, these rules fire as well. Eventually the cycle reaches a steady state where some new conclusion may have been reached. This new conclusion becomes the output of the system [16].

Some CDS systems have adopted the MYCIN strategy of using expert system technology to encode much more complex knowledge models, and then to reason against the model as new data arrived. One theoretical advantage to an expert system based system as compared to a large if-then-else MLM is that complex decision logic can be represented with simple statements that can be maintained more or less independently of each other. In contrast, a large MLM may require that the entire clinical logic be maintained as a deeply nested, executable script. An expert system can also separate the clinical facts (the information model) from the procedural knowledge to apply the facts to a specific clinical situation [49]. Because of this scalability of knowledge capture using declarative rules, some CDS implementers believe that expert-system approaches are better for highly complex decision support. However, the "knowledge engineering" process to create a comprehensive knowledge model for non-trivial clinical domains can be difficult. When engineering an expert system, it can be difficult to guarantee that any given rule-base can account for all the cases that the logic needs to cover. An incomplete rule base can lead to gaps in coverage that are hard to detect. Thus, many of the published uses of expert system CDS have focused on complex use-cases for specific disease states, for example tuberculosis diagnosis [38], heart failure [46], liver disease [30], and lung disease [29].

### 1.5.1   Using Guideline-Based CDS to Expand the Breadth of Clinical Coverage

Another Arden-based approach to simplifying complex clinical models is to leverage a *guideline-based* technique that separates the clinical problem into a series of linked clinical decisions. The overall guideline can be arbitrarily long and complex, but each specific decision can be relatively straightforward. Guideline Interchange Format (GLIF) [6, 40] is an example of an early standard that was proposed to implement this approach. GLIF utilized a flow-chart metaphor that strung decisions together using branching logic that captured the sequence of necessary decisions. Arden MLMs defined the clinical logic for each decision node. Of course, the use of Arden Syntax brought forward the "curly brace" problem described elsewhere.

Several other guideline-modeling languages have been developed, including PROforma [9], SAGE [52], and GEM [18]. These approaches to guideline modeling also decompose complex clinical scenarios into simpler steps. Some of these tools (e.g., SAGE and PROforma) included "guideline execution engines" as part of their design. These tools were designed to incorporate the guideline's logic directly into the clinical workflow, addressing the limitations of Arden-based GLIF by using the guideline engine itself to "execute" the decision logic. This might have solved the "curly brace" issue, but did not solve the harder problem of the lack of standards to integrate the guideline engine itself into the EHR.

Another problem is that a typical clinical guideline might naturally evolve over long periods of time, crossing multiple encounters, and involving numerous providers. For this to work in an EHR, the current state of the guideline would need to be preserved for future encounters, and the EHR would need some way to ensure that the treating clinicians are aware that the patient is being managed under one or more "active" guidelines. This level of integration is difficult to achieve within typical EHR workflows that tend to be driven by ad hoc navigation, in which the clinician has full control over the next decision and actions. Also, long-running guidelines can be brittle – they often don't account for patients that "fall off the path" or have co-morbidities that might generate conflicting recommendations. For these reasons, delivering a comprehensive guideline execution engine remains a challenge for CDS experts and for EHR vendors.

New approaches are being taken by a number of developers to address these limitations and move towards the vision of comprehensive guideline engines by deploying what might be called "*mini-guidelines*". In this approach, specific isolated steps of an overall guideline can be independently invoked based on patient context, using triggers such as admitting diagnosis, recent lab results, or algorithmic risk predictors. These mini-guidelines can assist with a series of more or less independent high-value decisions, even in the absence of a more coordinated guideline flow. Informaticists at Vanderbilt were among the first to build this type of focused guideline support into their "Wiz Order" computerized provider order entry (CPOE) system [36]. In a similar fashion, Cerner deploys a venous thromboembolism (VTE) prophylaxis mini-guideline that is triggered when a patient has data that suggest high risk for VTE. The mini-guideline is triggered by a traditional CDS rule, but instead of a simple alert, the mini-guideline engages the provider in a short conversation to ensure that the right prophylaxis is chosen. The conversation (see Fig. 1.1) occurs in a pop-up window, and can capture additional data before pushing suggested orders into the provider's order-entry workflow.

Intermountain Healthcare (Salt Lake City) has developed a large set of evidence-based clinical guidelines that they call "care process models (CPM)" [10]. These CPMs were initially deployed to the bedside using paper forms, which succinctly described the key decisions that needed to be made and captured the parameters that drove the provider's decision. The resulting data was fed into a continuous quality model that then informed revisions of the CPM logic. These paper-based processes have made significant improvements on system quality, while simultaneously controlling costs [27]. Cerner is now working with Intermountain to convert these paper CPMs into a series of EHR-based mini-guidelines, each of which will be triggered by specific patient contexts. The data captured by the CDS conversations will be used as input to a continuous quality process to ensure that the decision advice stays current and robust.

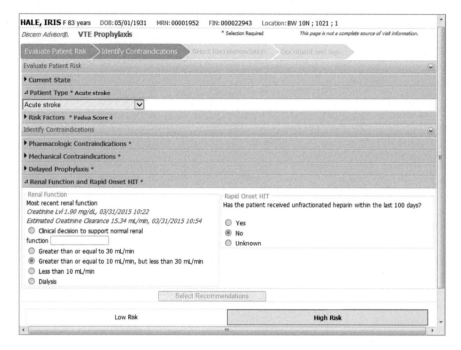

**Fig. 1.1** Screenshot from venous thromboembolism mini-guideline

## 1.6 Diagnostic Decision Support

Not all CDS is related to alerts and reminders. Historically CDS alerts have focused on treatment issues, but it can be equally valuable to focus decision support on the diagnostic process that comes before treatment – *diagnostic decision support*. The problem being addressed is that the optimal workup of a complex problem may be as much of a cognitive challenge to the clinicians as the treatment and management of the problem itself.

*Differential diagnosis* systems have been a favorite target of informatics research from the earliest days of computer patient records. Differential diagnosis decision support starts with information about the current patient and produces a list of alternate diagnoses that might account for the patient's presentation. One of the very first such tools was the INTERNIST-1 system [35], developed at the University of Pittsburgh. Other notable differential diagnosis systems include QMR [34], DxPlain® [2], PEPID™, and Isabel© [54]. These systems start with facts about the patient, potentially including patient history, physical findings, and diagnostic test data. They use a variety of algorithms to sift through a large database of diseases to see which diseases best explain the findings of the targeted patient. For example, the INTERNIST-1 algorithm included three parameters that linked findings to diseases: IMPORT (the importance of the finding in the abstract,) EVOKS (the evoking strength between the finding and any particular disease,) and FREQ (the frequency of the finding given the presence of a particular disease.) Typically these systems are able to rank the choices that best explain the presenting patient's data, and most can prioritize the diseases that would be most dangerous to misdiagnose.

Until recently, a problem shared by most of these systems is that they required the clinician to manually enter the relevant history, findings and lab data. With the availability of natural language processing systems, it has recently become possible for the EHR to automate the extraction of this data from the provider's note, making it much easier to invoke the differential tool. In general, these systems appear to be well accepted by students and doctors in training, who can test their growing skills against the computer's knowledge. However, more experienced clinicians have observed that the systems are brittle, in that sometimes a small change in the findings input can have a surprisingly large effect on the diseases presented in the differential. For example, in one system that this author evaluated, the difference between entering a finding of "fever" versus "high fever" had a dramatic affect on the differential presented (McCallie, personal observation, June 2000).

Numerous formal assessments of differential diagnostic systems have been performed. A recent study [5] evaluated 23 systems capable of some type of diagnosis support, but found only four systems considered robust enough for general use. The best of the four scored moderately well (case score 69 out of a possible 100) on a set of difficult cases. Viewing a list of alternate diagnoses may help prevent premature closure of the physician's thought process, but some evaluations have raised concerns about the potential for diagnostic confusion introduced by seeing a large list of alternatives [3]. Since most of the displayed alternatives will be incorrect, the large list of diseases could trigger unnecessary additional workup, resulting in higher expense or even harm. Nonetheless, findings-driven, differential diagnosis systems are enjoying a renaissance and may well find a routine place in the CDS toolkit.

Another growing use of diagnostic decision support involves *appropriateness screening* where CDS is used to recommend the most cost-effective diagnostic strategy. These rules are usually applied to high-cost diagnostic tests, such as expensive or invasive radiologic studies. The rules seek to ensure that the clinician starts a workup using the least expensive, least invasive test, before escalating to more costly or dangerous tests. Much of the initial work in this area has been applied to radiology procedures, resulting in creation of the ACR Appropriateness Criteria (ACRAC), developed in the mid-1990s by the American College of Radiology [13]. Initially, the criteria were presented as reference text, but numerous computerized versions have been deployed that can intervene in the CPOE process. The ACR now offers ACRAC as a web service [1] that can be embedded into any EHR. The approach has been so successful that the Centers for Medicaid and Medicare (CMS) recently announced that reimbursement for radiologic procedures would require appropriateness screening, starting in 2017 [45].

## 1.7  Knowledge Portability: Standards for Clinical Decision Support

Due to the inherent limitations of Arden Syntax, early CDS systems were usually deployed inside locally created EHR systems, with the consequence that most of the knowledge content tended to be developed and deployed by the same team that created the EHR software. Many early CDS systems used proprietary knowledge representations that were tuned to the local system's database engine and to the EHR's workflow. However, as the history of Arden System shows, informatics researchers have put substantial effort into creating standard formats to encode and share clinical knowledge. The task of developing such standards is decidedly non-trivial. As noted earlier, adoption of the Arden Syntax was stymied by the "curly brace" problem. Different EHR systems have idiosyncratic database models and use different databases (SQL, MUMPS, etc.) Additionally, even if the same database engine was used, implementations usually built locally developed, non-standardized clinical vocabularies to represent the clinical facts about the patient. Absent national vocabulary standards, it was common for different organizations to use different codes for the same lab tests or medications, for example. Only recently have widely accepted standards for lab test names – LOINC® [25], and medications – RxNorm [39] emerged. Adding to the challenge is the fact that there is no standard clinical workflow that different EHRs follow. Each vendor implements workflows that fit their assumptions about their customers. This means that rules that work well in one vendor's workflow might be unhelpful or have poor usability in a different organization's implementation of the same EHR, or in a different vendor's product. Nonetheless, the informatics and standards communities have continued to seek appropriate standards for encoding "executable knowledge" in a vendor neutral way. It has been estimated that an average, academic medical center will deploy as many as 2,000 MLM-like rules [19]. The work of developing and maintaining such a comprehensive set of rules can be very expensive. If standard libraries were available, costs would diminish and best practices could be more widely shared.

One approach to standardizing CDS knowledge has been to focus on standards for encoding the specification of the clinical knowledge itself, as a precursor to standardizing an "executable" form of the knowledge. For example, GEM [18] is a standard for using XML to encode human-readable guidelines. Guidelines that follow the GEM encoding are theoretically more readily translatable to computerized form. Work done by the multi-stakeholder CDS Consortium [11] took a similar layered encoding approach to CDS rule specifications [7]. The CDS Consortium defined a 4-layer model, where the top layers focused on human readable specification and the lower layers focused on executable forms of the value sets and rule logic.

## 1.8  Standard Development Organizations' Efforts

HL7 has a long history of developing candidate standards for various aspects of CDS. HL7 took over maintenance of the Arden Syntax standard in 1998 [20]. HL7 experts found the "curly brace" problem to be unsolvable using the existing

Arden approach, and so began efforts to create new CDS standards that were based on the HL7 Version 3 Reference Information Model (RIM) [21]. By building CDS standards on top of the V3/RIM model, HL7 believed that it could create a more comprehensive CDS approach that addressed the "curly brace" problem.

One HL7 V3-based attempt was the GELLO Expression Language [51]. GELLO is an object-oriented expression language that was designed to access and compute clinical data. GELLO logic and data access is expressed in terms of the abstract information model that underlies the V3 RIM. The RIM is based on six "backbone" classes from which the broad array of healthcare concepts is to be derived: Act, Participation, Entity, Role, Act Relationship, and Role Link [21]. Since the RIM is intended to represent all clinical data, the belief was that GELLO expressions could access and manipulate any necessary clinical data via the RIM. However, since the RIM itself was not suitable for direct manipulation via GELLO expressions, an abstract "virtual medical record" (vMR) was defined. The vMR sits above the RIM, and expresses aggregates of commonly used clinical data via a template mechanism defined to represent common clinical entities, such as "all active problems" or "reason for admission". The complexities that underlie the RIM are intended to be hidden behind the vMR definitions.

The RIM and the vMR templates are by definition expressed in a vendor-independent way – they propose a universal abstraction of the data model. By defining the data access logic in GELLO using the constructs of the vMR, the expression logic capturing the clinical goal can remain vendor and database independent. In theory, a medical logic rule encoded in GELLO could run against the clinical data in any vendor's system as long as the vendor is able to express proprietary data models in terms of the vMR.

In essence, the GELLO/vMR approach moves the "curly brace" problem out of the Arden-style expression logic and puts the work onto the mapping of the vMR to the actual clinical database in use. This should make GELLO-encoded clinical decision rules a vendor independent way to share clinical knowledge bases. However, the RIM has not proven to be a very efficient or practical representation of the complexity of real-world clinical data as evidenced by the small number of vendors who have deployed RIM-based native databases or have implemented a vMR mapping over non-RIM EHR databases. Since the vMR templates are defined in terms of the RIM, the dearth of RIM-based EHRs has caused the original vision of the CDS encoded with GELLO and the vMR to remain unproven.

## 1.9 Government Initiated Standards Efforts

In part due to the absence of widespread uptake of GELLO and the vMR, the Office of the National Coordinator for Health IT (ONC) launched Health eDecisions (HeD) as a major Standards & Interoperability (S&I) project in 2013. The goal of the Health eDecisions project was "to define and validate standards that enable CDS sharing at scale" (ONC [37]). The HeD group's work focused on two main use-cases. The first use-case, "CDS Artifact Sharing" aimed to address and refine standards for encoding CDS logic that could be imported into vendor products. The second use-case, "CDS Guidance as a Service" focused on invoking remote CDS services, and is discussed in more detail in Chapter 28. Health eDecisions evaluated several existing CDS standards and decided to retain the vMR approach, but to replace GELLO with a new expression language known as ECA, which stands for "Event, Condition, Action" (ONC [37]). An ECA expression is an XML data structure that captures the if-then-else logic of any particular rule in the form an Abstract Syntax Tree (AST) representation of the logic. The ECA elements use XML query expressions to connect to the vMR for access to the necessary data elements. The HeD team believed that an AST representation of the decision logic would be relatively easy for vendors to parse and execute as part of their native (proprietary) rule systems.

Despite a few successful pilots, vendor enthusiasm for HeD has been muted. In part, this is because few vendors are able to provide vMR mappings over their own data models, for the reasons noted above. Perhaps a more important issue is that the HeD/ECA approach does not address the complexities of workflow, trigger logic, or the other aspects of usability that lead to "alert fatigue." This means that most ECA-encoded rules would probably have to be re-written in terms of the vendor's native rules engine anyway, which defeats many of the goals of the HeD vision of a universal CDS standard that vendors could automatically import into their client's systems.

Notwithstanding the lack of initial uptake of the HeD approach, several HL7 standards teams are moving to re-define the vMR and ECA approaches to better align rule logic with the standards used to define clinical quality measures (CQM.) The approach is based on the assumption that CDS rules are often used to prompt clinicians towards achieving higher clinical quality outcomes, so it makes sense to use a similar knowledge specification standard to define the quality measures and the rules that support attainment of the quality outcomes. To that end, work is underway at HL7 to define QUICK – the QUality Improvement and Clinical Knowledge model [22]. QUICK has replaced the vMR with a new abstract data model that harmonizes the vMR with an existing quality standard known as the Quality Data Model (QDM.) QUICK also proposes to replace ECA with a new expression language known as Clinical Quality Language (CQL), which attempts to capture lessons learned from previous attempts at encoding decision logic such as Arden, GELLO, and ECA. This new set of standards will be able to use HL7's emerging data access Application Programming Interface (API) standard known as FHIR – Fast Healthcare Interoperability Resource [23] as a way to specify a more direct access to an EHR's clinical data, without requiring the overhead of a RIM mapping. FHIR specifies a library of standard clinical "resources" that can be readily mapped to existing EHR data models. FHIR resources roughly correspond to the data content of vMR templates, but avoid the complexity of mapping through the RIM intermediary. The potential role of FHIR in CDS is discussed in more detail in Chapter 28.

## 1.10   Discussion

In this chapter, we have described the more common approaches in use by mainstream vendor products to deliver routine CDS. These systems are dominated by Arden-like, script-based "if-then-else" alerts and reminders, with occasional use of expert-system tools and other specializations. We described a number of CDS standardization efforts, yet most CDS knowledge is still being coded to vendor-proprietary formats, especially for data access to the EHR record. Despite noted limitations, the major vendor systems do cover significant clinical ground, especially around well-understood areas such as drug-drug and drug-lab interactions, best practice notifications, and health mainte-nance reminders. As we have seen, the cognitive burden of "alert fatigue" remains a challenge, though some of the burden can be reduced by careful attention to alert deliv-ery. Some best practices for alert management discussed and summarized here are:

- Maximize alert accuracy by using a robust clinical decision model, minimizing false-positive interruptions.
- Prioritize the alert for urgency and importance, to ensure that the most important data is noticed.
- Route the alert to the optimal target, which may not be the currently active user.
- Deliver the alert in the least disruptive way, ranging from:

  - "Full-stop" interruptive alerts for critical messages.
  - Ambient alerts, delivered in a non-interruptive way for medium priority knowledge relevant to the current workflow.
  - Asynchronous reminders delivered outside the current workflow for messages that are suitable for non-urgent follow-up.

The process of standardizing CDS knowledge artifacts is complex and remains unfin-ished. The efforts described in this chapter fall into what might be called the "Arden era" because the most widely used CDS knowledge models are specified using the if-then-else logic described by the Arden Syntax. As noted above, a major limitation of the Arden Syntax approach is the inability to specify a standard way to define access to the clinical data in the EHR. To address this, informaticists have tried to specify data access standards using data intermediaries based on the HL7 V3 RIM, most notably the vMR. For the most part, these approaches have not enjoyed widespread vendor support. Chapter 28 intro-duces what might be called the "FHIR era" in which clinical data access can be defined in terms of a simplified resource-oriented model, accessed via the vendor-neutral FHIR API. In addition, Chapter 28 introduces some innovative approaches including CDS as a service, cloud-based delivery, knowledge models based on statistical techniques such as machine learning, as well as CDS delivered via standards-based plug-in "SMART apps."

## References

1. ACR. ACRSelect. 2014. http://www.acrselect.org/solution.html. Accessed 25 Mar 2015.
2. Barnett GO, Cimino JJ, Hupp JA, Hoffer EP. DXplain. An evolving diagnostic decision-support system. JAMA. 1987;258:67–74.

3. Berner ES, Webster GD, Shugerman AA, et al. Performance of four computer-based diagnostic systems. N Engl J Med. 1994;330:1792–6. doi:10.1056/NEJM199406233302506.
4. Bleich HL. Computer evaluation of acid-base disorders. J Clin Invest. 1969;48:1689–96. doi:10.1172/JCI106134.
5. Bond WF, Schwartz LM, Weaver KR, et al. Differential diagnosis generators: an evaluation of currently available computer programs. J Gen Intern Med. 2012;27:213–9. doi:10.1007/s11606-011-1804-8.
6. Boxwala AA, Peleg M, Tu S, et al. GLIF3: a representation format for sharable computer-interpretable clinical practice guidelines. J Biomed Inform. 2004;37:147–61. doi:10.1016/j.jbi.2004.04.002.
7. Boxwala AA, Rocha BH, Maviglia S, et al. A multi-layered framework for disseminating knowledge for computer-based decision support. J Am Med Inform Assoc. 2011;18 Suppl 1:i132–9. doi:10.1136/amiajnl-2011-000334.
8. Bryant AD, Fletcher GS, Payne TH. Drug interaction alert override rates in the meaningful use era: no evidence of progress. Appl Clin Inform. 2014;5:802–13. doi:10.4338/ACI-2013-12-RA-0103.
9. Button DR, Fox J. The syntax and semantics of the PRO forma guideline modeling language. J Am Med Inform Assoc. 2003;10:433–43.
10. Byington CL, Reynolds CC, Korgenski K, et al. Costs and infant outcomes after implementation of a care process model for febrile infants. Pediatrics. 2012;130:e16–24. doi:10.1542/peds.2012-0127.
11. CDS Consortium. 2013. http://www.cdsconsortium.org/dissemination.asp. Accessed 9 Jan 2015.
12. Carspecken CW, Sharek PJ, Longhurst C, Pageler NM. A clinical case of electronic health record drug alert fatigue: consequences for patient outcome. Pediatrics. 2013;131:e1970–3. doi:10.1542/peds.2012-3252.
13. Cascade PN. The American College of Radiology. ACR appropriateness criteria project. Radiology. 2000;214(Suppl):3–46. doi:10.1148/radiology.214.1.r00ja493.
14. Duke JD, Li X, Dexter P. Adherence to drug-drug interaction alerts in high-risk patients: a trial of context-enhanced alerting. J Am Med Inform Assoc. 2013;20:494–8. doi:10.1136/amiajnl-2012-001073.
15. Duke JD, Morea J, Mamlin B, et al. Regenstrief Institute's medical gopher: a next-generation homegrown electronic medical record system. Int J Med Inform. 2014;83:170–9. doi:10.1016/j.ijmedinf.2013.11.004.
16. Feigenbaum E, Barr A. The handbook of artificial intelligence, vol I. Addison-Wesley, Boston; 1986.
17. Frame PS, Zimmer JG, Werth PL, Martens WB. Description of a computerized health maintenance tracking system for primary care practice. Am J Prev Med. 1991;7:311–8.
18. Hajizadeh N, Kashyap N, Michel G, Shiffman RN. GEM at 10: a decade's experience with the guideline elements model. AMIA Annu Symp Proc. 2011;2011:520–8.
19. Halamka J. Life as a healthcare CIO: decision support service providers. 2010. http://geekdoctor.blogspot.com/2010/06/decision-support-service-providers.html. Accessed 13 Jan 2015.
20. HL7. HL7 standards product brief – arden syntax V2.7. 1998. http://www.hl7.org/implement/standards/product_brief.cfm?product_id=2. Accessed 17 Mar 2015.
21. HL7. Version 3: Reference Information Model (RIM). 2012. http://www.hl7.org/implement/standards/product_brief.cfm?product_id=77. Accessed 17 Jan 2015.
22. HL7. Clinical quality information. 2014. http://www.hl7.org/Special/committees/cqi/index.cfm. Accessed 17 Mar 2015
23. HL7. FHIR. 2014. http://www.hl7.org/implement/standards/fhir/. Accessed 18 Dec 2014.
24. Hripcsak G. Arden syntax for medical logic modules. MD Comput. 1991;8(76):78.
25. Huff SM, Rocha RA, McDonald CJ, et al. Development of the Logical Observation Identifier Names and Codes (LOINC) Vocabulary. J Am Med Inform Assoc. 1998;5:276–92. doi:10.1136/jamia.1998.0050276.
26. Huser V, Rasmussen LV, Oberg R, Starren JB. Implementation of workflow engine technology to deliver basic clinical decision support functionality. BMC Med Res Methodol. 2011;11:43. doi:10.1186/1471-2288-11-43.

27. James BC, Savitz LA. How intermountain trimmed health care costs through robust quality improvement efforts. Health Aff (Millwood). 2011;30:1185–91. doi:10.1377/hlthaff.2011.0358.
28. Jenders RA, Hripcsak G, Sideli R V, et al. Medical decision support: experience with implementing the Arden Syntax at the Columbia-Presbyterian Medical Center. Proc Annu Symp Comput Appl Med Care.1995;19:169–73.
29. Kar A, Miller GE, Sheppard SV. PULMONOLOGIST: a computer-based diagnosis system for pulmonary diseases. Int J Biomed Comput. 1987;21:223–35.
30. Lucas PJ, Janssens AR. Development and validation of HEPAR, an expert system for the diagnosis of disorders of the liver and biliary tract. Med Inform (Lond). 1991;16:259–70.
31. McCoy AB, Thomas EJ, Krousel-Wood M, Sittig DF. Clinical decision support alert appropriateness: a review and proposal for improvement. Ochsner J. 2014;14:195–202.
32. McDonald CJ. Action-oriented decisions in ambulatory medicine. New York: Year Book Medical Publishers, Chicago – London; 1981.
33. McDonald CJ, Hui SL, Smith DM, et al. Reminders to physicians from an introspective computer medical record. A two-year randomized trial. Ann Intern Med. 1984;100:130–8.
34. Miller R, Masarie FE, Myers JD. Quick medical reference (QMR) for diagnostic assistance. MD Comput. 1986;3:34–48.
35. Miller RA, Pople HE, Myers JD. Internist-1, an experimental computer-based diagnostic consultant for general internal medicine. N Engl J Med. 1982;307:468–76. doi:10.1056/NEJM198208193070803.
36. Miller RA, Waitman LR, Chen S, Rosenbloom ST. The anatomy of decision support during inpatient care provider order entry (CPOE): empirical observations from a decade of CPOE experience at Vanderbilt. J Biomed Inform. 2005;38:469–85. doi:10.1016/j.jbi.2005.08.009.
37. ONC S&I. Health eDecisions Homepage. 2013. http://wiki.siframework.org/Health+eDecisions+Homepage. Accessed 17 Mar 2015.
38. Osamor VC, Azeta AA, Ajulo OO. Tuberculosis-Diagnostic Expert System: an architecture for translating patients information from the web for use in tuberculosis diagnosis. Health Inform J. 2014;20:275–87. doi:10.1177/1460458213493197.
39. Parrish F, Do N, Bouhaddou O, Warnekar P. Implementation of RxNorm as a terminology mediation standard for exchanging pharmacy medication between federal agencies. AMIA Annu Symp Proc. 2006;1057.
40. Peleg M, Boxwala AA, Bernstam E, et al. Sharable representation of clinical guidelines in GLIF: relationship to the Arden Syntax. J Biomed Inform. 2001;34:170–81. doi:10.1006/jbin.2001.1016.
41. Phansalkar S, van der Sijs H, Tucker AD, et al. Drug-drug interactions that should be non-interruptive in order to reduce alert fatigue in electronic health records. J Am Med Inform Assoc. 2013;20:489–93. doi:10.1136/amiajnl-2012-001089.
42. Raschke RA, Gollihare B, Wunderlich TA, et al. A computer alert system to prevent injury from adverse drug events: development and evaluation in a community teaching hospital. JAMA. 1998;280:1317–20.
43. Ridgely MS, Greenberg MD. Too many alerts, too much liability. 2012. http://www.rand.org/pubs/external_publications/EP201200144.html. Accessed 17 Mar 2015.
44. Riva G. Ambient intelligence in health care. Cyber Psychology Behav. 2003;6:295–300. doi:10.1089/109493103322011597.
45. RSNA. New law mandates use of imaging appropriateness criteria. 2015. http://rsna.org/NewsDetail.aspx?id=12360. Accessed 30 Mar 2015
46. Seto E, Leonard KJ, Cafazzo JA, et al. Developing healthcare rule-based expert systems: case study of a heart failure telemonitoring system. Int J Med Inform. 2012;81:556–65. doi:10.1016/j.ijmedinf.2012.03.001.
47. Shah NR, Seger AC, Seger DL, et al. Improving acceptance of computerized prescribing alerts in ambulatory care. J Am Med Inform Assoc. 2006;13:5–11. doi:10.1197/jamia.M1868.
48. Shortliffe EH, Davis R, Axline SG, et al. Computer-based consultations in clinical therapeutics: explanation and rule acquisition capabilities of the MYCIN system. Comput Biomed Res. 1975;8:303–20.

49. Shwe M, Sujansky W, Middleton B. Reuse of knowledge represented in the Arden syntax. Proc Annu Symp Comput Appl Med Care. 1992;16:47–51.
50. Smith M, Murphy D, Laxmisan A, et al. Developing software to "track and catch" missed follow-up of abnormal test results in a complex sociotechnical environment. Appl Clin Inform. 2013;4:359–75. doi:10.4338/ACI-2013-04-RA-0019.
51. Sordo M, Boxwala AA, Ogunyemi O, Greenes RA. Description and status update on GELLO: a proposed standardized object-oriented expression language for clinical decision support. Stud Health Technol Inform. 2004;107:164–8.
52. Tu SW, Campbell JR, Glasgow J, et al. The SAGE guideline model: achievements and overview. J Am Med Inform Assoc. 2007;14:589–98. doi:10.1197/jamia.M2399.
53. Van der Sijs H, Aarts J, Vulto A, Berg M. Overriding of drug safety alerts in computerized physician order entry. J Am Med Inform Assoc. 2006;13:138–47. doi:10.1197/jamia.M1809.
54. Vardell E, Moore M. Isabel, a clinical decision support system. Med Ref Serv. 2011;30:158–66. doi:10.1080/02763869.2011.562800.
55. Wagner MM, Tsui FC, Pike J, Pike L. Design of a clinical notification system. Proc AMIA Symp. 1999;989–993.
56. Yu VL, Buchanan BG, Shortliffe EH, et al. Evaluating the performance of a computer-based consultant. Comput Methods Prog. 1979;9:95–102.

# Chapter 2
# Electronic Health Record Features, Functions, and Privileges That Clinicians Need to Provide Safe and Effective Care for Adults and Children

**Dean F. Sittig, Christopher A. Longhurst, Elise Russo, and Hardeep Singh**

**Abstract** This chapter will describe and discuss key requirements to enable clinician-users of electronic health records (EHRs) to deliver high-quality, safe, and effective care. We frame these requirements as "rights" and "responsibilities." The "rights" represent not merely desirable, but also important EHR features, functions, and user privileges that clinicians need to perform their job. Each "right" is accompanied by a corresponding clinician duty or "responsibility," without which the ultimate goal of improving healthcare quality might not be achieved. The issues discussed are generalizable to clinicians who care for adults and children using electronic health records across the globe. We recognize that healthcare presents complex and often unique challenges for the design and operation of health information

Adapted from:

Sittig DF, Singh H. Rights and responsibilities of users of electronic health records. CMAJ. 2012;184(13):1479–83. doi:10.1503/cmaj.111599.

Sittig DF, Singh H, Longhurst CA. Rights and responsibilities of electronic health records (EHR) users caring for children. Arch Argent Pediatr. 2013;111(6):468–71. doi:10.1590/S0325-00752013000600003.

D.F. Sittig, PhD (✉)
University of Texas Health Science Center at Houston's School of Biomedical Informatics and the UT-Memorial Hermann Center for Healthcare Quality & Safety, Houston, TX, USA
e-mail: dean.f.sittig@uth.tmc.edu

C.A. Longhurst, MD, MS
Division of Systems Medicine, Department of Pediatrics, Stanford University School of Medicine, Stanford, CA, USA

Information Services, Stanford Children's Health, Menlo Park, CA, USA
e-mail: CLonghurst@stanfordchildrens.org

E. Russo, MPH • H. Singh, MD, MPH
Houston Veterans Affairs Center for Innovations in Quality, Effectiveness and Safety, Michael E. DeBakey VA Medical Center, Houston, TX, USA

The Section of Health Services Research, Department of Medicine, Baylor College of Medicine, Houston, TX, USA
e-mail: elise.russo@bcm.edu; hardeeps@bcm.edu

© Springer International Publishing Switzerland 2016
C.A. Weaver et al. (eds.), *Healthcare Information Management Systems: Cases, Strategies, and Solutions*, Health Informatics,
DOI 10.1007/978-3-319-20765-0_2

technology-related facilities and EHRs worldwide. Addressing these rights and responsibilities comprehensively will be challenging, but we need to make the care delivered using electronic health record systems safer and more efficient.

**Keywords** Electronic health records • Physicians/ethics • Social responsibility • Decision support systems, clinical • Electronic health records/ethics • Electronic health records/standards • Health care quality • Medical informatics • Information systems

## 2.1 Introduction

Over the last 10 years the governments of Australia [1], Canada [2], United Kingdom [3], Belgium [4], Denmark [5], and most recently the United States of America [6], have all made long-term, multi-billion dollar investments in health information technologies (HIT), including electronic health records (EHRs). The primary goal of these initiatives is to transform the collection, display, transmission, and storage of patient data with the aim of improving citizens' health, while a secondary goal is to use this data to design improvements in their health care delivery systems. However, each of these initiatives has experienced significant challenges, including the poor fit between technology and clinical workflow that often leads to larger than expected disruptions in usual clinical processes [7]. These disruptions often result in safety concerns that are now emerging in several countries and for which there does not seem to be an immediate solution [8–11]. Several studies have also raised concerns about reduced clinician productivity and increased workload related to processing electronic information [12]. Moreover, the guaranteed costs of EHRs borne by clinicians (e.g., monetary or required changes in workflow) appear to outweigh the direct benefits to clinicians, while both patients and payers appear to benefit greatly [13,14]. Thus, EHR-enabled healthcare must facilitate the provision of features and functions that clinicians require to provide high-quality, cost-effective care, and the regulatory environment must support these provisions [15].

Based on emerging literature and our experiences in clinical informatics-focused health services research [16–23], we propose recommendations on a variety of topics to overcome many challenges faced by clinician EHR users. If adopted, these recommendations will provide assurances to clinician EHR users that EHRs will deliver the features and functions they require for safe and effective healthcare. In the second half of the chapter, we also take into account and propose a separate set of recommendations for children because of the differences involved in using an EHR when caring for children as opposed to adults. EHRs are often introduced as part of system redesign initiatives to improve safety and efficiency of long standing work processes, and thus some degree of workflow disruption is necessary. However, our recommendations address problem areas that are not easy to manage or may have long-term unintended consequences. The areas addressed here arise directly from our recently developed eight-dimension socio-technical model of safe and effective EHR use [24].

To encourage debate about these recommendations between clinicians and other stakeholders involved and to ensure that the regulatory environment will support them, we propose these recommendations as clinician-oriented, "professional rights." The "rights" represent not merely a desirable, but also an important set of EHR features, functions, and user privileges that clinicians need in order to provide the highest quality, safest, and most cost-effective care. Practicing clinicians are often at a relative disadvantage when negotiating EHR-related issues with other stakeholders, for example, healthcare administrators, HIT vendors, governments, insurance companies, other payers, or policy makers. A set of "rights" for clinicians is also essential to "level the playing field" so that EHRs, or the governmental or institutional policies that result from the aggregate data collected by them, do not restrict the freedom and ability of clinicians' to practice medicine in an open and safe manner [25]. Nevertheless, each "right" is accompanied by a corresponding clinician duty or responsibility, without which the ultimate goal of improving health care quality might not be achieved [26]. While these "rights" are clearly not of the same magnitude or universal importance as the United States Constitution's first ten amendments [27] or the Hippocratic Oath [28], these "rights" can reduce the potential impact of unintended adverse consequences on patient care and clinicians' livelihood [29]. We propose that these "rights" should be a foundation upon which HIT designers, developers, implementers, policy makers, and most importantly, users, can co-create a new age of computer-assisted healthcare [30].

## 2.2 Recommendations for Professional "Rights" and Responsibilities

### 2.2.1 Uninterrupted EHR Access

As clinicians and healthcare organizations begin to rely on computer-based patient records, extended EHR outages can pose a significant risk to their patients' health as well as the operation of the organization itself [31]. Therefore, clinicians have the right to access a certified EHR via a secure, network-attached device 24 hours-per-day, 7 days-per-week, 365 days-per-year. While no device can be 100 % reliable, EHR vendors, institutions, and clinicians must work together to design, implement, and use fail-safe equipment and downtime processes to protect data.

Clinicians have the responsibility to review all EHR data pertinent to their patient's medical history [32] (such as previously abnormal test results that might be buried in the EHR) while ensuring that EHR use does not replace the time-honored tradition of observing, listening to, and examining patients [33].

### 2.2.2 Ability to See All Data Required to Provide Safe and Effective Care

Unavailable or missing clinical information is a fertile ground for medical errors [34]. Thus, clinicians have the right to see all electronically captured clinical data pertaining to their patients in order to provide safe and effective care [35]. Amid concerns about patient privacy, some have argued that patients, or clinicians, should be able to "hide" specific data such as, alcohol/drug treatment or psychiatry notes [36], or even to "opt-out" of having their data available, www.thebigoptout.com [37]. However, this practice of limiting full access to patient data introduces additional, and we believe, unnecessary ambiguity and liability [38].

Clinicians have the responsibility to routinely use multiple strategies to protect the integrity of sensitive data such as creating strong passwords, logging off the system when done, and accessing only records of patients under their care.

### 2.2.3   Access to a Succinct Patient Summary

Current EHRs contain a wealth of clinical data, and as more Accountable Care Organizations (ACOs) are created and organization- or EHR vendor-specific, community-wide Health Information Exchanges come on-line, the amount of data available for review will grow exponentially, creating a potential for relevant information to be overlooked [39]. Clinicians thus have the right to EHRs that provide succinct summaries of their patients' medical problems, medications, laboratory test results, vital signs, and progress notes [35]. Some EHRs currently have "summary" views that arrange data by type: for example, all laboratory results in one place, and time-organized data displayed on different screens that show most recent data followed by previous data [40]. However, problem-oriented summaries that combine data from different sources related to a specific problem on one screen should also be tested and implemented because they might facilitate better information processing and exert a lower cognitive load [41,42].

To facilitate appropriate information gathering by other health care providers and for aggregate data collection, clinicians have the responsibility to maintain accurate, up-to-date problem lists using a controlled clinical terminology (e.g., SNOMED-CT) and to link them with corresponding diagnostic and treatment elements through the EHR [43].

### 2.2.4   Ability to Override Computer-Generated Alerts

Clinicians receive an excess of computer-generated alerts, many of which are considered unnecessary [44], causing fatigue, and some of which disrupt workflow because they cannot be overridden [45]. Clinicians have a right to override, but not permanently disable, any computer-generated clinical alert, except those prohibiting events that should never occur (e.g., ordering promethazine as intravenous push by peripheral vein [46]). Disallowing overrides, except in extreme circumstances, implies that computers have access to more accurate data and greater medical knowledge and expertise than clinicians. In reality, computers are often not able to interpret or convey the clinical context for many reasons: unavailable or inaccurate data; errors in logical processing (e.g. software bugs); situation-specific clinical exceptions, as when a user's request for blood transfusion is denied by Clinical Decision Support (CDS) intervention that did not capture active bleeding since last hemoglobin result [47]; and, user-interface limitations, such as in limited screen space available to show most recent laboratory results near medication order [48].

To prevent the possibility of critical information being ignored, clinicians have the responsibility to justify overrides and be accountable for decisions by agreeing to have their actions reviewed [49]. Clinicians also have a responsibility to participate on CDS oversight committees and work with other stakeholders to review, redesign, test, re-implement, or remove CDS interventions judged ineffective [50].

### 2.2.5 Explanation of Computer-Generated Clinical Interventions

A multitude of advanced CDS interventions are necessary if EHRs are to generate the improvements in healthcare quality, safety, and effectiveness that everyone expects [51]. Nevertheless, clinicians have the "right" to a clear, evidence-based rationale for all computer-generated clinical alerts or reminders at the point of care. For instance, it is insufficient to remind a clinician that a patient is due for a screening mammogram without also displaying the date and result of the previous test and a link to the clinical logic, as in, *all women over age 50 should have a mammogram every 2 years* [52].

Clinicians have the responsibility to consider computer-generated clinical interventions encountered in the EHR and use clinical judgment to assess their appropriateness in the patient's clinical context [53]. Either blindly following or ignoring CDS interventions can lead to errors [15].

### 2.2.6 Compensation for Technology-Mediated Care

With the widespread adoption of new technologies such as e-mail, personal health records, and video conferencing, clinicians are being asked to provide clinical consultations in ways for which reimbursement mechanisms are not well developed. Clinicians, therefore, have the right to receive compensation or workload credit for provision of healthcare mediated by HIT, be that through secure messaging or non-visit consultations based on EHR review, regardless of their or the patient's geographic location [54].

Clinicians have the responsibility to use state-of-the-art hardware, software, and procedures to ensure that communication remains confidential [55] and that all interactions are accurately documented for medico-legal purposes [56]. In addition, they should clarify their availability and policies regarding expected response times, so patients are not misled into expecting real-time responses to asynchronous communication [57].

### 2.2.7    Ability to Review Discrepancies in Performance-Measurement Data

EHR-based performance measurement is inevitable. Current data collection and measurement methods are not fail-safe and often measure what is easy to measure [58]. To correct discrepancies, clinicians have the right to review all EHR-based processes used to generate reports that further inform policy decisions or performance-measurement. All computer-based measurements should have unambiguous exclusion criteria and allow clinicians to identify patients for whom the measure does not apply; for example, no diabetic foot exams on patients with bilateral below-the-knee amputations [59]. Often, the first iterations of these computer-generated quality reports have errors which can lead to questions of the validity of the measures [60]. If needed, clinicians should be able to work with data analysts who have access to queries, data extracts, and statistical methods used to generate measurement reports. In addition, proactive collaboration with stakeholders such as the organizational leadership will help ensure that calculation, interpretation, and application of these performance measures are valid.

To ensure continuous quality improvement, clinicians have the responsibility to review the feedback they are provided on their performance and act on valid feedback.

### 2.2.8    Freedom to Report Errors

There are increasing reports of errors created by HIT (e-iatrogenesis) [61–63]. However, vendor contract clauses might prohibit error-reporting, at least in the US [64]. Clinicians must have the right to report EHR-related errors to the vendor and the organization that implemented the system, as well as to external organizations, such as AHRQ-approved Patient Safety Organizations (PSOs), and to expect errors to be investigated and resolved in a timely manner [65,66]. EHR errors can lead to substantial harm because of the large number of patients potentially affected; thus, error reports should be publically available so that others can learn from them as well [67].

Clinicians also have the responsibility to report, help investigate, and learn from these EHR errors.

### 2.2.9    Appropriate Access to Training and Assistance

State-of-the-art EHRs are complex tools designed to facilitate the entry, storage, review, interpretation, and transmission of patient data. Clinicians have the right to receive training in all EHR features that enable these processes, and to access online instruction and real-time assistance via telephone and remote computer support while caring for patients. Training should include refresher courses to meet evolving functionality.

Clinicians have the responsibility to maintain a high level of user proficiency with the same level of diligence as other clinical skills. To improve efficiency and safety, clinicians must learn to type, complete EHR training, and demonstrate competence in use of all functions required to care for patients (e.g., enter orders, add problems to the problem list, initiate referrals). Finally, clinicians are responsible for asking for help when they reach limits of their proficiency, for example electronically entering a complex steroid taper [68].

## *2.2.10   Access to EHRs That Fit Routine Clinical Workflows*

Embedding EHRs with computer-based provider order entry and real-time, point-of-care clinical decision support interventions fundamentally changes the way clinicians coordinate their work activities, communicate, and collaborate to deliver high-quality, safe, and effective healthcare [69]. Clinicians have the right to a safe, effective, and usable EHR that contains evidence-based, problem- and task-specific order sets and documentation templates designed to fit their clinical workflows [70].

Clinicians have the responsibility to ensure that they have done everything their partially automated documentation shows they have done. For instance, to generate new notes, they should avoid copying and pasting previous notes that are not relevant. Furthermore, clinicians have a responsibility to work with EHR vendors and local information technologists, in much the same way as they have successfully worked with various pharmaceutical manufacturers, medical device, and monitoring companies, to design, develop, and implement data entry, review, and CDS tools and to modify previous paper-based workflows to overcome limitations of EHRs [71]. Clinicians should either be compensated or given some type of educational or certification credit for their time spent working with information technology professionals to optimize these EHR systems.

## 2.3   Children and Neonates

As mentioned earlier, establishing a safe and effective electronic health record-enabled healthcare delivery system is complex and challenging. In addition to support from executive leadership, a robust EHR from a reputable vendor, and access to knowledgeable and committed information technology professionals, clinician support is instrumental in overcoming the challenges. While there is an increasing breadth of knowledge about good clinical practices needed to address EHR implementation and use in the general population, including the ten "rights" described above, clinicians responsible for the care of neonates, children, and adolescents face a unique set of additional challenges. For example, children have unique EHR requirements related to dosing of medications, as well as specific needs related to their growth and development that the EHR needs to facilitate [72].

Because of the unique circumstances involving the safe and effective care of children and the fact that most children are not cared for in facilities where the EHR has been designed exclusively for children, we propose these "pediatric amendments" to the above "Rights and Responsibilities of Users of EHRs" [73]. All previously identified rights and responsibilities still apply, along with these new pediatric-specific items discussed below.

### 2.3.1  Support for Medication Prescribing in Children

The epidemiology of harm associated with medication prescribing for neonates and children is very different from that of adult patients. Both hospitalized and ambulatory pediatric patients are at higher risk of harm from drug dosing errors than from drug-drug interactions [74,75]. Clinicians seeing pediatric patients have the right to both inpatient and ambulatory electronic prescribing systems that are safer and more effective for children and include weight-based dosing recommendations, age appropriate dosing calculators, dose-range checking, and pediatric-specific drug-drug interaction alerts [76,77].

Clinicians seeing pediatric patients have the responsibility to consistently and reliably document patient weights and should maintain familiarity with medication dosing guidelines, for example, to mitigate the "propensity of [clinicians] to over rely on automated advice" [78]. Several studies have documented that incorrect clinical decision support recommendations can cause clinicians to change from a correct to an incorrect course of action. These so-called "negative consultations" are one way to demonstrate "automation bias" [79].

### 2.3.2  Electronic Display of Growth Charts

Visual display of patient information is an important decision support tool. Clinicians should have the right to view their young patients' anthropometric data using growth charts [80] that display age-based percentiles for weight, height, head circumference, and body mass index (BMI) within their EHR [81].

All of these age-appropriate displays require up-to-date, accurate data capture; therefore, clinicians have the responsibility to record or facilitate the recording of patient's height, weight, and head circumference. Additionally, they should use this information to apply the appropriate age-specific clinical guidelines and provide copies of these charts to parents.

### 2.3.3 Child-Friendly, EHR-Equipped Exam Room

While not a specific feature or function of the EHR, clinicians caring for children have the right to an EHR-equipped exam room that is designed using appropriate human factors principles [82]. For example, rooms should have a layout that provides adequate room for the patient, a parent, and the clinician to move around [83]. In addition, keyboards and touchscreens should be cleaned and disinfected on a regular basis [84]. Finally, the computer, if wall-mounted, should be sturdy enough to withstand a child swinging from the support arm.

Clinicians have the responsibility for positioning the monitor so that he/she, as well as the parent and the patient, can see the screen simultaneously. This is particularly important in pediatrics, as children cannot rationalize the use of a computer in the exam room and may unintentionally misinterpret the intention [85].

### 2.3.4 User Interface That Supports Correct Identification of Patients

Several studies have suggested that pediatric patients in general and neonates in particular are at higher risk for misidentification because of naming issues during the newborn period and siblings being treated simultaneously at pediatric visits [86]. Clinicians who see these patients have a right to an EHR user interface which minimizes wrong-patient errors. Such functionality may include limiting users to one open chart at a time, availability of patient pictures within the EHR, and including additional patient verification processes with computerized order entry systems [87,88].

Electronic systems themselves may actually carry the unintended consequence of increasing the risk for "wrong-patient" type errors [89]. Users of these systems have a responsibility to ensure that processes are setup to capture patient photographs in the EHR so as to stay timely and current, and that misidentification errors are appropriately reported and fixed.

### 2.3.5 An EHR That Supports Adolescent Confidentiality

Although exact legal requirements vary, most countries acknowledge that adolescents have the right to keep mental, behavioral, and sexual healthcare confidential from their parents or guardians. Unfortunately, many commercial EHR's do not yet provide the functionality needed to respect these legal and ethical positions [90]. Pediatric users have the right to EHR software which includes default settings for adolescent privacy, customizable point-of-care privacy controls for clinicians, clear on-screen labeling of confidential data elements, patient-adjustable proxy access capabilities for patient portals, and suppression capabilities for specific items on post-visit summaries, bills, and post-visit surveys. In addition, adolescent privacy standards must be built into health information exchange data sharing agreements. These privacy standards should not limit any authorized clinician from seeing patient information; rather they are intended to help adolescents maintain their right to privacy as they make the difficult journey from being cared for by their parents to independent adulthood.

Clinicians seeing adolescent patients have the responsibility to understand local adolescent confidentiality regulatory requirements. They should also review the entire patient experience from registration to post-clinic surveys to ensure that the adolescent's confidentiality is maintained in light of these requirements.

### 2.3.6   EHR Content That Supports Pediatric Practice

To deliver appropriate preventive well-child care, pediatricians have the right to an EHR with content that supports the care of children. This includes appropriate decision support rules for timely preventive care, such as administration of immunizations and linkages to immunization registries, as well as content for pediatric normative values (e.g. laboratory test values) that frequently change with age [91]. Furthermore, EHRs must be optimized to support recording of quality measures for pediatrics.

Pediatricians have the responsibility to review decision support rules (e.g. do they match local vaccination schedules) and record key data that would lead to the generation of appropriate decision support.

## 2.4   Setting the Groundwork for Future Debate

Although this chapter lays the groundwork for future debate, it has several limitations. First, we do not specifically outline who might enforce these clinician "rights" and responsibilities or what alternatives could be pursued if these conditions are not met. However, we believe it is premature for us to do so at this conceptualization stage without further debate and agreement amongst clinical stakeholders, researchers, and policymakers. Second, we focus only on rights and responsibilities of users, but other EHR-related stakeholders might have different sets of rights and responsibilities which we did not cover in this chapter. Third, we recognize that even with consensus regarding the necessity of these "rights," delivering them in the next 3–5 years will be difficult using today's technology and in today's socio-political and economic environments. For example, two authors (DFS and HS) recently developed recommended practices for safe and effective EHR use in the form of the Safety Assurance Factors for EHR Resilience (SAFER) guides [92] with support from the US Office of the National Coordinator for Health Information Technology (ONC) [93]. Following their release in January 2014, the Electronic Health Record Association published a 27-page document [94] detailing their concerns that many of the recommendations are "beyond the current capabilities of HIT." Our goal, however, for putting forth such recommendations and for proposing EHR users' rights and responsibilities is to lay the foundation for a long-term agenda, that must begin now, to provide clinicians access to safe, effective, and easy to use EHRs that support their cognitive and physical work processes. Furthermore, the care of children and neonates presents complex challenges for the design and operation of healthcare facilities and EHRs worldwide. Similarly, for clinicians to provide the highest quality, safe, and effective care to children, EHRs providing care to children must be properly designed and configured, and clinicians must use them correctly. Finally, we recognize that achieving high-quality and affordable healthcare is a complex, socio-technical endeavor. Thus, these clinician rights might not be the perfect solution because there are many competing and often opposing views of the best way to accomplish this endeavor; however, most of the recommendations in this chapter represent basic EHR functionality that every EHR should provide. Moreover, safety requires innovation, and the current status quo will not improve standards of safety unless new functionalities evolve over time. The goal of these rights and responsibilities is to create a starting point to bring stakeholders together to discuss what's best for our patients, and not create regulation, policy, or guidelines. Therefore, we strongly recommend that EHR vendors, healthcare organizations, and clinicians come together and begin working to make them a reality, as soon as possible.

In addition, other stakeholders in this debate, including payers, administrators, policy makers, and patients, are also entitled to an equally important and valid set of "rights." Payers, administrators, and/or policy makers, for example, have the right to mandate use of EHR-related functions that promote patient safety (e.g., order entry); prohibit use of EHR-related functions that jeopardize patient safety (e.g., use of a non-secure, web-based calendar to facilitate clinician workflow [95] or use of text messaging for order entry [96]); enforce specific rules and regulations (e.g., reprimand users for unauthorized access to patient data); create new CDS interventions to encourage efficient, effective, evidence-based care; and evaluate clinicians' performance using EHR data. Likewise, patients have the right to access their data, have any data entry errors corrected, obtain a list of everyone who has viewed their data, confidentially communicate electronically with their providers, and request that certain data not be used for purposes other than research or public health benefit without their written consent [97]. In the event that one group's rights infringe upon those of another group, we are optimistic that organizations and the constituents they represent will participate in an open, constructive debate on these "rights" and reach consensus [98]. Following ratification, relevant stakeholders (e.g., EHR vendors, EHR implementers, professional boards, hospital committees, users, patients, and government agencies) can work together to design and implement EHRs and the corresponding policies, procedures, and regulations required to ensure these "rights."

## 2.5   Summary

We have developed a draft set of professional "rights" and responsibilities for clinician EHR-users in an effort to unite clinicians on key challenges they are currently facing while using EHRs. We make no claims regarding the prioritization of these "rights," rather we believe that taken together they form an important set of EHR features, functions, and user privileges that clinician users need to enable them to practice high-quality, safe, and effective medicine. These recommendations are generalizable to many clinicians and EHRs across the globe, and if turned into reality, can stimulate EHR adoption and use in a more efficient and safe manner. Moreover, organizations that provide their clinicians with state-of-the-art EHRs and grant them the professional "rights" identified along with the additional "pediatric amendments" could see dramatic improvements in clinician usage of their EHRs. This will lead us closer to the ultimate goal of improving the quality, safety, and effectiveness of care delivered to adults and children.

We acknowledge that our recommendations do not specifically outline who will enforce these "rights" and responsibilities or what alternatives will be pursued if these conditions are not met. However, we believe that healthcare organizations should begin working with their EHR vendors to implement these recommendations. In addition, clinicians must begin to accept their "responsibilities," which may add to their already over-extended workload. Therefore, we recognize that further debate and agreement is needed to figure out who should make these changes and how they will be implemented. We recognize that high-quality, affordable healthcare is a complex, socio-technical problem and that there are many competing and often opposing views of the best way to accomplish this task. In addition, we recognize that there are other stakeholders in this debate, most importantly, patients who are also entitled to a set of "rights" which may conflict with one or more of the clinicians' "rights." In that event, we are optimistic that medical societies and the clinicians they represent will participate in an open, constructive debate on these "rights" and reach consensus. Following ratification, relevant stakeholders (e.g., EHR vendors, EHR implementers, professional boards, hospital committees, users, patients, and government agencies) can work together to design and implement EHRs and the corresponding policies, procedures, and regulations required to ensure these "rights."

## References

1. Health Connect Implementation Strategy v2.1. 2005. http://www.health.gov.au/internet/hconnect/publishing.nsf/Content/archive-docs/$file/implementation.pdf.
2. EHRS Blueprint: an interoperable EHR framework. 2006. *https://knowledge.infoway-inforoute.ca/EHRSRA/doc/EHRS-Blueprint.pdf*,(Version 2).
3. House of Commons Public Accounts Committee. The National Programme for IT in the NHS: progress since 2006. 2009. Second Report of Session 2008–2009.

4. France FR. eHealth in Belgium, a new "secure" federal network: role of patients, health professions and social security services. Int J Med Inform. 2011;80(2):e12–6. doi:10.1016/j.ijmedinf.2010.10.005. doi:S1386-5056(10)00176-0 [pii]; Retrieved from PM:21035383.

5. Protti D, Johansen I. Widespread adoption of information technology in primary care physician offices in Denmark: a case study. Issue Brief (Commonw Fund). 2010;80:1–14. Retrieved from PM:20232528.

6. Health Information Technology for Economic and Clinical Health Act (HITECH). Public Law 111–5, 123 Stat 226, 2009.

7. Westbrook JI, Braithwaite J. Will information and communication technology disrupt the health system and deliver on its promise? Med J Aust. 2010;193(7):399–400. doi:wes10686_fm [pii]. Retrieved from PM:20919970.

8. Harrington L, Kennerly D, Johnson C. Safety issues related to the electronic medical record (EMR): synthesis of the literature from the last decade, 2000–2009. J Healthc Manag. 2011;56(1):31–43. Retrieved from PM:21323026.

9. Magrabi F, Ong MS, Runciman W, Coiera E. An analysis of computer-related patient safety incidents to inform the development of a classification. J Am Med Inform Assoc. 2010;17(6):663–70. doi:10.1136/jamia.2009.002444. doi:17/6/663 [pii]; Retrieved from PM:20962128.

10. Sittig DF, Singh H. Defining health information technology-related errors: new developments since to err is human. Arch Intern Med. 2011;171(14):1281–4. Retrieved from http://archinte.ama-assn.org/cgi/content/abstract/171/14/1281.

11. Meeks DW, Takian A, Sittig DF, Singh H, Barber N. Exploring the sociotechnical intersection of patient safety and electronic health record implementation. J Am Med Inform Assoc. 2014;21(e1):e28–34. doi:10.1136/amiajnl-2013-001762. Retrieved from PMID: 24052536.

12. Poissant L, Pereira J, Tamblyn R, Kawasumi Y. The impact of electronic health records on time efficiency of physicians and nurses: a systematic review. J Am Med Inform Assoc. 2005;12(5):505–16. doi:10.1197/jamia.M1700. doi:M1700 [pii]; Retrieved from PM:15905487.

13. Johnston D, Pan E, Walker J, Bates D, Middleton B. The value of computerized provider order entry in ambulatory settings center for information technology leadership. 2003.

14. Sprivulis P, Walker J, Johnston D, Pan E, Adler-Milstein J, Middleton B, et al. The economic benefits of health information exchange interoperability for Australia. Aust Health Rev. 2007;31(4):531–9. doi:ahr_31_4_531 [pii]. Retrieved from PM:17973611.

15. Sittig DF, Singh H. Eight rights of safe electronic health record use. JAMA J Am Med Assoc. 2009;302(10):1111–3. Retrieved from http://jama.ama-assn.org.

16. Ash JS, Sittig DF, Poon EG, Guappone K, Campbell E, Dykstra RH. The extent and importance of unintended consequences related to computerized provider order entry. J Am Med Inform Assoc. 2007;14(4):415–23. Retrieved from PM:17460127.

17. Campbell EM, Sittig DF, Ash JS, Guappone KP, Dykstra RH. Types of unintended consequences related to computerized provider order entry. J Am Med Inform Assoc. 2006;13(5):547–56. Retrieved from http://www.jamia.org/cgi/content/abstract/13/5/547.

18. Hysong SJ, Sawhney MK, Wilson L, Sittig DF, Esquivel A, Watford M, et al. Improving outpatient safety through effective electronic communication: a study protocol. Implement Sci. 2009;4:62. doi:10.1186/1748-5908-4-62. doi:1748-5908-4-62 [pii]; Retrieved from PM:19781075.

19. McMullen CK, Ash JS, Sittig DF, Bunce A, Guappone K, Dykstra R, et al. Rapid assessment of clinical information systems in the healthcare setting. An efficient method for time-pressed evaluation. Methods Inf Med. 2010;50(2):299–307. doi:10.3414/ME10-01-0042. doi:10-01-0042 [pii]; Retrieved from PM:21170469.

20. Singh H, Naik A, Rao R, Petersen L. Reducing diagnostic errors through effective communication: harnessing the power of information technology. J Gen Intern Med. 2008;23(4):489–94. doi:10.1007/s11606-007-0393-z. Retrieved from PM:18373151.

21. Singh H, Thomas EJ, Sittig DF, Wilson L, Espadas D, Khan MM, et al. Notification of abnormal lab test results in an electronic medical record: do any safety concerns remain? Am J Med.

2010;123(3):238–44. doi:10.1016/j.amjmed.2009.07.027. doi:S0002-9343(09)00956-5 [pii]; Retrieved from PM:20193832.

22. Singh H, Thomas EJ, Mani S, Sittig DF, Arora H, Espadas D, et al. Timely follow-up of abnormal diagnostic imaging test results in an outpatient setting: are electronic medical records achieving their potential? Arch Intern Med. 2009;169(17):1578–86. Retrieved from PM:19786677.

23. Sittig DF, Wright A, Osheroff JA, Middleton B, Teich JM, Ash JS, et al. Grand challenges in clinical decision support. J Biomed Inform. 2008;41(2):387–92. Retrieved from PM:18029232.

24. Sittig DF, Singh H. A new sociotechnical model for studying health information technology in complex adaptive healthcare systems. Qual Saf Health Care. 2010;19 Suppl 3:i68–74. Retrieved from http://qualitysafety.bmj.com/content/19/Suppl_3/i68.abstract.

25. Bambas L. Integrating equity into health information systems: a human rights approach to health and information. PLoS Med. 2005;2(4):e102. doi:10.1371/journal.pmed.0020102. doi:05-PLME-PF-0080 [pii]; Retrieved from PM:15839742.

26. Good Medical Practice: the duties of a doctor registered with the General Medical Council. Med Educ. 2001;35(Suppl 1):70–78.

27. Burns R. Introduction to a more perfect union: the creation of the United States Constitution. Washington, DC: Published for the National Archives and Records Administration by the National Archives Trust Fund Board; 1986.

28. The Hippocratic Oath. 2012. http://www.nlm.nih.gov/hmd/greek/greek_oath.html.

29. Sittig DF, Ash JS. Clinical information systems: overcoming adverse consequences. Sudbury: Jones and Bartlett Publishers, LLC.; 2009.

30. Stead WW, Searle JR, Fessler HE, Smith JW, Shortliffe EH. Biomedical informatics: changing what physicians need to know and how they learn. Acad Med. 2011;86(4):429–34. doi:10.1097/ACM.0b013e3181f41e8c. Retrieved from PM:20711055.

31. Campbell EM, Sittig DF, Guappone KP, Dykstra RH, Ash JS. Overdependence on technology: an unintended adverse consequence of computerized provider order entry. AMIA Annu Symp Proc. 2007;2007:94–8. Retrieved from PM:18693805.

32. Singh H, Hirani K, Kadiyala H, Rudomiotov O, Davis T, Khan MM, et al. Characteristics and predictors of missed opportunities in lung cancer diagnosis: an electronic health record-based study. J Clin Oncol. 2010;28(20):3307–15. doi:10.1200/JCO.2009.25.6636. doi:JCO.2009.25.6636 [pii]; Retrieved from PM:20530272.

33. Verghese A. Culture shock – patient as icon, icon as patient. N Engl J Med. 2008;359(26):2748–51. doi:10.1056/NEJMp0807461. doi:359/26/2748 [pii]; Retrieved from PM:19109572.

34. Smith PC, Raya-Guerra R, Bublitz C, Parnes B, Dickinson LM, Van Vorst R, et al. Missing clinical information during primary care visits. JAMA J Am Med Assoc. 2005;293(5):565–71. Retrieved from http://jama.ama-assn.org/cgi/content/abstract/293/5/565.

35. American College of Obstetricians and Gynecologists. Patient safety and the electronic health record. Committee opinion no. 472. Obstet Gynecol. 2010;116:1245–7.

36. Popovits RM. Confidentiality law: time for change? Behav Healthc. 2010;30(4):11–3. Retrieved from PM:20491322.

37. Greenhalgh T, Hinder S, Stramer K, Bratan T, Russell J. Adoption, non-adoption, and abandonment of a personal electronic health record: case study of HealthSpace. BMJ. 2010;341:c5814. Retrieved from PM:21081595.

38. Blumenthal D, Squires D. Giving patients control of their EHR data. J Gen Intern Med. 2015;30 Suppl 1:42–3. doi:10.1007/s11606-014-3071-y. Retrieved from PMID: 25480725.

39. Sittig DF, Singh H. Legal, ethical, and financial dilemmas in electronic health record adoption and use. Pediatrics. 2011;127(4):e1042–7. doi:10.1542/peds.2010-2184. doi:peds.2010-2184 [pii]; Retrieved from PM:21422090.

40. Laxmisan A, McCoy AB, Wright A, Sittig DF. Clinical summarization capabilities of commercially-available and internally-developed electronic health records. Appl Clin Inf. 2012;3(1):80–93. doi:10.4338/ACI-2011-11-RA-0066. Retrieved from PM:22468161.

41. Feblowitz JC, Wright A, Singh H, Samal L, Sittig DF. Summarization of clinical information: a conceptual model. J Biomed Inform. 2011;44(4):688–99. doi:10.1016/j.jbi.2011.03.008. doi:S1532-0464(11)00059-1 [pii]; Retrieved from PM:21440086.

42. Powsner SM, Wyatt JC, Wright P. Opportunities for and challenges of computerisation. Lancet. 1998;352(9140):1617–22. doi:10.1016/S0140-6736(98)08309-3. doi:S0140-6736(98)08309-3 [pii]; Retrieved from PM:9843122.
43. Samal L, Linder JA, Bates DW, Wright A. Electronic problem list documentation of chronic kidney disease and quality of care. BMC Nephrol. 2014;4(15)):70. doi:10.1186/1471-2369-15-70. Retriced from PMID: 24885821.
44. Isaac T, Weissman JS, Davis RB, Massagli M, Cyrulik A, Sands DZ, et al. Overrides of medication alerts in ambulatory care. Arch Intern Med. 2009;169(3):305–11. Retrieved from PM:19204222.
45. Strom BL, Schinnar R, Aberra F, Bilker W, Hennessy S, Leonard CE, et al. Unintended effects of a computerized physician order entry nearly hard-stop alert to prevent a drug interaction: a randomized controlled trial. ArchIntern Med. 2010;170(17):1578–83. doi:10.1001/archinternmed.2010.324. doi:170/17/1578 [pii]; Retrieved from PM:20876410.
46. Grissinger M. Preventing serious tissue injury with intravenous promethazine (phenergan). P T. 2009;34(4):175–6. Retrieved from PM:19561855.
47. Lepage EF, Gardner RM, Laub RM, Golubjatnikov OK. Improving blood transfusion practice: role of a computerized hospital information system. Transfusion. 1992;32(3):253–9. Retrieved from PMID: 1557808.
48. Horsky J, Kuperman GJ, Patel VL. Comprehensive analysis of a medication dosing error related to CPOE. J Am Med Inform. 2005;12(4):377–82. Retrieved from PMID: 15802485.
49. Kuperman GJ, Bobb A, Payne TH, Avery AJ, Gandhi TK, Burns G, et al. Medication-related clinical decision support in computerized provider order entry systems: a review. J Am Med Inform Assoc. 2007;14(1):29–40. Retrieved from PM:17068355.
50. Wright A, Sittig DF, Ash JS, Bates DW, Feblowitz J, Fraser G, et al. Governance for clinical decision support: case studies and recommended practices from leading institutions. J Am Med Inform Assoc. 2011;18(2):187–94. Retrieved from PM:21252052.
51. Linder JA, Ma J, Bates DW, Middleton B, Stafford RS. Electronic health record use and the quality of ambulatory care in the United States. Arch Intern Med. 2007;167(13):1400–5. doi:10.1001/archinte.167.13.1400. doi:167/13/1400 [pii]; Retrieved from PM:17620534.
52. U.S. Preventive Services Task Force. Screening for breast cancer: recommendation statement. Ann Intern Med. 2009;151(10):716–26. Update retrieved from http://www.uspreventiveservicestaskforce.org/Page/Document/UpdateSummaryDraft/breast-cancer-screening1.
53. McCoy AB, Waitman LR, Lewis JB, Wright JA, Choma DP, Miller RA, Peterson JF. A framework for evaluating the appropriateness of clinical decision support alerts and responses. J Am Med Inform Assoc. 2012;19(3):346–52. doi:10.1136/amiajnl-2011-000185. PMID: 21849334.
54. Stone JH. Communication between physicians and patients in the era of E-medicine. N Engl J Med. 2007;356(24):2451–4. doi:10.1056/NEJMp068198. doi:356/24/2451 [pii]; Retrieved from PM:17568026.
55. Ruotsalainen P. Privacy and security in teleradiology. Eur J Radiol. 2010;73(1):31–5. doi:10.1016/j.ejrad.2009.10.018. doi:S0720-048X(09)00582-8 [pii]; Retrieved from PM:19914020.
56. Marguet CG, Springhart WP, Preminger GM. New technology for imaging and documenting urologic procedures. Urol Clin North Am. 2006;33(3):397–408. doi:10.1016/j.ucl.2006.03.002. doi:S0094-0143(06)00034-6 [pii]; Retrieved from PM:16829273.
57. Byrne JM, Elliott S, Firek A. Initial experience with patient-clinician secure messaging at a VA medical center. J Am Med Inform Assoc. 2009;16(2):267–70. doi:10.1197/jamia.M2835. doi:M2835 [pii]; Retrieved from PM:19074303.
58. Ofri D. Quality measures and the individual physician. N Engl J Med. 2010;363(7):606–7. doi:10.1056/NEJMp1006298. Retrieved from PM:20818853.
59. Persell SD, Dolan NC, Friesema EM, Thompson JA, Kaiser D, Baker DW. Frequency of inappropriate medical exceptions to quality measures. Ann Intern Med. 2010;152(4):225–31. doi:10.7326/0003-4819-152-4-201002160-00007. doi:152/4/225 [pii]; Retrieved from PM:20157137.
60. Kern LM, Malhotra S, Barron Y, Quaresimo J, Dhopeshwarkar R, Pichardo M, Edwards AM, Kaushal R. Accuracy of electronically reported "meaningful use" clinical quality measures: a

cross-sectional study. Ann Intern Med. 2013;158(2):77–83. doi:10.7326/0003-4819-158-2-201301150-00001. Retrieved from PMID: 23318309.

61. Myers RB, Jones SL, Sittig DF. Review of reported clinical information system adverse events in US Food and Drug Administration databases. Appl Clin Inform. 2011;2:63–74. doi:10.4338/ACI-2010-11-RA-0064.

62. Menon S, Singh H, Meyer AN, Belmont E, Sittig DF. Electronic health record-related safety concerns: a cross-sectional survey. J Healthc Risk Manag. 2014;34(1):14–26. doi:10.1002/jhrm.21146. PMID: 25070253.

63. Meeks DW, Smith MW, Taylor L, Sittig DF, Scott JM, Singh H. An analysis of electronic health record-related patient safety concerns. J Am Med Inform Assoc. 2014;21(6):1053–9. doi:10.1136/amiajnl-2013-002578. Retrieved from PMID: 24951796.

64. Koppel R, Kreda D. Health care information technology 'vendors' "hold harmless" clause. JAMA J Am Med Assoc. 2009;301(12):1276–8. Retrieved from http://jama.ama-assn.org/content/301/12/1276.short.

65. Goodman KW, Berner ES, Dente MA, Kaplan B, Koppel R, Rucker D, et al. Challenges in ethics, safety, best practices, and oversight regarding HIT vendors, their customers, and patients: a report of an AMIA special task force. J Am Med Inform Assoc. 2011;18(1):77–81. Retrieved from http://jamia.bmj.com/content/18/1/77.abstract.

66. Middleton B, Bloomrosen M, Dente MA, Hashmat B, Koppel R, Overhage JM, Payne TH, Rosenbloom ST, Weaver C, Zhang J. Enhancing patient safety and quality of care by improving the usability of electronic health record systems: recommendations from AMIA. J Am Med Inform Assoc. 2013;20(e1):e2–8. doi:10.1136/amiajnl-2012-001458. Retrieved from PMID: 23355463.

67. Walker JM, Carayon P, Leveson N, Paulus RA, Tooker J, Chin H, et al. EHR safety: the way forward to safe and effective systems. J Am Med Inform Assoc. 2008;15(3):272–7. doi:10.1197/jamia.M2618. doi:M2618 [pii]; Retrieved from PM:18308981.

68. Singh H, Mani S, Espadas D, Petersen N, Franklin V, Petersen LA. Prescription errors and outcomes related to inconsistent information transmitted through computerized order entry: a prospective study. Arch Intern Med. 2009;169(10):982–9. doi:10.1001/archinternmed.2009.102. doi:169/10/982 [pii]; Retrieved from PM:19468092.

69. Campbell EM, Guappone KP, Sittig DF, Dykstra RH, Ash JS. Computerized provider order entry adoption: implications for clinical workflow. J Gen Intern Med. 2009;24(1):21–6. Retrieved from PM:19020942.

70. Wright A, Sittig DF, Carpenter JD, Krall MA, Pang JE, Middleton B. Order sets in computerized physician order entry systems: an analysis of seven sites. AMIA Annu Symp Proc. 2010;2010:892–6. Retrieved from PM:21347107.

71. Koppel R, Metlay JP, Cohen A, Abaluck B, Localio AR, Kimmel SE, et al. Role of computerized physician order entry systems in facilitating medication errors. JAMA J Am Med Assoc. 2005;293(10):1197–203. Retrieved from PM:15755942.

72. Spooner SA. Special requirements of electronic health record systems in pediatrics. Pediatrics. 2007;119(3):631–7. doi:10.1542/peds.2006-3527. doi:119/3/631 [pii]; Retrieved from PM:17332220.

73. Sittig DF, Singh H. Rights and responsibilities of users of electronic health records. CMAJ. 2012. doi:10.1503/cmaj.111599. cmaj.111599 [pii], Retrieved from PM:22331971.

74. Kaushal R, Bates DW, Landrigan C, McKenna KJ, Clapp MD, Federico F, et al. Medication errors and adverse drug events in pediatric inpatients. JAMA J Am Med Assoc. 2001;285(16):2114–20. doi:joc01942 [pii]. Retrieved from PM:11311101.

75. Kaushal R, Goldmann DA, Keohane CA, Christino M, Honour M, Hale AS, et al. Adverse drug events in pediatric outpatients. Ambul Pediatr. 2007;7(5):383–9. doi:10.1016/j.ambp.2007.05.005. doi:S1530-1567(07)00090-1 [pii]; Retrieved from PM:17870647.

76. Harper MB, Longhurst CA, McGuire TL, Tarrago R, Desai BR, Patterson A. Core drug-drug interaction alerts for inclusion in pediatric electronic health records with computerized prescriber order entry. J Patient Saf. 2014;10(1):59–63. doi:10.1097/PTS.0000000000000050. Retrieved from PM:24522227.

77. Stevens LA, Palma JP, Pandher KK, Longhurst CA. Immunization registries in the EMR Era. Online J Public Health Inform. 2013;5(2):211. doi:10.5210/ojphi.v5i2.4696. ojphi-05-211 [pii]. Retrieved from PM:23923096.

78. Goddard K, Roudsari A, Wyatt JC. Automation bias: a systematic review of frequency, effect mediators, and mitigators. J Am Med Inform Assoc. 2012;19(1):121–7. doi:10.1136/amiajnl-2011-000089. doi:amiajnl-2011-000089 [pii]; Retrieved from PM:21685142.

79. Goddard K, Roudsari A, Wyatt JC. Automation bias: empirical results assessing influencing factors. Int J Med Inform. 2014;83(5):368–75. doi:10.1016/j.ijmedinf.2014.01.001. [doi]. Retrieved from PMID: 24581700.

80. Rosenbloom ST, Qi X, Riddle WR, Russell WE, DonLevy SC, Giuse D, et al. Implementing pediatric growth charts into an electronic health record system. J Am Med Inform Assoc. 2006;13(3):302–8. doi:10.1197/jamia.M1944. doi:M1944 [pii]; Retrieved from PM:16501182.

81. Lowry S, Quinn M, Ramaiah M, Brick D, Patterson E, Zhang J. et al. A human factors guide to enhance EHR usability of critical user interactions when supporting pediatric patient care national institutes of standards and technology: US Department of Commerce. 2012. Retrieved from: http://www.nist.gov/healthcare/usability/upload/NIST-IR-7865.pdf.

82. Freihoefer K, Nyberg G, Vickery C. Clinic exam room design: present and future. HERD. 2013;6(3):138–56. Retrieved from PM:23817912.

83. Henriksen K, Dayton E, Keyes MA, Carayon P, Hughes R. Understanding adverse events: a human factors framework. 2008. doi:NBK2666 [bookaccession]. Retrieved from PM:21328766.

84. Neely AN, Sittig DF. Basic microbiologic and infection control information to reduce the potential transmission of pathogens to patients via computer hardware. J Am Med Inform Assoc. 2002;9(5):500–8. Retrieved from PM:12223502.

85. Toll E. A piece of my mind. The cost of technology. JAMA J Am Med Assoc. 2012;307(23):2497–8. doi:10.1001/jama.2012.4946. doi:1187932 [pii]; Retrieved from PM:22797449.

86. Gray JE, Suresh G, Ursprung R, Edwards WH, Nickerson J, Shiono PH, et al. Patient misidentification in the neonatal intensive care unit: quantification of risk. Pediatrics. 2006;117(1):e43–7. doi:117/1/e43 [pii];10.1542/peds.2005-0291 [doi]. Retrieved from PM:16396847.

87. Hyman D, Laire M, Redmond D, Kaplan DW. The use of patient pictures and verification screens to reduce computerized provider order entry errors. Pediatrics. 2012;130(1):e211–9. doi:10.1542/peds.2011-2984. doi:peds.2011-2984 [pii]; Retrieved from PM:22665415.

88. McCoy AB, Wright A, Kahn MG, Shapiro JS, Bernstam EV, Sittig DF. Matching identifiers in electronic health records: implications for duplicate records and patient safety. BMJ Qual Saf. 2013;22(3):219–24. doi:10.1136/bmjqs-2012-001419. doi:bmjqs-2012-001419 [pii]; Retrieved from PM:23362505.

89. Levin HI, Levin JE, Docimo SG. "I meant that med for Baylee not Bailey!": a mixed method study to identify incidence and risk factors for CPOE patient misidentification. AMIA Annu Symp Proc. 2012;2012:1294–301. Retrieved from PM:23304408.

90. Anoshiravani A, Gaskin GL, Groshek MR, Kuelbs C, Longhurst CA. Special requirements for electronic medical records in adolescent medicine. J Adolesc Health. 2012;51(5):409–414. doi:S1054-139X(12)00335-7 [pii];10.1016/j.jadohealth.2012.08.003 [doi]. Retrieved from PM:23084160.

91. Spooner SA, Classen DC. Data standards and improvement of quality and safety in child health care. Pediatrics. 2009;123 Suppl 2:S74–9. doi:10.1542/peds.2008-1755E. doi:123/Supplement_2/S74 [pii]; Retrieved from PM:19088233.

92. Sittig DF, Singh H, editors. SAFER electronic health records: safety assurance factors for EHR resilience. Oakville: Apple Academic Press; 2015.

93. Office of the National Coordinator for Health Information Technology. Safety Assurance Factors for EHR Resilience (SAFER) Guides. 2014. Available at: http://healthit.gov/safer/.

94. HIMSS Electronic Health Record Association. 2014. Comments on SAFER guides. Available at: http://www.himssehra.org/docs/SAFER%20Guides%20Comments%20Final.pdf.

95. Department of Veterans Affairs Monthly Report to Congress on Data Incidents. 2010. Retrieved from: http://www.va.gov/ABOUT_VA/docs/monthly_rfc_nov2010.pdf.

96. The Joint Commission. Texting orders. 2011. Retrieved from: http://www.jointcommission.org/standards_information/jcfaqdetails.aspx?StandardsFaqld=401&Programld=1.
97. Smith, M. Patient's bill of rights: a comparative overview (PRB 01-31E). Government of Canada: Depository Services Program; 2002. Retrieved from: http://dsp-psd.pwgsc.gc.ca/Collection-R/LoPBdP/BP/prb0131-e.htm.
98. Beard L, Schein R, Morra D, Wilson K, Keelan J. The challenges in making electronic health records accessible to patients. J Am Med Inform Assoc. 2012;19(1):116–20. doi:10.1136/amiajnl-2011-000261. doi:amiajnl-2011-000261 [pii]; Retrieved from PM:22120207.

# Chapter 3
# The Journey to Usability: A Vendor's Perspective

James T. Ingram

**Abstract** To successfully utilize the full functionality of a mission-critical application such as an electronic health record (EHR), it is imperative to be flexible, intuitive, feature-rich and scalable. On a foundational level, having access to an application running with high-speed connections and fast processing speeds with an easily accessible network on a device suitable to the clinicians' choice and for the environment desired is the expectation of most users. But when it comes to usability, can the subjective become a science? Vendors, certification bodies, insurance payers, federal policy organizations and the Institute of Medicine think so, and have been working to reconcile the two-way street of adherence to training and implementation with design and workflow best practices. The additional challenge for the EHR software vendors has been the interoperability of all the components within a clinical setting to achieve optimal efficiency and results. Continued challenges grow as care coordination, quality reporting and more detailed coding lead to user options in the areas of data recognition and/or sophisticated voice recognition that capture discrete codified information. For those of us in the medical Information Technology (IT) space, ensuring that the parallel tracts of hardware, communications, networks, browsers and software applications lead to an effective EHR requires constant balance. Users must reconcile the reality of "clicks" with the need for availability of data without becoming overwhelmed. Together, the challenge of advancing mutually beneficial solutions in a highly regulated and standards-based environment has truly been monumental. This review looks at the past leading up to our current status and what is on the near and far horizon of gains in EHR usability.

**Keywords** History of ambulatory EHR • Usability impacted by hardware • Software • Regulations and features • Training and user engagement

J.T. Ingram, MD, FACS
Chief Medical Officer, Clinical Informatics, Greenway Health, Inc., Carrollton, GA, USA
e-mail: jim.ingram@greenwayhealth.com

© Springer International Publishing Switzerland 2016                                      39
C.A. Weaver et al. (eds.), *Healthcare Information Management Systems:*
*Cases, Strategies, and Solutions*, Health Informatics,
DOI 10.1007/978-3-319-20765-0_3

## 3.1   Introduction

To fully grasp the usability issues within an EHR system, you must have an under-standing of the developmental history of an EHR. There have been many changes over the past two to three decades within the United States (US) healthcare system. The Institute of Medicine (IOM) called for paperless medical records in 10 years in a publication in 1991 [13]. President George W. Bush, in the State of the Union address in January 2004, announced, "By computerizing health records, we can avoid dangerous medical mistakes, reduce costs, and improve care. To protect the doctor patient relationship and keep good doctors doing good work; we must elimi-nate wasteful and frivolous medical lawsuits" [4], the goal being to provide every citizen in the US with a personal electronic medical record. The intensity of that effort was accelerated by President Obama in February of 2009 when he signed into law the American Restoration and Recovery Act and Health Information Technology for Economic and Clinical Health (HITECH) Act, which provided financial and technical assistance to practices implementing an EHR [2].

Since then, there has been a significant, if not dramatic, change in the develop-ment and implementation of electronic health records. For many years there was a mounting frustration for healthcare workers dealing with a paper-centric world while many other industries had learned to function efficiently and effectively in an electronic environment. This only heightened the desire for a modernized approach for complete patient management within a software application.

In the 1980s and early 1990s, the business tools used in physicians' offices on a daily basis had become highly sophisticated, but our patient clinical documentation lagged behind and still was still paper-based. Some physicians began to embrace some basic forms of electronic document capture for direct patient care. It became obvious to many that expanding to a more sophisticated system that allowed the clinical side of the practice to be as effective as the practice management was desir-able. But most clinicians had concerns as to how an EHR was going to capture all the details of a highly variable patient documentation environment.

As physicians became more exposed to other industries that were embracing internet based applications, they were developing an increased interest in having similar applications in clinical medicine. The securities and banking world led the way towards web browser-based applications; the world of clinical medicine, how-ever, was lacking that ability to modernize for a variety of reasons. So, the idea of having an internet accessible application where the practice records, both financial and clinical, were housed at a remote server and therefore out of the direct control of the practice was concerning for physicians and administrators. This was new for practices and initially a major concern because the practice would literally come to a standstill if the access stopped. Additionally, all the practice data were in the hands of someone else, which left physicians very uncomfortable. However, as more practices became comfortable with companies that offered remote applica-tions, the resistance was been much less. Currently, the trend is towards a distribu-tive network of servers or Cloud technology. If those other business institutions could effectively deal with the security and privacy issues, then it seemed reasonable for healthcare to be able to do the same.

But to achieve a highly usable EHR application within a practice, a major basic need is having an IT workforce that understood medical practice workflow and requirements. How to get the EHR application at the point of care without interfering with the delivery of care was paramount. Early on, the networking and wireless capabilities were very limited and the cost in many ways was especially challenging for smaller practices. For some small practices, it was just cost-prohibitive to implement an EHR.

With the introduction of tablets and portable laptops, many practices saw the advantages of these tools. But these devices were bulky and heavy with a short battery life, which made them a challenge to use at the point of care. Also, their function was compromised by generally poor wireless connections within the physical plant of a practice. Many traditional paper-based practices had a physical layout that was not conducive to good wireless communications or having adequate workspace for the larger desktop computers near the exam rooms. Even when hard wired to their internet service, the internet service provider (ISP) were not reliable, requiring practices to invest in a higher-speed, more expensive T1 connection.

In addition, the software was primarily designed for desktop PC use, so having a smaller-form tablet caused more usability issues. Issues like font size, scalability and page loading over the wireless caused many users to become frustrated. So early on, only the committed, tech-savvy users embraced the new world of EHRs. Despite frustrations, these early adopters saw the advantages of the electronic health record.

Additionally, regulatory elements such as Health Insurance Portability and Accountability Act (HIPAA) were and continue to be a significant force in how an EHR potentially handles privacy and security in the protection of personal health information. And above all, patient safety is paramount in the EHR world – we need to protect, validate and act on reliable medical information to provide the utmost in patient care.

As a physician, my natural focus within my practice was to find an efficient workflow to handle the needs of my patients and at the same time provide a usable, functional document for my patient visits. Documentation requirements and needs have exploded over the last few decades. Initially the main focus of a clinical document was to provide a "note" for future reference about the patient's condition. But we all know this has been expanded to deal with coding and billing needs as well as medicolegal needs and payer audits. And now, there is an increased need for discrete data for Meaningful Use and other quality analytics. So the physician in the trenches finds himself and his staff documenting a variety of things that are not considered germane to the care of the patient.

My, and many of my colleagues', criticism of the early experience with an EHR has been that the technology did not allow me to be as efficient as I thought I was in the paper world. It has been hard for clinicians to straddle the proverbial EHR fence when adopting an EHR, still having one foot in the paper world and one foot in new the EHR world. EHRs seemed restrictive and inflexible when it came to the demands within a clinical practice. So the challenge seemed to be that an EHR had to have the same flexibility as a paper record. That seemed reasonable until one realized that paper records had their own challenges in that not only were they bulky and disorganized, but only one person could have access to them at a time. Additionally, they often got misplaced, took up significant space and had to be maintained for at least 10 years by law, and there was a high paper/resource cost to "open" a chart on a new patient.

Despite the general frustration with EHRs over the years, many clinicians, when asked, would not return to paper. As of 2013 according to a National Center for Health Statistics (NCHS) Data Brief [8], nearly 80 % of physician practices in the US had at least a basic EHR. Acute care hospitals by 2013 have a 59 % adoption rate of a basic EHR, with 94 % being a certified EHR, according to an Office of the National Coordinator (ONC) Data Brief in May, 2014 [5].

The goal of this chapter is to explain how the components of an EHR interact to impact usability and how they have changed over time. As with most changes that occur within an industry, demand, regulations, law, and technology drive the innovation and improvements. No user wants to use, and no vendor wants to design and build, an unusable product. The over-arching desire is to have a fully functional EHR that incorporates the features needed to join the patient and providers in a comprehensive care record.

## 3.2 The Journey Up Until Now

So, how has usability been impacted over the years? There are multiple forces impacting the world of EHRs. Reviewing the developmental history of electronic medical records over the previous two to three decades gives us a better understanding of the complexity of the topic of usability.

When EHRs, formerly known as EMRs (electronic medical records) and before then, CPRs (computerized patient records), started gaining popularity in the early 1990s, their focus was obviously much more rudimentary than it is now. Practice management (PM) systems had existed for approximately a decade and filled a significant need for most ambulatory practices. The PM applications were growing in sophistication with the enhanced requirements for billing and claims management. The realization that the clinical side of practice was still in a paper world provided a strange dichotomy as the clinicians became more knowledgeable about computers.

The challenge has always been based on the argument that it is hard to capture the amount of variability within a clinical visit in an electronic format. However, at the same time, many ambulatory practitioners used some types of forms to capture information, and others dictated their visit encounters. As I took a more critical view of this argument, I began to realize there were many things I did in my practice that were very repetitive on a daily basis. When conditions such as the Flu or sinusitis, gallstones or a routine health visit are the concern, then a narrative can easily be repeated with relatively little variation from the previous patient with the same issue. This situation lends itself nicely to having a symptom- or diagnosis-based template to easily compile the patients' medical history information and their current complaints along with a standard set of orders and instructions for that patient. However, for a certain percentage of patient visits, depending on the specialty, an argument can be made that there are situations in which a more detailed and complex narrative is needed to capture the nuances of the patient's problems. Many clinicians still used commercial or self-made forms, or used a set of dictation templates that their transcriptionists inserted into the documentation. Despite the documentation purists in the medical world, a ubiquitous statement in medical training was "common things happen commonly, so when you hear hoof beats, don't always think of zebras." Using this argument, many EHRs have focused on some type of template-based application for the clinical side. Build a system that allows common frequent tasks to be performed effectively and efficiently, but leave enough flexibility for the exceptions in documentation and workflow.

In the paper world, trying to get information out of the collective set of medical records in a practice was a significant, laborious challenge. Individual records had to be "pulled," then meticulously reviewed and the expectant data elements compiled in order to get a view of a group of patients. So most physicians only had a supposition of how they effectively practice on a population basis. How did their management of a diabetic patient compare to that of their peers? With an EHR, now clinicians have the ability to understand practice patterns and treatment of a population of patients. Population health management now becomes more likely in the EHR world.

More physicians could see the advantage of making the clinic side as efficient as the practice side had become. A good example of this was when a drug named Vioxx by Merck became available in May, 1999, a non-steroidal anti-inflamatory drug, Vioxx became a very popular prescription for patients with discomfort from musculo-skeletal problems, such as arthritis. There were studies, such as VIGOR, that raised concerns about the increased incidence of heart attacks and deaths directly related to the drug [10]. Greener stated that there were an estimated 88,000 heart attacks and 33,000 deaths from Vioxx [6]. Using this example, if more physicians were able to compile their information, perhaps the fact that Vioxx was a dangerous drug could have been verified earlier. In a paper-based practice, the physicians had no clear understanding of which patients were on this drug. Someone within the practice would have had to literally look through each patient's paper record to identify and verify whether the patient had received Vioxx. Now in an EHR, a report can quickly be run on those patients. This feature alone has without a doubt improved patient safety. This example only illustrates the usefulness of being able to extract valuable information out of an EHR; the challenge is still the inputting of data into a system. But this will slowly resolve as more systems are interoperable through the sharing of discrete codified data.

Additionally, outside of the office or clinic, there was no access to patient information. So, many decisions when dealing with a patient afterhours were made by memory or inadequate feedback from the patient or a relative. This was especially true when one was covering for a large number of colleagues and had never met or cared for the patients previously. Certain physicians, such as obstetricians, were forced to have paper charts available for their near-term pregnant patients at the hospital's labor and delivery department. The potential of losing the charts or having them compromised in some way was real.

With more discrete data being accumulated, there is a perception, if not a demand from outside agencies that these data should be readily accessible to them. This has put an increasing demand on clinicians and staff to record even larger amounts of data that may not directly impact or improve patient care. The incentive payments vortex draws practices and physicians into an ever increasing requirement for advanced reporting. Grant-based programs, such as Federally Qualified Health Care (FQCH) clinics and Community Health Clinics (CHC), add another layer of demographic data collection and reporting that is usually not part of most practices' information needs. Unfortunately, there may be an unrealistic expectation that the potential availability of all these data implies some level of clinical effectiveness. So, are EHRs more uniformly able to provide clinically relevant data with which to accurately assess the effectiveness of treatment of a patient and the level of competence of medical staffs?

PM systems became the first obvious step on practices' electronic journeys. There were many data points to capture regarding demographics, insurance plan details, scheduling, coding and billing for claims. Electronic claims filing requirements made an electronic PM system mandatory for practices while the clinical side still maintained a paper record, but we still had PM needs within the paper record also. To the casual observer, it was apparent that there were two worlds in the ambulatory practices.

For the most part, employees in the front office were stationary and could easily use a desktop computer to effectively do their work. However, the clinical staffs were constantly on the move between exam and procedure rooms. They needed mobility in the computer systems that just wasn't available at that time. Additionally, there were external elements in our world: payers, legal, hospitals, medical consultants and regulatory agencies still needed or required a paper document. Communication among medical environments was all paper-based, with mail and fax as the only electronic link.

Early EMRs were focusing on documenting the visit. But it became obvious early that a computer could perform additional functions such as Evaluation and Management (E&M) coding and alerts/reminders. So within a short time it became obvious that there are multiple other needs within a clinical setting that a computer could facilitate. At the same time, hospitals were exposed to a variety of systems that allowed electronic capture of information in various departments. Inventory control was the principal need, followed by pharmacy needs and laboratory as well as clinical documentation needs. Once the hospitals entered into the era of computerized physician order entry (CPOE), the demands on the IT infrastructure increased as a result of patient care needs and safety. All of us who lived through those transitions remember the challenge of CPOE. What now came to the forefront was the development of IT shops within the acute care situations. Hospitals, as they added more modules to their software, were requiring more sophisticated IT staffs. However, in the ambulatory environment, there was a paucity of local IT companies that could help practices with their computer and network needs.

As the IT infrastructure moved from individual PCs to a local network, there became an added level of expertise that many practices did not have or did not want to develop. Many locales around the country did not have expertise in the surrounding vicinity to assist the practices in establishing a good IT strategy.

Wireless (Wi-Fi) standardization started in 1997 with the IEEE (Institute of Electrical and Electronics Engineers) version 802.11. The most common version was 802.11b, but it had limited use in clinics because bandwidth was small, so most EHR applications required more bandwidth to be useful. However, several upgraded versions were needed to get to the level at which the EHR requirements could be handled. Wireless technology started to provide the mobility and, along with the development of tablets, gave the clinician staff some workflow flexibility. With improving communications speeds and more convenient mobile devices, there was more interest in EHR adoption.

Another important need was to be able to visualize radiographic imaging outside of the radiology suite and within the ambulatory clinic. DICOM (Digital Imaging and Communications in Medicine) and PACS (Picture Archiving and Communication System) systems were developed and provided a significant advantage in handling patients' radiographic imaging. This opened the door to telemedicine, whereby radiologists could be in remote locations from where the imaging was performed and still render a specialist interpretation. Now, other areas are expanding in the telemedicine field, with online consultations with peers as well as commercial ventures in providing online medical consultation to consumers.

As most of our world has become very mobile, the demand for increased mobility in the medical world has developed. For the most part, most of the legacy EHR software was not web browser-type technology. There was a significant reliance on Remote Desk Top (RDP) for connecting clinic sites remote from the main office or for use by clinicians at home while on call; this was mostly a PC-based, DOS to VB script-type software development, which was not as compatible with the mobile environment that users wanted. There are many factors at play at this point in the journey. The rudimentary networks; weak, evolving wireless networks; and early browser-based software with early tablet hardware all had an impact on the user's experience.

Most of the practice management systems in early 1980s were DOS-based with a slow evolution to Windows-based technology. When my company approached the problem in the early 2000s, we were dealing with early browser-based functionality. It had many of the looks of a typical Internet application of the time, but lacked a lot of the functionality that Windows products were able to deliver. Users were becoming more comfortable with surfing the internet but still wanted some of the Window functionality.

It became obvious to some of us as vendors that a browser-based approach was able to provide an effective solution for the future with increased mobility to the user and increased flexibility to the practices. As more upgraded versions of Hypertext Markup Language (HTML) became available, the enhancements of capabilities increased dramatically for application. Today, many EHR applications are HTML-based, with more becoming Cloud-focused. With a more cloud-based approach, updating applications becomes much more reasonable and timely. With less dependence on a Thick Client-based application, the hardware infrastructure for a practice becomes much more cost-effective and more flexible in the type of form factors that are available for a user. So it becomes much easier for smaller practices to keep current with the most recent version and features of their EHR product.

When looking at the path of the journey of usability over the course of the maturation of the EHR, there should be an appreciation of the multifactorial impact on the EHR development. Perhaps a train analogy would be representative of this. As the engine and caboose starts off, multiple cars get added, such as the Certification Commission for Healthcare Information Technology (CCHIT) certification, eRx, patient portal, claims eligibility, alerts and reminders, quality reporting, Meaningful Use (MU) reporting, etc. The vendors find themselves constantly trying to add a more powerful engine to pull the weight of all these "cars" so we can deliver everything in an efficient, timely fashion. In short, we want to build an application that is as perfect as can be, in which a caregiver can deliver medical care to the patient with the utmost efficiency and effectiveness and with the most value at the least cost to the payer.

## 3.3   The Hardware/Communications

The continued challenge for EHR vendors with a variety of hardware options is that the program have the ability to scale to size as well as deal with different device operating systems. With the different form factors increasingly available to the end-user comes the challenge for the user to find the appropriate use for their device in the current setting. Trying to use a smart phone inside a clinic when you would be looking up the results, or reading documentation or relying on point and click functionality is very difficult. However at the same time, the increasing capacities and changing size options constantly impact how vendors and users are expecting to use the device and EHR application in different environments. Improved speech technology is making voice documentation of a patient document much more effective. The smart phone's best use appears to be outside the clinic for limited functions such as coding visits for rounds in the hospital, dictating messages for the staff or memos for the chart, or eRx prescribing.

Basically there are four options for putting clinical information into an EHR – typing, handwriting recognition, point-and-click and dictation via speech recognition or transcription. Since many clinicians over the years have used dictation, there is an interest in continuing that for speed and capturing the essence of the patient encounter. The challenge with speech recognition over the years has been that it is purely speech-to-text. When the speech was translated to text, the computer systems could only store as text. When there is a need for discrete data, text alone is not a viable option. The text must be processed through a Natural Language Processing (NLP) engine. This is a reasonable option when the data can be obtained after the fact, for instance when looking at a large number of documents and searching for certain textual elements.

The challenge is using speech recognition, and then having it run through a speech-understanding engine to produce an Extensible Markup Language (XML) document, which can be processed by different engines for evaluation and management (E&M) coding and alerts and reminders. M*Modal's speech recognition technology [7] allows speech to be rendered as a text document, but also with a CDA/XML document in the background. This functionality can make significant impact on future EHR functionally with regards to discrete data. Then a clinician can focus on the patient's management. The documentation is created by importing historical medical information and dictating the elements of the visit that are specific to the patient's complaint, compiling this into a readable document; and exporting components of the document to the super bill, laboratory test orders, prescriptions, correspondence and as responses to alerts and reminders. This will significantly enhance the usability of EHRs and the discrete data capture for clinical analytics.

Now with RFID (radio frequency identification), Bluetooth and Near Field Communication (NFC), device-to-device interoperability is becoming an emerging area in medicine. Passing medical information between devices when a patient presents to a physician's office or hospital and pulling that information into a practice EHR would be of great value in keeping medical records current and portable.

Even with the most current hardware capabilities within the clinic, network design, internet speeds, wireless speed and connectivity add another layer to the usability challenge. Wireless devices within the ambulatory space require excellent connectivity to avoid loss of critical information. Wireless routers have markedly improved over the last decade, but the demand for handling higher speeds and more bandwidth is also growing. Also, cell phone carriers are often hampered by the volume of local calls in high peak times as well as user access to cell connections. There is a movement in some areas of the country to allow the higher cellular bandwidth emergency frequencies to be open for medical use. This comes at a time when more sophisticated home healthcare is being provided with demands to have an always-on connection through which to access images and lab results when Wi-Fi connections are not feasible or available.

In the hardware world, specifically in the hand-held devices, the rapid design and functional changes over recent years have been aggressive. New and faster tablet designs are providing greater usability options for the mobile user. Much of this change has come out of the environment of human factor design and ergonomics. The computer hardware world deals with ergonomics in a very obvious way. The human-computer interface makes a huge difference in the comfort and acceptance of a user. This obviously extends to the software application used on the device.

So, the reality is that future medical practices will be limited by a variety of elements such as devices, connectivity, security, software and input issues. Although adoption of an EHR has been hindered at times as a result of these limitations, medicine has continued to move forward with EHRs. When there is a fundamental change in a well-embedded process, such as there is in medicine, there will be definite challenges of adoption and utilization.

## 3.4  Software Development

EHR vendors have had significant challenges in this area. With the last 20–30 years the advancement of software programs has been tremendous. As new vendors enter the EHR world utilizing the newest software languages, the older applications are challenged to keep their relevance with respect to design and look. Vendors have faced real challenges in dealing with rapidly changing software languages. Moving from client-based to browser-based software as well as cloud-based options has kept the industry on its toes. At the same time, hospitals and practices have been at the mercy of the vendors' capabilities to update their software. There are well-known applications based on MUMPS software developed out of Massachusetts General Hospital (MGH) in the mid 1960s that have been popular and are still effective. However, more user-friendly and modern designs are gaining strength and popularity.

Web browser maturity has opened up the EHR environment to move from the premise based, older code-based systems to a cloud-based, internet-connected environment. With this option comes concern over protection of PHI (patient health information) and basic security issues as a whole. More and more experience to date with cloud technology has decreased the privacy and security concerns regarding electronic health records, but hasn't completely eliminated the concern. As Microsoft became more dominant in the software world, VBScript became a more commonplace code base for healthcare applications.

Applications that can take advantage of Application Program Interfaces (APIs) are showing up on the radar in greater numbers. This expands EHR vendors' capabilities by opening up the environment for development compatible focused applications by others that can connect with the parent EHR and share information in a bi-directional way. This way, the primary application can control and certify the applications to be included in a software marketplace to fit the need of the users. The best of breed of these applications rise to the top in popularity, similarly to the way the Apple or Google stores function.

The extension of the API approach improves interoperability between EHR applications, which is a significant need in dealing with patient's medical information and portability. Interoperability has been a significant obstacle, and several approaches have been tried, including health information exchange (HIE) and health internet service provider (HISP). The Agency for Healthcare Research and Quality (AHRQ) at HHS had contracted with a group of scientists, the JASON group, which published a report in April 2014 entitled "A Robust Health Data Infrastructure" – commonly called the JASON report – with a revision November, 2014 [1].

In conjunction with the software coding world is another component related to effective use of the application. An area that has developed over the years is the environment of human factor design and ergonomics.

## 3.5   Usability

What is Usability?

Usability is the effectiveness, efficiency and satisfaction with which specific users can achieve a specific set of tasks in a particular environment. [11]

Usability has been a major issue in the EHR industry, with opinions on the topic being varied. In reality, this is no different than with any software application. Many EHR users in various roles have felt that many applications have failed to achieve the goal of a highly intuitive application that a physician and staff can implement and use to achieve the highest usability in the shortest time frame. This goes for both inpatient and ambulatory applications. There are so many different types of users with varying capabilities, training, and needs and expectations using EHRs, it is no wonder at this point in EHR development history that a complex application fails to achieve the ultimate usability goal. Regardless of whether it is a pure inpatient or an ambulatory application, or a combination of both, there are just too many variables involved in the pursuit of a "perfectly usable EHR." Despite this environment, the user expects a highly usable application that works on any device, anywhere at any time with the highest speed. This is a highly desirable goal, however it is impractical in common practice environments of the day.

When you look at the variety of medical and surgical specialties, as well as allied health specialties, there are an overwhelming number of workflows needed, not counting the different medical environments such as acute care hospitals, nursing homes, hospice, ambulatory surgical centers, clinics and more. The workflows can be highly variable, even within the same practice. So when EHR designers are working on a particular feature, for instance ePrescribing, there can be some real consistency obtained because the workflow is generally similar for most physicians writing for medications. However, when looking a feature like Tasking, there is such variability in how clinics handle passing information/tasks to each other that it becomes a huge challenge to design a facile feature that works well for everyone who touches it.

In product design, sometimes there are options in the application for a less rigid workflow, allowing some short cuts or alternate paths toward the same end. But at the same time, patient safety concerns or possible quality reporting concerns may very rigidly require a single path to completion of a task. In the transition to an EHR for seasoned physicians and other healthcare workers, the restrictions are often considered a feature of poor usability. To the EHR vendor, there is a lack of consensus on the workflow and necessary elements needed within the feature for it to be an effective tool.

To understand usability from the vendors' perspective, you need to take into account the process of software development in the healthcare space. The vast majority of EHR companies started as small, agile development shops on a mission to build an application that would interface with a practice management application, generally built by another company. Many times, the clinical expertise had great intentions in providing subject matter expertise, but often there was some misinterpretation of the needs or workflow requirements. Then, more features were added as the demands and needs from the user community grew.

Practically, there is no uniform industry standard tool that the product team could run the application through that gave them feedback on usability. Because of this, most companies relied on the user stories to develop an application and UAT (User Acceptance Testing). The UAT generally came once the application feature was nearly complete. Experienced users, for the most part, would be asked to perform defined test-case scenarios primarily to flush out bugs in the application. This process at times would expose a suboptimal, but acceptable workflow in the users' hands. The goal of UAT was to fix bugs and get the applications into general release, and not necessarily to change the workflow, especially if it markedly impacted the release date. Unfortunately, with the best of intentions, more issues were often identified once the application came into general release, when many more different types of users started working the application in different clinical situations. Perhaps nowhere has this been more obvious than in the compressed stages of Meaningful Use. Again, usability is impacted and distracts from the user's experience with the application.

In 2009, the AHRQ published a monograph on "Electronic Health Record Usability: Interface Design Considerations" [3]. Their concerns about EHR adoption were in part focused on usability and informational design issues. Perhaps at the time of the publication, a challenge for EHR designers and developers was the lack of effective usability tools for testing as well as the inexperience of the industry in understanding workflows in both hospitals and clinics. Personal experience in this area only highlighted a translational gap between the development team and the clinicians. Often a feature or need that I thought was effectively relayed to the development team was misconstrued and potentially became an ineffective workflow. Other times, different teams worked on components of a complex workflow that when merged together became an awkward process.

In many of the earlier EHR products, the resources for the master design and architecture of a product just weren't available. Some of the products included both practice management and clinical (EHR) either as an interfaced or an integrated application. The original scope of the earlier EHR systems was primarily focused on documentation. The overall product development mindset was that of build-as-you-need-it or build-as-requested. Soon the EHR took on increased complexity because practices started to appreciate the level of integration and sophistication of features and capabilities they wanted. This soon led to many vendors having backlogs of customer-desired features. When you add the interest by the EHR user world, the governmental agencies of Centers for Medicare and Medicaid (CMS) and ONC, requirements-based groups like SureScripts and First Data Bank (FDB), and the ancillary interest groups such as Institute of Medicine (IOM), NQF and others, the demands for features and requirements on the EHR vendors becomes immense. The noise, so to speak, of the demands from so many different users, practice types and outside partnered vendors added many layers of complexity to an EHR that could not help but impact usability.

There has been no major formula for usability in the EHR industry. As the complexity and the sophistication of needs increased along with expansion of features to include patient-centric needs, the usability issues have increased with EHRs. Vendors on their own have dealt with trying to improve their usability with staffs that are designers, focus-user groups and general feedback from their users. But again, challenges surrounding feature priorities and regulatory demands often push some of the little usability items to the back of the line.

When EHRs were increasing in numbers, there were two issues starting to play out. First, each vendor was developing their approach to the EHR environment, therefore there was an inconsistency between the features and functions. Second, trying to interact with each other or with a common third party such as clinical laboratories was a challenge for vendors owing to a lack of standards. Since the federal government had a vested interest in promoting EHRs, there was move to help develop standards and certifications.

CCHIT became active as an organization granted by the ONC. More than 250 volunteers provided expertise in setting up the requirements for an EHR. The goal was to set up minimal standards for an EHR; subsequently, a certification process was set in place for vendors to obtain. In the early phases, usability was left to the design of the EHR vendor. Towards the end of CCHIT certification era, a usability score was given to applications that went through the process. Although this was a reasonable first step towards trying to emphasize usability, it really did not have an impact.

Additionally, The Healthcare Information Technology Standards Panel (HITSP) [9], a private and public collaborative, was formed to develop and harmonize standards for sharing information in the healthcare ecosystem, and was disbanded in April, 2010. Its areas of interest covered a wide range of the interoperability needs for EHR. These recommendations covered the information-handling requirements of all types of stakeholders. Again, this was all reasonable, but expanded the scope and requirements for an EHR.

The mission is to not to delve deeply into the science of usability, as far as specific testing modalities, but to give a broad understanding of all the components that impact the usability of an EHR. The areas of heuristic evaluations, UAT-User acceptance testing, cognitive walkthroughs and other modalities are well documented elsewhere along with the challenges in their utilization in the EHR industry.

The next phase of usability focus came with the Strategic IT Advanced Research Projects (SHARP) grants funding by ARRA and administered by the ONC. Fifteen million dollars in grants in four specific domains were awarded, one SHARP-C was Patient-Centered Cognitive Support, focus in areas of Clinical Decision Support and Usability centered at the University of Texas-Houston in the National Center for Cognitive Informatics and Decision Making in Healthcare, headed by Jaijie Zhang, PhD.

Some of the focus of the grant was on work by Dr. Zhang and his team of researchers from numerous universities in a usability lab, along with the development of tools for EHRs to run testing on while in development. Efforts by vendors have always had usability as a major emphasis, but many challenges have complicated these efforts over time.

There are a variety of options for usability testing. In recent years, more definitive work has been done in a variety of academic labs with a focus on how to automate testing. Traditionally, in the EHR realm, the focus was on an internal review of usability, perhaps followed by focused user testing moving on to Beta testing. A challenge for vendors has been the impossibility of testing in all of the varied environments available to users, whether thick client, thin client, multi-tenet, third party hosting, RDP or Citrix, to name a few. Many companies have tried to limit the environment to one, such as a hosted solution, but then there are challenges there. Usually it is the connection of devices that has posed the problem, most commonly scanners and printers but also clinical devices such as ECG and lab devices.

An enhanced usability lab was available to focus on workflow designs for enhanced usability in both acute care and ambulatory environments. Over the course of the project, software tools were developed specifically to help in measuring and improving usability, and are now available for the EHR vendor community. The TURF (Toward a Unified Framework) Project project was an approach to develop EHR usability guidelines and standards [14]. From this project, an application is now available for comparison testing of workflows within an EHR.

Most vendors of sophisticated, complex software applications would probably agree that usability is always a challenge. Limitations in the native software coding environment, forms factors, and operating systems, to name a few, restrict options and workflow design.

Don Norman, PhD, has been a prominent force in the world of design. His user-centered design concept has had a major impact on a variety of products and industry. He played a prominent role on the SHARP-C advisory panel. His books, The Design for Everyday Things and The Invisible Computer have been a model for any designer in all types of disciplines and fields. The tendency in many software companies is to focus more on the development side and less on the design side when it comes to usability constraints. The lack of an overall design methodology often leads to less than optimal usability features.

Trying to wrap your hands around the usability needs of an EHR user can be very challenging. Often users tend to focus on a very particular action within an EHR that is causing them angst in their daily use. When you combine this complaint with those of other users, you may see a significant variance in the issues and how users prioritize them. An action's role within a practice as well as the frequency of its use also has an impact. Sometimes usability issues center around a rarely used feature that nevertheless plays a significant role in the workflow and or patient safety.

EHR vendors certainly focus on their users' needs for features and usability. It's the challenge that comes with the turf and has its ups and downs for all EHR companies. But the real issue when thinking about usability is that it is a process that occurs over time. We tend to focus on a specific action, but it really is a process. As a feature is enhanced or matured, there are changes that can make it more usable. Usability at times is like looking at a piece of art – the person looking at it can tell you that its good or bad, but there tends to be a spectrum from good to bad. Often the vendor leaves certain features at a state or stage that needs further work. The minimal requirements are in place, but a more mature design or added components can make the feature much more usable to the end user.

Perhaps one thing that may not come into view in the usability spectrum is training. As with any commercial software application, especially a complex EHR application, whether hospital or ambulatory, the users must have a clear understanding of the application and the feature that takes them through an effective workflow. When an experienced practice or clinical worker begins his or her exposure to a new EHR application, the issue is not his or her business or clinical capabilities. The issue is his or her willingness to learn a new system. It is easy to criticize a system which forces a user into a workflow that is different from what they are used to, particularly in a practice coming from a paper-based system. Many practices have not clearly documented their workflows, so often there is noticeable disagreement within the business or clinical areas as to how they can do "best practice" on a certain task, whether it be something like scheduling on the practice side or perhaps clinical tasking on the clinical side. So, when the implementation starts with an EHR, the trainers may have a challenge in getting the users on the same page for a particular feature. The practices that manage the change effectively become much more successful in their implementation.

## 3.5.1  Change Management

The one area involving the human factor that impacts all of us in our daily lives, and certainly has become a huge factor in implementing an EHR effectively, is change management. If we lived in a perfect practice world with an EHR application beyond reproach, clinicians as well as staff would still have to deal with change effectively, inside and outside of the practice walls.

When you are introducing a sophisticated application into an active practice, a couple of important points become very apparent early. First and foremost, how effective is the practice leadership in guiding their team through the change? Have they engaged the team in the necessary training and preparation well before "go-live" to ensure as successful an implementation as possible? There have been various vendor options for training both in the mechanisms of training, such as web-based, on-site, on-page training, off-site and conference type, as well as cost and mixtures of training. This only means that there is not a perfect way to train a user that sticks for every user.

Much has been written and discussed over the years about change management in different environments, but I would argue that the medical world, which is very experienced with change, is not as accepting or prepared for effective change. The resistance to change can be significant when egos, ownership and attitude come into play. In part, it could come from the attitude that anything to do with treating patients, such as a new medication regime or a procedure, is reasonable to learn about, but if it involves the business of medicine, then it is best left up to the staff to figure out.

Basic human nature has a significant impact on the success of an EHR implementation. Inquisitiveness and flexibility and an eagerness to learn, regardless of the type of user, have a huge impact. But this is no different than in other situations, like sports teams. When practices focus on success through effective leadership, it will follow – especially in implementation.

Being part of the vendor world now, I became aware of this when two practices of the same specialty, in nearby locations with similar provider and staff numbers, went "live" on an application in the same week. They had on-site training by two experienced trainers. However, they had two different outcomes: one had embraced the change and prepared effectively and became very self-sufficient in a short time, while the other practice struggled and took much longer and felt that their experience was not good. Regardless of an EHR vendor's efforts in their design of the application features, users within a practice still require adequate training and significant understanding of their roles and tasks to get the most out of an application. Practice users must understand that there is a continuum of learning for an EHR because requirements change and features are added or enhanced all the time. Vendors have learned that once practices are on-boarded to an application, it's a must that they maintain the most current upgrade, because being orphaned on a version or not keeping up with the new features just handicaps the practice in so many ways.

This perspective on usability may be getting a little beyond what most readers would consider when speaking of usability, but it is worth mentioning. Practices, as well as any vendor in the EHR space, face this challenge. Change is inevitable, so how we handle it does impact usability in many ways. Usability in its purist sense may be at the atomic level, concerning the location of an icon, the color of a section of a page, or how to make a choice by point and click. I would argue that usability is so much broader, and involves so many things that impact the user's experience.

Change management is a challenge for vendors also, so the point is that it impacts whether the end user can effectively use the application in a meaningful way. Awareness of change is a major concern in developing an application and training its users successfully.

### 3.5.2 Challenges and Destination

So far the discussion has included the expected issues in any software application development with some particular needs and requirements within the healthcare space. The most challenging and somewhat unpredictable are the external forces that play an instrumental role in the impact on the doctor-patient relationship, for example the Social Security Act of 1965, two amendments to which launched Medicare and Medicaid and brought the government into the mixture as a payer. As medicine expanded its capabilities in providing more sophisticated treatments and procedures through the next decades, it also caused an increase in the cost of care. Obviously, the advancement of medicine prolongs the wellness and the health of the patient population. We are touching on this to highlight the challenge of addressing the needs in a software application of all three groups – patients, caregivers and payers.

The shift of fee-for-service model to a value-based model is certainly gaining momentum as the payers start rewarding caregivers for delivery of quality care to the patient. Pulling the providers together as a care team, as in Patient Centered Medical Home (PCMH) and Accountable Care Organization (ACO) model, or earlier quality data gathering programs like Provider Quality Reporting Initiative (PQRI) and Provider Quality Reporting System (PQRS) or the Comprehensive Primary Care Initiative (CPCI), are all attempts to communicate between the caregivers for the betterment of the patient. What this means for vendors is that a significant amount of resources, expertise and time is spent trying to stay ahead of the curve on the programs and requirements mandated by the payers. Often they are in conflict to the types of information they want. This impacts usability in two ways; first, it often changes the priority of projects that the vendor wants to include or modify in the application to enhance usability, and secondly, the requirements may require a redesign, re-factoring to potentially accommodate a small segment of caregivers.

The healthcare IT space has ballooned with a host of specialty applications that provide a specific need for the practice. So, as most of the major EHR vendors focus on core required and needed functionality, there are ancillary needs that may start off as a "nice to have," but may become "must have." Looking back, one remembers that being able to have prescription writing capability within an EMR was a "nice to have." Subsequently, alerts and reminders, followed by clinical decision support (CDS), and the feature sets have continued to explode in popularity.

CDS was interesting to me, since everyone felt the need for it, but there were so many flavors and strengths of decision support that it was hard to compare apples to oranges. Caregivers were complaining about "alert fatigue," and there was little option to stratify the alerts by role so that an individual user got the type of alerts he or she needed to care for the patient. There were attempts by different medical associations to do a best practice approach and recommend certain CDS, but those sometimes ran counter to other associations' thoughts. Also, content vendors were becoming more common with increased interest in and capabilities for connecting with an EHR. In order to facilitate pulling in medical and patient-related education, features like the "Info button" and the "blue button" became part of the EHR experience or the purpose of linking to CDS materials.

Because of the disparity of techniques and need for linking EHR and CDS-type features, there was an increasing demand from vendors to standardize the access to CDS. Certain agencies, like the NQF, have worked diligently to pull all this together. Trying to get to a universally available CDS electronic format (XML) so that content vendors can publish and EHR applications can consume CDS content is still much needed. This has become even more of a problem with Meaningful Use because of the inconsistency in the quality measures required for incentive reporting.

There has been an outcry from physicians and other healthcare workers who do not like EHRs. This is understandable when you take the whole development, scope and breadth of the EHR into consideration. Modern medicine is a complex, challenging system to work in. So many forces come into play and impact the user at the point of care that it's not hard to be frustrated with most EHRs in their current state of functionality.

While great strides have been taken to continually improve the experience, at the same time it has been extremely challenging for vendors to "keep it between the ditches," so to speak. The vast majority of healthcare workers are in a similar position of not wanting to return to a paper medical record. There is a light at the end of the tunnel. Usability will improve across the board with newer technologies, devices and design. More systematic software organization and development processes, early coordinated User Acceptance Testing, usability tools for automated testing, and better design considerations are all becoming a necessary focus for vendors.

On the other hand, users have a responsibility to fully engage in the implementation process, train themselves on the software and learn to give constructive criticisms by working with their vendors. Practices need to have both practice management and clinical advocates in the leadership. The certification agencies and standards organizations also need to aggressively work with the vendors to accelerate work in the interoperability arena. Many of these organizations have found themselves being outrun by the needs and demands within the EHR user world.

Allowing the medical world to be part of the National Broadband Plan [12] promoted by the Federal Communications Commission (FCC) would benefit our healthcare delivery. With this expansion of broadband coverage into medical ecosystems, there could be better delivery of care into ancillary facilities such as nursing homes, remote clinic locations and home healthcare, allowing higher speeds and a higher volume of data transfer.

Hopefully, the essence of the challenges within the EHR has been captured in this chapter. Just like any ecosystem, EHRs have been impacted by myriad forces from many directions which, without a doubt, has in turn impacted usability at the point of care for the healthcare worker. The industry recognizes this, and is working diligently to improve the experience.

The future looks bright for modernizing the US healthcare information technology world, which will have a significant impact on the delivery of high-quality and good-valued medicine with improved patient safety and outcomes for our population.

# References

1. A Robust Health Data Infrastructure. JASON Group for AHRQ, April, JSR-13-700; 2014.
2. American Recovery and Reinvestment Act of 2009, Public Law 111-5, Feb. 17, 2009.
3. Armijo D, McDonnell C, Werner K. Electronic health record usability: interface design considerations, AHRQ Publication No. 09(10)-0091-2-EF. Rockville: Agency for Healthcare Research and Quality; 2009.
4. Bush GW. Address before a joint session of the Congress on the State of the Union. 2004.
5. Charles D, Gabriel M, Furukawa M. Adoption of electronic health record systems among U.S. non-federal acute care hospitals: 2008–2013, ONC Brief, No. 16, many 2014, 1–9.

6. Greener M. First do no harm. Improving drug safety through legislation and independent research. EMBO Rep. 2008;9(3):221–4. doi:10.1038/embor.2008.17.
7. Handler J. Creating smarter healthcare IT: putting the doctor back in the driver's seat. M*Modal Communication. 2013.
8. Hsiao C, Hing E. Use and characteristics of electronic health record systems among office-based physician practices: United States, 2001–2013, NCHS Data Brief, No. 143, 1–7 Jan 2014.
9. The Healthcare Information Technology Standards Panel (HITSP) http://www.hitsp.org/.
10. Prakash S, Valentine V. Timeline: the rise and fall of Vioxx. 2007. http://www.npr.org/templates/story/story.php?storyId=5470430.
11. Schoeffel R. The concept of product usability. ISO Bull. 2003;34:6–7.
12. The National Broadband Plan. 2010. FCC 17 Mar 2010.
13. Wolfe A. Institute of Medicine report: crossing the quality Chasm: a new health care system for 21st century. Policy Polit Nurs Pract. 2001;2(3):233–5.
14. Zhang J, Walji MF. TURF: toward a unified framework of EHR usability. J Biomed Inform. 2011;44(6):1056–67. /jbi.2011.08.005.

# Chapter 4
# Snapshot at Mid-stride: Current State of EHRs and Their Use by Clinicians from a CMIO's Perspective

Thomas H. Payne

**Abstract** Electronic health records (EHRs) are now approaching mainstream in healthcare, after years in which their use was limited to academic centers and early adopters. We'll begin by defining terms and setting the context, and then describe design, functionality, advantages and challenges to EHRs from the perspective of the IT Medical Director of a large academic medical center with multiple facilities and multiple EHRs. Though the transition from paper to electronic records is difficult, in this chapter we'll review why we believe it is worth the effort: current and potential advantages to EHRs over paper are substantial and are very likely to grow. We'll also review some of the story of adoption of technology in aviation, and lessons this holds for healthcare information technology: improvements in flight deck design, checklists, and other innovations contributed to the unparalleled safety record in aviation to which healthcare can aspire.

**Keywords** Electronic health records (EHR) • Electronic medical records (EMR) • CPOE (computerized practitioner order entry) • Usability • Aviation

## 4.1 Introduction

Like Muybridge's nineteenth century stop action photographs of a galloping horse, viewing the current state of EHRs is a snapshot in a period of rapid change. Adoption of EHRs has risen dramatically since 1999, changing care processes with it. We work with electronic records as never before, using almost exclusively commercial EHR vendor products.

T.H. Payne, MD
Medical Director, Information Technology Services and Department of Medicine,
University of Washington, Seattle, WA, USA
e-mail: tpayne@u.washington.edu

© Springer International Publishing Switzerland 2016
C.A. Weaver et al. (eds.), *Healthcare Information Management Systems:
Cases, Strategies, and Solutions*, Health Informatics,
DOI 10.1007/978-3-319-20765-0_4

The reception to this change has been mixed. Not surprisingly, early adopters and technologically-avid providers find much to like. But the transition from paper records to commercial EHRs extends far beyond early adopters to those in the rest of the bell-shaped curve, many of whom are unenthusiastic. This reflects in part the difficulty faced by EHR vendors in matching electronic tools to highly complex and varied healthcare workflows, but also this mixed reception by providers exposes weakness in EHR usability, time requirements, and altered interaction between patient and provider. Commercial EHRs largely show their design origins in the paper medical record: using a chart tab metaphor seen in paper charts, and an orientation around laboratory, radiology and other sources of data, rather than a problem-oriented medical record [1]. Most EHRs are oriented around encounters as required by payers rather than around the continuous life of a person. Drop-down menus and radio buttons from 1990s are the norm, and typing skills are expected. Use of voice to create notes is rising, and some have adopted the ultimate user-interface aid: another human being (scribe) who handles interaction with the EHR while the clinician interacts with the patient [2]. What does the use of scribes tell us about the user interface of the current generation of EHRs?

Should it be surprising that this transition is difficult? The history of adoption of technology of other industries is instructive: Aviation struggled mid-century to improve safety, but over decades adapted flight deck design to human strengths, developed checklists, refined teamwork, and adopted blameless reporting of near-misses before achieving the unparalleled safety we experience today.

Yet despite these challenges we have largely made the difficult transition from paper to EHRs and laid the foundation for the promise of EHRs. 'Promise' is the best word, for in early efforts at clinical decision support such as avoiding drug-drug interactions, alerts are mostly overridden; widespread exchange of information isn't here yet; and the goal of liberating patient and provider from duplicate data entry and excessive time requirements are all ahead of us.

Before we can exchange electronic information our information must be in electronic form. Decision support tools rely on accurate electronic information to be credible and useful. We can now share the record among the provider team, and increasingly with people who come to us for care.

In this chapter we will cover these themes in greater detail: EHR design and functionality, advantages to EHRs and their current problems, and what we might learn from other industries to help us in this work.

## 4.2   Background

Let's begin this review of the current state of EHRs with definitions and an understanding of the context. The term EHR is most commonly applied to the collection of functionality and computing systems used to create a record of a person's health and illness and to assist health care providers in delivering care. In this sense EHRs go beyond a record, and become a means to order, schedule, arrange and communicate care. So an EHR is a system or collection of systems, to do all this and more. Other terms have been applied to these systems, beginning (at least in my career) with computer-based medical record systems, followed by the computer-based patient record and electronic medical record. Why 'health' instead of 'medical' as the middle term? Most people are healthy and not hospitalized nor in a clinic. Some feel there are other differences between EMRs and EHRs, that the latter represents the record collected from all locations of care while the former is institution-based, but in my experience EHR and EMR are used to mean the same thing. In this paper I will use EHR since it is more common today.

Since the American Recovery and Reinvestment Act (ARRA) was passed in 2009, [3] there has been rapid growth in adoption of EHRs in US ambulatory and hospital care settings where Americans receive care as a result of Meaningful Use incentives programs [4]. Adoption of EHR systems in hospitals has more than doubled since 2009. Attesting to Meaningful Use requirements carries substantial financial benefit—up to $44,000 per eligible provider and far more for eligible hospitals. This is a period of enormous change in use of EHRs, particularly in the US. Other countries, notably the United Kingdom, made such a transition in primary care long ago [5].

The process of certification of EHRs has accelerated from early efforts such as Certification Commission for Healthcare Information Technology (CCHIT) [6]. To receive ARRA incentive payments, eligible hospitals and providers must use a certified EHR. Some have argued this presents a difficult barrier to use of highly functional EHRs, while others feel the barrier is not high enough. This has introduced a government role of influencing EHR functionality in a new way, in providing guidance on what EHRs should offer to users. Again, some argue the government role is too great and others see greater need for government involvement in oversight of these tools which are so important in influencing how care for Americans is delivered.

## 4.3   Current EHR Design Paradigm

As mentioned above, EHR design has converged around a traditional representation of medical charts familiar to those who have used paper charts. Information is arranged largely by source, such as imaging, laboratory, and notes, using a tab metaphor. The term 'skeuomorphism' means that design elements are derived from earlier forms to achieve the same objective, such as the leather rim to a calendar that has appeared in electronic calendaring applications. In EHRs, the tab metaphor mimics what was found in traditional paper charts and so stands as a classic skeuomorphism example. Designing the EHR to look like the paper chart has the advantage of greater familiarity to new clinician users accustomed to paper charts; the transition to the electronic replacement is therefore more familiar and possibly simpler. Among the disadvantages are that applying the old design paradigm may limit possible improvements that are possible when it is no longer necessary to bind paper pages of a chart together.

Familiar paradigms used in EHRs are drop down menus, radio buttons, and other visual designs that date back to early graphical user interfaces in the 1990s. It is remarkable how similar these design elements are between EHRs from different vendors. Vendors have been careful not to copy designs from competitors nor to make their designs easily available to others who may be tempted to copy them; nevertheless what vendors produce is surprisingly similar with the consequence that the strengths, limitations and weaknesses of our current major EHR design paradigms are shared.

Another design element shared by EHRs in the United States (US) is orientation around an encounter and the tasks, procedures and/or tests performed within that encounter, [7] because that is how payment is organized in the US, rather than around the continuous record of a patient's care and it's outcomes. Features to address billing requirements permeate both ordering and documentation functionality.

The navigational designs of EHRs are different enough that it can be confusing for clinicians who have to move from one EHR to another across the range of EHRs that are used in clinics, hospitals and different healthcare organizations [8]. Renting a car or borrowing a friend's bike is a simple matter for most because the fundamentals of operating a car or bike are very similar from one model to another. Not so when going from one vendor EHR to another. Finding scanned images, writing admission or transfer orders, creating and saving a progress note, dictating an operative note can be profoundly different when moving from one EHR to another. And this navigational confusion can remain even after clinicians have completed the (usually mandatory) training for each vendor's product. Interestingly, here is another example where aviation can teach us: Once pilots are certified to fly one Boeing aircraft (767), certification to fly a different one (757) required hours, not days of pilot training, because the flight decks were deliberately designed to be similar [9].

The current marketplace EHRs are commonly developed with graphical user interface presentation layer tools available for the Microsoft Windows operating system, resulting in a 'Win32' application. (This dependence on Win 32 severely limits screen design, navigation and presentation of data back to clinicians. User friendly and more powerful options from web technologies aren't reflected in the graphical interfaces and screens unless user is taken out of the EHR.) However in large organizations this Win32 application is delivered to the device used by the bedside clinician using terminal servers such as Citrix which avoid the need to install several applications and supporting files on hundreds or thousands of end-user devices [10].

Not all commercial EHR products are the same, however, and some are very different. In some EHRs, the workstation screens with which the clinician interacts most often are web applications that do not require Citrix. This means they can be accessed as easily as web applications, without the extra effort required to log in to Citrix, and to configure the device to use Citrix. Some EHRs have dramatically different designs that do not follow the tab metaphor, and which use touch screens and other alternatives to the mouse and keyboard. But market penetration of these newer systems is modest at the moment, and they tend to be in the ambulatory/clinic market rather than acute care.

## 4.4 EHR Functionality

EHR functionality is broad, spanning those high level functions listed in Table 4.1. Table 4.1 list reinforces the point that an EHR is more than a record, though serving as the medico-legal record for hundreds of millions of people remains an extremely important role. EHR functionality as listed in Table 4.1 is roughly divided into three categories: reviewing and understanding patient data and the story; assisting clinician workflow; and, entering data and orders into the record. Clinicians spend most of their time entering information and so these are the areas of functionality that receive the most attention. Writing notes, entering data, and entering orders are an essential part of care delivery, and these areas largely depend on use of the mouse and keyboard at present. The time required to do so varies by aptitude and computer skill of the clinician, skills that do not overlap closely with clinical skill.

Doctors, nurses and pharmacists sometimes are not skilled at using computing devices and are sometimes embarrassed by this as though it represents a failing on their part rather than a natural variation in aptitude for various tasks. Skills that characterize excellent clinicians–judgment, the ability to listen, empathize, reason, interact with others, and procedural skill–are far more important than typing speed and facility with mouse and screen.

### 4.4.1 Reviewing Information

Reviewing patient information is an important foundation for decision making, but it is increasingly complex given the enormous rise in information stored in EHRs, and what is becoming available from other medical devices and data generating sources [11]. We are reaching or surpassing our ability to absorb this information

**Table 4.1** EHR functionality[*]

| | |
|---|---|
| Message box (proprietary names vary but functionality similar) | Billing<br>   Professional fee<br>   Facility fee |
| Results review (lab, path, imaging, notes) | Quality metrics, dashboards |
| Documentation (direct entry, structured/ unstructured, dictation, mixed) | Electronic communication<br>   With team<br>   With patients |
| Order management | Patient monitoring review |
| Patient summary displays | Patient support |
| Medication administration record | Population health |
| Bar code medication administration | External resources |
| Patient lists, schedule, rounding/handoff tools | Administrative |

[*]Each of these areas of functionality can offer decision support, and should address security and compliance with law and regulation

[12] and so results review functionality is more important than ever. The advantages of EHRs come into play here: search can be more sophisticated than it used to be, graphical representations and summarization of data can potentially aid and speed comprehension and pattern recognition. And one of the holy grails of EHRs to supplement human decision-making with computerized clinical decision support is possible on a small scale, and more complex support seems within reach.

### 4.4.2  Workflow

Workflow in healthcare is highly complex, in part because the healthcare setting is many times unpredictable and chaotic. The irregular and sometimes unpredictable nature of workflow surprises those new to healthcare and those from outside healthcare who study it. Thirty minutes on hospital rounds with interruptions, code blues, families arriving, interpreters not being available, and unexpected emergencies—all of these make the task of matching EHR functionality to workflow extremely difficult. Add to this the multitude of specialists, bedside clinicians, therapists, and technologists involved in a patient's care and requirements of work hour limitations for residents so care is transferred from one person to another more often, and the need to help with workflow has never been greater. Functionality to help support workflow includes: rounding and sign out applications; [13] patient lists, messaging and telephony functionality; scheduling and referral applications; and, importantly a rapidly growing sets of tools to help manage collections (populations) of patients with common conditions and attributes. Developing applications to support workflow is a fruitful area for advance, and though it is related to other functionality such as documentation, order entry, and results review, it is growing separately too.

### 4.4.3  Order Entry and Documentation

Clinicians, and especially physicians, spend more time using documentation and order entry than any other functions. These are special cases of EHR functionality because clinicians spend more time in these activities than in others [14]. Computerized practitioner order entry (CPOE–sometimes the P is for physician, provider, or prescriber) is defined as the entry of orders into an electronic system by the person responsible for the order [15]. This is in contrast to writing the order on a piece of paper which is then transcribed into an electronic system by someone else. The main driver for the move to CPOE is the potential to guide ordering at the moment the order is formulated. If you are alerted that the person is allergic to penicillin just when you are about to order penicillin, you can change the order immediately. Similarly when a new drug requires monitoring, you can respond to automated prompts to order that monitoring too—so called corollary orders [16]. These advantages are harder to achieve if you write an order on paper or communicate your order verbally, and expect someone else to transcribe the order into the computer system for you. Errors can result in the transcription step and the availability of clinical decision support (CDS) is reduced. The time required to enter orders is an important barrier to broad acceptance of CPOE, especially when single, simple orders are entered frequently, such as in the outpatient setting. But it may be there is a middle ground that preserves both safety and efficiency and so CPOE is under scrutiny.

Designing functionality to enter orders is highly complex and carries higher risk for harm than other functionality. Systems to enter orders for medications that can be both life-sustaining but also toxic requires extremely careful design, which must give opportunities for double- or triple-checking before the drug reaches the patient. The act of ordering must be as rapid as possible while remaining safe, because it will be used for tens of thousands of orders on thousands of patients each day, every day of the year. CPOE design is highly complex. There are no shortage of ideas on how to improve this process from users, but each enhancement must meet the same exacting safety standards as the original application, and each change in design must be learned and used by clinicians who may be fatigued and distracted. Designing safe, efficient CPOE is difficult.

Clinicians, and especially physicians, spend a large part of their day documenting care [17]. There are many ways to enter notes into an electronic system, including dictation, typing, using a template or using a scribe. Each has its advantages and disadvantages, including time spent, cost, training requirements, how easily the notes are understood by others, and whether their contents can be used to support decision support. Tools to create notes comprised of separate, selectable codes are used frequently, an approach known as *structured documentation*. Some prefer to create notes using narrative text rather than structured documentation, or a combination of the two. Fortunately advances in natural language processing [18] make it increasingly possible to extract the meaning contained in narrative text, so that use of structured documentation tools to create a note—awkward for some—is not required for all purposes. The transition from paper to electronic documentation is often quite difficult and involves workflow and technical barriers that must be addressed [19].

There is much more functionality to be created, including better tools to help manage care of populations, to coordinate care across the health maintenance, acute care, post-acute care, and in home and community settings.

Health information technology beyond EHRs has grown as other healthcare processes and workflows adopt IT, such as imaging, pharmacy, personal health records, [20] and including the very visible difficulties in public enrollment in healthcare coverage [21].

## 4.5 Advantages Achieved

The most obvious and likely most important advantage of EHRs is that the contents of the medical record and EHR functionality is in electronic form rather than paper. This means that it can be available to more than one person at the same time, in geographically distant locations. This is referred to as multiple simultaneous access and may seem a self-evident and minor point to those who have not wasted time looking for a paper chart or waited until a colleague was finished with it before beginning your work. And once you use the electronic chart, penmanship no longer obscures content.

When information is in electronic rather than paper form, it is possible to leverage computing technologies to analyze, supplement, summarize and display it in ways not possible with paper. When the record is in electronic form, we can ride the enormous wave of computer science technology in which computing power doubles every 18 months to do important and useful things with the information in the EHR. Finding patterns, looking for risks for heritable disease, trending hematocrits and serum creatinine, use natural language processing to find markers of care quality or tap the clinician on the shoulder when needed, all these things and more are available today and are progressively improving. None of this could happen easily with a paper record.

Alerts and reminders have been an early and remarkable success of EHRs. Since the 1970s the value of reminders based on simple rules has been recognized [22]. Preventive and chronic care is more reliably delivered with these aids [23]. Medication safety is improved: CPOE was associated with a 55 % reduction in serious adverse medication events in a frequently-cited 1998 JAMA study [24].

With the transition from paper to EHRs, we now can have simultaneous access that includes patients who have growing interest and ability to access their record [25, 26]. Though possible with the paper record, it might require several weeks' wait and considerable cost to do so. Early efforts to measure quality are based on electronic information [27].

Perhaps the most important advances made possible by EHRs are those that could not in any practical sense occur with a paper record. Given the life long data captured over time for a population, it is now possible to gather information on thousands of people to better understand their health and health needs, and in some sense to "manage" the population. The cost to pull a paper record and review it to gather information would make following a million people to assess preventive care impossible. With big data analytics, health service research such as, projecting costs of care and designing alternative reimbursement strategies based on risk and health status of the population are now possible. While improving population health does not require large health IT and EHR investments, the information gathered from EHRs can help target resources and use them more efficiently.

## 4.6    Clinician Complaints, and the Potential to Address Them

These advantages make it very rare that once institutions have moved from paper records to EHRs that they go back to paper. However the rich functionality of EHRs and its effect on workflow is profound. Change of any kind—let alone change this dramatic—is usually not without problems. Is it surprising that clinicians find fault with the current generation of EHRs? Complaints are sometimes vociferous and impassioned to match the emotion-laden process of delivering health care [28–30]. The major theme is that using an EHR to do the tasks of documentation and orders takes longer than it used to using a paper chart, [31] where an order could be quickly written or given verbally, and documentation could be dictated or quickly written. With the EHRs, time in the exam room or at the bedside that previously could be used to listen and talk with a patient is now spent clicking, typing and addressing endless requirements to capture more information or click buttons attesting that you have met some requirement. The most touching example of what effect this can have is a child's diagram of her doctor facing the computer rather than her [32]. Clinicians will often express their frustration in statements such as, "This is not why I went to medical school/nursing school." The user interface is almost always criticized as being unintuitive and complex, and recommendations for improving usability abound [33]. Speed in refreshing screens or accepting orders is of the essence—there is no such thing as too much speed or performance. Popup alerts are not helpful and can lead to missing one important alert in a string of 100 that are not helpful—so called alert fatigue [34]. Training occupies much more time than it seems that it should yet most clinicians learn only a small fraction of the functionality of their EHR and many of their requests for new functionality are already in place in the application they are using.

Clinician users provide lots of feedback, some of which fits the term complaint, but more of which is in the form of a suggestion, proposed enhancement, or idea for a change. The challenge for anyone who has received this feedback is the diversity of opinion, some of which is diametrically opposed to what others want, and the challenge in deciding which improvements to undertake is enormous. This must also be balanced with the understanding that users may not really know what they want; sometimes the best new design is not reactive to user feedback but rather based on carefully observing what users do. And improvements take time which may be better spent addressing performance problems or fixing true problems, the cause of which may run more deeply and require more effort than those who discover the problem appreciate.

Structures to address the user suggestions dilemma include user groups, conferences, wikis, web application suites, and personal relationships with key opinion-leader users. Of course the effort to incorporate these proposed improvements and enhancements needs to be balanced against the need for developers to meet regulatory and mandatory changes such as Y2K, ICD-10, and to address requirements of government incentive programs such as Meaningful Use and changes in reimbursement structures such as Accountable Care Organizations.

CDS' potential to aid care greatly exceeds what has been achieved today. CPOE alerts for drug-drug interactions are overridden with high frequency and this has not yet changed [35]. The rules that trigger many CPOE alerts are often too simple and do not include data—such as patient kidney function, age and other characteristics—that could mean the difference between helpful CDS and an annoying popup that is overridden [36]. Diagnostic decision support, an early area of promise in artificial intelligence, [37] has not yet been carefully integrated into most EHRs despite high frequency of diagnostic errors [38, 39]. One of the barriers to greater use of CDS is dispersion of data needed for accurate advice, sometimes in different EHRs or in scanned or narrative text content not yet available for accurate extraction.

Much of the data that is needed to simplify search, CDS, and quality measurement is within the record, but in narrative text. For example, in a note, a clinician may list diseases being considered in the differential diagnosis and CDS could be invoked to propose other diseases to be added to that list. But these data are not 'computable' in their narrative text form. Natural language processing (NLP) is used increasingly to make this natural, narrative content accessible to automated tools so that the computing system 'understands' what is contained in the narrative text [18]. Since early work in applying NLP to small section of the note, it is finding application for identifying problem statements [40], assisting in billing rule compliance [41], and identifying need for further action in radiology reports [42]. Today uses of NLP in EHRs are not common, but much more can be done by unlocking the information within narrative text and using it to make CDS more useful, and measurements of quality more detailed.

Are vendors villains or angels? Of course they are neither. Some make enormous profits, usually years after they have assumed large risks and devoted herculean effort to achieve a toehold in the marketplace. Dissatisfaction with those profits does not always take into account that early effort nor the technical, interpersonal and organization skill required and nurtured to achieve what the vendor now enjoys. We should also remember that those who think they have a better idea are free to develop EHRs to compete, just as current vendors did.

Most Americans receive care from providers who use commercial EHRs. Very few organizations use EHRs they developed and maintain themselves, though such examples still exist [43]. The wide marketplace has also begun to consolidate, with some vendors subsuming others.

## 4.7   Learning from Other Industries. The Case of Aviation

Healthcare is complex, involves highly variable patient circumstances and characteristics, is unpredictable and involves highly trained and experienced professionals. Another risk-prone, high stakes, highly technical field is aviation, from which many claim there are lessons for healthcare. But every flight is about the same, the argument goes, every plane is the same, and what happens on a flight is the same—transporting people from one runway to a nearly identical runway somewhere else. For these reasons other industries, including aviation, have few lessons for health IT. Thus runs the narrative used to argue against learning from other industries.

The trouble with these arguments against learning from aviation is that they are not accurate. Aviation had a difficult history beginning with an accident rate that we now know only from history books and articles. Planes are highly complex and were from the beginning. Pilots have been very intelligent for the most part. An inspection of a single summary statistic, shown in Fig. 4.1, introduces an interesting story. Something, or many things, happened between the left and the right ends of this curve resulting in a state that we hope for healthcare today: dramatic rise in safety to the point where it is sometimes taken for granted today. Think about your local airport: planes land and take off every hour of every day. Do you recall seeing an accident? A fatal accident?

The aviation system includes more than the plane. It is the people in the plane, the thousands of other planes in the air around it, barely predictable and powerful weather patterns, and physical forces that pose high risk to human life: speed, thin air, and highly flammable materials. How has aviation done it? It is not a miracle and it is (and was) not simple. Aviation has adopted standardization, reporting and careful analysis not just of fatal accidents, but of all accidents, and also near misses. Aviation uses central repository to gather all reports of near misses and accidents, and to share about these events across proprietary and national boundaries. There is cooperation between competitors where cooperation makes sense for safety benefiting all, but there is fierce competition in other areas leading to a tough marketplace and many consumer options. Sharing safety data does not impair competition. Designing a flight deck includes psychologists, engineers, standards organizations and regulators [44, 45]. Checklists in aviation are refined and their use ingrained. Regulators are empowered with substantial power—including the ability to halt flights and ground aircraft—because governments and their citizens realize this can improve safety.

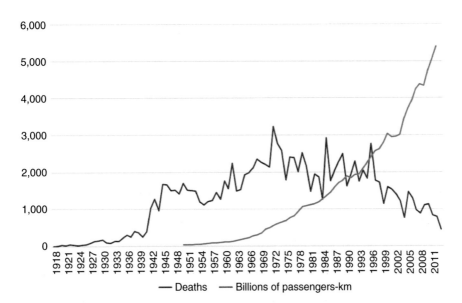

**Fig. 4.1** Number of yearly fatalities due to air transport crashes and billions of passengers-Km, 1918–2009 (Dr. Jean-Paul Rodrigue, Dept. of Global Studies & Geography, Hofstra University, New York, USA. Used with permission. Data source: Aircraft Crashes Record Office, Geneva (http://www.baaa-acro.com/))

Contrast this with the highly variable EHR user interface seen by a physician who may move from office to hospital, to ICU, or to a different hospital. In general in healthcare there is voluntary and so spotty reporting [46] and collected results not widely shared and there is no national central collection. Designs that can impact safety are regarded as proprietary and sometimes contractually precluded from being shared with others. How did check lists begin? Answer: with a fatal accident [47]. It seems we have much to learn from the aviation history and this is just one example of human endeavor that has latent lessons for our new field [48].

## 4.8   Summary

Healthcare organizations and practitioners have largely made the transition from paper to EHRs. Ahead of us is enhancement, maintenance, new approaches and paradigm shifts and careful gentle refinement of what seems to work and where the risk of change must be balanced against the likelihood of new harm that change might introduce.

EHRs are complex systems, with diverse functionality, woven into the even more complex fabric of the process of maintaining and improving health. From the early efforts to develop EHRs decades ago, we now see them applied to the care of most Americans and broadly across the globe. The transition to using EHRs is almost always difficult, but we persist because of their potential to achieve our hopes for them: That they can address those parts of information management at the limits of human ability, leaving us to concentrate on what humans do best. At this snapshot in our longer story, those hopes are not yet achieved. Perhaps those reading these words will move us closer.

## References

1. Weed LL. Medical records that guide and teach. N Engl J Med. 1968;278(11):593–600.
2. Gellert GA, Ramirea R, Webster SL. The rise of the medical scribe industry: implications for the advancement of electronic health records. JAMA. 2014. doi:10.1001/jama.2014.17128 [Epub ahead of print].
3. Steinbrook R. Health care and the American recovery and reinvestment act. N Engl J Med. 2009;360:1057–60.
4. Centers for Medicare & Medicaid Services. Medicare & Medicaid EHR Incentive Program. Meaningful use stage 1 requirements overview 2010. https://www.cms.gov/Regulations-and-Guidance/Legislation/    EHRIncentivePrograms/downloads/MU_Stage1_ReqOverview.pdf. Accessed Jul 2013.
5. Payne TH, Detmer DE, Wyatt JC, Buchan IE. National-scale clinical information exchange in the United Kingdom: lessons for the United States. J Am Med Inform Assoc. 2011;18(1):91–8. PMID: 21134976.
6. HealthIT.gov. About the ONC HIT certification program. Available at http://www.healthit.gov/policy-researchers-implementers/about-onc-hit-certification-program. Accessed 24 Jan 2015.

7. Cimino JJ. Improving the electronic health record—are clinicians getting what they wished for? JAMA. 2013;309(10):991–2.
8. Payne TH, Fellner F, Dugowson C, Liebovitz DM, Fletcher DS. Use of more than one electronic medical record system within a single health care organization. Appl Clin Inform. 2012;3:462–74.
9. Personal communication, Frank Ruggerio, Boeing commercial airplanes (retired).
10. Payne TH, Beckton KA. Architecture of clinical computing systems. In: Payne TH, editor. Practical guide to clinical computing systems. Design, operations, and infrastructure. 2nd ed. London: Academic; 2015.
11. Schiff GD, Bates DW. Can electronic clinical documentation help prevent diagnostic errors? N Engl J Med. 2010;362(12):1066–9.
12. Stead WW, Searle JR, Fessler HE, et al. Biomedical informatics: changing what physicians need to know and how they learn. Acad Med. 2011;86:429–34.
13. Van Eaton EG, McDonough K, Lober WB, Johnson EA, Pellegrini CA, Horvath KD. Safety of using a computerized rounding and sign-out system to reduce resident duty hours. Acad Med. 2010;85(7):1189–95.
14. Oxentenko AS, West CP, Popkave C, Weinberger SE, Kolars JC. Time spent on clinical documentation: a survey of internal medicine residents and program directors. Arch Intern Med. 2010;170:377–80.
15. Sittig DF, Stead WW. Computer-based physician order entry: the state of the art. J Am Med Inform Assoc. 1994;1:108–23.
16. Overhage JM, Tierney WM, Zhou XH, McDonald CJ. A randomized trial of "corollary orders" to prevent errors of omission. J Am Med Inform Assoc. 1997;4:364–75.
17. Block L, Habicht R, Wu AW, Desai SV, Wang K, Silva KN, Niessen T, Oliver N, Feldman L. In the wake of the 2003 and 2011 duty hours regulations, how do internal medicine interns spend their time? J Gen Intern Med. 2013;28(8):1042–7. doi:10.1007/s11606-013-2376-6. PubMed PMID: 23595927, PubMed Central PMCID: PMC3710392.
18. Nadkarni PM, Ohno-Machado L, Chapman WW. Natural language processing: an introduction. J Am Med Inform Assoc. 2011;18(5):544–51.
19. Payne TH, tenBroek AE, Fletcher GS, Labuguen MC. Transition from paper to electronic inpatient physician notes. J Am Med Inform Assoc. 2010;17:108–11.
20. Tang PC, Ash JS, Bates DW, Overhage JM, Sands DJ. Personal health records: definitions, benefits, and strategies for overcoming barriers to adoption. J Am Med Inform Assoc. 2006;13:121–6.
21. Brill S. Code red. Last fall, a hastily assembled group of tech wizards arrived in D.C. to revive HealthCare.gov. Time. 2014;183(9):26–36.
22. McDonald CJ. Protocol-based computer reminders, the quality of care and the non-perfectability of man. N Engl J Med. 1976;295:1351–5.
23. Shojania KG, Jennings A, Mayhew A, et al. Effect of point-of-care computer reminders on physician behaviour: a systematic review. CMAJ. 2010;182:E216–25.
24. Bates DW, Leape LL, Cullen DJ, Laird N, et al. Effect of computerized physician order entry and a team intervention on prevention of serious medication errors. JAMA. 1998;280:1311–6.
25. Mandl KD, Kohane IS. Tectonic shifts in the health information economy. N Engl J Med. 2008;358(16):1732–7.
26. Delbanco T, Walker J, Darer JD, Elmore JG, Feldman HJ, Leveille SG, et al. Open notes: doctors and patients signing on. Ann Intern Med. 2010;153:121–5.
27. Roth CP, Lim YW, Pevnick JM, Asch SM, McGlynn EA. The challenge of measuring quality of care from the electronic health record. Am J Med Qual. 2009;24(5):385–94.
28. Verdon DR. Physician outcry on EHR functionality, cost will shake the health information technology sector. Med Econ. 2014;91(3):18–20, 27.
29. Hyman P. The day the EHR died. Ann Intern Med. 2014;160:576–7.
30. Sinsky CA, Beasley JW. Texting while doctoring: a patient safety hazard. Ann Intern Med. 2013;159(11):782–3.

31. McDonald CJ, Callaghan FM, Weissman A, et al. Use of internist's free time by ambulatory care electronic medical record systems. JAMA Intern Med. 2014;174(11):1860–3.
32. Toll E. A piece of my mind. The cost of technology. JAMA. 2012;307(23):2497–8.
33. Middleton B, Bloomrosen M, Dente MA, Hashmat B, Koppel R, Overhage JO, Payne TH, Rosenbloom ST, Weaver C, Zhang J. Enhancing patient safety and quality of care by improving the usability of electronic health record systems: recommendations from AMIA. J Am Med Inform Assoc. 2013;20(e1):e2–8.
34. Carspecken CW, Sharek PJ, Longhurst C, Pageler NM. A clinical case of electronic health record drug alert fatigue: consequences for patient outcome. Pediatrics. 2013;131(6):e1970–3.
35. Bryant AD, Fletcher AS, Payne TH. Drug interaction alert override rates in the meaningful use era: no evidence of progress. Appl Clin Inform. 2014;5:802–13.
36. Payne TH. Electronic health records and patient safety: should we be discouraged? BMJ Qual Saf. 2015;24(4):239–40.
37. Miller RA, Pople HE, et al. INTERNIST-1: an experimental computer-based diagnostic consultant for general internal medicine. N Engl J Med. 1982;307:468–76.
38. Schiff GD, Hasan O, Kim S, et al. Diagnostic error in medicine: analysis of 583 physician-reported errors. Arch Intern Med. 2009;169(20):1881–7.
39. Singh H, Sittig DF. Advancing the science of measurement of diagnostic errors in healthcare: the Safer Dx framework. BMJ Qual Saf. 2015. doi:10.1136/bmjqs-2014-003675. pii: bmjqs-2014-003675, [Epub ahead of print].
40. Meystre S, Haug PJ. Natural language processing to extract medical problems from electronic clinical documents: performance evaluation. J Biomed Inform. 2006;39:589–99.
41. Payne TH, Garver-Hume A, Kirkegaard S, Sweeney J, Ash M, Kailasam KK, Hall CL, Sinanan MN. Group improves coding with natural language processing. MGMA Connex. 2011;11(9):15–7.
42. Yetisgen-Yildiz M, Gunn ML, Xia F, Payne TH. A text processing pipeline to extract recommendations from radiology reports. J Biomed Inform. 2013;46(2):354–62.
43. Geissbühler A, Miller RA. A new approach to the implementation of direct care-provider order entry. Proc AMIA Annu Fall Symp. 1996;689–93.
44. Spenser J. The airplane. 9. Flight deck. New York: HarperCollins; 2008.
45. Jacobsen A, Graeber D, Weidemann J. Crew station design and integration. In: Salas E, Maurino D, editors. Human factors in aviation. 2nd ed. Burlington: Academic; 2010.
46. Hazell L, Shakir SA. Under-reporting of adverse drug reactions: a systematic review. Drug Saf. 2006;29(5):385–96.
47. Gawande A. The checklist manifesto. How to get things right. New York: Henry Holt and Company; 2008.
48. Haynes AB, Weiser TG, Berry WR, et al. A surgical safety checklist to reduce morbidity and mortality in a global population. N Engl J Med. 2009;360(5):491–9.

# Chapter 5
# The Evolution of EHR-S Functionality for Care and Coordination

George R. Kim, Krysia Warren Hudson, and Colette Ann Miller

**Abstract** The purpose of electronic health record systems (EHR-S) functionalities is to improve patient safety by reducing medical errors that lead to harm and to facilitate the measurement of care quality by providing access to process and outcomes data. Through collaborative standards development, the definition and translation of health-care work into specific system functionalities for improving clinical data capture, communication and coordination has evolved from technical "wish lists" into commercially available products that meet the needs of multiple stakeholders: patients, clinicians, managers, systems developers, payers and regulatory agencies. Important technical drivers in the development and adoption of EHR-S functionalities have been: (a) progressive regulatory requirements for reporting quality measures and (b) lessons learned from deployment of EHR systems and other health information technology. A growing area of attention and challenge for health IT functionality development is in supporting longitudinal care coordination for patients with complex and chronic disease across time, providers and resources. Work in this domain has focused on (a) aligning and connecting Patient Centered Medical Homes and Medical Neighborhoods via data/communication standards to facilitate health information exchange (HIE) and (b) building the information infrastructures to facilitate the collection and reporting of quality measures related to care processes and outcomes.

**Keywords** Electronic health record systems • Health information technology • Standards development • Clinical information functionalities • Meaningful use •

G.R. Kim, MD (✉)
Division of Health Sciences Informatics and Armstrong Institute for Patient Safety and Quality, Johns Hopkins University School of Medicine, Baltimore, MD, USA
e-mail: gkim9@jhmi.edu

K.W. Hudson, DNP, MSN, RN, BC
Department of Acute and Chronic Care, Johns Hopkins University School of Nursing, Baltimore, MD, USA
e-mail: khudson2@jhu.edu

C.A. Miller, MSN, RNC-Nic
Baccalaureate Program, Johns Hopkins University School of Nursing, Baltimore, MD, USA
e-mail: cmille96@jhu.edu

© Springer International Publishing Switzerland 2016    73
C.A. Weaver et al. (eds.), *Healthcare Information Management Systems: Cases, Strategies, and Solutions*, Health Informatics,
DOI 10.1007/978-3-319-20765-0_5

Certified electronic health record technology • Patient centered medical home •
Medical neighborhoods • Health information exchange • Care coordination •
Analytics • Quality measurement • Patient safety • Healthcare redesign

## 5.1 Introduction

The functionalities of electronic health record systems (EHR-Ss) and other health
information technologies are determined by clinical and regulatory needs: to streamline and standardize care delivery, to facilitate access to information across the continuum of patient care and to provide measures of care quality. Rooted in patient
safety, EHR-S functionalities have been articulated and realized through standards
development processes and guided by the requirements of diverse clinical practice.
They have also been shaped by lessons learned from implementation and from the
evolution of healthcare science, practice, business and regulation. An important area
of ongoing in developing EHR-S and health IT functionality is in care coordination
through the Patient Centered Medical Home.

The goals of widespread adoption of electronic health record systems (EHR-S)
and other health information technology (health IT) are:

- Assurance of reliable and consistent high-quality (i.e., safe, effective, patient-
  centered, timely, efficient and equitable) patient care delivery and
- Access to accurate and timely clinically-based measures of the quality and outcomes of care

Together, these support the overall Triple Aim [52] of redesigning and optimizing
health care into a highly-reliable [18], continually learning [23] collaborative system.

As the availability of electronic clinical information has grown, health IT functionalities have evolved to meet the needs of multiple stakeholders. Clinical data
functionalities have grown from possibilities (what systems can do) to user needs
(what they should do) to requirements (what they must do). As the scope of patient
care continues to expand to include continuity of care over time and multiple stakeholders (including patients as partners in their own care), EHR system functionalities must also continue to evolve to assure and measure care.

## 5.2 History: EHR System Functionality, Patient Safety and Standardization

In 2003, the Institute of Medicine (IOM) Committee on Data Standards for Patient
Safety recommended key capabilities for EHR systems to promote patient safety,
care quality and efficiency [22]. They recommended categories of functionalities
(Health Information and Data, Result Management, Order Entry/Management,
Decision Support, Electronic Communication and Connectivity, Patient Support,

Administrative Processes and Reporting, Reporting and Population Health Management) that provided a framework for software development, with the goal of increasing reproducibility, completeness and accountability of health services.

The IOM identified overall aims of EHR-S functionalities as:

- Improving patient safety
- Supporting the delivery of effective patient care
- Facilitating chronic disease management
- Improving efficiency
- Feasibility (to be available within a reasonable period of time for purchase/implementation) [22], pp. 5–6.

The IOM recommendations were incorporated into Health Level Seven's EHR-S Functional Model (HL7 EHR-S FM, Fig. 5.1), with an eye to increasing primary use (Care Provision, Care Provision Support) and reuse (Population Health Support, Administrative Support) of health data, incrementally. The FM serves as a base on which to extend functionality recommendations.

Since the 2003 report, the evolution and progressive availability of functionalities for EHR-S and other health IT have been the subject of ongoing collaboration and negotiation among clinicians, systems developers and regulatory agencies to define a framework for clinical IT functionalities and roles within the healthcare infrastructure. This has led to the development of:

- Functional profiles (shepherded by Health Level Seven [43] and other clinical and technical organizations (Integrating the Healthcare Enterprise (IHE) and the Health Information Management Systems Society (HIMSS), among others)) for EHR systems, championed by physician groups, to translate unmet clinical needs into usable technical requirements for implementation and evaluation
- Certification for EHR technologies and products to provide recognition and assurance in meeting clinical, administrative and regulatory functions
- Financial incentives (with subsequent penalties for non-participation) for eligible providers (and hospitals) through the enactment of the Health Information Technology for Economic and Clinical Health (HITECH) Act (of 2009) for adoption and Meaningful Use (MU) of Certified Electronic Health Record Technologies (CEHRT)

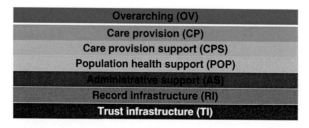

**Fig. 5.1** The HL7 Electronic Health Record System Functional Model (EHR-S FM) (HL7 EHR-System Functional Model, Release 2, April 2014; copyright and used with permission from HL7 International. All rights reserved)

- Accountability programs in the form of incremental electronic measures for HIT adoption, performance and clinical outcomes, linked to regulatory reporting requirements, quality/safety reporting and remuneration
- Communications and interoperability standards and networks to connect and coordinate care and information providers
- Collective quality improvement initiatives to measure, support and control care processes and outcomes on patient, service and population levels
- Recognition of the importance of incorporating the adaptive, organizational and teamwork components of care and coordination in safety and quality assurance and improvement and into the development and successful deployment of health IT systems

## 5.3 Drivers of EHR System Functionality in Patient Care

Health IT functionality is the result of ongoing negotiation among multiple stakeholders: clinicians (physicians and nurses), system developers/vendors, administrators, payers, standards development organizations, regulatory agencies, safety officers, researchers and patients. Success in negotiations requires active leadership and collaboration by the stakeholder groups to manage feasibility, viability and sustainability of health IT development (See [87 plus its associated textbook] for an example). In general, the progression of realizing health IT functionality requires:

- Articulation and specification of what user needs into technical (system and workflow) requirements for design and implementation. This requires organization of and active input by clinicians/users and informed analysis by developers who understand the needs of clinical information work
- Design and implementation of technical solutions into available products for purchase/incorporation. This requires mutual prioritization by customers (practice leaders/clinical users), vendors/developers and other stakeholders (payers, regulatory agencies) to evaluate and make products available for clinical use
- Adoption and incorporation of products/tools into clinical work. This requires acceptance and active use by users/customers, continuous support by developers and systems and reinforcement by organizations and regulators/payers

The negotiation and prioritization of specific functionalities are informed and influenced by:

- Unmet clinician needs
- Experience and lessons learned from implementation

### 5.3.1 Unmet Clinician Needs

Basic EHR-S functionalities empower clinicians to:

- Organize care

  - Identify patients correctly and link the right patient to the right information
  - Create work lists for session-based clinical tasks

- Document care

  - Capture and store records for reference, communication and coding
  - Provide a reliable legal record of care

- Order and manage therapies and tests

  - Prescribe, dispense and deliver medications/tests correctly and safely
  - Track, review and respond to results (test results, consultations) in a timely and facilitated fashion

- Make informed decisions

  - Use evidence and data to support timely choices, decisions and actions
  - Implement evidence-based guidelines and protocols

Expanding the HL7 EHR-S FM, a growing number of clinician groups and other stakeholders have articulated additional information functionality needs for specialty-based clinical workflows. Some of these needs have been translated into functionalities that have been incorporated into the HL7 model, while others are varying stages of development. In some cases, vendors have implemented special functionalities into standalone "niche" products.

Specific EHR-S functionalities that go beyond the HL7 EHR-S FM have been articulated for different specialties, with each effort being led by a coalition of physicians, IT developers, standards development organizations and regulators. These include:

Behavioral Health:
The HL7 Behavioral Health Functional Profile [46, 62] supports mental health-specific templates that integrate with the medical electronic record to allow documentation and attestation by different provider types (psychiatrists, psychologists, social workers) for full psychiatric (Axis I-V) diagnosis (according to the Diagnostic and Statistical Manual (DSM)) with robust support for coding and billing.

Child Health:
EHR-S functionalities for child health were first articulated in 2001 and updated in 2007 [82] with incorporation into the HL7 EHR-S FM as the Child Health Functional Profile [42] with implementation as a Children's Electronic Health Record Format (as part of the Child Health Insurance Program Reauthorization Act (CHIPRA)). Specific functionalities include:

- Immunization management (point-of-care decision support and forecasting, tracking aids for lapsed vaccines, linkage to office and regional immunization information systems),

- Growth tracking (special charts (such as for premature infants), graphical representation and calculations of body parameters such as BMI)
- Universal weight/surface-area based medication dosing (with pediatric dosing options for age and school-day regimens) for inpatient and ambulatory prescribing
- Standards for handling patient identification at the beginning of life (prenatal and newborn identifiers and clinical data, linkage to mother, name changes, ambiguous gender)
- Connection of EHR-S data among medical homes, hospital nurseries, school health offices, health information exchanges (immunization registries, hearing screening registries) and other child health care stakeholders

Adolescent Medicine:
Adolescent medicine health information functionalities focus on control and maintenance of privacy and confidentiality of encounter data while retaining advantages (tracking, billing, health information exchange) of EHR systems. Inherent conflicts in achieving this include:

- Recognition and preservation of the legal status of adolescents' health information vs. parental rights to access knowledge of services rendered (billing functionality)
- Customization of confidentiality (and access to patient information) according to local jurisdictional law according to patient status (such as for emancipated minors)
- Electronic sharing of adolescent health information and confidentiality issues regarding sensitive health issues (sexuality and pregnancy, sexually transmitted infections, HIV, mental health and substance abuse) and when data must be shared among different services [6, 13]

These conflicts present barriers in articulating needs as technical requirements and pose continuing challenges in successful implementation of adolescent-appropriate EHR-S functionalities [9].

Obstetrics and Gynecology:
Obstetrics and gynecology, characterized as both a medical and surgical specialty and as both hospital and office-based, "requires data fields and image displays unlike any other…discipline…" An effort by the American Congress of Obstetricians and Gynecologists to articulate its special needs [96] has included functionalities for:

- Pregnancy-specific immunization management
- Fetal development tracking with normative growth and laboratory data
- Medication management: Gynecologic oncology dosing
- Patient identification: Assisted reproductive technology (tracking sperm, egg donors) and multiple gestations
- Privacy: reproductive history and choice, contraception, abortion
- Flow sheets:

  - Pregnancy management with trimester-specific screening, medication requirements, laboratory testing and counseling and decision support

- Chemotherapy management
- Clinical documentation
- Guideline-based clinical decision support
- Displays for fetal age, biophysical profiles and imaging (still, video) management, fetal heart rates, non-stress testing

- Interoperability with specific electronic clinical tools: (biopsies, hysteroscopy, colposcopy, urodynamics, ultrasound, cystoscopy)
- Support for genetic, pre-pregnancy and assisted reproductive technologies, cord blood banking
- Medico-legal records management

As incentives increase the adoption of EHR-Ss in obstetrics-gynecology practice, there are still barriers to implementation of some of these functionalities.

Geriatrics:

The medical care of older adults poses vulnerabilities to errors that may lead to harm for this population of patients. Risks include:

- Multiple chronic and acute conditions of varying complexity and duration with input from multiple providers and caregivers
- Complex care and care transitions [89] related to hospitalization
- Polypharmacy and its co-morbidities [29]
- Functional (cognitive, communication, depression, nutrition, social) status issues that impact on health [16, 32, 33] and that put patients at risk for inpatient readmission and increased morbidity/mortality
- Hospitalization in settings where expertise in geriatric needs is scarce

Many of these functions are served by previously articulated EHR-S functionality, with the principal issue/barrier/problem being the implementation of existing guidelines. Screening tools, such as EHR-S checklists/templates and other decision support can help to identify patients at risk to guide appropriate care and link human expertise as needed [63]. Health IT supports for care coordination may help address geriatric care challenges.

Oncology:

Clinical Oncology Requirements for the EHR (CORE) is a 2009 document created collaboratively between the American Society of Clinical Oncology (ASCO) and the National Cancer Institute (NCI) (who lead in the effort to improve all aspects of oncology care and its safety). A consensus statement outlined oncology needs of EHR-S technology, which includes support for:

- "A treatment plan to be shared with patients and other care providers;
- A treatment summary to be shared with patients and their care teams;
- The use of calendars that patients and their care teams can use to organize the care process;
- Safe chemotherapy administration [94, 95]
- Use of decision support tools, such as ASCO and National Comprehensive Cancer Network (NCCN) guidelines" American Society for Clinical Oncology [5]

Oncology-specific functionalities include:

- Common core data elements to support oncology care and research
- Detailed analysis of functions to support chemotherapy and drug management.

    - Facilitation of electronic chemotherapy orders
    - Interface with pharmacy systems
    - Redundancy of nursing and pharmacy electronic safety checks of chemo-therapy orders

- Standardized order sets with dose calculators with clinical decision support based on patient height, weight and test results
- Special features to support patient safety and comfort
- Coordination of care

    - Scheduling functions for physician visits, laboratory and radiology testing, patient education and training, infusions and injections
    - Calendar and reminder functions for patients
    - Patient portals
    - End-of-life care management tools

- Oncology practice and research support

    - Inventory control and billing functions linked to operational bar-coding/RFID
    - Patient matching to prescribed medications and samples
    - Tools for summarization, communication and reporting [5], p. 5–6.

Anesthesiology:

Adoption of anesthesia information management systems (AIMS) has increased because of increased functionality and decreased costs of available systems, but also because of increased regualtory reporting requirements. AIMS are usually standalone systems that must interoperate with monitors, anesthesia machines and hospital information systems. Systems must also be ergonomic with respect to available working space of the operating suite. In addition, anesthesia EHR-S functionalities should include:

- Structured collection and sharing of preoperative data for assessment and risk-stratification
- Manual intraoperative charting and automatic transcription from monitors and ventilators
- Continual real-time access to and organized display of accumulating anesthe-sia data
- Reminders for intraoperative tasks (drug dose times)
- Provision for tracking performance and practice data for quality and safety improvement [30]

Ophthalmology:

Clinical ophthalmology, as a medical and surgical discipline, is centered on the anatomy and physiology of the eyes (and brain). Clinical assessments are frequently graphical and photographic: anatomic drawings, diagrams and images. Vital signs are ophthalmology-specific: intraocular pressure, visual acuity and examinations are performed by teams, in sequences that employ specialized imaging and measurement tools with unique and sophisticated graphical outputs not used elsewhere. The high level of clinical graphical data requires the use of picture archiving and communications systems (PACS, requiring Digital Imaging and Communication in Medicine (DICOM) standards).

Because care is rendered in parallel by teams, a patient record must be simultaneously accessible by all team members when a patient receives care. The American Academy of Ophthalmology (AAO) promotes best practices ("Preferred Practice Patterns") as templates for clinical data collection and management. The AAO has articulated desired ophthalmologic EHR-S functionalities to guide purchasers and to promote the standardization process. Specific functionality for ophthalmology EHR-S technology includes:

- Seamless linkage and integration of the EHR-S to ophthalmologic instruments and devices using defined standards (i.e., DICOM)
- Standards for interoperability of ophthalmologic and other health data within EHR systems
- Representation of ophthalmologic concepts within a reference terminology
- Summarization of ophthalmologic data for pre-visit review in high-volume practices
- Tools (other than a mouse) that facilitate the creation and annotation of clinical drawings for the record [20]

Dermatology:
Dermatology is also characterized as both a surgical and medical subspecialty with a heavy reliance on clinical images (photographs and diagrams). Its practitioners interact closely with other specialists, such as pathologists and surgeons. Dermatology-specific EHR-S functionalities form an adjunct to larger profiles and include: tools that:

- Facilitate the management and annotation of visual documents (photographs and diagrams)
- Connect the EHR-S to tools that can import such data (dermatoscopes)
- Permit rapid structured communication of skin lesion descriptions and classifications (to surgeons, as in Mohs procedures)
- Allow simultaneous access to records by multiple personnel (such as scribes) and
- Streamline work via connectivity to mobile technology such as tablets [56]

Dentistry and Oral Health:
The information technology needs for dentistry and oral care have been described [11, 75] and several themes which distinguish this field have emerged:

- Dentistry provides primary care to patients of all ages. Payment for services is typically separate from other forms of health insurance which all patients may not have.

- Dental records are separate from medical record, in paper and electronically. There may be other separated documents of care, such as orthodontic records. In addition, data for consultations for some oral surgical procedures may be contained in the medical (non-dental) record in some institutions.
- Dental radiographic technology and the documentation of oral anatomy and pathology have special technical needs and terminologies that are not found or used elsewhere.
- Special relationships exist between dental care and chronic disease (such as diabetes mellitus) that require incorporation into longitudinal care protocols.
- There is variable integration of dental and medical electronic records when both exist.

Emergency Medicine and Trauma Care:
The information technology needs of emergency medicine have been long articulated within the HL7 functionality framework, with a focus on patient throughput:

- Patient tracking and registration
- Task and order management
- Clinical documentation and all stages of patient management
- Management of roles of different workers [44].

The care of trauma patients requires special information workflows that bridge emergency departments to field settings. Use of tools in low-resource settings has been explored to support:

- Checklist generation
- Clinical scoring (for trauma severity)
- Wireless data transfer to electronic registries (i.e., trauma databases) [92].

Other Medical Subspecialties:
Cardiology [90] and gastroenterology (in particular GI endoscopy [58, 91]) are two domains in which clinicians have identified specific workflows, data elements and vocabularies for use in EHR-S and other health IT to meet the needs of practitioners in care, quality assurance and research. With the increasing dependence of patient care on technology to standardize clinical information workflows and to collect information for quality/safety and remuneration of services, the articulation of information functionality needs will continue to expand and evolve.

## 5.3.2   Experience from Implementation

Standards-based system functionalities are silent as to their implementation. As electronic functionalities are implemented and deployed, they change workflows and may create competing priorities which in turn may require redesign of those workflows or system re-implementation (at additional cost, effort and time).

### 5.3.2.1   Workflow Conflicts

The standardization of tasks may create non-alignments between user goals and/or organizational performance. Examples include:

- Security practices versus user convenience (timed lockouts after periods of non-use requiring re-entry of credentials)
- Safety practices versus provider efficiency (opening records on multiple patients for parallel work during care) [15]
- Technology versus workspace needs (pharmacy tracking (medication cabinets) may crowd anesthesiologists and nurses occupying the same operating room space around a patient)
- Attention needed for technology versus clinical needs (requirement of clinician to enter orders into a system [34] vs the use of scribes [2]
- Mobile technology used for portable charting that also introduces a vector for nosocomial infections

### 5.3.2.2   Nursing Workflows

Nursing activities involve direct care and interaction with patients. Workflows are information-intensive, parallel and highly interruptive. In general, health IT functionality, design and implementation do not match nursing tasks well, resulting in unexpected (and frequently unresolved) workarounds [79].

- Patient handoffs ideally are individualized, nurse to nurse and patient by patient, with time for questions and reflection. However, busy units, changing patient loads, time constraints, cross-coverage and management needs make centralized unit reports (away from the patient) the norm.
- Nursing work lists within most EHR-S products omit informal information and tools: nursing assessments, patient summaries, scheduling functions and/or customization (i.e., level of detail of tasks, according to the nurse's experience).
- Bar-coding medication administration (BCMA) decreases nursing errors [74], but increases the number of steps in the process [8]. Workarounds have been observed, such as duplication of patient bar-codes to a common location that reduce the number of steps [26].
- Mobile devices (cell phones and pagers) are used by nurses to reduce noise (overhead paging) on floors, but are not used to their full clinical potential because of institutional constraints and concerns for misuse.

### 5.3.2.3   Patient Safety

Inpatient patient misidentification rates are an indicator of hospital quality [50] and its reduction is a current (2015) National Patient Safety Goal [54]. The problem of assurance of patient identification becomes more complex as data from multiple electronic sources are combined for direct care and care coordination. The Office of the National Coordinator has a set of recommended safety practices [40] that include adaptive and behavioral practices by users.

#### 5.3.2.4 Clinical Documentation

EHR-S enhanced documentation has resulted in "note bloat" (superfluous negatives and copy-pasting/copy-forwarding) and in increased time spent by clinicians in documenting care. The American College of Physicians has published a position paper that outlines the problems and suggested system functionalities and practices (including physician leadership and user education specifically for electronic documentation) [59].

The implementation of ICD-10 for coding will bring higher specificity to diagnoses, and may further increase the time needed for provider documentation, and pushback by providers and care organizations has delayed its implementation requirement in the US. Recently the Centers for Medicare and Medicaid Services (CMS) stated it would help make the ICD-10 transition less disruptive by not deny claims solely on the basis of insufficient specificity for up to a year to help facilitate implementation of ICD-10 [98].

#### 5.3.2.5 Integration and interoperability

Integrated (defined as combined "software components, hardware components, or both into an overall system" [51], p. 41) single-vendor systems may limit functionality implementation, resulting in failure to meet the needs of some users. Standalone systems may provide solutions, but depend on interoperability (defined as "the ability of two or more systems or components to exchange information and to use the information that has been exchanged" [51], p. 42) with enterprise and business systems. Some institutions may combine the enterprise and standalone systems with one tradeoff being that clinicians may need to master multiple EHR systems and their interfaces. Governance may be complex with differential impacts on organizational culture [87].

A 2014 KLAS report revealed that 25 % of polled ambulatory practices are considering replacement of current systems due to financial, regulatory or political (hospital affiliation) issues [57]. Although there are efforts to reduce the time and cost of interoperability among systems [45], challenges persist [3].

### 5.3.3 New Needs

#### 5.3.3.1 New Data Types

In addition to EHR-S functionalities for rendering image and signal data, systems will need to manage genetic/genomic and pedigree data, which pose technical, administrative, legal and ethical issues. EHR-S functionalities for handling personal genomic data include the ability to: (a) store and share it in a clinically computable and usable format, (b) link to phenotypic information and (c) display and link findings and test results [64] to patient-directed information and decision tools. These functionalities are needed in several clinical domains: obstetrics/gynecology, pediatrics and oncology, among others.

Another challenge (and opportunity) lies in how patients can report and share their personal health data. Stage 3 Meaningful Use will incorporate patient-generated health data (PGHD) [86] into standard healthcare information flows which will pose many implementation challenges: technical, operational, legal, cultural and educational [78, 80]. Such "patient-facing" technologies hold great promise in increasing patient engagement for improving care quality, research and policy [27, 47].

### 5.3.3.2   Emergent/Adaptive Clinical Systems

A persistent problem of systems functionality development processes is that they are locked into a standards/contracts based "task-artifact" (clinician-to-developer-to-user) cycle which creates a continual lag in meeting user needs in the face of rapidly changing clinical (and regulatory) demands [88]. This results in persistent dissatisfaction and pushback from clinicians and physician groups on meeting initially specified regulatory deadlines for implementation (ICD-10 for example, and Meaningful Use Stage 2).

A recent development has been the pilot of an emergent clinical information system, the design approach that gives clinicians complete control over Web-based systems by providing

- Design tools that do not require programming
- Automatic real-time conversion of designs into executable clinical information systems
- Real-time iteration to facilitate problem identification and solution [12].

### 5.3.3.3   Usability and Patient Safety

Growing recognition of the importance of cognitive and usability of EHR-S and health IT in clinical workflow, system design and error reduction (especially in critical care [73]) has led to research and new approaches in design, implementation and deployment. Workflows that have been studied include: clinical summarization, problem list management and clinical comprehension [93].

New hazards posed by poorly designed or deployed health IT within the already complex delivery of care has been a concern of the health and regulatory community [53], with the consensus that even with regulation and standardization, safety of health IT is multi-factorial and dependent on human users (i.e., beyond functionality alone) [55]. Unsafe health IT and unsafe use of health IT persist, with barriers to detecting and reporting on such problems [67].

#### 5.3.3.4   Information Assurance

The progressive dependence of healthcare practice on EHR systems and other health IT has made information assurance (confidentiality, integrity and availability) of data, interfaces, applications and networks essential to maintaining healthcare operations:

- Tradeoffs between convenience and security persist as theft/loss of laptops and removable media with protected health information (PHI) remains the leading cause of data breaches [84] with a recent report that the root cause of health care breaches are shifting from accidental to intentional [97]. Concerns for cybercrime involving health data has led to progressive requirements for health data security training for all users and to proactive institutional risk assessment and management [39] as standard practice [31] which may be overwhelming to some organizations [61].
- Poor documentation practices (copy-pasting, over-documentation, etc.) threaten the integrity of clinical content and require training and monitoring.
- The interplay between sociotechnical health information infrastructures and high-reliability IT networks have created lowered tolerances to prolonged system crashes that may paralyze institution-wide clinical work flow [10] (and create additional burdens of data recovery).

## 5.4   EHR System Functionality in Care Coordination

Care coordination has been identified as a national strategy priority for improving healthcare quality [85]. A 2012 cross-sectional study of US office-based physicians revealed that measures of care continuity (completion rates of consultation requests, hospital discharge summaries and consultant reports) were low, even when practices had an EHR-S. Over a third did not routinely receive needed patient information, with over half not receiving it electronically. EHR-S technology only slightly improved receipt of needed information [48].

Care coordination is defined as "a function that helps ensure that the patient's needs and preferences for health services and information sharing across people, functions, and sites are met over time…[maximizing] the value of services delivered to patients by facilitating beneficial, efficient, safe, and high-quality patient experiences and improved healthcare outcomes" [49]. From a management perspective, it is "the organization of…activities between two or more participants involved in a patient's care to facilitate…appropriate delivery of health care services…marshalling of personnel and other resources needed to carry out all required patient care activities and…managed by the exchange of information among participants responsible for different aspects of care" [66, p 6].

## 5.4.1 Framework for Care Coordination

### 5.4.1.1 The Medical Neighborhood

Care coordination (described in the AHRQ Care Coordination Measures Atlas (Fig. 5.2)) bridges gaps between providers (services, goods, participants, information) and requires pragmatic and proactive organization of resources and services with respect to the patient. Centered on the **health care home** (aka "medical home" or "patient-centered medical home" (PCMH) [69]), the **medical neighborhood** includes "the constellation of…clinicians providing health care services to patients within it,…community and social service organizations and State and local public health agencies" [83] that connect and communicate with each other (Fig. 5.3).

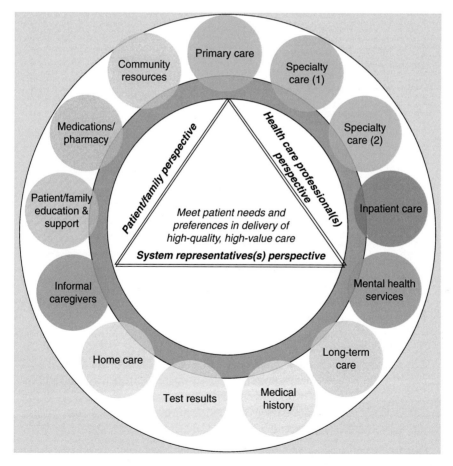

**Fig. 5.2** Conceptual structure of care coordination [66] (Reprinted with permission of the Agency for Healthcare Research and Quality)

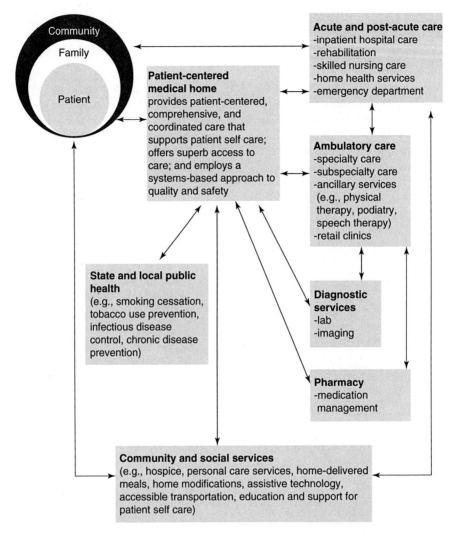

**Fig. 5.3** Information Flows in a Medical Neighborhood [83] (Reprinted with permission of the Agency for Healthcare Research and Quality)

High functioning medical neighborhoods encourage collaboration through well-defined (via formal agreements) and shared infrastructures, resources and information (Fig. 5.3) with "regular communication, collaboration, and shared decision-making across various actors in the system" through effective use of information and communication technologies [68]. Care coordination is characterized by:

1. _**Individualized management**_ by teams and centralized in the healthcare home, with
2. _**Specific plans**_ for tracking and follow-up,

3. **_Well-defined_ transitions of care, communication, coordination and collaboration** inclusive of clinicians, patients, families and others involved in ongoing care of the patient, and
4. **_Strongly-linked_ community services and resources** that align and facilitate care

Expected outcomes of high-functioning medical neighborhoods include improved patient safety and satisfaction with reduced costs and utilization and improved population health [83 pp. 7, 9.].

### 5.4.1.2   The Medical Home

To support the IHI Triple Aim (Improve the patient experience, Improve population health, Reduce the cost of healthcare [52]), and other HIT functionalities must support the medical home. Functions that Patient Centered Medical Homes (PCMHs) must provide include: 24/7 access and continuity to care and medical advice by patients, team-based care, population health management, care planning/management (including medication management/prescribing), test and referral tracking and performance measurement and improvement (Fig. 5.4). PCMHs must facilitate communication and collaboration with other members of the medical neighborhood (Fig. 5.3) and with health information exchanges (HIE).

NCQA provides certification to PCMH organizations that meet stringent criteria and to EHR-S and other health IT products aligned to their needs [70].

Still, availability of an EHR-S and patient infrastructure are not enough. Health homes and their medical neighborhoods must themselves be high functioning with dedicated case management in partnership with engaged primary care providers [76]. For patients with complex and chronic health problems, comprehensive periodic needs assessments with updated individualized plans/summaries by a knowledgeable care team that uses HIT optimally are essential [76], pp. 11–12. A framework for coordination support has been described [77, 81] for:

- Coordination within care teams

  - Documentation using structured (and searchable) clinical data for decisions
  - Summarization tools to view and share patient data and trends over time
  - Comprehensive care plan tools to provide accountability over different aspects of care

- Coordination across care teams

  - Interoperability to handle data from multiple sources, reducing the need for multiple entry
  - Tools for medication reconciliation
  - Tracking and loop closure functions for test results, referrals and consultations

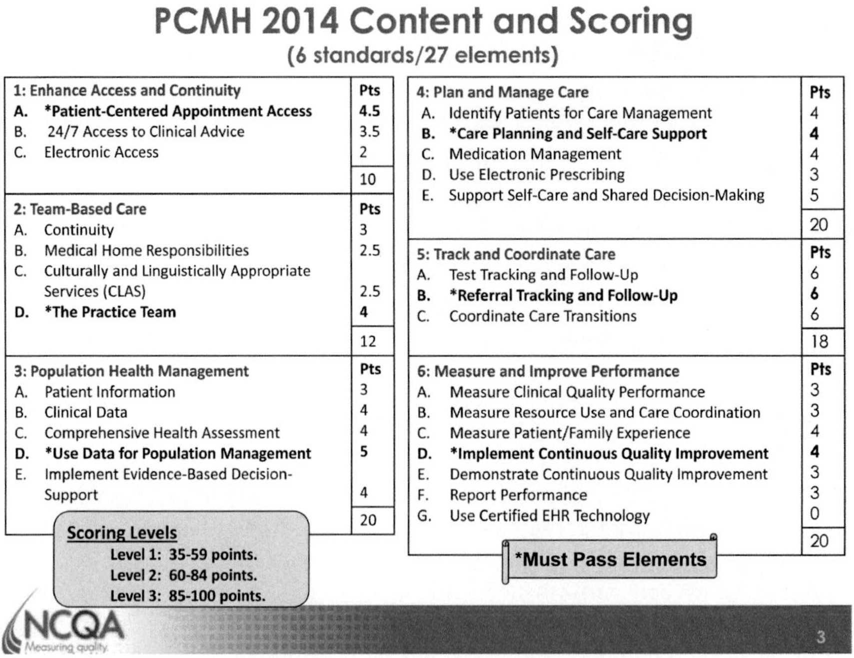

## PCMH 2014 Content and Scoring
### (6 standards/27 elements)

| 1: Enhance Access and Continuity | Pts | | 4: Plan and Manage Care | Pts |
|---|---|---|---|---|
| A. *Patient-Centered Appointment Access | 4.5 | | A. Identify Patients for Care Management | 4 |
| B. 24/7 Access to Clinical Advice | 3.5 | | B. *Care Planning and Self-Care Support | 4 |
| C. Electronic Access | 2 | | C. Medication Management | 4 |
| | 10 | | D. Use Electronic Prescribing | 3 |
| | | | E. Support Self-Care and Shared Decision-Making | 5 |
| 2: Team-Based Care | Pts | | | 20 |
| A. Continuity | 3 | | | |
| B. Medical Home Responsibilities | 2.5 | | 5: Track and Coordinate Care | Pts |
| C. Culturally and Linguistically Appropriate | | | A. Test Tracking and Follow-Up | 6 |
| Services (CLAS) | 2.5 | | B. *Referral Tracking and Follow-Up | 6 |
| D. *The Practice Team | 4 | | C. Coordinate Care Transitions | 6 |
| | 12 | | | 18 |
| 3: Population Health Management | Pts | | 6: Measure and Improve Performance | Pts |
| A. Patient Information | 3 | | A. Measure Clinical Quality Performance | 3 |
| B. Clinical Data | 4 | | B. Measure Resource Use and Care Coordination | 3 |
| C. Comprehensive Health Assessment | 4 | | C. Measure Patient/Family Experience | 4 |
| D. *Use Data for Population Management | 5 | | D. *Implement Continuous Quality Improvement | 4 |
| E. Implement Evidence-Based Decision- | | | E. Demonstrate Continuous Quality Improvement | 3 |
| Support | 4 | | F. Report Performance | 3 |
| | 20 | | G. Use Certified EHR Technology | 0 |
| | | | | 20 |

**Scoring Levels**
Level 1: 35-59 points.
Level 2: 60-84 points.
Level 3: 85-100 points.

**\*Must Pass Elements**

NCQA
Measuring quality

3

**Fig. 5.4** Patient Centered Medical Home Criteria (Reproduced with permission of the National Committee for Quality Assurance (NCQA) [99]

- Coordination between care teams and community resources
  - Tracking patient use of community resources
  - Facilitated communication with community resources
- Continuous familiarity with a patient across time
  - Listing of all members of the care team
  - Ability to share information with the patient and the team simultaneously
- Continuous proactive and responsive action between visits
  - Disease/condition specific decision support (reminders/alerts)
- Patient-centered care
  - Patient portals and personal health records

Other factors important to care coordination success are:

- Active engagement of patients in their own care with direct communication among patients, providers and specialists
- Dedicated teams with stratified approaches dependent on the complexity of care required
- Business models with incentives that support and reward care coordination eHealth Initiative [49, p. 6].

### 5.4.1.3 The Care Coordinator

The designated individual or team responsible for identifying a patient's care plan goals, coordinating services and providers and helping the patient to navigate the medical system is essential. Ideally, coordination is an integrated multi-disciplinary team that includes one such designee who works in close partnership with the patient, the provider and services [24]. A major aim is to engage the patient in all aspects and decisions of care. The American Nurses Association promotes the training and essential role of registered nurses in providing excellence in care coordination [4].

## 5.4.2 Health IT to Support Care Coordination

EHR systems and other health IT form the information infrastructure and mechanisms by which:

1. Care coordination activities are documented, communicated, managed and tracked
2. Performance measures are defined, collected and managed

The roles of EHR and other health IT systems are to: (a) assure, simplify and reduce the burden of data collection and sharing, (b) provide access to *clinical* details not available otherwise for care and quality and performance measures and (c) generate views of aggregated longitudinal patient data over time and providers [66, p. 28]. At the PCMH (practice) level, this translates into EHR-S functionalities:

- Decision support (condition-specific reminders, alerts) for clinicians and care coordinators to manage and track tests, results, referrals and consultant reports for individual patients
- Dashboards that facilitate care coordinators to follow up on the care of individuals and groups of patients (completion of prescriptions, testing, referrals, communications, patient reports, seasonal care (i.e., immunizations))
- Report specification and generation tools for multiple users and uses: clinical tracking, practice monitoring and improvement, patient outreach, regulatory measures and research.

### 5.4.2.1 Health Information Exchange (HIE) and Early Notification

HIE refers to (a) electronic sharing of healthcare information across and among organizations and (b) an organization that provides this functionality to stakeholders. The goal of HIE is to provide timely access to data for high-quality patient-centered care that prevents unnecessary duplication and to prevent abuses.

For definition (a), there are currently three standards [41]:

- The Direct Standard: for secure electronic transfers between providers for care coordination [38]

- The NHIN CAQH CORE X12: for providers to query and request electronic clinical information about a patient between providers [35]
- Consumer-mediated exchange: an example of which is the Blue Button Initiative [21, 37] to empower patients to access their medical information securely from a Web portal.

For definition (b), one example is a collaborative Early Notification System (ENS) Program which provides notification of an admission/transfer/or discharge about patients in Maryland and Delaware [19, 28] to enrolled providers. This program supports transitional care management (TCM) to reduce hospital readmissions [7]. Another example is Maryland's Prescription Drug Monitoring Program (PDMP) [25] using its CRISP HIE (http://crisphealth.org/). The PDMP helps to identify patients seeking controlled substances by prescription from multiple providers, preventing morbidity and promoting appropriate services to patients in need.

### 5.4.2.2    Care Plan Documentation Standards

Much work has been done by several standards development organizations (HL7, IHE, HITSP) to define a structure for an interoperable electronic document for Care Coordination (the Care Plan, a shared, consensus-driven, comprehensive blueprint of concerns and interventions by multiple providers and the patients). The Care Plan formalizes data fields and values (Fig. 5.5) for use in electronic records and transactions.

### 5.4.2.3    Performance Measurement Tools

The National Quality Forum (NQF) has endorsed a Care Coordination Framework [71] that identifies an evolving set of coordination measures that includes (but is not limited to): (a) the healthcare home, (b) a proactive plan of care and follow-up, (c) communication, (d) information systems and (e) transitions/hand-offs. In addition, NQF has developed the Quality Data Model (QDM) [17], a formal, standardized framework for enabling structured authoring (via its Measure Authoring Tool, https://www.emeasuretool.cms.gov/) of logically consistent electronic eMeasures (or eCQM). The QDM defines categories of information, their context of use and relationships to other information to allow automated capture of data from HIT such as EHR-Ss Health [36, 65]; http://public.qualityforum.org/hitknowledgebase/Pages/Knowledge%20Base%20Home.aspx.

EHR-based measures, some with formal (QDM) specification, have been identified in Meaningful Use (of Certified Electronic Health Technology) core and menu objectives (Stages 1 and 2) and clinical quality measures [66], pp. 31–34. Current

## LCC Care Plan Exchange: Conceptual Workflow

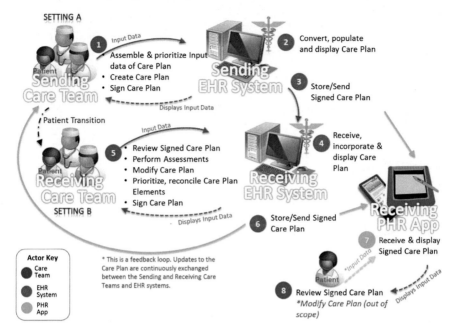

**Fig. 5.5** Conceptual Workflow of a Care Plan (Reproduced, courtesy of HealthIT.gov, Office of the National Coordinator) [100]

Meaningful Use objectives for which eMeasures are currently specified (although not implemented) include Clinical Quality Measures:

- Closing the Referral Loop: Receipt of a Specialist's Report
- Follow-Up Care for Children Prescribed ADHD Medication
- Diabetic Retinopathy: Communication with the Physician Managing Ongoing Diabetes Care
- Home Management Plan of Care: Document Given to Patient/Caregiver

### *5.4.3   Challenges*

#### 5.4.3.1   Inclusion of External Care

As more patients receive care in "nontraditional settings" (retail clinics, urgent care centers, school and work clinics), a question that has arisen is: "What is the capacity for these settings to connect with the medical home?" This forms a basis for a recent initiative by NCQA to assess these sources of health care as "visible" parts of the medical neighborhood [72].

#### 5.4.3.2 Management of Inherent Complexity

The challenges of care coordination are long-standing. Even with new approaches, infrastructures and information tools [14], there are inherent complexities in coordinating and optimizing care and health that make success elusive:

- Accountable care organizations' (ACOs') call to engage patients in their care
- Changing patient behaviors
- Medication reconciliation [60] and problem list management [1].

## 5.5 Conclusion

EHR systems and other health IT technologies are now a part of mainstream healthcare. The evolution of system functionalities has resulted from ongoing negotiations among clinicians and systems developers to meet the growth of clinical information workflow needs. Two important drivers that have increased adoption of EHR-S technology and stimulated development of functionalities are federal regulations (quality measures reporting and Meaningful Use incentives/penalties) and lessons learned from implementation.

Care coordination, as a means to improve transitions and longitudinal care of patients across time, providers and resources, is a national healthcare strategy goal. The management of care trajectories through a medical neighborhood by Patient Centered Medical Homes (PCMHs) requires dedicated nurse-led multi-stakeholder teams and appropriate business models to sustain them. The development of EHR-S and health IT functionalities for care coordination have focused on (a) tools to assure completion of tasks, (b) interoperability standards for health information exchange (HIE) among stakeholders and (c) infrastructures to measure care processes and outcomes.

The starting point and the final arbiter in any functionality of health information tools is how it impacts on the quality of patient care: its safety, effectiveness, efficiency, equity and patient-centeredness.

## References

1. AHIMA. Problem lists in health records: ownership, standardization and accountability; 2012. URL: http://library.ahima.org/xpedio/groups/public/documents/ahima/bok1_050158. pdf. Last accessed 11 Feb 2015.
2. AHIMA. Using medical scribes in a physician practice. J AHIMA. 2012;83(11):64–. URL: http://library.ahima.org/xpedio/groups/public/documents/ahima/bok1_049807. hcsp?dDocName=bok1_049807. Last accessed 6 Feb 2015.
3. American Medical Association. 15 questions to ask before signing an EMR/EHR agreement, AMA, 2008-11. URL: http://www.himss.org/files/HIMSSorg/content/files/Code%20 93_15%20questions%20to%20ask%20before%20signing%20an%20EMR-EHR%20agree-ment_AMA.pdf. Last accessed 23 Mar 2015.

4. American Nursing Association. The value of nursing care coordination: a white paper. June 2012.
5. American Society for Clinical Oncology, National Cancer Institute, caBIG, NCI Community Cancer Centers Program. Clinical Oncology Requirements for the EHR (CORE); 2007. p. 2.
6. Anoshiravani A, Gaskin GL, Groshek MR, Kuelbs C, Longhurst CA. Special requirements for electronic medical records in adolescent medicine. J Adolesc Health. 2012;51(5): 409–14.
7. Audacious Inquiry. DHIN launches encounter notification system for two medicaid managed care organizations; (2015). URL: http://ainq.com/case_study/encounter-notification-system-for-two-medicaid-mcos/. Last accessed 15 Feb 2015.
8. Bargren M, Lu D. An evaluation process for an electronic bar code medication administration information system in an acute care unit. Urol Nurs. 2009;29(5):355–67.
9. Bayer R, Santelli J, Klitzman R. New challenges for electronic health records: Confidentiality and access to sensitive health information about parents and adolescents. JAMA. 2015;313(1):29–30. doi:10.1001/jama.2014.15391.
10. Berinato S. All systems down. Computerworld; 2003. URL: http://www.computerworld.com/article/2581420/disaster-recovery/all-systems-down.html. Last accessed 17 Mar 2015.
11. Bertaud-Gounot V, Chaumeil B, Ehrmann E, Fages M, Valcarcel A. Computerizing the Dental Office. In: Venot A, Burgun A, Quantin C, editors. Medical informatics, e-Health: fundamentals and applications. Paris: Springer-Verlag France; 2014. p. 365–403.
12. Bishop RO, Patrick J, Besiso A. Efficiency achievements from a user-developed real-time modifiable clinical information system. Ann Emerg Med. 2015;65(2):133–42.e5.
13. Blythe MJ, Del Beccaro MA, Committee on Adolescence; Council on Clinical and Information Technology. Standards for health information technology to ensure adolescent privacy. Pediatrics. 2012;130(5):987–90.
14. Burns LR, Pauly MV. Accountable care organizations may have difficulty avoiding the failures of integrated delivery networks of the 1990s. Health Aff (Millwood). 2012;31(11): 2407–16.
15. Campbell EM, Sittig DF, Ash JS, et al. Types of unintended consequences related to computerized provider order entry. J Am Med Inform Assoc. 2006;13(5):547–56.
16. Campbell SE, Seymour DG, Primrose WR, ACMEPLUS Project. A systematic literature review of factors affecting outcome in older medical patients admitted to hospital. Age Ageing. 2004;33(2):110–5.
17. Centers for Medicare & Medicaid Services, Office of the National Coordinator for Health Information Technology. Quality data model, Version 4.1.1., September 16, 2014. URL: http://www.healthit.gov/sites/default/files/qdm_4_1_1.pdf. Last accessed 5 Jan 2015.
18. Chassin MR, Loeb JM. High-reliability health care: getting there from here. Milbank Q. 2013;91(3):459–90.
19. Chesapeake Regional Information System for our Patients (CRISP). CRISP Encounter Notification System (ENS). URL: http://crisphealth.org/CRISP-HIE-SERVICES/Encounter-Notification-System-ENS. Last accessed 15 Feb 2015.
20. Chiang MF, Boland MV, Brewer A, Epley KD, Horton MB, Lim MC, McCannel CA, Patel SJ, Silverstone DE, Wedemeyer L, Lum F, American Academy of Ophthalmology Medical Information Technology Committee. Special requirements for electronic health record systems in ophthalmology. Ophthalmology. 2011;118(8):1681–7.
21. CMS.gov. The Blue Button initiative, Jan 2013. URL: http://www.cms.gov/Research-Statistics-Data-and-Systems/Files-for-Order/NonIdentifiableDataFiles/BlueButtonInitiative.html. Last accessed 10 Feb 2015.
22. Committee on Data Standards for Patient Safety. Key capabilities of an electronic health record system: letter report. Washington, DC: National Academies Press; 2003.
23. Committee on the Learning Health Care System in America; Institute of Medicine; Smith M, Saunders R, Stuckhardt L, et al., editors. Best care at lower cost: the path to continuously learning health care in America. Washington (DC): National Academies Press (US); 2013 May 10. URL: http://www.ncbi.nlm.nih.gov/books/NBK207218/. Last accessed 1 Feb 2015.

24. Craig C, Eby D, Whittington J. Care coordination model: better care at lower cost for people with multiple health and social needs. IHI innovation series white paper. Cambridge, MA: Institute for Healthcare Improvement; 2011.
25. CRISP. (no date b) The Maryland Prescription Drug Monitoring Program (PDMP). URL: http://crisphealth.org/CRISP-HIE-SERVICES/Prescription-Drug-Monitoring-Program-PDMP. Last accessed 10 Feb 2015.
26. Debono DS, Greenfield D, Travaglia JF, Long JC, Black D, Johnson J, Braithwaite J. Nurses' workarounds in acute healthcare settings: a scoping review. BMC Health Serv Res. 2013;11(13):175. doi:10.1186/1472-6963-13-175.
27. Deering MJ. Issue brief: patient-generated health data and health IT. Office of the National Coordinator of Health Information Technology, Dec 2013.
28. Delaware Health Information Network. Another DHIN "First": DE & MD are first HIEs to exchange ADT information. The DHIN Dialogue, June 2014. URL: http://www.dhin.org/sites/default/files/DHIN%20Dialogue%20June%202014_0.pdf. Last accessed 15 Feb 2015.
29. Evans DC, Cook CH, Christy JM, Murphy CV, Gerlach AT, Eiferman D, Lindsey DE, Whitmill ML, Papadimos TJ, Beery 2nd PR, Steinberg SM, Stawicki SP. Comorbidity-polypharmacy scoring facilitates outcome prediction in older trauma patients. J Am Geriatr Soc. 2012;60(8):1465–70.
30. Ehrenfeld JM, Rehman MA. Anesthesia information management systems: a review of functionality and installation considerations. J Clin Monit Comput. 2011;25(1):71–9.
31. Federal Trade Commission. Consumer information – medical identity theft; 2012. URL: http://www.consumer.ftc.gov/articles/0171-medical-identity-theft. Last accessed 11 Mar 2015.
32. Greysen SR, Covinsky KE. Functional status – an important but overlooked variable in the readmissions equation. J Hosp Med. 2014;9(5):330–1.
33. Greysen SR, Hoi-Cheung D, Garcia V, Kessell E, Sarkar U, Goldman L, Schneidermann M, Critchfield J, Pierluissi E, Kushel M. "Missing pieces" – functional, social, and environmental barriers to recovery for vulnerable older adults transitioning from hospital to home. J Am Geriatr Soc. 2014;62(8):1556–61.
34. Han YY, Carcillo JA, Venkataraman ST, Clark RS, Watson RS, Nguyen TC, Bayir H, Orr RA. Unexpected increased mortality after implementation of a commercially sold computerized physician order entry system. Pediatrics. 2005;116(6):1506–12.
35. HealtheWay. Exchange specifications; 2015. URL: http://www.healthewayinc.org/index.php/resources/exchange-specifications. Last accessed 10 Feb 2015.
36. Health Information Technology Research Center (HITRC). Continuous Quality Improvement (CQI) strategies to optimize your practice: Primer. The National Learning Consortium, April 30, 2013. URL: http://www.healthit.gov/sites/default/files/tools/nlc_continuousqualityimprovementprimer.pdf. Last accessed 5 Jan 2015.
37. HealthIT.gov. Blue Button; 2014. URL: http://www.healthit.gov/patients-families/your-health-data. Last accessed 10 Feb 2015.
38. HealthIT.gov. Direct basics: Q&A for providers; 2014. URL: http://www.healthit.gov/sites/default/files/directbasicsforprovidersqa_05092014.pdf. Last accessed 10 Feb 2015.
39. HealthIT.gov. Health information privacy and security: a 10 step plan; 2013. URL: http://www.healthit.gov/providers-professionals/ehr-privacy-security/10-step-plan. Last accessed 11 Mar 2015.
40. HealthIT.gov. The patient identification SAFER guide. The Office of the National Coordinator. January 2014. URL: http://www.healthit.gov/safer/guide/sg006. Last 20 Jan 2015.
41. HealthIT.gov. (May 12, 2014). What is HIE? URL: http://www.healthit.gov/providers-professionals/health-information-exchange/what-hie#query-based_exchange. Last accessed 10 Feb 2015.
42. Health Level Seven Child Health Functional Profile Workgroup Pediatric Data Standards Special Interest Group (PeDSSIG). Health level seven. Child health functional profile, final version 1.0. National Institute of Standards and Technology. Functional Profile Registry; 2007.

43. Health Level Seven International (No date). HL7 Standards – Section 4: EHR Profiles. URL: http://www.hl7.org/implement/standards/product_section.cfm?section=4. Last accessed 2 Jan. 2015.
44. HL7. Emergency Department Information Systems (EDIS) Functional Profile, April 2007. URL: http://www.hl7.org/documentcenter/public_temp_A4DB3F90-1C23-BA17-0C1B2021CE42201A/wg/emergencycare/EDIS%20FP%20R1.pdf. Last accessed 17 Mar 2015.
45. HL7 (no date). FHIR Specification. Health Level 7. URL: http://www.hl7.org/implement/standards/fhir/index.html. Last accessed 23 Mar 2015
46. HL7 EHR Work Group & The Behavioral Health Profile Working Group. HL7 EHR behavioral health functional profile, Release 1, 2008 (reaffirmed Apr 2014).
47. Howie L, Hirsch B, Locklear T, Abernethy AP. Assessing the value of patient-generated data to comparative effectiveness research. Health Aff. 2014;33(7):1220–8.
48. Hsiao CJ, King J, Hing E, Simon AE. The role of health information technology in care coordination in the United States. Med Care. 2015;53(2):184–90.
49. eHealth Initiative. Centering on the patient: how electronic records enable care coordination. eHealth Initiative; 2011.
50. Hughes DM. Patient identification. In: Agrawal A, editor. Patient safety: a case-based comprehensive guide. New York: Springer; 2014. p. 3–18.
51. IEEE Std 610.12-1990, IEEE standard glossary of software engineering terminology; 1990.
52. Institute for Healthcare Improvement. IHI Triple aim initiative. 2009. URL: http://www.ihi.org/Engage/Initiatives/TripleAim/pages/default.aspx. Last accessed 1 Feb 2015.
53. Institute of Medicine. Health IT and patient safety: building safer systems for better care. URL: http://www.iom.edu/Reports/2011/Health-IT-and-Patient-Safety-Building-Safer-Systems-for-Better-Care.aspx. Last accessed 17 Apr 2015.
54. The Joint Commission. National patient safety goals. 2015. URL: http://www.jointcommission.org/standards_information/npsgs.aspx. Last accessed 20 January 2015.
55. The Joint Commission. Sentinel Event Alert # 54. Safe use of health information technology. Issue 54, March 31, 2015. URL: http://www.jointcommission.org/assets/1/18/SEA_54.pdf. Last accessed 17 Apr 2015.
56. Kaufmann MD, Desai S. Special requirements for electronic health records in dermatology. Semin Cutan Med Surg. 2012;31(3):160–2.
57. KLAS. One out of four ambulatory EMRs are in danger of being replaced. KLAS Press Room, Aug 2014. URL: http://www.klasresearch.com/News/PressRoom/2014/Ambulatory%20EMR%20Perception%202014. Last accessed 10 Feb 2015.
58. Korman KY, Delvaux M, Bidgood D. Structured reporting in gastrointestinal endoscopy: integration with DICOM and minimal standard terminology. Int J Med Inform. 1998;48:201–6.
59. Kuhn T, Basch P, Barr M, Yackel T, Medical Informatics Committee of the American College of Physicians. Clinical documentation in the 21st century: executive summary of a policy position paper from the American College of Physicians. Ann Intern Med. 2015. doi:10.7326/M14-2128. [Epub ahead of print] PubMed.
60. Lehnbom EC, Stewart MJ, Manias E, Westbrook JI. Impact of medication reconciliation and review on clinical outcomes. Ann Pharmacother. 2014;48(10):1298–312.
61. Levinson DR. Not all recommended safeguards have been implemented in hospital EHR technology, OEI-01-11-00570. Department of Health and Human Services, Office of the Inspector General, December 2013. URL: http://oig.hhs.gov/oei/reports/oei-01-11-00570.pdf. Last accessed 17 Mar 2015.
62. Lopez NI. Implementing a behavioral health electronic medical record. Health information management systems society; 2007.
63. Malone ML, Vollbrecht M, Stephenson J, Burke L, Pagel P, Goodwin JS. Acute Care for Elders (ACE) tracker and e-Geriatrician: methods to disseminate ACE concepts to hospitals with no geriatricians on staff. J Am Geriatr Soc. 2010;58(1):161–7.
64. Marsolo K, Spooner SA. Clinical genomics in the world of the electronic health record. Genet Med. 2013;15(10):786–91.

65. McDonald K, Schultz E, Chapman T, et al. Prospects for care coordination measurement using electronic data sources (Prepared by Stanford University under subcontract to Battelle on Contract No. 290-04-0020--AHRQ SQI-II) AHRQ Publication No. 12-0014-EF. Rockville: Agency for Healthcare Research and Quality; 2012.

66. McDonald KM, Schultz E, Albin L, Pineda N, Lonhart J, Sundaram V, Smith-Spangler C, Brustrom J, Malcolm E, Rohn L, Davies S. Care Coordination Atlas Version 4 (Prepared by Stanford University under subcontract to American Institutes for Research on Contract No. HHSA290-2010-00005I). AHRQ Publication No. 14-0037- EF. Rockville: Agency for Healthcare Research and Quality; 2014.

67. Meeks DW, Smith MW, Taylor L, Sittig DF, Scott JM, Singh H. An analysis of electronic health record-related patient safety concerns. J Am Med Inform Assoc. 2014;21:1053–9.

68. Meyers D, Peikes D, Genevro J, et al. The roles of patient-centered medical homes and accountable care organizations in coordinating patient care AHRQ Publication No. 11-M005-EF. Rockville: Agency for Healthcare Research and Quality; 2010.

69. National Committee for Quality Assurance. Patient-Centered Medical Home Recognition; 2014. URL: http://www.ncqa.org/Programs/Recognition/Practices/PatientCenteredMedical HomePCMH.aspx. Last accessed 5 Jan 2015.

70. National Committee for Quality Assurance (NCQA) (no date). PCMH Prevalidation Program. URL: http://www.ncqa.org/programs/recognition/Practices/patientcenteredmedicalhomep-cmh/pcmhprevalidationprogram.aspx. Last accessed 10 Feb 2015.

71. National Quality Forum (NQF). Preferred practices and performance measures for measuring and reporting care coordination: a consensus report. Washington, DC: NQF; 2010.

72. NCQA. News release: NCQA seeks early adopters for connected care evaluation program, February 5, 2015. URL: http://www.ncqa.org/Newsroom/NewsArchive/2015NewsArchive/NewsReleaseFebruary52015.aspx. Last accessed 11 Feb 2015.

73. Patel V, Kaufman D, Cohen T, editors. Cognitive informatics in health and biomedicine case studies on critical care, complexity and errors. London: Springer-Verlag London Limited; 2014.

74. Poon EG, Keohane CA, Yoon CS. Effect of bar-code technology on the safety of medication administration. N Engl J Med. 2010;362:1698–707.

75. Powell V, Dim FM, Acharya A, Torres-Urquidy MH, editors. Integration of medical and dental care and patient data. London: Springer-Verlag London Limited; 2012.

76. Rich E, Lipson D, Libersky J, Parchman M. Coordinating care for adults with complex care needs in the patient-centered medical home: challenges and solutions. White Paper (Prepared by Mathematica PolicyResearch under Contract No. HHSA290200900019I/HHSA29032005T). AHRQ Publication No. 12-0010-EF. Rockville: Agency for Healthcare Research and Quality. 2012. p. 16–18.

77. Samal L, Hasan O, Venkatesh AK, et al. Health Information technology to support care coordination and care transitions: data needs, capabilities, technical and organizational barriers, and approaches to improvement. Boston: National Quality Forum; 2012.

78. Santana MJ, Haverman L, Absolom K, Takeuchi E, Feeny D, Grootenhuis M, Velikova G. Training clinicians in how to use patient-reported outcome measures in routine clinical practice. Qual Life Res. 2015;24(7):1707–18.

79. Sengstack P. System design supporting workflow vs nursing process: a paradigm shift? ANIA Newsl. 2012;27(3):5–6.

80. Shapiro M, Johnston D, Wald J, Mon D. Patient-generated health data: White Paper. Prepared for the Office of Policy and Planning, Office of the National Coordinator, Apr 2012.

81. Singer SJ, Burgers J, Friedberg M, Rosenthal MB, Leape L, Schneider E. Defining and measuring integrated patient care: promoting the next frontier in health care delivery. Med Care Res Rev. 2011;68:112–27.

82. Spooner SA, Council on Clinical Information Technology, American Academy of Pediatrics. Special requirements of electronic health record systems in pediatrics. Pediatrics. 2007;119(3):631–7.

83. Taylor EF, Lake T, Nysenbaum J, Peterson G, Meyers D. Coordinating care in the medical neighborhood: critical components and available mechanisms. White Paper (Prepared by

Mathematica Policy Research under Contract No. HHSA290200900019I TO2). AHRQ Publication No. 11-0064. Rockville: Agency for Healthcare Research and Quality; 2011.
84. Thomson L. Health care data breaches and information security: addressing threats and risks to patient data. In: Peabody A, editor. Health care IT: the essential lawyer's guide to health care information technology and the law. Chicago IL, American Bar Association; 2013. p. 253–67.
85. U.S. Department of Health and Human Services. Report to Congress: National strategy for quality improvement in health care; 2013. URL: http://www.ahrq.gov/workingforquality/nqs/nqs2013annlrpt.pdf. Last accessed 5 Jan 2015.
86. Van Doornik, W. Meaningful use of patient-generated data in EHRs. J AHIMA84. 2013;10:30–5. http://library.ahima.org/xpedio/groups/public/documents/ahima/bok1_050394.hcsp?dDocName=bok1_050394. Last accessed 11 Feb 2015.
87. Walker JM, Komar MJ. Special purpose software. In: Walker JM, Bieber EJ, Richards F, editors. Implementing an electronic health record system. London: Springer-Verlag London Limited; 2005. p. 134–40.
88. Wears RL. Health information technology and victory. Ann Emerg Med. 2015;65(2):143–5.
89. Weiner M, Callahan CM, Tierney WM, Overhage JM, Mamlin B, Dexter PR, McDonald CJ. Using information technology to improve the health care of older adults. Ann Intern Med. 2003;139(5 Pt 2):430–6.
90. Weintraub WS, Karlsberg RP, et al. ACCF/AHA 2011 key data elements and definitions of a base cardiovascular vocabulary for electronic health records: a report of the American College of Cardiology Foundation/American Heart Association Task Force on Clinical Data Standards. J Am Coll Cardiol. 2011;58(2):202–22.
91. WEO committee for standardization and terminology. Minimal Standard Terminology for Gastrointestinal Endoscopy MST 3.0. Organization Mondiale Endoscopia Digestive (OMED), 2008. URL: http://www.worldendo.org/mst.html. Last accessed 30 Sept 2013.
92. Zargaran E, Schuurman N, Nicol AJ, Matzopoulos R, Cinnamon J, Taulu T, Ricker B, Garbutt Brown DR, Navsaria P, Hameed SM. The electronic Trauma Health Record: design and usability of a novel tablet-based tool for trauma care and injury surveillance in low resource settings. J Am Coll Surg. 2014;218(1):41–50.
93. Zhang J, Walji M, editors. Better EHR: usability, workflow and cognitive support in electronic health records. Strategic Health IT Advanced Research Projects (SHARPC), The National Center for Cognitive Informatics and Decision Making in Healthcare (NCCD). 2014.
94. Shulman LN, Miller RS, Ambinder EP, Yu PP, Cox JV. Principles of Safe Practice Using an Oncology EHR System for Chemotherapy Ordering, Preparation, and Administration, Part 1 of 2. Journal of Oncology Practice. 2008;4(4):203–6.
95. Shulman LN, Miller RS, Ambinder EP, Yu PP, Cox JV. Principles of Safe Practice Using an Oncology EHR System for Chemotherapy Ordering, Preparation, and Administration, Part 2 of 2. Journal of Oncology Practice. 2008;4(5):254–7.
96. McCoy MJ, Diamond AM, Strunk AL, et al. Special requirements of electronic medical record systems in obstetrics and gynecology. Obstet Gynecol. 2010;116(1):140–3.
97. Ponemon Institute. Fifth Annual Benchmark Study on Privacy & Security of Healthcare Data. Sponsored by ID Experts. May 2015. https://www2.idexpertscorp.com/fifth-annual-ponemon-study-on-privacy-security-incidents-of-healthcare-data [Accessed 20 July 2015].
98. Stack SJ. CMS to make ICD-10 transition less disruptive for physicians. AMA Wire, 6 July 2015. http://www.ama-assn.org/ama/ama-wire/post/cms-icd-10-transition-less-disruptive-physicians [last accessed 20 July 2015].
99. National Center for Quality Assurance. Patient Centered Medical Home Criteria, 2014. http://www.ncqa.org/Programs/Recognition/RelevanttoAllRecognition/Recognition Training/PCMH2014Standards.aspx [Last accessed: April 2015].
100. Office of the National Coordinator. Standards and Interoperability Framework. Longitudinal Coordination of Care Interoperable Care Plan Exchange Use Case v2.0. 23 July 2013. http://wiki.siframework.org/file/view/LCC%20Care%20Plan%20Exchange%20Use%20Case%20Final.pdf/442230840/LCC%20Care%20Plan%20Exchange%20Use%20Case%20Final.pdf [last accessed 10 February 2015].

# Chapter 6
# Great Promises of Healthcare Information Technology Deliver Less

Ross Koppel

**Abstract** Healthcare Information Technology (HIT) continues to hold immense promise for reducing medical errors, collecting instant and vast data from across medical providers, increasing efficiency, improving clinician and patient satisfaction, sharing data, guiding clinicians with up-to-date findings, and facilitating teamwork within and across professions. Yet, almost everywhere clinicians find this technology frustrating and falling short of its promised benefits. In this chapter I examine the reasons for this chasm between promises and reality. In doing so, I review the many benefits of healthcare Information Technology (IT), the origins of electronic health records in both academic and commercial settings, government policies intended to spur the economy and encourage implementation of healthcare IT, the forces influencing those policies, vendor contracts, in addition to the role of the Office of the National Coordinator of Healthcare IT and of other offices in the Bush and Obama administrations. I also explore the barriers to establishing data standards, interoperability, full and transparent evaluations of EHRs and similar technologies, sharing of problematic EHR screen shots, and rapid remediation of healthcare IT-linked difficulties. Healthcare IT, despite its problems, provides many and essential benefits, and will continue to improve. To that end, I offer suggestions for bringing the promise and reality closer together.

**Keywords** Healthcare IT • EHRs • Usability • Healthcare policy • Regulation

## 6.1 Introduction

Healthcare IT was conceived in hope of reducing errors, increasing efficiency, improving clinician and patient satisfaction, sharing data, improving patient safety, guiding clinicians via evidenced-based medicine, and facilitating teamwork within and across professions [1, 3, 5, 8, 12, 24, 31, 39, 46, 53]. Yet, everywhere clinicians

R. Koppel, PhD, FACMI
Department of Sociology, and Center for Clinical Epidemiology and Biostatistics, and LDI
Wharton School, University of Pennsylvania, Philadelphia, PA, USA
e-mail: rkoppel@sas.upenn.edu

© Springer International Publishing Switzerland 2016     101
C.A. Weaver et al. (eds.), *Healthcare Information Management Systems:*
*Cases, Strategies, and Solutions*, Health Informatics,
DOI 10.1007/978-3-319-20765-0_6

often complain that HIT fails to provide these benefits and even creates barriers to achieving these benefits [1, 3, 5, 8, 12, 14, 15, 22, 24, 31, 39, 40, 46, 53]. How could HIT fall so short of its promises? In this chapter, we seek to explore the reasons for this disparity between hope and reality, and to offer suggestions for bringing the two closer together.

Healthcare IT (HIT) includes Electronic Health/Medical Records (EHR/EMR), Computerized Provider Order Entry (CPOE – usually a part of EHRs/EMRs) Barcoded Medication Administration (BCMA), Pharmacy IT, Computer Decision Support (CDS), radiographs and image transfer, and electronic prescribing (eRx), among other technologies. Collectively and individually HIT offers advantages that include:

- Freedom from unreadable and confusing handwriting
- Speed and instant access to and from the pharmacy, other record systems, labs, everywhere
- The ability to compare prescriptions that might interact in unwanted ways
- Reductions in duplicate orders, tests, and procedures
- Order formats that require specification of patient, route, dose, schedule/time, and formulation
- Facilitating continuity of care
- Ubiquity – immediate sharing of all information across the hallway and the nation
- Multiple and simultaneous access
- Ability to incorporate natural language processing, and
- Ability to mine the vast oceans of data generated by digital data, which could advance medical knowledge in ways that would otherwise take decades to accomplish.

Computerization was to provide all of these benefits – not only as improvements to the former paper-based systems that dominated medicine for a few hundred years,[1] but, more important, with the myriad functions and features only possible with computerization. This distinction between improvement and new developments is worth exploring. For example, one could improve paper-based medication ordering by structuring a computer template to "require" the physician to specify the medication's route, schedule, dose, et cetera. In contrast, a computer can list all of the available doses, formulations, routes, and ensure all relevant information is specified according to the patient's weight, age, pregnancy, comorbidities, drug allergies, and other medications (drug-drug interactions) before the order is submitted. Another comparison may be helpful: one could type a medication order rather than handwrite it, thus alleviating the handwriting problem, but even with many carbon copies, instant and ubiquitous transmission and access across the institution or the nation is not possible without computers, nor are the aforementioned checks for weight, age, pregnancy, etc.

---

[1] We note that paper-based systems were themselves essential and valuable efforts to improve the practice of medicine and the safety of patients.

## 6.2    Understanding the Gap Between Potential and Real

So how did this extraordinary technology generate the level and range of disappointments experienced by so many clinicians and healthcare IT scholars? [3, 5, 12, 14, 24, 25, 30, 31, 34, 36, 39, 47, 53]. To answer this question, we start with a very brief look at the genesis of these software systems, and important, at the recent governmental efforts to require their use. There are two interwoven roots.

### 6.2.1    Enterprise-Wide HIT: For Hospitals and Healthcare Systems

Most EHRs (a term we use to include EMRs) were either developed by clinician-informaticists or were substantially modified from billing systems to form the software that combines orders, notes, lab reports, etc. Some of the difficulties we now face are a result of software's origins in transaction-based foci and reporting systems for payments or for governmental needs.

Most early influential systems were:

- Octo Barnett's COSTAR (COMPUTER-STORED AMBULATORY RECORD) system, started 1971 – with the Harvard Community Health Plan
- Stead and Hammond's TMR (The Medical Record) at Duke, started as GEMISCH (Generalized MIS for Community Health) started in 1969
- Clem McDonald's RMR (Regenstrief Medical Record) at Regenstrief Institute of Health Care and the Indiana University's School of Medicine, from 1973
- Homer Warner's HELP system at LDS in Salt Lake City Utah, earlier the Kaiser Permanante (KP) system developed by Morrie Collen and started in 1963 with IBM 1440s
- Shepard and Levy Simborg and Blum's Johns Hopkins Hospital (JHH) system
- Also there were many single-specialty as well as general-screening systems developed as in the 1950s, such as Don Lindberg installing IBM terminals for capturing nursing data at the University of Missouri (~1954) (C. Kulikowski, personal communication. February 26, 2015) [7].

Very few systems were built de novo by commercial firms. An example of one of these "exceptions" is the early commercial system by Technicon, called TDS, introduced at El Camino Hospital in Mountain View, CA in the mid-1970s. Indeed, most of the pioneering enterprise-wide systems have been bought or absorbed by commercial vendors who sell them to hospitals for considerable sums, ranging from several million dollars to several hundred million dollars. Those amounts do not include the cost of implementation, linkages to other systems, consultants, customization, building order sets or computer decision support rules, and the hundreds of other steps needed to make the systems function within a hospital or healthcare system. Implementation, in fact, costs three-to-five times the price of the software.

Thus, an EHR vendor selling a system to a very large hospital complex – for example a system for a complex of four hospitals plus clinics, labs, pharmacy IT, et cetera – might charge $350 million for the software, and then the hospital complex will spend $1.3 billion in implementation costs, for a total bill of almost $1.7 billion just to implement. Ongoing software maintenance fees, hardware, networks, staff resources and training all add to the total cost of ownership and these EHR costs runs into the multimillions of dollars annually.

There are only a few remaining, homebuilt pioneer systems at major academic centers (e.g., Beth Israel -Deaconess, Vanderbilt), but almost all healthcare institutions have implemented or are implementing commercial systems that were probably created years ago at major academic medical centers or from billing software. The days of homebuilt enterprise-wide systems, so essential to the development of medical informatics, have largely disappeared.

### 6.2.2  Small Practice EHRs

There is a common joke that every doctor who had a brother-in-law with a garage and with knowledge of *vis-i-calc* (an early spreadsheet software program) built an EHR. There are in fact over 6,000 certified EHRs or EHR modules listed with the federal government's Office of the National Coordinator of Healthcare IT and with the Centers for Medicare and Medicaid (CMS). However, very few of these are actually in use by more than one physician or practice.

No matter how the HIT systems came to be, a key concern is: do they do what we need them to do? Do they improve care and all of the other benefits they promise? How much to they succeed in that effort? And if not as successful as anticipated, why not?

As we shall illustrate, the HIT systems, although dramatically superior to paper in so many ways, are not what clinicians hoped they would be, nor what they certainly could be. Below we explore the reasons for these difficulties, from creation of vendor-friendly policies, to reluctance to agree on data standards, to refusal to allow public review of usability, to use of inadequate workarounds on interchange of data, to pricing, to lack of transparency on screenshots involving patient safety dangers, to the myriad of other factors.

## 6.3  Policy Creation and Capture

The horror of medical error is so great, the complexities of care so daunting, the need to train clinicians in new rotations so constant, and the vulnerabilities of aging and sick patients so challenging, that we have sought solutions in computational technology. What other mechanisms can help move, sort, track, analyze and compare the quantities of data? None! It is that need and hope that inspired the founders of HIT, and that then empowered the sellers of that technology to request and receive: (1) A regulatory-free environment from the FDA, leaving only the CMS/ONC leaders who were aggressively promoting HIT as an essential panacea for healthcare's ill; and (2) Subsidies, mandates and encouragements that quickly became a crusade flying with the banners of efficiency, patient safety, cost reductions, speed, improved measurement, up-to-date guidance, and provider control. That these magnificent goals were either unproven or profoundly contested never impeded the ardor of HIT's supporters, nor the dollars in subsidies, nor the demands that healthcare providers and hospitals purchase these systems. We developed policies based on faith in the technology absent empirical evidence of the policies' wisdom or efficacy.

One consequential event in the formation of policy – and an example of the assumptions and uncurious faith that distorted perceptions and research – was the seminal article by Jha et al. [21] that found United States' hospitals required subsidies for HIT purchases, incentives to continue HIT use, certification of HIT systems, better IT departments, and fewer technophobic physicians. A review of the survey instrument on which that New England Journal of Medicine paper was written, however, reveals the authors asked no questions about usability, data standards, interoperability, unfriendly user interfaces, clunky software, irrational choices in menus, lost laboratory results, and non-responsive vendors. The only options the hospital respondents were offered were about the needs for subsidies, incentives, certifications, better IT departments, and fewer technophobic physicians. While not intentionally biased, it nevertheless assumed HIT is beneficial, and that any impediments must be found among users and their institutions. Interestingly, the senior ("anchor") author of that paper was David Blumenthal, who would soon become the head of the agency, Office of the National Coordinator of Healthcare IT (hereafter, ONC) that created the regulations and oversaw the HIT industry. The ONC implemented the policies that were supported by the findings of Jha et al.'s [21] research.

In 2008, it's also true that one of the major goals of the Obama administration at that time was to thwart the rampant recession inherited from the previous administration by infusing America with money for the purchase of HIT. Helping implementation of HIT was perceived as a double win: (1) helping to save the economy, and (2) saving lives and healthcare dollars with the miracle of computerization and digitization of healthcare information. It is also true that the $24–34 billion in stimulus and incentive spending – and, far more important, the trillions of dollars required of hospitals and clinicians to buy and install the systems – was beneficial to the economy. But another side of that equation is unresolved and even more essential: would it have been better to require data standards, interoperability and usability standards as part of the incentive and subsidy package? Was there a way of supporting purchase of HIT systems while also encouraging interoperable and useful HIT? And could this be done in a way that would neither stifle innovation nor require usability metrics not responsive to the needs of clinicians or to other stakeholders? I argue that it would have been possible to achieve far more than we realized from the existing policies. How?

1. *Data Standards* – the format one uses to record the collected medical information: There were several available ontologies and data standards for defining almost all of the measures used in medicine in 2009. We could have chosen one and insisted that any system that could receive incentives and subsidies had to use that data standard. Without data standards, interoperability becomes almost impossible. Of course, there could have been a flexibility built into that process. For example, any system could be installed in 2009–2010 but that system had to incorporate the unified data standards within a year.

   Perhaps worse, without unified data standards we cannot share information across systems; we fail to achieve real interoperability. The systems create towers of Babel and those towers become isolated from each other; a noisy but deaf city.

2. *Interoperability:* sending information from one system to another – has been mastered in electronics and almost every other industry for over 40 years, often for several hundred. The major barrier in HIT was the aforementioned lack of a unified standard and the refusal of vendors to select a method of data transmission. Again, selecting any of the available methods in 2009 would have enabled the transmission and collection of medical information – a core, but still missing, virtue of HIT. Several arguments are offered for the industry's inability or refusal to create its own interoperability protocols or for its lack of agreement on existing interoperability protocols:

   - Vendors benefit from sales of entire suites of products, e.g., the linked software programs of CPOE, pharmacy IT, the electronic medication administration recording systems (eMARs), etc. By not allowing a vendor's software and/or hardware to interact with other vendors' systems, a vendor ensures sales of a combined package.
   - A related argument: by selling one system, say, the CPOE, to a hospital, vendors can be assured that additional purchases will be in their same product lines.
   - Because these systems are so expensive, because implementing them is three to five times more than just the initial software and hardware costs, and because the implementation process takes 3–5 years, opportunities for buyer remorse is limited or made unacceptable. The buyer is locked in; often wed to that system for a decade. The vendors thus seek to capture market share as soon as possible, and are encouraged to rush HIT products to market before they are sufficiently tested. Aggressive marketing and subsidies also obscured or prevent objective discussion of HIT's merits and challenges. The vast funds involved, and the consequential career implications of those participating in HIT purchases enhance intimidation of critics and those who report problems with the technology [36]. The general faith in technology and the sincere desire to see HIT improve medical workflow encourages so many to define critics as technophobes, incompetents, and non-team players.

- Data loss threats: lack of interoperability makes switching HIT systems peril-ous, with dangers of massive data loss, which would be a catastrophic failure for healthcare institutions. A variant of this is when a current vendor offers to sell you your own data in non-machine readable formats, i.e., as millions of PDF pages. (This is a true case.) They thus add injury to insult by demanding the hospital or practice pay for this printing function when it could obviously be sent via a digital medium, and therefore more usable in the next HIT system.

  As with data standards, the ONC could have offered flexibility in the tim-ing of an interoperability requirement. Thus, for example, any system would be acceptable to purchase in 2009–2010, but all systems would have to be able to use an agreed-upon exchange protocol within a year of installation.

3. *Usability*: defined as ease of use, ability to learn, effectiveness, efficiency, error tolerant, engaging, and responsive [35]. As we discuss below, usability is mea-surable and the rules for better vs. worse usability are well known [23, 29, 35]. In fact, the National Institute of Standards and Technology (NIST) was appointed by the enabling law in 2008–2009 to conduct usability testing, but was circum-vented, or rendered toothless by the then ONC leadership and others who were primarily focused on encouraging implementation of EHRs. This circumvention (discussed below) was extended to allow bypassing the ONC-funded University of Texas at Houston's usability program, even after it was anointed as a major program for the HIT industry. Submission of HIT software to UT Houston's evaluation labs was not mandated and UT Houston's offer of assistance for usability measurement and improvement was not integrated into any of the ONC's or CMS' core requirements.

*Regulatory Creation and Capture with Enforced Markets:* One reason for the continuing disappointing performance of HIT systems is found in what economists call "regulatory capture" – where the enterprises (businesses) that are theoretically regulated by an agency gain control of the regulatory agency or processes. Sometimes this is called "the foxes guarding the henhouse". Although with HIT, it might better be called, the foxes are architects of the hen house.

## 6.4    Certification and Testing Processes

Vendors secured the best of both worlds for themselves. Healthcare providers and hospitals were required to buy the HIT systems to receive subsidies and incentives (worth billions), and would be penalized in reduced payments for Medicare and Medicaid services if they failed to use the HIT systems. This created a captured market where vendors competed to scoop up market share and were often protected from competitive pressures to make the software responsive to healthcare providers' needs once the sale was made. In addition, "certification," a process whereby EHRs or their components were "certified" to complete specific functions, was designed in such a way that all vendors found a process that almost always resulted in approval. For example, although the reality of medical care is that providers have little time to order a medication or a lab test, the certification process is conducted without time constraints. Thus, to continue this not so hypothetical example, a certification "test," that might involve modifying a medication order schedule, which should ordinarily take a few seconds, would nevertheless pass even if it took several hours and required the assistance of a team of the vendor's engineers.

Perhaps more disconcerting is the in vitro unrealities of these tests. That is, they are conducted apart from the organization in which these programs will operate. And the context, as the vendors are quick to remind all when discussing usability, can be all important in determining how a program will function. Nevertheless the tests are in isolated test beds with none of the usual interferences or contextual realities in which they must eventually work.

## 6.5   Scaling Back the Functionality

Vendors were instrumental in creating the legislation and regulations under which they were supposed to operate. Consider the following: The requirements that HIT vendors' software had to meet were consistently scaled back from the time that functional requirements were first suggested to their eventual publication with full regulatory authority. Often the vendors would insist that they were iteratively seeking to minimize their software's regulatory requirements (called "Meaningful Use," or "MU") on behalf of their clients, claiming that the providers did not have the skills or capability to meet the requirement. But in almost all cases, the underlying reason was that the software was insufficiently robust or so poorly designed or inflexible such that meeting the requirements was impossible [43].

For example, time lines for meeting criteria were repeatedly pushed back or eliminated from the upcoming deadline. Lists of requirements were cut from 20 to 16, and then made "flexible" via revisions that required only meeting, a modest portion of the several original requirements.

Three examples illustrate this constant retreat from functionality: Although subject to CMS audits, providers are not required to show proof of their use of the HIT, but rather to only "attest" to the fact that their software could perform those functions and that they were using those functions for a given percent of the actions, e.g., they "attested" that their software could send out digital prescriptions (eRx) and that they were sending at least 50 % of their prescriptions via eRx [6].

The use of attestation rather than submission of direct proof that the stated function was used in X percent of cases was necessitated by the difficulties of sending even the digital information to the government – in itself an indication of the problems with the software. As noted CMS has the right to back up the attestation process with audits. Moreover, the government has found cases where vendors' software accidently exaggerated the functionality or exaggerated the number of patients for whom the functionality was claimed; [6, 41, 43, 52] or where providers were inaccurately – for reasons other than software errors – claiming cases where they had not in fact met those requirements [41]. Another issue of required function-alities' reductions is seen in this example about negotiations over what an EHR must do. Specifically, this situation emerged over whether or not the ONC should require EHR software to allow a user (e.g., an MD or nurse) to search a patient's *entire* record for some needed information, or should just require the software to only search the one screen currently displayed to the user? One would assume that a clinician would want to be able to search the entire record, not just the one screen in front of him or her. However, in this instance, the legacy software employed by the EHR vendor apparently made the more complete search function problematic.

Rather than improve or conform the software to make such (full) searches pos-sible, the vendor sent a note to all its clients that asked them to request only limited searches. That is, the vendor asked the clients to demand regulations that would hobble their own abilities and EHR systems rather than fix the systems to allow a full search. How do we know this? Because several providers sent in the vendor-suggested text to the government but failed to remove the vendor's stage directions (as in, "remove these instructions and insert your name here.") Thus, because these documents were filed with the government, we could see them in the public record. The relevant section read:

> *"Informational Comments for Organizations Using Epic (remove before submitting to ONC)"* [emphasis added] "…your requests for a chart search feature, and our desire to see this certification criterion removed does not mean we don't want to develop such a feature. In a future version of Epic… However, if this criterion stays in the Final Rule, we worry we'll have to divert attention from future chart search features you've requested to focus on a simplified, less valuable version of the feature to meet certification". [19]

## 6.6   FDA Exemption for EHR Vendors

Our last example of regulatory non-oversight is observed in the recent requests of the Federal committee that oversees policies about HIT. Some historic context is needed: In 1997, the HIT industry, via its trade association, Healthcare Information and Management Systems Society (HIMSS), plus several other organizations including the American Nursing Association and the American Medical Informatics Association (AMIA) – but not the American Medical Association – met with the FDA to request that the HIT industry be made effectively exempt from FDA over-sight. The industry and its partners argued that FDA oversight might retard innova-tion by the vendors. Vendors were therefore not required to submit their products for examination a priori or for post-market analysis, and no clinical trials were needed either before use or during use. Vendors could report known errors to the FDA's list-ing of medical device problems, the "Manufacturers and Users Facility Device Experience" (MAUDE) data base, but no testing or other requirements were demanded. In contrast, for example, pre- and post-market analysis is required for even an electronic stethoscope – which is a stethoscope that amplifies the sound, a trivial technology compared to the millions of lines of computer code in an EHR or the EHR's myriad connections to other IT systems.

Then, recently, at the end of 2014, the industry and its allies on the Health IT Policy Committee and Health IT Standards Committee of the ONC asked for further reduction of oversight from the FDA, again urging greater "flexibility" and, critically here, a view that HIT is "low risk." To me, what is surprising about this request is that the industry feels it necessary to ensure continued non-regulation because it has achieved an effective regulation-free environment since 1997. As one wag asked: "What's less regulation than zero?"

### 6.6.1  Hold Harmless and Non-disclosure Clauses in Vendor EHR/CPOE Contracts

In 2009, Koppel and Kreda [28] published an article in JAMA about two clauses found in vendor HIT contracts. One clause prohibited clinicians from publicly displaying screen shots of EHRs or CPOEs even if they felt those screen shots illustrate a danger to patient safety, e.g., illustrated how a medication listing was confusing or wrong, or how a drop-down menu continued beyond (below) the screen but that the fact that the menu continued below was not evident (thus leading clinicians to make an inappropriate choice) or that a drug name was truncated and misleading. This offered vendor protection against display of vendor screen images even if they involve patient safety. A part of that clause also prohibited clinicians from speaking pejoratively about the vendor's product. The second clause, "hold harmless," said that the vendor was not responsible for any errors committed because of their products even if the vendor had been repeatedly informed that the product was defective in some way. For example, if the software displayed a wrong weight for a child patient because of some software glitch, the vendor was not responsible – the vendor was "held harmless." The legal logic of the clause is that the vendor merely creates a "tool" used by a learned intermediary – a physician, nurse, pharmacist, physical therapist – who has both immediate bedside knowledge of the patient and has esoteric medical knowledge. Therefore that learned intermediary has the authority to take whatever information is shown and make a considered professional judgment, including realizing that the information shown to him or her via the software is incorrect. To be clear, the medical professional/user can inform the vendor of the error, and can inform the vendor and fellow users via its customer chat rooms or Listservs. The professional can also show the possibly faulty screen shot to his/her fellow professionals standing next to her. But if she/he were to send that screen shot to a publicly available website, say, for example, a blog, then both that professional and his/her hospital or practice would be liable for massive monetary compensation to the vendor.

Since the publication of JAMA 2009 article, the IOM, the JASON report sponsored by the government, and the ethics committee of AMIA have called for removal of those clauses [2, 13]. In contrast, the ONC, CMS, and HIMSS have never demanded that those clauses be removed. In fact, some key staff members of the ONC and HIMSS insist that the clauses do not exist even though HIMSS' EHRA (EHR Association…a HIMSS subgroup comprised of the largest manufacturers of EHRs) say they exist but are only found in a few vendors' contracts. (Note: there is good reason to believe that those "few" vendors represent a large proportion of all EHRs sold.) No vendor has published their contracts to allow public review of their documents by attorneys. We also note that vendors receive many thousands of reports about their software and have mechanisms for classifying those reports into various categories. Generally reports involving patient safety are addressed with all possible dispatch; and nothing here should be interpreted to suggest that vendors are inattentive to patient safety issues. That's not the issue here. Rather, we are discussing the vendors focus on their liability for any problems their software may cause. The non-disclosure clause, while separate from the hold harmless clause, perpetuates healthcare professionals' inability to learn about possibly faulty software and to engage in speedy accommodations to their workflow processes, software customizations, or other steps that could facilitate patient safety and clinician security. The non-disclosure language in vendor contracts works against the full exposure of potentially harmful software.

## 6.6.2 The Office of the National Coordinator

I argue that the ONC, from its very beginning, has viewed its primary role as encouraging the purchase and use of HIT. It routinely publishes data cheering the number of EHRs sold and focuses on extolling the virtues of HIT via its publications, programs, funding, and reports. It actively solicits stories of successful implementations even though there are data to suggest that up to 70 % of software implementations are failures [50]. Indeed, the ONC often funds HIT-enthusiasts but has been far less generous to those who are less-than-enthusiastic about the software – as if we only learn from our successes and not from our difficulties. In its several publications that discuss HIT-related errors, it often focuses on technophobic clinicians or on problematic implementations [27]. Even when it supports work on patient safety and HIT, it has worked to avoid regulation and to concentrate on the almost infinitesimal proportion of errors that are more accessible and reported [42, 48]. This approach contrasts to the majority of HIT-related errors that pertain to medication ordering errors, which are extraordinarily difficult to determine because patients are often old, sick (sic), suffering from 3 to 5 comorbidities, and are on another 10 to 13 other medications. In addition, the patients' homeostatic systems are trying to keep them alive or are failing at that task. Good things happen to patients when we do many things incorrectly and bad things happen to patients when we do everything correctly. Last here, we note that if physicians or others realize they've ordered the wrong drug, they quickly act to stop that order [32]. It is by definition only the unknown errors that are most at risk of causing patient harm.

The ONC commissioned the JASON group to study HIT and patient safety. JASON issued a report based on the 2013 meetings [16]. In 2014, the ONC's Health IT Policy Committee and Health IT Standards Committee published its recommendations based on the 2014 JASON report. The ONC's committee rejected those JASON recommendations that directed the ONC to focus their MU efforts primarily on interoperability. The ONC's committee also did not address the JASON recommendation to demand removal of the two clauses – hold harmless and non-disclosure – discussed above. (Full disclosure: JASON was again commissioned in 2014 by the ONC, AHRQ and The Robert Wood Johnson Foundation to issue another report. I was among the academics who briefed the JASON group on the topic.)

## 6.7 Usability as a Contentious Reality in EHR Development

For many years, vendors insisted usability was a subjective and unmeasurable concept. Vendors accepted some of the usability literature, such as agreeing that usability is dependent on:

1. The training and skill of the user
2. The implementation of specific systems in specific settings
3. The history of HIT use in any setting and by any user
4. The relationship of a specific system to the other IT systems with which it must interact
5. The physical environment (e.g., lighting, noise levels, quality of display screens).

One might add that vendors would probably accept other usability factors, such as: the frequency and degree of changes made by the host organization and by the vendor; and, the degree of data interoperability with IT systems that are both exogenous to the host organization and to the IT systems within the host organization.

All of these factors absolutely influence usability, often profoundly. But none of them should be allowed to obscure the reality that usability is intimately dependent on the *design* of the system. Moreover, none of these factors means that usability is not measurable. Indeed, there are well-documented scientific methods for measuring usability, including measures that incorporate and acknowledge the other factors that affect use [17]. As a thought experiment consider automobile safety. No one would deny that a car's performance and braking ability are influenced by road conditions, the driver's skill, and the driver's alertness. Yet it would be absurd to insist that basic automobile design decisions do not seriously affect a car's stability, safety and braking effectiveness. In contrast to the automobile analogy, HIT vendors have, until recently, defended their lack of focused attention on usability by reiterating the mantra that usability is subjective, too theoretical, or essentially unmeasurable. Some vendors have claimed that there is only scant proof of the relationship between usability and safety. At the same time, and apparently without irony, several vendors also note they have employed usability experts and that their own tests find their systems to be very usable.

The issues here are several fold: you can't add usability to a poorly designed EHR or CPOE system; usability must be baked in from the beginning; testing usability (and iteratively improving usability) is an expensive, extensive, and ongoing process. One can't test an EHR in one environment with a limited set of clinicians, and then call it finished. True tests would involve several environments plus scores, or even hundreds, of clinicians of the variety that must use the system. Moreover, and more important, improvements and testing of usability are never "done" [23, 35]. The systems must interact with other IT systems that are constantly changing as well as new environments, e.g., patients with differing diseases, new clinicians with different training, new equipment, and new requirements.

The EHR vendor association, (EHRA), a subsection of HIMSS discussed above, and HIMSS itself, admits that usability is the primary challenge and the major barrier to wider acceptance of EHR systems [9]. The frequent complaints by clinicians about clunky, slow, unfriendly systems has become undeniable. And blaming physicians as hopeless technophobes is no longer a fully viable strategy. All vendors now pay homage to the importance of usability, but few appear to be willing to address the steps needed to consider redesigns based on usability essentials [9].

For one example, consider evaluations of EHR usability. When the current legislation subsidizing and incentivizing the purchase of EHRs was formulated (HITECH), the law appointed the National Institute of Standards and Technology (NIST) as the agency that would test EHRs usability. Vendors were to submit their systems to NIST. However, by the time the regulations were enacted: (1) vendors were allowed the option of submitting their systems or not submitting their systems for evaluation, and (2) vendors are not required to inform the public whether or not they did so. Also, (3) NIST is prohibited from telling the public if or if not a vendor has submitted their system for usability evaluation, and (4) NIST is not allowed to show their evaluations to other vendors, but can only show the evaluation to the vendor who submitted its system. In other words, neither vendors nor, more important, clinicians have the ability to compare usability across systems – and can't even see the usability testing results of any system nor can they even know if a system was evaluated.

## 6.8   Is HIT's Development or Use Based on Evidence?

In this section we explore an intriguing question, but one usually avoided, ignored, or assumed. We ask: Is healthcare information technology (HIT) evidence-based? To what extent is HIT designed, built/or implemented on a foundation of evidence derived from systematic evaluation of what works and what fails to work, or of where HIT may be more or less effective, or of the necessary conditions for HIT to work at all [27]?

*Structure:* The section has three parts: First, we ask what types of evidence would be needed for HIT to be "evidence-based." Second, we briefly note the absence of evidence and provide a list of reasons and rationales frequently offered for or assumed when purchasing and implementing systems. We also note that a general *absence of hard evidence* of efficacy does not mean HIT is without support. There are many studies by advocates and others attesting to its value; and some devotes insist HIT's benefits are self-evident. One major problem is that HIT's effectiveness is wickedly hard to measure. Indeed, the third section enumerates the many difficulties in trying to measure HIT's impact and costs.

### 6.8.1  Is HIT Evidence-Based? To Answer the Question We Must Unpack It: Evidence of What?

- Is the *design* or *construction* of HIT based on evidence of what is most efficient and effective in practice?

    - Is navigation within and among software screens evaluated and modified to be the least burdensome and most intuitive? Are clicking and scrolling reduced to the minimum? Do clinicians know "where they are" and how to get to where they are going, or at least, how to get back?
    - Is usability of the systems – as measured via human factors research – tested and progressively improved?
    - Are displays of information in graphic and textual form carefully assessed? Are they tested on a wide range of users in many real-life settings?
    - Are observations of clinicians' use of HIT systematically analyzed as to how information can be amassed and analyzed with minimum distractions and minimum unnecessary cognitive burdens?

- Are differing systems evaluated when *implemented* in situ across similar settings? Or are implementations of the same system evaluated in dozens or hundreds of various medical settings, also, by definition, in situ? If such comparisons are available, are they routinely provided to potential purchasers?

    - Are we assessing various methods of implementation, incorporating facility design, number of clinicians, number of intersecting offices, expertise of the IT team, etc.?
    - At what point is an implementation fairly evaluated? Six months after the "go live" date? A year after the "go live" date? After the third upgrade? After each patch or version is installed?
    - In light of HIT vendors' reasonable statements that each implementation is an essential element of that system's safety and effectiveness, is it sensible to evaluate HIT systems independent of their implementations? And given that concern, is "certification" of an "isolated" HIT system a futile exercise?

- Are evaluations based on Randomized Controlled Trials (RCT) or double blind RCTs? Is RCT possible with "evidence" from HIT use?

- Are clinical decision support (CDS), order sets, disease protocols, or dosage alerts built on the latest medical knowledge? Is CDS examined to ensure it achieves:

  - Reduced alert fatigue by careful titration of alerts to only the most essential?
  - Presentation of alerts in ways that align with clinical workflow and thought-flow?
  - Presentation of information in alerts that is relevant to the user at the point-of-care and the time of decision?
  - Easy access to additional information on how the alerts are determined?

- Are there evaluations of the connections among the many IT systems that are linked to the CPOE or EHR systems? Not only is each connection a vulnerability to the overall system, but because many of the other IT systems interact with each other separately from the EHR, there are factorial interactions and vulnerabilities. The core HIT systems are embedded in a network of other systems, each of which potentially affects many other elements of the network. Is the network evaluated synergistically? Is there evidence of one of HIT's most basic promises: Interoperability, or proof that HIT is capable of interoperability – sharing information in usable formats with interpretable data? Do HIT systems permit sharing data across a region, across town, across the hallway, or across the room?

- Is there a reliable calculation of the return-on-investment (ROI) in HIT? Are there savings in time, in staff, in avoided errors, and in fewer repeated tests and laboratory orders? Is the ROI the basis of the decision to use HIT or is it a *post hoc* justification? Implicit in this question is that one knows the cost of HIT and its implementation. As we shall see, this is a wickedly difficult figure to determine.

- Is there evidence of improved patient safety from HIT? Improving patient safety is one of the central claims of HIT; are there consistent and systematic data to support this claim?

- In the evaluations, are there statistical controls for:

  - Training of clinicians – a critical issue, because of the role of teaching hospitals, "voluntary" attendings, clinicians who practice in different hospitals or offices with differing EHRs and CPOE systems?
  - Patient loads and acuity?
  - History of technology use in each institution and by each clinician user?

## 6.8.2  Alas, Usually Missing

Answers to all of these questions are usually missing. Why they are missing is discussed below. But understand, *"missing" or" not provided" data does not mean that HIT programs and implementations are without value or that purchase decisions are uninformed or wrong.* "Missing" also does not mean that compelling evidence is not forthcoming. What "missing" means, rather, is that much of HIT's development, selection, and implementations are based on:

- Legacies of earlier systems
- What others tell us may have worked elsewhere
- What we think makes sense
- What we can afford
- What vendors recommend
- What many – usually differing clinicians and leaders within our institutions – have compromised upon
- What customers have told vendors
- What we've read
- Subsidies and incentives by governments
- Regulations
- Decisions of larger institutions with which we are affiliated
- How much time and energy we have to customize the systems
- The legal and technical limits of customization
- Other IT systems with which we must currently connect, and
- On our best judgments as problems emerge.

Many of the decisions involving development, selection, and implementation are made with great thought and consideration, with earnest debate, with careful reading of the available literature, and with the advice of consultants. But few are evidenced-based in the way we conceptualize serious evaluation or the scientific method.

*Also, the lack of evidence in building or implementing HIT does not mean these systems are ineffective.* Although there is little *systematic* research, many HIT systems appear to work for several functions: As pointed out above, EHRs can enable physicians and patients to maintain a complete, and omnipresent medical record. CPOE systems allow physicians and other health care professionals to enter medication orders directly into a computer system, avoiding handwriting or transcription errors, and speeding orders to pharmacies and laboratories. CDS provides information to physicians or nurses when they order or administer medications, for example, warning that the proposed dose exceeds the normal range or that the patient is listed as being allergic to a proposed drug. These systems help physicians and nurses to order and administer medications in a timely fashion. Many of these technologies, also, may reduce redundant tests and procedures.

So, lack of scientific evidence [8, 12, 24, 31, 39, 46, 53] and the mountain of conflicting evidence [1, 3, 5, 14, 15, 21–25, 35, 47] for the many HIT features and elements noted above do not negate HIT's benefits to patients and healthcare providers. Humans built bridges before trigonometry and calculus. We covered wounds before the germ theory of disease. Moreover, just as much of all-but-modern medical practices were based on theories we now hold as absurd (e.g., humors, blood surfeit, and demonic possession) and were "supported" by dubious evidence of efficacy, physicians nonetheless often achieved successful outcomes. We shall continue to invest trillions in HIT systems because they are usually better than paper, because we so dread medical errors, and because the complexity of medical care is so daunting.

## 6.9   Why Do We Not Yet Have Evidenced-Based HIT?

There are many reasons we lack consistent and valid evidence of HIT's efficacy. Measurement of HIT's efficacy is hard; its measurement in situ is even harder. Consider the messy reality of medical practice. In general, the real world applicability of evidence-based medicine (EBM) is frequently overstated. Our research model is the clinical trial, where studies are conducted with carefully selected samples of patients to observe the effects of the medicine or treatment without additional interference from other conditions. Unfortunately, the clinical trial model differs from actual medical practice because hospitals and doctors' waiting rooms are full of elderly patients suffering from several co-morbidities and taking about a dozen or more medications, (some unknown to us). It is often a great leap to apply findings from a study under "ideal conditions" to the fragile patient. So physicians must then balance the "scientific findings" with the several vulnerabilities of real patients. Clinicians are obliged to constantly deal with these messy tradeoffs, and the utility of evidence-based findings is mitigated by the complex challenges of the sick patients, multiple medications taken, and massive unknowns. This mix of research with the messy reality of medical and hospital practice means that evidence, even if available, is often not fully applicable. *When applied to HIT*, very similar factors come into play. No two hospitals or practices are the same; every CPOE system must be installed into an existing network of other IT systems, workflows, clinician experience, etc.

### 6.9.1   Evidence for HIT's Effects

Added to these limitations of EBM just discussed, are additional challenges of measuring HIT's *impact* independent of the many other factors that co-vary with it. The number and complexity of variables involved in medical settings and in medical care are staggering and each HIT implementation is unique. (As the saying goes, "you've seen one EHR implementation, you've seen one EHR implantation.") HIT training among interns, senior physicians, nurses, and the myriad of other clinicians varies dramatically. There are constant flows of professionals and students. Medical practice is also a teaching practicum. The number and criticality of interactions with other systems (within an institution and across the globe) is usually unknown and often far more nuanced than anyone suspects de novo. A list of factors that affect HIT's influence in any institution, while not infinite, is beyond most users' comprehension [15, 22, 25, 36, 47].

Moreover, this list does not begin to include the promised outcome measures (e.g., reduced errors, efficient billing, ward acuity measures, nursing personnel needs, cost and time savings, inventory control), which are certainly as complex and varied as the context, patient types, and users.

## 6.9.2  Randomized Controlled Trials

The gold standard of research is the randomized controlled trials method (RCT). Even better is the double-blind study, where neither subjects nor researchers know which is the test intervention and which is the placebo or standard intervention. Such research designs are impossible to imagine for HIT. Double-blind, or even single-blind research designs would require all of the participants' active involvement in not examining the type of system they would be obliged to use for a year or two. Also, can anyone believe that a large hospital system and its clinicians can spend 300 million dollars and 4 years (plus a billion dollars) implementing an EHR about which the clinicians are not fully informed? Then one also must assume the implementation is followed by a few years of evaluation of the EHR-in-use while also keeping everyone in the dark? More basic, for the reasons enumerated in the two paragraphs directly above (on obtaining similar settings, linkages, staff, IT, etc), the research design requirements for RCT are extremely difficult to enact in the real world.

In what amounts to "an act of faith", we have assumed that *more* HIT generates *better* and safer healthcare. This assumption has been assisted by massive efforts by vendors, vendor trade associations, lobbyists, legislators, policy experts, business groups, governmental agencies charged with encouraging HIT use, insurance carriers hoping HIT will reduce costs, academics, and many healthcare providers [4, 9, 11, 18, 20, 22, 25, 30, 34, 36, 47]. The lobbying and marketing budget of vendors is many millions of dollars. As with any faith, expressing doubts about HIT's benefits is viewed as heretical [37] and possibly career limiting.

## 6.9.3  Evidence for CDS

While few doubt the eventual value of CDS, most CDS alerts are generally ignored or overridden because they are viewed as useless or just annoying. Override rates are as high as 97 % [26, 44, 45] – a reality that makes the evaluation of CDS inherently problematic. Does one count only actions based on the small percent of alerts that generate change, and ignore the vast bulk of alerts that generate only annoyance or rage? And even then, does one count only those actions that are associated with beneficial change, and discount those CDS-inspired actions that result in new or additional errors (a non-trivial occurrence). Any evaluation, moreover, should reflect the distractions, interruptions in work flow, cognitive burden, and errors associated with the many overridden/ignored alerts and recommendations. CDS alerts are in fact, the most hated feature of HIT. Measuring their efficacy is therefore challenging and efforts at systematic assessments are disappointing. In one major study, Metzger and colleagues [38] found that CDS detected only 53 % of all medication orders that would have resulted in fatalities and caught from 10 to 82 % of orders that would have caused serious adverse events. Drugs prescribed for a wrong diagnosis were caught only 15 % of the time (that is, in ideal cases in which the computer already had the patient's record and could "know" that the drug was inappropriate), and drugs that were wrong for a patient of a given age were intercepted only 14.1 % of the time. Nevertheless, CDS remains on everyone's list as a central, critical feature of HIT benefits.

## 6.9.4   Data Standards

We discussed data standards above. Here with note only that another problem with lack of unified data standards and data formats limits or prevents creation of evidence of HIT's efficacy across differing facilities and HIT systems. Proprietary interests, legacy systems, and existing capital investments make agreement on standards difficult. But without unified data standards and data formats, we create a tower of Babel within each medical facility, and we severely attenuate the utility of HIT.

## 6.9.5   Customization

Customization is a double-edged sword. On the one hand, each institution and each clinician is promised with (and flattered by) the ability to make significant modifications to the system(s). And indeed there are excellent reasons why customization is needed. On the other hand, customization is used as a marketing ploy, and creates massive problems. It makes upgrades and patches far more difficult than they need be, it attenuates systematic collection of evidence of HIT's efficacy, and it endangers patients and healthcare when clinicians must practice across differing HIT systems, each with different ways of viewing data, ordering medications, arranging problem lists, etc. Customization is thus often a perverse benefit: a workaround for integration of IT systems that should be but are not designed for interaction; perpetuating a laissez faire digital environment of autonomous silos when interoperability is the absolute requirement for better care and patient safety.

## 6.9.6   Return on Investment

To calculate return on investment (ROI), one needs to know the cost of the investment and the economic value of the "return." With most of HIT, we have neither, or at least neither with reliable estimates. In 2013, the RAND corporation published a report that seriously questioned the economic savings from HIT they previously estimated [25]. In addition, the new publication brought to light the fact that their previous RAND report of 2005, so effective for HIT promoters, was in fact supported by HIT vendors Cerner and GE. Vendors and system developers have long provided favorable analyses of ROI [25, 36]. But these are generally self-justification, incomplete arithmetic, marketing, or acts of faith transubstantiated into numbers [8, 12, 24, 31, 53] because:

1. One has little idea how much these systems cost in total
2. There will be unknown additional needed personnel in IT, in medical, nursing, or pharmacy informatics
3. Each hospital HIT upgrade requires about 40,000 person hours to implement and test [22]
4. Few if any organizations predict such costs [49, 51]
5. As outlined above, we seldom know the outcomes of HIT's use;
6. The cost of the systems is not disclosed and often obscured or modified via joint marketing agreements, reductions on future upgrades or add-ons, fees for demonstrations to other potential clients;
7. Healthcare providers suffer dramatic productivity losses when the HIT is newly implemented; and many of those losses continue for years [30, 45].

## 6.10  Conclusion

Evaluation of HIT is often hard to measure, always nuanced, and profoundly complex. Unintended side effects (both good and bad) as well as intended effects are often discovered slowly, and only with vigilance, thoughtful examination, and openness to surprises. Policymakers, health care executives, and clinicians must gain a balanced understanding of the powers, problems, and implications of the technology if they are to assess evidence of its efficacy. But as daunting a challenge as that is, there are no viable alternatives. The often oversold technology – a belief assiduously nurtured by an HIT industry with much to gain – does not negate the significant benefits HIT offers. And as HIT evolves, it will be of even greater value to patients, clinicians, and budgets. Ironically, the extravagant hype, the rush to market, and the reluctance to measure its problems and effects may be more of a danger to its continued growth than are its multifaceted failures. The continuing, and well-orchestrated, chorus of promises may deafen the industry's ability to hear its customers and to recognize their needs. Patient safety, which has so much to benefit from good HIT, will suffer until the healthcare experts and the HIT industry are willing to carefully evaluate the evidence of these systems, and then use that evidence to improve them.

## 6.11  Recommendations for What Healthcare Institutions and Clinicians Should Do?

At last, we come to an opportunity to suggest positive actions. Clinicians and healthcare IT staff should not accept HIT vendors' assessments of their own HIT without independent investigation. Even though systematic evaluation of HIT is remarkably difficult, it is not impossible. A recent study by Duke et al. [10] compared the efficacy of two types of CDS alerts using a randomized study of physicians. Although the findings showed no improvements with either method, the work illustrates rigorous evaluation methodology in a circumscribed but potentially valuable area of EHR functionality. However, there are several new studies (supported by ONC) that show serious advantages to CDS, including important safeguards in dosing and avoidance of several drug-drug interactions [42].

These recommendations are offered with reservations about their probability of implementation. Nevertheless, we should at least try.

1. Establish clear metrics for HIT's core functions. This will require separate examinations for CPOE, EHRs, pharmacy IT, etc. The tests must include time-at-task as well as completion of the task. In the United States, the HIT certification process has been an open-book test with unlimited time, making it remarkably dissimilar to real clinical environments. Unlike testers, clinicians do not have an hour to enter each medication order.

2. If, as vendors insist, HIT is dramatically altered once implemented, then the testing must be conducted both in vitro (in laboratory settings) and in situ (in actual field conditions – a hospital, clinic or office).

   If we need interim test-bed settings (e.g., a "standard" set of hospital linkages to other IT systems, a "standard" workflow environment), than this should be established. At least a realistic test bed is a better guide than only an abstract and isolated test.

3. Recognize the need for multi-method testing procedures: Discovering how HIT works in reality requires the full range of research techniques and data sources [30]. Koppel et al.'s study of CPOE [31] employed surveys, observations, focus groups, shadowing of physicians and nurses, one-on-one interviews with many different kind of staff, expert interviews (with IT and hospital leaders), and shadowing of pharmacy personnel as they used the system. Koppel and colleagues' study of medication barcoding administration [33] used all of these methods plus analysis of almost half a million scans of patient IDs and medication IDs, vendor interviews, review of vendor specifications, and interviews with dozens of hospital and IT leaders from throughout the nation.

4. Require data standards. Without unified data standards and data formats, achieving interoperability is nearly impossible. Without both, HIT's utility – and the ability to evaluate HIT's utility – is profoundly attenuated. Note that several organizations and groups are actively involved in providing data standards and semantic interoperability. The need for data standards does not mean there is a need for new standards. Some of those standard-setting organizations include the association publishing this chapter, The International Medical Informatics Association, along with others: HL7, the International Health Terminology Standards Development Organization, which owns and administers the rights for SNOMED CT, etc.

5. Establish consistent usability tests for every major screen and function. These should include careful examinations of system navigation, way finding, and ability to determine where in the system one is. Improvement of HIT will only be achieved if it is based on careful and unbiased evaluation of HIT design,

implementation, training, and use. While acknowledging evaluations cannot reach the level of RCTs, they will still be far better than the current slate of marketing hype, ad hoc testimonies, and self-analyses. We must listen to the frustrations of clinicians and of local IT personnel, and then act constructively to address those problems. Denying those frustrations, or failure to examine HIT's flaws, is counterproductive and will condemn patients to unsafe care and condemn clinicians to unnecessary burdens and stress.

6. Evaluate graphic presentations of data. HIT offers extraordinary abilities to convert numeric data to easily viewed formats. But confusing and poorly annotated graphic displays are worse than none at all.

7. Use the tests to help vendors improve their products and to help healthcare providers select the best products for their needs. Do not allow proprietary interests to influence the assessment process or the distribution of findings. However, vendors should have the ability to annotate and dispute any reports offered by clinicians and testing services.

8. Make these evaluation processes transparent.

9. Publish the findings.

10. Do not allow hidden contractual agreements, (e.g., joint sales agreements, fees for demonstrating a product, or fees for attesting to the excellence of a product) to distort colleagues' judgments. It's permissible to reimburse hospitals and clinicians to talk with potential customers, but those customers must know if money or goods are being provided as compensation [2]. Transparent pricing and clear reporting of implementation and training costs would help providers make better informed judgements about these expensive systems. The vast funds and personnel involved and the patient safety consequences demand nothing less.

# References

1. Aarts J, Ash J, Berg M. Extending the understanding of computerized physician order entry: implications for professional collaboration, workflow and quality of care. Int J Med Inf. 2007;76:S4–13.
2. Agency for Healthcare Research and Quality (AHRQ). A robust health data infrastructure. Prepared by: JASON, The MITRE Corporation. AHRQ Publication No. 14-0041-EF April. 2014.
3. Ash J, Sittig D, Poon E, et al. The extent and importance of unintended consequences of computerized physician order entry. JAMIA. 2007;14:415–23.
4. Berger R, Kichak J. Computerized physician order entry: helpful or harmful? JAMIA. 2004;11:100–3.
5. Campbell E, Sittig D, Ash J, et al. Types of unintended consequences related to computerized provider order entry. JAMIA. 2006;13:547–56.
6. Centers for Medicare and Medicaid Services. Data and reports. 2015. http://www.cms.gov/Regulations-and-Guidance/Legislation/EHRIncentivePrograms/DataAndReports.html. Accessed 2 Apr 2015.
7. Collen M. A brief historical overview of hospital information system (HIS) evolution in the United States. Int J Med Inform. 1991;29(3–4):169–89.

8. Chaudhry B, Wang J, Wu S, Maglione M, Mojica W, Roth E, Morton SC, Shekelle PG. A systematic review: impact of health information technology on quality, efficiency, and costs of medical care. Ann Int Med. 2006;144(10):742–52.
9. Craven C, Koppel R, Weiner M. Information and evidence failures in daily work: how they can affect the safety of care. In: Zipperer L, editor. Patient safety: perspectives on evidence, information and knowledge transfer. Farnham: Gower Publishing; 2014.
10. Duke JD, Li X, Dexter P. Adherence to drug-drug interaction alerts in high-risk patients: a trial of context-enhanced alerting. JAMIA. 2013;20:494–8.
11. Electronic Health Record Association. Health Information Management Systems Society (HIMSS); 2015. http://www.himssehra.org/ASP/index.asp. Accessed 5 Apr 2015.
12. Garg A, Adhikari N, McDonald H, Rosas-Arellano MP, Devereaux PJ, Beyene J, Sam J, Haynes RB. Effects of computerized clinical decision support systems on practitioner performance and patient outcomes: a systematic review. JAMA. 2005;293(10):1223–38.
13. Goodman K, Berner E, Dent M, Kaplan B, Koppel R, Rucker D, Sands D, Winkestein P. Challenges in ethics, safety, best practices and oversight regarding HIT vendors, their customers, and patients: a report of an AMIA special task force. JAMIA. 2011;18:77e81.
14. Han Y, Carcillo J, Venkataraman S, Clark R, Watson S, Nguyen T, Bayir H, Orr R. Unexpected increased mortality after implementation of a commercially sold computerized physician order entry system. Pediatrics. 2004;116:1506–12.
15. Harrison M, Koppel R, Bar-Lev S. Unintended consequences of information technologies in health care: an interactive socio-technical analysis. JAMIA. 2007;14:542–9.
16. Health IT Policy Committee. JASON report task force final report. 15 Oct 2014. http://www.healthit.gov/facas/sites/faca/files/Joint_HIT_JTF_JTF%20HITPC%20Final%20Report%20Presentation%20v3_2014-10-15.pdf. Accessed 4 Apr 2015.
17. Healthcare Information Management Systems Society. HIMSS EHR usability task force. Defining and testing EMR usability: principles and proposed methods of EMR usability evaluation and rating. 2009. http://www.himss.org/files/HIMSSorg/content/files/himss_definingandtestingemrusability.pdf.
18. Healthcare Information Management Systems Society. http://www.himss.org/ASP/aboutHimssHome.asp. Accessed 25 Dec 2012.
19. Healthy4U Blog. Healthcare vendor epic caught red handed: ghost writing and using customers as stealth lobbyists. Did ONC ignore this? August 2012. http://healthy4uaz.blogspot.com/2012/08/health-it-vendor-epic-caught-red-handed.html#. Accessed 3 Apr 2015.
20. Hillestad R, Bigelow J, Bower A, et al. Can electronic medical record systems transform health care? Potential health benefits, savings, and costs. Health Aff. 2005;24:1103–17.
21. Jha AK, Desroches CM, Campbell EG, et al. Use of electronic health records in U.S. Hospitals. N Engl J Med. 2009;360:1628–38.
22. Jones S, Koppel R, Ridgely S. AHRQ guide to reducing unintended consequences of HIT implementation and use. 2011. www.ucguide.org. Accessed 21 Jan 2013.
23. Kannry J, Kushniruk A, Koppel R. Meaningful usability: health information for the rest of us. In: Ken O, editor. Medical informatics: an executive primer. 2nd ed. Chicago: Healthcare Information and Management Systems Society; 2011. p. 53–74.
24. Karsh B-T, Weinger MB, Abbott PA, Wears RL, et al. Health information technology: fallacies and sober realities. JAMIA. 2010;17:617–23.
25. Kellermann AL, Jones SS. What it will take to achieve the as-yet-unfulfilled promises of health information technology. Health Aff. 2013;32(1):63–8.
26. Koppel R. The marginal utility of margin guidance: commentary on Ridgely and Greenberg. J Health Law Policy. 2012;l5(2):311–8.
27. Koppel R. Keynote chapter: is HIT evidenced-based? International medical informatics yearbook. Stuttgart: Schattauer Publishers; 2013.
28. Koppel R, Kreda D. Healthcare information technology vendors' "Held Harmless clauses—implications for patients and clinicians. Commentary. JAMA. 2009;301(12):1276–8.
29. Koppel R, Kreda DA. Healthcare IT usability and suitability for clinical needs: challenges of design, workflow, and contractual relations. Stud Health Technol Inform. 2010;157:7–14.

30. Koppel R, Gordon S. First, do less harm: confronting the inconvenient problems of patient safety. Ithaca: Cornell University Press; 2012.
31. Koppel R, Localio AR, Cohen A, Strom BL. Neither panacea nor black box: responding to three journal of biomedical informatics papers on computerized physician order entry systems. J Biomed Inform. 2005;38(4):267–9.
32. Koppel R, Leonard CE, Localio AR, Cohen A, Auten R, Strom B. Identifying and quantifying medication errors: evaluation of rapidly discontinued medication orders submitted to a computerized physician order entry system. JAMIA. 2008;15(4):461–5.
33. Koppel R, Wetterneck T, Telles JL, Karsh BT. Workarounds to barcode medication administration systems: their occurrences, causes, and threats to patient safety. JAMIA. 2008;4:408–23.
34. Koppel R, Majumdar SR, Soumerai SB. Electronic health records and quality of diabetes care." Editor's correspondence. NEJM. 2011;365:2338–9.
35. Kushniruk A, Monkman H, Tuden D, Bellwood P, Borycki E, et al. Integrating heuristic evaluation with cognitive walkthrough: development of a hybrid usability inspection method. In: Courtney KL, editor. Deriving quality in informatics: fulfilling the promise. Amsterdam: Ios Press; 2015. p. 221–5.
36. Madara JL. Open letter to office of the national coordinator of HIT Chair, Dr. Farzad Mostashari on the American Medical Association's position on "Meaningful Use" regulations. 2013. http://www.ama-assn.org/resources/doc/washington/stage-3-meaningful-use-electronic-health-records-comment-letter-14jan2013.pdf.
37. McCormick D, Bor D, Woolhandler S, Himmelstein D. The effect of physicians' electronic access to tests: a response to Farzad Mostashari. Health Affairs Blog. March 12, 2012: http://healthaffairs.org/blog/author/dmdbswdh/. Accessed 25 Dec 2012.
38. Metzger J, Welebob E, Bates DW, Lipsitz S, Classen DC. Mixed results in the safety performance of computerized physician order entry. Health Aff. 2010;29(4):655–63.
39. Nebeker J, Hoffman JM, Weir CR, et al. High rates of adverse events in a highly computerized hospital. Arch Int Med. 2005;165:1111–6.
40. Office of the National Coordinator (ONC). EHR incentives & certification – HealthIT.gov. 2010. www.healthit.gov/providers-professionals/ehr-incentives-certification. Accessed 2 Apr 2015.
41. ONC. Key health alliance: regional extension assistance center for HIT: eligible hospitals: pre-attestation and audit checklist tool. 2013. http://www.healthit.gov/sites/default/files/eh_preat-testationauditchecklisttool_07182013.pdf. Accessed 2 Apr 2015.
42. ONC. Safer assurance factors For EHR resilience. Jan 2014. http://www.healthit.gov/safer/safer-guides. Accessed 4 Apr 2015.
43. ONC. EHR incentives and certification: what is meaningful use. Health IT.gov. 2015. http://www.healthit.gov/providers-professionals/ehr-incentives-certification. Accessed 3 Apr 2015.
44. Ridge MS, Greenberg MD. Too many alerts, too much liability: sorting through the malpractice implications of drug-drug interactions clinical decision support. J Health Law Policy. 2012;15(2):257–96.
45. Riskin L, Koppel R, Riskin D. Re-examining health IT policy: what will it take to derive value from our investment? JAMIA. 2015;22:459–64. doi:10.1136/amiajnl-2014-003065. Perspective.
46. Shulman R Singer M, Goldstone J, et al. Medication errors: a prospective cohort study of hand-written and computerised physician order entry in the Intensive Care Unit," Critical Care. 2005;9:R516–21.
47. Silverstein S. Contemporary issues in medical informatics: good health IT, bad health IT, and common examples of healthcare IT difficulties. 2015. http://cci.drexel.edu/faculty/ssilverstein/cases/?loc=home. Accessed 7 Apr 2015.
48. Sinsky CA, Hess J, Karsh B, Keller JP, Koppel R. Comparative user experiences of health IT products: how user experiences would be reported and used [Internet]. Washington (DC): Institute of Medicine; 2012 Sept. http://www.iom.edu/Global/Perspectives/2012/~/media/Files/. Accessed 4 Apr 2015.

49. Spencer J, Koppel R, Ridgely MS. AHRQ Guide to reducing unintended consequences of HIT implementation and Use, 2011. www.ucguide.org. Accessed 13 May 2011.
50. Smith SW, Koppel R. Healthcare information technology's relativity problems: a typology of how patients' physical reality, clinicians' mental models, and healthcare information technology differ. JAMIA. 2014;21(1):117–31.
51. Terry KJ. Doctors' 10 Biggest Mistakes When Using EHRs. Medscape business of medicine. 1 May 2013. http://www.medscape.com/viewarticle/803188. Accessed 4 Apr 2015.
52. Wachter R. RIP meaningful use born 2009 – died 2014??? The Healthcare Blog. 2014. http://thehealthcareblog.com/blog/2014/11/26/rip-meaningful-use-2009-2014/.
53. Wears R, Berg M. Computer technology and clinical work: still waiting for Godot. JAMA. 2005;293(10):1261–3.

# Chapter 7
# Ten Reasons Why Interoperability Is Difficult

Margo Edmunds, Douglas Peddicord, and Mark E. Frisse

**Abstract** In this chapter, we define interoperability simply as the electronic sharing of information among systems. We describe ten barriers to interoperability, including technical, financial, organizational, legal, and cultural factors that affect information-sharing, and provide a perspective on the policy and practical challenges of building infrastructure under the Health Information Technology Clinical Health Act (HITECH). We close by making some observations about what has been learned and how those lessons might apply to future policy goals.

**Keywords** Health information technology (Health IT) • Health Insurance Portability and Accountability Act (HIPAA) • Health Information Technology Clinical Health Act (HITECH) • Interoperability • Meaningful use • Public-private collaboration

## 7.1 Introduction

The Health Information Technology and Clinical Health Act (HITECH) was enacted as part of the American Recovery and Reinvestment Act of 2009 (ARRA), more commonly known as the stimulus package. It provided $30 billion in financial incentives for clinicians and hospitals to adopt electronic health records (EHRs). HITECH was also described as a down payment on healthcare reform, because it was hoped that the "meaningful use" of EHRs by providers would help to improve care coordination, quality, and safety; make it easier for patients to access their own health information; and also would improve population and public health.

M. Edmunds, PhD (✉)
Department of Evidence Generation and Translation, AcademyHealth,
1150 17th Street, NW, Suite 600, Washington, DC 20036, USA
e-mail: margo.edmunds@academyhealth.org

D. Peddicord, PhD
President, Washington Health Strategies Group, Washington, DC, USA

M.E. Frisse, MD, MS, MBA
Department of Biomedical Informatics, Vanderbilt University Medical Center,
Nashville, TN, USA

© Springer International Publishing Switzerland 2016
C.A. Weaver et al. (eds.), *Healthcare Information Management Systems:
Cases, Strategies, and Solutions*, Health Informatics,
DOI 10.1007/978-3-319-20765-0_7

The Patient Protection and Affordable Care Act (ACA), signed into law in March 2010, provided comprehensive health reform, with health coverage expansions, insurance market reforms, and provisions to develop national strategies to improve quality and patient engagement and reduce disparities. The ACA assumed that EHRs or Health IT (health information technology) more broadly were being adopted so that information could easily flow across clinical settings and organizations and drive quality improvement, improve the availability of data for research, and improve administrative efficiencies.

The two pieces of legislation – HITECH and ACA – were the largest investment in healthcare in the nation's history, and they were intended to stimulate technology evolution and innovation. And while their combined intent and goal was to use information technology to enable improvements in the quality of care and flow of information to the right person at the right time, in reality their implementation unfolded separately, on parallel and independent tracks, with different federal agencies and stakeholder groups, different sources of support and resistance, and vastly different media coverage.

Policies can either stimulate technology evolution in proactive ways, or arise as a reaction to emergent changes in the market [1]. For example, when the photocopy machine and the Internet reached the market, Congress reacted to protect copyrights and intellectual property through laws such as the 1998 Digital Millennium Copyright Act [2].

In contrast, the massive HITECH investment might be seen as Congress being proactive about stimulating the market toward electronic information exchange. There was no great demand for EHRs among healthcare providers at the time, although some early adopters, professional societies, and policymakers were raising alarms about the quality and inefficiencies of a paper-based system. After the Institute of Medicine released the *Quality Chasm* report in 2001 calling for EHRs and technology-supported quality improvements, there had been discussion in policy and clinical circles about the importance of coordinating care because that was better for patients. But there was no corresponding market demand for interoperability among clinical systems or settings to allow care coordination to take place more easily.

This chapter is being written during the comment period for the draft nationwide interoperability roadmap released by the Office of the National Coordinator for Health IT (ONC). Given that interoperability refers to the generation and flow of electronic health information, and electronic health records (EHRs) are a key source of that information, we think it is useful to ask the following question:

Why did it take more than 20 years (from the 2001 IOM *Quality Chasm* report) and a $30–40 billion dollar investment in 2009 by the Federal government in "meaningful use" (MU) to finally reach a "tipping point" in the last year or two, where a majority of physicians and hospitals had deployed some type of EHR?

The use of check image capture for deposits went from less than 5 % of banks in 2004 to 95 % in 2015. Why is it taking so long for clinicians and healthcare delivery systems to achieve interoperability? We suggest the following reasons.

## 1. Healthcare information is complex.

The vision and promise of HITECH are that clinical information from patient records will be shared electronically among clinicians from different specialties, organizations, and geographies in real time, at the point of care, to improve the quality of care and make it safer for patients. Moreover, the electronic clinical data will be aggregated and "reused" by clinical and health services researchers, public health officials, and other third parties in a way that preserves patient privacy but also makes it possible to accelerate the learnings from comparative effectiveness research (CER) and patient-centered outcomes research (PCOR), improve population health planning, and improve consumers' access to their own personal health information for self-management.

Some have likened the HITECH investments to the early days of automating financial services in the 1980s and have compared the public's initial resistance to ATMs to the provider community's challenges in implementing EHRs. While there are many organizational, philosophical, technology literacy, usability, and other challenges to clinicians using EHRs, there is also exquisite complexity in clinical data. Computer processing requires data to be structured, complete, unambiguous, and validated [3]. Clinical data rarely meet those criteria.

In 1999, the California Healthcare Foundation issued a 5-year forecast on the future of the Internet in healthcare, aiming to "sift through the hype" and focus on the expectations of consumers to find health information online and "change the balance of power" in the practice of medicine as well as encouraging practitioners to share information about clinical practice and individual patients [4]. Since the time of that forecast, clinicians are using EHRs but they are not routinely sharing information with other clinicians. In addition, the balance of power has not shifted to patients, and the majority still do not have ready access to their own personal health information. No one has talked about the hype cycle in a long time, but the underlying cultural issues about provider-to-provider and provider-patient information sharing still have not been addressed.

## 2. Financial incentives were not aligned for EHR adoption.

Notwithstanding the argument that EHRs could, among other things, reduce duplicative tests and procedures and thereby reduce health care costs, it made little sense for a physician to spend $50,000 or a hospital several million dollars, when such savings would accrue to insurers and health plans – the payers, in other words – and not to the provider organization that made the investment in the EHR. In fact, the physician practice or hospital would likely lose revenue when duplicative tests or procedures were avoided. The MU provider incentives helped somewhat to offset the costs of the investment, but did not cover the actual costs.

Policy influencers like the Institute of Medicine (IOM) and leaders in academic medical centers took the position that EHR adoption was rather like a social responsibility, something that physicians and hospitals would do for the good of patients and of the health care system, if not for themselves. This turned out to be a very big ask, not unlike expecting banks to install ATMs for customer convenience, but expecting them to also keep personal tellers available. The balance shifted when the United States Congress, while saving the economy with an economic stimulus, invested in the future of health care with HITECH. In effect, it took Federal dollars to do what misaligned financial incentives and inaccurate policy assumptions could not – actually drive EHR adoption. Since another stimulus is not likely, it is difficult to foresee what incentives will move health systems and providers to share health information with patients and with each other.

### 3. **Health care delivery does not function like a free market.**

Again, the financial incentives in the health care system are not aligned in ways that encourage the sharing of health data between and across physicians, hospitals, plans, payers, researchers and patients. Today hospitals and doctors vie for business in an extremely competitive marketplace and they are loathe to "lose" patients to other providers or plans. As with EHR adoption, the burden (of creating health data that is structured, standardized and computable, and systems that can exchange data electronically) falls on providers, while the "benefits" of data exchange to any stakeholder other than the payer, and perhaps the patient, are intangible.

Unlike a true market, patients have almost no ability to encourage (or force) information exchange that might benefit them. For a variety of reasons, patients do not – and cannot – behave like consumers in a competitive marketplace. For example, the selection of health plans is largely made by employers, and the choice of hospitals for procedures depends on where the health plan has a contract and the insured individual's physician has privileges, not on where the patient would prefer to go. Consumer choice might apply to healthy individuals preferring to go to providers who have converted to EHRs, but that opportunity is still relatively rare.

### 4. **No one was in charge of change management.**

Anyone who has been involved in rolling out an IT system knows that delays and failure to achieve objectives are common. The scale and complexity of the national infrastructure goals were unprecedented in healthcare, and so was the vision of having every clinician adopt an EHR that would be interoperable with other clinicians and health systems.

As mentioned above, it was assumed that financial incentives to adopt EHRs would move the market, but it was not acknowledged that healthcare does not function like free markets. The enormity of behavioral and organizational changes needed from bedside to administrative systems were not only underestimated, but largely ignored until providers began to complain about the poor design and quality of software and the amount of time required to do normal clinical activities, particularly documentation of clinic visits. This series of events was often described as a failure to make the business case for interoperability, but the use case for having a patient's information follow the patient across the system out into the community and home to improve the quality of care was also never clearly articulated.

From a policy perspective, ONC is more policy executor than policy maker, and as the title of the office indicates, its principal function is to coordinate. Congress, not ONC, has the power of the purse, and it is instructive to go back and look at the funding amounts in the stimulus package again. While hospitals and other providers were targeted with $30-plus billion in EHR incentives, ONC received only $2 billion for HIT infrastructure and standards development, workforce programs, research and demonstration projects, and the like. It was as though the infrastructure required to launch the ambitious healthcare overhaul was an afterthought.

While the ONC budget sounds like lot of money, it was passed through quickly to providers and other stakeholders and by FY 2015 ONC's budget had shrunk back to $60 million, about one-seventh as much as was allocated to the Agency for Healthcare Research and Quality (AHRQ.) Meanwhile, AHRQ's Health IT portfolio was continuing to fund research and build and disseminate evidence about the value of health information exchange to improve quality [5].

In short, the National Coordinator has a bully pulpit but has neither the money nor the authority to incentivize interoperable information exchange in a meaningful way. And Congress, whose members understood the need for a massive fiscal incentive to drive EHR adoption in 2009, now seem increasingly impatient with the fact that MU requirements in and of themselves will not be enough to ensure the interoperable exchange of health information [6].

## 5.  User-centered design is not a key part of IT industry culture.

Every clinical specialty has its own views and approaches to patient care, but this complexity was not well understood or appreciated by the developers of what are now known as legacy EHR systems. In most healthcare systems, purchasing decisions were made by operations and administrative leadership, and rarely involved clinical leadership and end-users of the systems for patient care. This disconnect has been one of the most vexing in the adoption of health IT, even among those who see the potential for Health IT to reduce harm and errors and improve patient quality.

Because the early health information systems developed from administrative billing systems, they were largely transaction-based. Interoperability means that the senders and recipients of data in each transaction understand the same data in the same way. The number of transactions in healthcare systems is unimaginably vast, and the original notion of health information exchange was largely confined to internal flow among departments within hospitals or health systems. Thus, vendors provided proprietary non-standardized systems to early adopters, and it was not unusual for departments within the same health system to acquire their own departmental systems that were incompatible with the EHR system.

It is perhaps easiest to see this disconnect among developers and users through the example of the EHR, the most ubiquitous tool for practicing clinicians. While some EHR vendors have taken a user-centered design approach, there are seemingly endless variations in screen layout, controls, color, and application flow for different EHR products. At the very least, this means that residents and other clinicians who are working in different settings must take time to learn each new software product. In time-sensitive circumstances, the differences in EHR layout and functionality can lead to preventable errors, which can have serious consequences for patients.

Recently, an AMIA task force recommended that an industry coalition develop a common user interface style guide for selected EHR functionalities [7]. A minimum set of design patterns could be shared among vendors to reduce the end-user burden and ultimately benefit patients. Human factors research could support the selection process, using an evidence-based approach to design, and best practices for system implementation and ongoing management could be learned from implementation research and evaluation.

A similar approach has been used successfully by the Continua Health Alliance, a global, non-profit open-industry association of healthcare and technology companies. Continua's mission is to promote interoperable personal connected health solutions that connect products of diverse vendors, supported by a product interoperability certification program developed in collaboration with government regulatory agencies. Continua's end-users include clinicians and health systems as well as individual patients and caregivers, who use interoperable devices for remote monitoring of their chronic healthcare conditions and other telehealth applications. The Continua business case for interoperability is that products by different vendors are being used together in the marketplace, and it is in every company's best interest for their products to be interoperable with products made by competitors.

### 6. Technology literacy in healthcare has lagged behind other industries.

From the perspective of the IT industry, health informatics education is vital because "most end users are technically unsophisticated, do not understand the development life cycle, and are simply unable to perform the sort of scrutiny that is demanded of them" [3]. With the exception of a very small number of clinician informaticians, some of whom developed "home-grown" information systems in their own institutions and many of whom were trained by the National Library of Medicine, the majority of clinicians have viewed Health IT as something that interferes with patient care rather than supporting it, in part because most EHRs do not match the usability and functionality of other consumer software

The recent implementation of meaningful use has had a profound impact on the adoption of EHRs and discussion of the goals and potential value of interoperable systems. Vendors and providers have generally felt that meaningful use criteria have been too difficult to meet, while patient groups and payers have tended to push for faster adoption. Some have been concerned that the focus on meaningful use criteria has diverted attention from quality improvement and efficiency agendas of their own institutions.

Meanwhile, continuing education training efforts for providers, such as AMIA's 10×10 program, will add to the number of informaticians who are experienced users of EHR systems and who understand the underlying infrastructure issues. Taking an optimistic view, the increasing attention to user-centered design criteria will help to improve the EHR products available and begin to reduce the user-developer gap.

### 7. The business case for RHIO's and local health information exchange was not appreciated.

At the time ONC was created, the terms RHIO (Regional Health Information Organization) and HIE (Health Information Exchange) were used interchangeably. The work of David Brailer at the Santa Barbara County Data Exchange had drawn national attention, along with work in Indianapolis and a few other communities that had been building information infrastructure for several years. The national preoccupation was with building a national infrastructure comprised of "a network of networks," and it led to an assumption that the only way to bring aggregated data to the point of care was to have a hierarchical system in place [8].

Recognizing the essential need for EHRs and other devices to communicate with one another as patients move from setting to setting, HITECH had followed the precedent of Medicaid legislation four decades earlier and provided grants to states to implement health information exchange infrastructures. At the time, these technologies were immature in most states, and both the low levels of funding and the many cultural and technical challenges presented by HIE led to disappointment.

However, the infrastructure implementation problems eventually made it apparent that most clinical information flows within a geographically-defined market, based on the referral patterns of local providers, and not at the state level. In practice, the majority of health information is exchanged in "point-to-point" transactions as part of the process of providing clinical care to individuals. We now know that there are significant geographic variations in how care is provided, in terms of practice and referral patterns and adoption of Health IT. We also have learned that organizational commitment and clinical leadership to transform clinical workflow and provide decision support have a more direct effect on practice patterns than national policy goals.

In general, HITECH chose a "push" effort that imposed detailed criteria for EHR use rather than a market "pull" mechanism based on accountable care organizations, bundled payments, and other approaches from the Affordable Care Act that are helping lead to standards harmonization and new industry alignments. However, the legislation's shortcomings with respect to health information exchange have led to a more distributed set of secure messaging standards to allow at least point-to-point communication.

Thus, well-intentioned as it may have been, the early view of interoperability was highly complex, unrelated to clinical incentives to improve quality of care, and ineffective in building support for health information infrastructure. Only the later introduction of financial incentives and guidelines and the promise of improved efficiencies and cost reductions were able to pique interest in further investments.

## 8. **HIPAA privacy requirements are so complex that their interpretations vary significantly across settings.**

It is indeed ironic that the Health Insurance and Portability and Accountability Act (HIPAA) regulatory framework has made information exchange difficult when the primary goal of HIPAA's Administrative Simplification provisions was to facilitate an electronic information environment.

HIPAA permits Covered Entities, and Business Associates working on their behalf, to use and disclose protected health information for purposes of "treatment, payment and health care operations." It could be argued that such discretionary uses and disclosures allow for the routine exchange of health data across Covered Entities for purposes including: consultation and coordination of care; outcomes evaluation, quality assessment and improvement activities; aggregation of health data to permit data analyses; and, a variety of other purposes.

But too often, the HIPAA rules are understood to mean that such uses and disclosures of health data can occur only within the walls of or under the clear control of a specific Covered Entity. In other words, the rules allow the use and disclosure of health data by a given hospital or doctor but do not allow the exchange of the data with another hospital or doctor, absent an authorization by the patient. Also, in the face of confusion on HIPAA rules, the common tendency is for organizations to deny legitimate patient data requests.

As a result, the achievement of interoperable data exchange is generally understood to require the consent of every individual whose protected health information is going to be exchanged, or asking an Institutional Review Board (IRB) to provide a waiver of individual consent. If we add in inadequate guidance on the topic of information exchange from the Office for Civil Rights, which enforces the HIPAA rules, it is no surprise that State and regional health information exchanges have had to devote enormous resources to the development of consent and governance models before they have even attempted to actually exchange data.

Given the experience of the HIEs, can we really expect that providers and other Covered Entities would over-ride their own risk-averse legal counsel and ignore the lack of financial incentives to exchange health information and invest in interoperability at this point? Fortunately, some multisite clinical data researchers are investing in HIE infrastructure for rapid-cycle innovation in care delivery and payment [9]. These innovative data stewardship and governance models eventually may lead to further innovations in the exchange of clinical data in real time as different health systems build trust in the value of HIEs to improve quality of care and the patient experience.

## 9. Health IT is a "team sport," but team members don't agree on strategy.

We have already discussed the disconnect between developers and end-users, inertia and vested interests involved in maintaining data siloes, and other barriers to interoperability. But the evolution of Health IT policy also is affected by differences of opinion about the role of government and the market in advancing the flow of health information.

In a few cases, notably e-prescribing, federal policy goals to improve quality and safety were aligned with industry trends to improve efficiency and reduce costs. By the mid-1980s, pharmaceutical manufacturers, wholesalers, retail stores, and payers had computerized their business model and by the early 1990s, 95 % of drug stores were submitting electronic claims [10]. Arguably, one of the reasons the e-prescribing incentive program was passed into law was that industry had already paid to develop an information infrastructure, and policymakers recognized that financial incentives could be effective in changing provider prescribing behavior.

Many observers and participants have noted that meaningful use planning was out of phase with the broad provider community and was led predominantly by vendors with technical expertise. The shortcomings of the vendor community in using common standards to promote interoperability have also been noted. Others have found that the actions of the Health IT Policy Committee and its approach to balancing policy goals with market trends and provider perceptions have represented the best possible leadership under very challenging circumstances.

Over time, the ability of healthcare systems to provide the right information at the right time in the right place will depend on finding agreement and alignment among policy-makers, healthcare providers, the software and medical device industries, payers, and other stakeholders. We hope that the alignment occurs around the goal of putting patients at the center of care, using technology to accelerate quality improvement and accountability.

10. **The Health IT community does not communicate clearly with Congress, the policy community, and the public about the goals of Health IT and interoperability.**

For many years, the Health IT community – informaticians, EHR users, product developers and vendors, health plans and payers, and others – made the argument that government needed to invest in the national health information infrastructure. For example, in 1991, the Institute of Medicine released a report on Computer-Based Patient Records and provided a blueprint for transitioning to EHRs. In 2001, the National Committee on Vital and Health Statistics (NCVHS) estimated the need for a 10-year $14 billion investment [11]. But notwithstanding the common belief that "HIT is bipartisan" and the vocal support of Congressional leaders ranging from Newt Gingrich to Tom Daschle, why did it take such a long time before the commitment of major dollars in the HITECH Act?

The short answer might be because the Health IT policy "campaign" was, like health care itself perhaps, uncoordinated and lacking in planning. While the policy target might have been an improved and more efficient electronically-enabled health care system, providers and vendors tolerated, if not actively encouraged, data silos by medical specialty, health system, geography, and other factors. In messaging to Congress, too often vendors have lobbied for vendors, hospitals for hospitals, and each physician specialty group for itself. There has never been a single unified voice representing the health care system, perhaps because it is not actually a system.

The current challenge for the HIT community is to talk clearly about the barriers to achieving interoperability and to provide positive answers to the question being posed by Congress: what has been accomplished with the HITECH funding? Where are the successes around the country, and why are some markets more amenable to health information exchange than others? It would be helpful, as well, to provide a clear vision of HIT policy goals and priorities in the interim period before broad implementation of ACOs and payment models in which information exchange not only makes economic sense but becomes a bedrock of care delivery.

## 7.2  Conclusions

It is important to remember that many EHRs are built on top of legacy systems with architectural platforms from the 1980s and mid-1990s. Thus, the go-forward plans for EHRs were being defined just as the Internet, mobile phones and web technologies were becoming a part of everyday life for the American public, including policy-makers and providers themselves. The tensions of developing flexible standards that meet expectations for accountability for public spending while encouraging innovation are significant, and we think they will continue to play out for some time.

The coupling of a financial stimulus effort with a highly prescriptive agenda emphasizing EHR adoption was a unique product of the economic recession and the new Obama Administration. To some extent, ARRA can be seen as an "arranged marriage" between a Keynesian stimulus effort designed to put more money into the economy quickly and a massive, comprehensive introduction of technology that significantly underestimated the degree of cultural and organizational change that would be required. From this perspective, the technology adoption goals of HITECH were overwhelmed by ARRA's overall requirement to expend funds quickly [12].

At the time HITECH passed, critics of federal intervention in the health IT market were vocal about their opposition to government spending for financial incentives on ideological grounds from the very beginning. Others later criticized the dominance of large technology firms and their creation and installation of proprietary systems that were not interoperable, making it difficult to meet the MU criteria even for those systems that were willing to exchange health data with their competitors.

Other implementation problems included small hospital systems and small group practices purchasing software from start-up firms that went out of business, lack of implementation and change management plans after software systems were installed, and the degree of customization of proprietary software making routine upgrades more costly than anticipated. Many of these problems reflected the extreme and quite mutual lack of understanding on the part of IT vendors and healthcare system leaders.

The consequences of coupling HITECH with a short-term economic stimulus required rapid introduction of "top down" detailed requirements that of necessity has led to "leaders and laggards." Well-financed, large care delivery organizations have been able to achieve goals relatively easily, although at great expense, and some early adopters have exceeded the national goals. The pace of adoption and transformation in smaller practices and rural environments has proven insufficient to protect providers from HITECH's initial penalties, but there is still time to encourage them to participate and support their participation.

We see many reasons why interoperability is hard to achieve, despite the good intentions of hundreds of people working on implementation. There are technical, organizational, and financial reasons it is taking a long time. Healthcare information is highly complex and unstructured, so it is very difficult to share across settings and systems even when providers want to share information. Many providers are reluctant to share data they view as proprietary. Financial incentives have not been aligned in a way that has encouraged many providers to adopt and implement EHRs, because they have to invest in systems that will make it easier for others to achieve cost savings (e.g., standardized electronic claims data reduces costs for payers).

While there is much to criticize, a case can also be made that we have learned a lot about what works and what doesn't work, and that we are closer to achieving interoperability than ever before. We hope that enlightened self-interest on the part of all public and private stakeholders will lead to the kind of innovation and transformation that will give us the healthcare system we want for ourselves and our families.

# References

1. Starr P. Remedy and reaction: the peculiar American struggle over health care reform. Revised edition. New Haven: Yale University Press; 2011.
2. Frisse ME, Tolva JN. The commerce of ideas: copyright in the digital era. Acad Med. 1996;71(1):45–53.
3. Benton T. Chapter 2: why interoperability is hard. In: Principles of health interoperability HL7 and SNOMED, health information technology standards. London: Springer; 2012. doi:10.1007/978-1-4471-2801-4_2.
4. Mittman R, Cain M. The future of the internet in health care: five-year forecast. Written by Institute for the Future for the California Healthcare Foundation. Menlo Park; 1999. Available at http://www.chcf.org/~/media/MEDIA%20LIBRARY%20Files/PDF/F/PDF%20forecast.pdf. Accessed on 20 Nov 2014.
5. AHRQ. Health information technology portfolio. 2014. http://www.ahrq.gov/cpi/portfolios/health-it/November 2014. Accessed 6 Mar 2015.
6. Thune J et al. REBOOT: re-examining the strategies needed to successfully adopt health IT. 2014.http://www.thune.senate.gov/public/index.cfm/2013/4/gop-senators-release-white-paper-on-health-it-cite-concerns.
7. Middleton B, et al. Enhancing patient safety and quality of care by improving the usability of electronic health record systems: recommendations from AMIA. J Am Med Inf Assoc. 2013;20(e1):e2–8. doi:10.1136/amiajnl-2012-001458. Published online 25 Jan 2013.
8. Miller R, Miller BS. The Santa Barbara care data exchange: what happened? Health Aff. 2007. doi:10.1377/hlthaff.26.5.w568. http://content.healthaffairs.org/content/26/5/w568.abstract?keytype=ef&siteid=healthaff&ijkey=HDkWYA8whH7QA.
9. McGraw D, Leiter AB. Pathways to success for multi-site clinical data research. eGEMs. 2013;1:Article 13. doi:http://dx.doi.org/10.13063/2327-9214.1041. Available at: http://repository.academyhealth.org/egems/vol1/iss1/13.
10. Starr P. Smart technology, stunted policy: developing health information networks. Health Aff. 1997;16:91–105.
11. National Committee on Vital and Health Statistics (NCVHS). Information for health: a strategy for building the national health information infrastructure. 2001. Available at http://www.ncvhs.hhs.gov/nnhiilayo.pdf.
12. Frisse ME. Health information technology: one step at a time. 2009. Health Affairs. http://content.healthaffairs.org/content/28/2/w379.abstract. Published online before print March 2009, doi:10.1377/hlthaff.28.2.w379. Health Aff. 2009;28(2):w379–84.

# Chapter 8
# The Evolution of Health Information Technology Policy in the United States

**Margo Edmunds, Douglas Peddicord, and Mark E. Frisse**

**Abstract**  The potential of Health Information Technology (Health IT) to transform the nation's healthcare system can only be realized through a realignment of competing priorities and interests in the public and private sectors. Consumers, clinicians, and health systems will benefit when health information flows more freely and is available at any point of care, but it has taken longer than anticipated to implement policies that develop Health IT infrastructure and operationalize the flow of health information. This chapter provides an overview of the development and implementation of Health IT policy, describing relatively recent federal laws, regulations, and other policies created to realize a federal information infrastructure consistent with a diverse array of federal, state, and private-sector priorities. We review the accomplishments of the Directors of the Office of the National Coordinator for Health IT (ONC) to illustrate the broad set of challenges faced by public-private sector collaboration and provide a narrative summary and timeline of key legislation that has created the current Health IT ecosystem. We conclude by identifying major trends and challenges that Health IT and health policy professionals will face in the years ahead.

**Keywords**  Health Information Technology (Health IT) policy • Health Insurance Portability and Accountability Act (HIPAA) • Health Information Technology for Economic and Clinical Health (HITECH) • Interoperability • Meaningful use • Office of the National Coordinator (ONC) • Public-private collaboration

M. Edmunds, PhD (✉)
Evidence Generation and Translation, AcademyHealth,
1150 17th Street, NW, Suite 600, Washington, DC 20036, USA
e-mail: margo.edmunds@academyhealth.org

D. Peddicord, PhD
President, Washington Health Strategies Group, Washington, DC, USA

M.E. Frisse, MD, MS, MBA
Department of Biomedical Informatics, Vanderbilt University Medical Center,
Nashville, TN, USA

© Springer International Publishing Switzerland 2016                                   139
C.A. Weaver et al. (eds.), *Healthcare Information Management Systems:
Cases, Strategies, and Solutions*, Health Informatics,
DOI 10.1007/978-3-319-20765-0_8

## 8.1   Introduction

### *8.1.1   Background and Policy Context*

Policies are courses of action that may be expressed through laws, regulations, public statements, budgets, position papers, actions, and other ways of communicating values. They may be voluntary, influenced by moral persuasion, or enforced through the rule of law, or by economic incentives and penalties. Policies may be created either as a response to a perceived need or as proactive measures that anticipate emerging needs. For example, administrative policies governing payment of medical claims were a reaction to the need for a national consensus on standardized payment when Medicare was introduced. Early pioneering work in the 1970s by Ed Hammond, Clem McDonald, Donald Simborg, and others served as a proactive foundation for subsequent widespread standards efforts.

The Health IT policy development process in the United States (US) is highly complex and poorly understood by most because it involves multiple stakeholders, including federal, state, and local government; private provider systems; academic institutions and professional organizations; independent research and policy organizations; philanthropies; standards development organizations; software and telecommunications industry associations; consumer organizations; and the media. Together with the number of players, the sheer size of the Health IT market is difficult to fathom, and there are many opinions on the role of government intervention in the market.

That said, we believe that the pace of Health IT adoption and the evolution of policies and regulations about interoperability of health systems can be better understood and appreciated when the policy and regulatory context is understood. This understanding will require an unmasking of some of the underlying infrastructures and tensions that come from shared power of different branches of government, the role of the private sector in policy development and implementation, and differences of opinion about what constitutes the public interest.

Individuals and organizations who seek to apply new technologies must navigate a complex and often incompletely understood array of binding and non-binding policies that may impact their own course of action. Encountering challenges or opportunities, these same individuals or organizations may seek to change policies to accommodate their concerns or interests. These pressure points are of particular concern as Health IT is both transformed and becomes more pervasive in traditional health care settings, in the home, in public places, and through wearable personal devices.

In this chapter we detail out the interrelations and interdependencies of the various public entities and policy bodies that have influenced Health IT legislation and its interpretation through regulations. We illustrate the interplay between public and private sectors through describing Health IT policy leaders, including the National Coordinators for Health IT, and by providing a timeline of key legislation and closely related policy-relevant events. We hope that a better understanding of the policy process will encourage citizen engagement in the policy process through position statements of professional societies, voluntary workgroups, public comments on draft regulations, and other means to contribute to policy decisions about legislation and regulation.

## 8.1.2 Overarching Health Policy Goals

There are many diverse and even polarized opinions about how the US healthcare delivery and payment systems can be transformed and improved. But there is general agreement on the national goals for access and quality as articulated by the Institute of Medicine (IOM) report *Crossing the Quality Chasm*: care should be safe, timely, efficient, effective, equitable, and patient-centered [18]. The IOM report viewed developments in information and communications technology as an integral component in achieving all six of these policy goals. At the time the *Quality Chasm* report was issued, the quality of existing, paper-based medical records was described as "embarrassing" and their redesign as a tool for care and information exchange was described as a "moon shot" [5].

In part, the emphasis on safety in the IOM report was a reaction to highly publicized deaths due to preventable medical errors [25], as well as a growing body of data demonstrating inexplicable geographic variations in clinical practice. For many policy-makers, early adoption of EHRs and automated clinical decision support systems brought the promise of safer care in hospitals and clinics by using evidence-based guidelines to standardize practice and reduce the "uneven and unpredictable quality of care provided at even the 'best' American institutions" [15].

Within months of the IOM report's publication, the September 2001 terrorist attacks and the anthrax attacks in Washington, DC and New York City accelerated Congressional interest in funding a health information infrastructure that could be used to improve healthcare quality and patient safety as well as support the more urgent goals of biosurveillance, emergency preparedness, and rapid response. The same information infrastructure that supports the flow of secure clinical information was envisioned to also generate future benefits to population health, by helping to aggregate standardized data for analytics and forecasting, targeting of resources, and research. Through a number of studies published by the IOM and elsewhere, policymakers and the public began to take note of geographic and other variations in access, quality, and cost of healthcare.

Not surprisingly, geographic and other variations also were found in the maturity of clinical information systems, the availability of broadband communications infrastructure, and attitudes toward sharing data electronically. However, with the exception of a few individuals, many of whom were members of the IOM, the "quality movement" in health policy and the movement promoting Health IT adoption diverged and became almost completely independent by the time the Affordable Care Act was passed in 2010.

Taken in a larger policy context, the current intense focus on adoption of electronic health records (EHRs) to promote patient safety and quality is a necessary but by no means sufficient component of information infrastructure and interoperability. In this chapter, our definition of infrastructure includes not only hardware and software, but also the regulatory environment and standards that promote interoperability, defined technically as the electronic exchange of health information within a secure computer network or more simply as the electronic sharing of information among systems. Infrastructure also includes organizations and people who develop, implement, evaluate, and use information systems and promote their use, or who choose to delay for financial, technological, or other reasons.

## 8.2   Policy Development in Public and Private Sectors

Under the United States Constitution, the Congress makes laws, the President and executive branch implement the laws, and the judicial branch interprets the laws. Because of the chapter's focus on implementation, we begin with a description of the executive branch.

### 8.2.1   Organization and Authority of the Federal Executive Branch

The President heads the executive branch of government, which has the responsibility to administer and implement laws. Executive branch activities include writing regulatory guidance to enforce the laws; developing budgets to support program activities and other policy priorities; and providing programmatic oversight.

The executive branch is organized into 15 Cabinet-level departments, including the Department of Health and Human Services (HHS), whose FY 2015 budget totaled $1 trillion [11]. HHS is the principal department that protects the health of all Americans, and it is organized into eight agencies or operating divisions that all have some responsibilities related to Health IT: the Agency for Healthcare Research and Quality (AHRQ); the Centers for Disease Control and Prevention (CDC); the Centers for Medicare and Medicaid Services (CMS); the Food and Drug Administration (FDA); the Health Resources and Services Administration (HRSA); the Indian Health Services (IHS); the National Institutes of Health (NIH); the Substance Abuse and Mental Health Services Administration (SAMHSA): and the Office of the Secretary (OS), where the Office of the National Coordinator for Health IT (ONC) is administratively housed.

Many HHS agencies collaborate with the Veterans Health Administration (VHA), part of the U.S. Department of Veterans Affairs (VA), and the largest integrated healthcare system in the U.S. The VA was an early adopter of electronic health records (EHRs) and developer of the consumer web portal known as Blue Button, which is being widely adapted by Medicare and many other programs.

Other agencies with responsibilities for information infrastructure and consumer protection include the Federal Communications Commission (FCC), which has invested in rural broadband infrastructure and which recently issued a joint report with the FDA and ONC on regulation of mobile health [16]; the Federal Trade Commission (FTC), which enforces the Health Breach Notification Rule for web-based businesses that are not covered by Health Insurance Portability and Accountability Act (HIPAA); the National Institute for Standards and Technology (NIST), a non-regulatory part of the U.S. Department of Commerce that advances measurement science to support technology innovation; and the President's Council of Advisors on Science and Technology (PCAST), administered by the White House Office of Science and Technology Policy, which advises the President and issues reports on policy issues, including Health IT.

In addition to these fully federal agencies, Congress has created two statutory agencies to advise the Secretary of HHS on health data and Health IT. They are the National Committee on Vital and Health Statistics (NCVHS) and the Health IT Policy Committee.

### 8.2.1.1   National Committee on Vital and Health Statistics (NCVHS)

Since 1949, the National Committee on Vital and Health Statistics (NCVHS) has been the statutory body advising the Secretary of HHS on key health data issues, including statistics, privacy, national health information policy, and policy implementation, including ways to facilitate interoperability and networking. The majority of NCVHS meetings are open to the public and most include invited testimony and presentations. Advice reflecting this public input is conveyed to the Secretary through letters that are posted on the HHS web site. The 18-member committee members include statistical and research experts from the private sector, including academia, delivery systems, foundations, and industry. Key federal staff come from the Assistant Secretary for Planning and Evaluation (ASPE) and the National Center for Health Statistics (NCHS), which is part of the Centers for Disease Control and Prevention (CDC).

Before HITECH created the Health IT Policy Committee, NCVHS was the primary source of national guidance on health information policy. In November 2001, NCVHS issued a strategy document for building the national health information infrastructure (NHII). The report identified personal health, providers, and population health as the three dimensions of health infrastructure and estimated that a 10-year investment of $14 billion would be needed across existing agencies and nongovernmental organizations. The report also called for better coordination of the nation's efforts across government and described its role as follows:

> The Government is called upon to help set the stage for private innovation, to catalyze change through visioning and standard-setting, and to help build incentives, in addition to performing such traditional governmental functions as providing material support, widening participation and access, and ensuring privacy and confidentiality protections. [30]

Much of the behind-the-scenes support for what became the Office of the National Coordinator came from the chairs and leadership of NCVHS, including Don Detmer, then the President and CEO of the American Medical Informatics Association; John Lumpkin, Senior Vice President at the Robert Wood Johnson Foundation; and many others. The NHII report later provided the basis for the National Health Information Network (NHIN), which was renamed and became a signature initiative of the Office of the National Coordinator (ONC) in 2004 during the Bush Administration.

### 8.2.1.2  The Health IT Policy Committee

Created by HITECH, the Health IT Policy Committee advises ONC on developing a policy framework for the development and adoption of a nationwide health information infrastructure. It is staffed by ONC and consists of several workgroups and subcommittees that hold virtual and in-person public meetings to address many issues from a variety of stakeholder perspectives, including provider, industry, and consumer views. For example, the Interoperability and Health Information Exchange workgroup makes recommendations to support care management and coordination through the electronic exchange of information.

Members of the policy committee include ex officio members from federal agencies as well as private-sector members from academia, delivery systems, EHR system developers, provider associations, consumers, caregivers, and many other relevant areas of expertise and experience. Similar to the process followed by NCVHS, the Policy Committee transmits its advice in formal letters to the National Coordinator.

The Policy Committee members have played an active role in approving the criteria for meaningful use, a security policy framework for EHRs, matching patients to their own health information in different systems, public trust in Health IT and Health Information Exchange (HIE), and many other key policy issues affecting adoption and implementation. All of their policy recommendations and transmittal letters are available online at www.healthit.gov.

## 8.2.2  Role of the Private Sector in Health IT Policy Development

In addition to the role of Congress in passing legislation and the executive branch of government in implementing it, advisory bodies play a major role in Health IT policy development. Some, including the National Committee on Vital and Health Statistics and the Health IT Policy Committee, are federally staffed and supported and have private-sector members who are appointed through a variety of means, including public and Congressional input. Others are private and independent, and the most noteworthy is the Institute of Medicine.

### 8.2.2.1 Institute of Medicine (IOM) of the National Academy of Sciences (NAS)

The Institute of Medicine (IOM) was founded in 1970 by the National Academy of Sciences, later renamed the National Academies (NAS), to provide independent advice to Congress and the executive branch on issues relate to health and science policy. Originally created by Congressional charter under President Lincoln, the NAS includes the National Research Council, which is an operating branch, along with the National Academy of Engineering (NAE), and the IOM. NAS, NAE, and IOM are all self-perpetuating elected membership organizations that convene expert committees to study and report on health, science, and technology policy issues and conduct public educational activities.

IOM studies are sometimes congressionally mandated or requested, and may also be requested and funded by federal agencies, philanthropies, or other private organizations. IOM committees are made up of members and non-members who reflect a broad array of opinions and expertise on the topic being studied. The IOM also sponsors roundtables, which convene discussions, organize workshops, and write issue briefs in areas of interest to the field, but without making consensus-based recommendations.

Over the years, IOM's reports have had a major impact on policy makers, the delivery system, and the research enterprise. Among many others, the subjects covered in these reports include: health care coverage [19]; patient safety and quality [23]; the role of Health IT in health system transformation [22]; and e-prescribing [21]. The *Quality Chasm* report mentioned at the beginning of this chapter clearly has been one of the most influential [19].

### 8.2.2.2 Other Private Sector Advisory Activities

Professional organizations such as the American Health Information Management Association (AHIMA), the American Medical Informatics Association (AMIA), the Alliance for Nursing Informatics (NIA), and the Health Information and Management Systems Society (HIMSS), also play a vital role representing their members' opinions and interests through providing testimony at Congressional hearings, meeting with Congressional members and staff to discuss policy issues, and submitting comments on draft reports and frameworks. For example, the 2015 ONC Interoperability Roadmap Draft Version 1.0 request for comments, currently open, is likely to receive hundreds of comments from stakeholders.

Private foundations, particularly The Robert Wood Johnson Foundation (RWJF), The California Healthcare Foundation (CHCF), The Commonwealth Fund (CWF), The John and Mary A. Markle Foundation, as well as The Aetna Foundation, The Kellogg Foundation, and The Kresge Foundation are all key players in health policy. These foundations have played an important role in Health IT policy development by convening advisory groups, funding programs and studies to build the evidence base on what works in implementation, and encouraging innovation. For example, the "Blue Button" technology that allows consumers to download their health information was jointly funded by a collaborative group involving the Markle Foundation and RWJF, and beta-tested and implemented by The Department of Veterans Affairs, The Department of Defense, and The Centers for Medicare and Medicaid Services (CMS) [13].

RWJF has funded several infrastructure projects to improve the flow of information across health care and public health settings. CHCF and Commonwealth have funded academic and think tank evaluation teams to learn best practices from the implementation of 17 Beacon Communities and the different phases of meaningful use criteria. The Markle Foundation, Engelberg Center for Health Care Reform at the Brookings Institution, and the Center for American Progress have collaborated on a series of public education events and public comments documents, and the Bipartisan Policy Center has also held public events as well as issued reports on Health IT, with support from health systems and industry payers.

### 8.2.2.3 Private Industry

In Health IT, policies often require adoption of standards for data representation and process flow. These standards generally arise through the deliberations and voluntary practices of industry-led consensus groups and are later embodied into law; such standards and policies are therefore a result of a perceived market "pull." When embodied into law, such policies change from a market "pull" adopted by some stakeholders to a mandatory "push" enforced on all stakeholders.

In the United States, the private, non-profit American National Standards Institute (ANSI) serves as a clearinghouse for national and international standards development efforts. A number of standards development organizations (SDOs) also play a critical role. Examples include: the ISO (International Organization for Standardization), responsible for many communication standards; the ASC (Accounting Standards Codification), responsible for many administrative transaction standards; HL7 (Health Level Seven), responsible for detailed clinical messaging standards; and NCPDP (National Council for Prescription Drug Programs), responsible for many standards pertaining to prescription drugs. These SDOs strive to coordinate their often overlapping interests to provide a coherent set of standards that have been incorporated into many Health IT policies.

Another example is Continua Health Alliance, a non-profit, open industry organization of technology, medical device, and healthcare industry leaders who are developing design guidelines and a certification program to promote interoperability among their diverse products. Continua focuses on Health IT that facilitates virtual visits or electronic connectivity outside of traditional office visits among patients, family members, and providers.

## 8.2.3 Key Legislation Influencing Health IT Policy

The major pieces of legislation governing Health IT are The Health Insurance Portability and Accountability Act (HIPAA) (1996), which was amended in the Health Information Technology for Economic and Clinical Health (HITECH) Act of 2009; the Medicare Prescription Drug, Improvement, and Modernization Act (also called the Medicare Modernization Act or MMA), passed in 2003; the Patient Protection and Affordable Care Act (ACA), 2009; and the Food And Drug Administration Safety And Innovation Act (FDASIA), which was passed in 2012.

### 8.2.3.1 Health Insurance Portability and Accountability Act (HIPAA)

In August of 1996, Congress passed the Health Insurance Portability and Accountability Act (HIPAA), also known as Kennedy-Kassebaum and then as Kassebaum-Kennedy, after two of its leading sponsors [4]. Title I of HIPAA protected continuity of care in the group and individual health insurance markets by ensuring that individuals could keep their coverage when they changed jobs. There was widespread public support for preventing "job lock," and it was one of two remaining issues from the Clinton health reform efforts that still had bipartisan support in Congress. The other issue was the State Children's Health Insurance Program (CHIP), which was authorized under the Balanced Budget Act of 1997. An 1998 IOM report on the CHIP program promoted the use of information technology for enrollment and clinical purposes as well as public reporting, consistent with other IOM reports and the new legislation, but also new for the Medicaid program and others in the children's health community who were implementing CHIP [14].

Title II of HIPAA, known as Administrative Simplification, required the establishment of national standards for electronic exchange of transactions relating to health care and payment for health care, including such functions as health plan enrollment and disenrollment, claims submission and payment, referral authorization, and the like. Broadly speaking, the goal was to facilitate the transition of the U.S. health care system from antiquated paper records and communications systems to an efficient electronic information environment.

The HIPAA legislation also called for promulgation of standards for the privacy of individually identifiable health information if Congress did not pass national health privacy legislation within 3 years. Accordingly, in 1999, responsibility for developing regulations governing health privacy passed to the Department of Health and Human Services.

In the period from 1999 to 2002, HHS reached out to a broad array of stakeholders, first under the Clinton and later the Bush Administration, for input into the health privacy standards that Congress had been unable to produce through the legislative process. These stakeholders included physicians and hospitals, insurers and health plans, researchers, pharmaceutical companies, patient groups, and many others. The resulting HIPAA Security and Privacy rules [45 CFR Part 164] provide *rights* to individuals (patients) and mechanisms for the exercise of those rights, while imposing *obligations* on Covered Entities (and Business Associates performing functions on their behalf) to protect the security and privacy of individually identifiable health information and to facilitate the individual's rights. Emphasizing the fundamental rights granted to individuals by HIPAA, the HIPAA Privacy and Security rules are enforced by the HHS Office of Civil Rights (OCR).

The Privacy and Security regulations have been modified once, at the direction of Congress. The modification was included in the HITECH Act of 2009 provisions aimed at strengthening HIPAA's privacy, security and enforcement requirements and broadening the reach of the rules.

The Privacy and Security rules have been highly efficacious in causing "*Covered Entities and Business Associates*" to devote significant resources to complying with a complex regulatory environment, which includes everything from the obligation to post a Notice of Privacy Practices to enormously expensive breach reporting requirements if electronic health data is "lost" or improperly accessed.

However, the rules appear to have been only marginally successful in making information available across providers delivering care and to patients seeking access to their own medical records. To some extent, these challenges are the result of immature technologies, but to a significant degree, they are also the result of a lack of consensus among providers and administrators of exactly what HIPAA requires and how it should be implemented. As a result, the achievement of interoperable data exchange is generally understood to require the consent of every individual whose protected health information (PHI) is to be transmitted, or securing a waiver of individual consent from an Institutional Review Board (IRB). Given inadequate guidance on the topic of information exchange from the Office for Civil Rights, which enforces the HIPAA rules, it is no surprise that state and regional health information exchanges have had to devote enormous resources to the development of consent and governance models before attempting to exchange data, and that most covered entities simply don't try. As a consequence of the complexity of the rules, sanctions, and penalties, some providers are resistant to fulfilling record requests, often on the advice of their attorneys. Thus, HIPAA is often seen by stakeholders, including legislators and other policymakers, as a barrier to information exchange, rather than the facilitator it was meant to be.

Some experts believe that the development of shared governance structures and data use agreements for multisite research can open up opportunities to support the freer flow of information across settings and help create the trust needed for learning health systems of the future [29]. From this perspective, it is the significant variability in interpretations of HIPAA that poses the main challenge in clinical data sharing, not the regulations themselves.

Others, however, believe that the "medical records" framework of HIPAA in which it is "covered entities" that create, maintain, and are responsible for health data, is increasingly outmoded in an era of wearables, patient-generated data, and health care-related applications developed outside of the traditional health care system and that a broad overhaul of health privacy regulations is called for. As of early

2015, it is difficult to believe that the current Republican Congress and Democratic President could accomplish such an undertaking.

### 8.2.3.2   e-Prescribing in the Medicare Modernization Act (MMA)

In 2003, the Medicare Modernization Act (MMA) included a new prescription drug benefit (Part D) and required drug plans participating in the new benefit to support electronic prescribing (e-prescribing, or e-rx). The e-prescribing provisions were designed to improve patient safety by reducing illegible handwritten prescriptions, providing alert and warning systems that reduce errors, and making it easier to include prescription drug information in electronic health records (EHRs). Sending a prescription directly to a pharmacy eliminates phone calls, faxes, and call-backs by clinical offices, and it was estimated that cost savings from ADEs and workflow efficiencies could total approximately $27 billion per year. It was also estimated that e-prescribing could eliminate more than two million adverse drug events (ADEs) a year, including 130,000 that were life-threatening. These changes also could increase patient adherence, by making it easier for patients to fill and pick up their prescriptions.

In 2005, HHS awarded $6 million to five teams for pilot projects [2] to test and evaluate initial standards for e-prescribing (e.g., medication history, formulary and benefits, prescription fill status notification, and others) and their interoperability with other standards. The pilot project evaluation found that provider uptake and satisfaction were generally good, and that clinical staff played a much larger role than prescribers themselves by preparing many of the orders for the prescribers' review and signatures. This finding led to an acknowledgement of the need for significant clinical workflow changes to move from paper to electronic order systems [31], although that point was apparently totally missed in the development of HITECH.

The MMA also authorized the creation of a Commission on Systemic Interoperability, charged with "developing a strategy to make healthcare information instantly accessible at all times, by consumers and their healthcare providers." In its 2005 report, the Commission provided many examples of individuals benefitting through "connected healthcare," and one of its recommendations was ensuring "an interoperable medication record for every American," including access to one's own prescription drug history [10]. With the growing use of medication data exchanges by pharmacies, pharmacy benefits managers, and health plans, such a goal seemed possible. But that same year, Hurricane Katrina showed the glaring weaknesses in infrastructure needed to share prescription drug information across pharmacy and clinic locations for thousands of people whose paper records had been destroyed by the storm [28].

In 2005, the Institute of Medicine undertook a Congressionally-mandated study of the prevalence of medication errors in order to develop a national agenda to reduce them. The report acknowledged that medication errors are both common and costly [20], and the resulting media attention made it easier for CMS to promote and encourage providers to participate in the e-prescribing program [41].

Two years later, an e-Prescribing Incentive Program was created by Congress in the Medicare Improvements for Patients and Providers Act of 2008 (MIPPA), authorizing a new financial incentive program for successful e-prescribers. After 5 years, providers who did not use e-prescribing for Medicare beneficiaries would receive lower Medicare reimbursements as a penalty. This is the same approach used by the Meaningful Use program under HITECH, beginning with incentives and then phasing in penalties for non-participation.

### 8.2.3.3    The Health Information Technology for Economic and Clinical Health Act (HITECH)

The Health Information Technology for Economic and Clinical Health (HITECH) Act was part of the $787 billion economic stimulus package passed as The American Recovery and Reinvestment Act (ARRA) of 2009. HITECH provided between $25 and $36 billion in incentive payments to promote the adoption and use of electronic health record (EHR) systems to improve healthcare quality, reduce costs through improved efficiencies, and also improve consumers' access to their personal health information.

To reconcile the rapidity mandated by HITECH with the concerns that federal funds would not be spent wisely, ONC and CMS worked together on a regulatory framework to ensure the value of IT investments to providers and patients. They named this set of financial incentives, certification requirements, and regulations *"meaningful use"* [9, 32]. The program was launched in 2011 and will continue through 2016. To receive an incentive payment, providers need to show that they are "meaningfully using" certified EHR technology. Eligible providers and organizations must show through their reporting that they are meeting certain measurement thresholds.

These measurements have been developed with extensive public involvement and comment and reflect a blend of policy goals and industry and provider readiness and capacity. The first round of certification (Stage 1) emphasized basic EHR functionality, and relatively wide adoption occurred. The second round of certifications (Stage 2) required a greater degree of communication with external entities, and these have not yet been as broadly accepted. Beginning in 2015, eligible professionals who do not successfully demonstrate meaningful use of EHRs will become subject to financial penalties, and this transition from incentives to penalties is catching some providers without certified systems. The third round (Stage 3) was released in March 2015, and it reflects a new emphasis on data flow and flexibility, reflecting both the successes and failures of the previous two stages [24]. Recent adoption figures show that more than half of physicians and more than 60 % of hospitals are using EHRs, which shows significant progress [1, 12].

Five years after HITECH was introduced, the consequences are not yet fully knowable. The legislation has led to an unprecedented degree of EHR adoption and serves as a critical foundation for future efforts to coordinate care. There is no doubt that the implementation of HITECH was hindered by the wide variation in the provider community in terms of experience with EHRs and health information exchange. However, evidence suggests that within a year of implementation most providers have improved workflow efficiency, appreciate the ability to access patient information from the office or remote locations, and do not want to return to paper [26].

Overtime, the slow rate of adoption at the state level led to the realization that the incentives for interoperability are primarily to support regional exchange within a geographic market, following the referral patterns of local providers. This may be one of the most important lessons from HITECH: developing a national plan such as the National Health Information Network (NHIN) from the top-down makes sense from a policy perspective, but in the end, all implementation is local. The incentives and business case for providers to invest in Health IT are based on their need for clinical information to flow between hospitals and other healthcare settings to take better care of the same patients as they move through the system, usually within a defined geographic area or market. The abstraction of a "national network of networks" is appealing intellectually but very difficult to operationalize.

As of spring 2015, concerns about HHS priorities and strategies to promote interoperability have been expressed by many, including the Government Accountability Office (GAO) [42], members of the provider community [37], and six US Senators [38]. All but the most ideological critics recognize the growing need for a comprehensive technology infrastructure capable of interoperability and information exchange in ways that assure care is both safe and financially account-able. However, interoperability is not exclusively a technical and legal challenge. Hospitals and health care organizations compete with each other for patients and staff, and there is no financial or other incentive for them to share information in a competitive marketplace. This fact about the healthcare market is rarely raised in policy discussions.

### 8.2.3.4   Food and Drug Administration Safety and Innovation Act (FDASIA)

Passed in 2012, FDASIA gives the Food and Drug Administration (FDA) authority to continue to collect user fees from the biomedical industry, as well as to regulate medical software. By request of the Secretary of Health and Human Services (HHS), the Health IT Policy Committee convened a stakeholder group to advise on a risk-based framework for regulating software, in collaboration with the FDA and the

Federal Communications Commission. A full report from the three agencies was released in the spring of 2014 [16].

The tri-agency report found that EHRs are relatively low-risk, and that full FDA regulation would not be helpful and could stifle innovation. However, the report recommended the creation of a new HIT Safety Center to improve the design, development, implementation, maintenance, and use of Health IT to prevent any future risks to patients. A federal contract is currently providing input about the Center's mandate and goals and a report will be issued later in 2015.

## 8.3 The Changing Policy Goals of the Office of the National Coordinator (ONC)

Earlier sections of this chapter have described federal responsibilities for Health IT, the role of the private sector in influencing and implementing policy, and the importance of the Office of the National Coordinator for Health IT (ONC) in serving as the focal point and channel for Health IT policy initiatives, which have involved an unprecedented level of public-private collaboration. We have deliberately provided a broad policy context because the complexity of the policy development process is poorly understood and often underappreciated, and because it continues to evolve under the influence of different stakeholders in the Health IT space. This section focuses on the Office of the National Coordinator (ONC) as a barometer of Congressional support for Health IT and as a reflection of the value of public-private collaborations. As will become clear, ONC leadership has played an important role in influencing provider and industry engagement, as well as informing public opinion and increasing awareness of the value of real-time information exchange to the clinical enterprise and to patients and caregivers.

### 8.3.1 The National Coordinators for Health IT (ONC)

The position of National Coordinator for Health IT was created by Presidential Executive Order in April 2004, and was legislatively mandated in 2009 in the Health Information Technology for Economic and Clinical Health Act (HITECH). Even at the time of the creation of the Office of the National Coordinator (ONC), it was recognized that the primary barriers to implementation of a nationwide health information infrastructure were not primarily technological, but were more related to leadership and organizational factors.

The role of the National Coordinator was seen as essential to the federal role of bringing together private and public stakeholders, and all levels of government [30]. It was also partly symbolic at the time it was created, in that the emerging field of Health IT began to coalesce once its importance was acknowledged by locating

ONC administratively in the Office of the Secretary of HHS. Over the next decade, each one of the National Coordinators brought a different leadership style and expertise, faced a different set of issues, and had different policy and implementation priorities that are arguably more visible in hindsight than they were at the time.

David Brailer, a physician entrepreneur and economist, was the first ONC director or "Health IT czar." He was appointed in May 2004 and agreed to stay in the position for 2 years, after which he planned to return to the private sector. Previously, Dr. Brailer had founded CareScience, a spin-off from the Wharton School of Business at the University of Pennsylvania and one of the first companies to use electronic health information to improve the quality of care. Dr. Brailer's credibility in launching the new federal office came not only from his deep knowledge of Health IT, but from his industry perspective and ability to frame the business case for Health IT in terms of bringing value from improved efficiencies and cost savings. Dr. Brailer was popular with the business media and was interviewed frequently. He often described the history of underinvestment in Health IT, with most hospitals spending 2–3 % of their budgets compared to 10 % for other industries, and appealed to industry to invest in the new field [8].

During the time Dr. Brailer served as National Coordinator, HHS formed a Federal Advisory Committee known as the American Health Information Community (AHIC), which met for the first time in November 2005. HHS also issued five contracts to convene a Health IT Standards Panel (HITSP); develop criteria and evaluation processes for certifying EHRs (Certification Commission for Health IT, or CCHIT); develop prototype architectures for the National Health Information Network (NHIN); identify security and privacy barriers in business and state laws; and measure the state of EHR adoption.

In September 2006, Robert Kolodner left the Veterans Health Administration (VA) to become the Acting National Coordinator, an appointment which was confirmed in April 2007. Dr. Kolodner, a psychiatrist, was well known in Health IT and informatics circles for his leadership in a variety of VA Health IT solutions, including My HealtheVet, a Personal Health Record for veterans, and VistA – the first successful large-scale Electronic Health Record implementation. Kolodner's appointment was reassuring to the field after Brailer's departure because he had a track record of demonstrating that implementation can be achieved at a large scale and that EHRs can improve workflow. He worked to continue to build support for EHRs among the provider community by appearing at conferences and publishing articles in provider journals, and was generally regarded as a good steward of the federal investments in the emerging field.

Before his appointment, Kolodner had already gone on public record supporting the national health information infrastructure [39], and his knowledge of government and years of experience in inter-agency collaboration helped ONC establish relationships with the Agency for Healthcare Research and Quality (AHRQ), which had been funding Health IT research and implementation projects, and with the Centers for Medicaid and Medicare Services (CMS). In retrospect, his most important contribution may have been building trust among the private-sector members of the American Health Information Community (AHIC) and the federal advisory body formed in 2005 to advise the Secretary of HHS on how to accelerate the adoption of Health IT. He served until the 2008 election and the change of administration.

After President Obama took office in 2009, David Blumenthal took a leave of absence from Harvard University to become the new National Coordinator. A practicing internist, health policy expert, and effective public speaker, Dr. Blumenthal had served as an advisor for the Obama campaign. He came from the highly interconnected environment of Partners HealthCare, the Harvard-affiliated health system that was an early adopter of Health IT, and the hallmark of his leadership at ONC was his sharing many examples of his first-hand clinical experience in seeing how Health IT improved the quality of care.

As director of Harvard's Institute for Health Policy, Dr. Blumenthal had been involved in IOM committees and other efforts to promote adoption of Health IT in the academic medical community. The tsunami of $27 billion in funding from HITECH included $2 billion in direct appropriation for ONC to set up a nationwide network of regional Health IT extension centers to provide technical assistance to local providers; launch Health IT training programs in community colleges; oversee the two Federal Advisory Committees Act committees created by HITECH (the Health IT Policy Committee and the Health IT Standards Committee), and establish testing and certification criteria for EHR. Also during Blumenthal's tenure, work began on defining criteria for meaningful use of certified EHRs, and after an extensive public comment period, the Stage 1 Final Rules were published in the Federal Register in July 2010. Through it all, Blumenthal built consensus with AHRQ and CMS, and kept the ONC focused on the value of providing quality care in a safe, secure environment. He returned to Harvard after his 2-year leave of absence to resume his academic appointment there.

The fourth ONC Coordinator, Farzad Mostashari, had been serving as a Deputy at ONC and was promoted in April 2011. He had come to ONC from the New York City Department of Health and Mental Hygiene, where he had served as Assistant Commissioner for the Primary Care Information Project and oversaw the adoption of Health IT by 1,500 providers in low-income communities. An epidemiologist with expertise in developing biosurveillance systems, Dr. Mostashari's appointment shifted the meaningful use discussion to include public health reporting and population health, which reflected the policy priorities of the Affordable Care Act (ACA). He was an energetic advocate for the use of "big data" for planning and research, and also for direct consumer access to personal health information through Blue Button, developed by the VA and adapted by the Medicare program.

By this time, the meaningful use incentives were starting to work and the majority of providers were adopting and using EHRs, although interoperability was still a long way away. After the American Medical Informatics Association (AMIA) issued a report on the unintended consequences of Health IT in terms of patient safety [6], ONC asked the Institute of Medicine to study the issue. The subsequent IOM [22] report suggested that a systems approach was required to monitor the impact of Health IT on patient safety, including a user-centered design approach to make software improvements that are a better reflection of workflow and use patterns. The

IOM also called for the creation of a new Health IT Safety Council to set safety standards, and advised against the Food and Drug Administration (FDA) being given those responsibilities. After the IOM report on Health IT and patient safety was released, ONC released a draft plan on how to make it easier to track and fix Health IT problems due to software malfunctions and systems errors and received more than 100 comments [35].

Dr. Mostashari announced his departure in August 2013 and became a Visiting Fellow at the Brookings Institution a few months later to focus on helping small clinical practices adopt Health IT. He did not make his reasons public, but HHS Secretary Kathleen Sebelius acknowledged his leadership in presiding over the enormously complex implementation of HITECH, linking meaningful use to population health goals, and increasing the focus on patients and families [7].

In December 2013, Karen DeSalvo, Health Commissioner from New Orleans, became the new National Coordinator, continuing the policy focus on public health reporting and population health. After the Ebola outbreak began in West Africa during the summer of 2014, Dr. DeSalvo was named the Acting Assistant Secretary for Health while continuing as National Coordinator. Industry leaders questioned whether it was possible for her to perform both positions and called for a full-time replacement at ONC, particularly in light of the recent departures of several senior ONC leaders [27]. As of spring 2015, Dr. DeSalvo was still holding both positions.

### 8.3.2  ONC's Draft Interoperability Roadmap

The Version 1.0 Interoperability Roadmap released by ONC for public comment in January 2015 [33] seeks to remedy some of the major criticisms of the meaningful use program, which many providers see as overly bureaucratic and burdensome [3] and some policy-makers see as too slow in achieving interoperability [40]. The stated goal of the roadmap is to ensure that individuals and their providers can get accurate, electronic health information when and how they need it to make informed decisions about healthcare. ONC's Interoperability Roadmap also calls for public and private stakeholders to collaborate around a core set of business and functional requirements to achieve a learning health system within 10 years. ONC's call for collaboration represents more of an aspirational goal than a mandate. This goal of collaboration would require a major shift in key stakeholders' willingness to share information for the public good as reflected in the policy goal of improvements in patient care and safety while also helping providers achieve cost-saving efficiencies.

Concurrently, ONC released an interoperability standards document to help clarify the technical infrastructure requirements for the learning health system. "Learning Health System" is a term first used by the IOM to reflect the use of data analytics to generate knowledge that is used to improve the quality and effectiveness of healthcare. The "open draft" document is non-regulatory and non-binding and describes a less prescriptive process for interoperability and implementation standards for clinical Health IT. It is intended to "begin a dialogue" with the provider community, the research community, and industry by supporting areas of consensus and agreeing on ways to harmonize standards to allow providers flexibility while accelerating interoperability and supporting health information exchange [34].

Together, these plans, particularly if coupled with a relaxation of meaningful use mandates and other HIT-related penalties, may shift attention back to what providers and patients think technology should do. And that goal is to promote the flow of information to the right person at the right time. It remains to be seen how many of the currently factionalized stakeholders will be able to work together to achieve this common goal.

## 8.4   What Lies Ahead?

This chapter is being finalized during the public comment period for ONC's January 2015 Interoperability Roadmap, which covers the next 10 years. From a broad policy perspective, we foresee that hospitals, physicians and other providers will increasingly be part of a "system" that takes on responsibility for the health and health care of individuals and groups and populations. These sociocultural shifts will happen concurrently as the US moves toward patient-centered and accountable care and payment models that reward quality and value and not merely tests and procedures. Healthcare organization and all stakeholders – providers, payers, patients, caregivers, and healthy consumers – will benefit from secure but highly accessible data exchange. Data exchange will happen at the point of care, as well as in other settings where analytics, discovery, health planning, and software systems development take place.

Many factors contribute to the problem of interoperability, of course, including that health data is multi-faceted and difficult to digitize, that the complexity of HIPAA and other regulatory constraints meant to protect patients have erected barriers to out-of-the-box problem solving, that vendor competition encourages data siloes, that basic usability problems are legion, etc. We have referred to these and many other obstacles throughout the chapter.

From our perspective, however, a key problem is that the ultimate end-users of health care – namely, patients and their caregivers – are still "missing persons" in the quest for interoperability. Patient advocacy groups are sometimes present during policy discussions, but even the Patient Centered Outcomes Research Institute (PCORI) created by the Affordable Care Act has not been able to address the problem of patients' inability to access their own personal health information. In all of the ambitious and even heroic efforts to implement HITECH, the goal of promoting patient access through meaningful use has not motivated industry and providers to develop systems that "talk to each other" in real time to improve patient care and access to their own information.

Other industry sectors – from banking and insurance to automotive and retail sales – understand consumer data as an asset, and monetization of such data as a part of a business's revenue stream. Health data is different, of course, not only because it may be far more sensitive than other consumer data but because it is shared with the business (the health care provider or payer) for a specific, confidential purpose (the delivery of care or payment for such care). There is a general expectation that the information will not be further used or shared, except for purposes such as research and public health analytics, which are typically seen as public goods.

Interoperable data exchange, even within a policy framework that protects confidentiality and individual privacy, represents a fundamental shift to the traditional expectations of all the stakeholders: providers, plans, payers and, most importantly, patients, families, and caregivers. In fact, interoperability and information exchange presume a more communitarian model of care, in which providers, patients, and caregivers are engaged in shared, evidence-based decision-making based on personal and family preferences and understanding of risks. We think that the challenges of the transformation to patient-centeredness in the provider community may be as much or more of a challenge than realigning financial incentives in the policy community.

The combined impact of federal and private-sector initiatives can make innovation even more likely, but only if goals are more closely aligned. The Blue Button initiative is a fine example of disruptive innovation that serves the interests of patients, families, and caregivers by improving their direct access to personal health information. Consumer healthcare is a rapidly growing market, and the demand for web portals, remote monitoring devices, and other devices will increase if proposed changes in Medicare payment policies for telehealth are implemented.

HITECH is the most recent and largest single national investment in Health IT, and its implementation has been a massive undertaking. There is no comparable initiative in the history of US healthcare, and the largely voluntary mobilization of private sector entities to engage in enlightened self-interest while serving the public interest has been unprecedented, and not without significant challenges.

To realize transformational change, health information technology and health policy goals must be aligned with industry trends and interests of the private providers. We recognize that without that alignment, the current state will be maintained. We firmly believe that those healthcare organizations that will thrive under the new reimbursement requirements, will be those early adopters that embrace the ability to share patient data with the individual patient and external entities that serve as their primary care and community/home care partners. We hope that the learning health systems of the future will find that it is to their competitive advantage to focus on the common goal of achieving patient-centric systems with interoperability across providers and systems. Once this end-point is reached, we will have achieved transformational change that benefits all.

## 8.5 Timeline of Key Events in Health IT Policy

Given the number of legislative, executive branch, and private-sector initiatives that have influenced Health IT policy over the years, we developed a timeline of events as a reference document. Timelines often illuminate the sequence of events in ways that narrative does not, and also illustrate the proverbial saying that "change takes time."

| Timeline of key events in Health IT policy | |
| --- | --- |
| January 1991 | Institute of Medicine releases *The Computer-Based Patient Record: An Essential Technology for Health Care*, with a blueprint for transitioning to CPRs, later known as Electronic Health Records (EHRs) |
| December 1991 | Congress passes the High Performance Computing and Communications Act of 1991, creating the National Research and Education Network (NERN) as a partnership of government, industry, and academia and leading to the National Information Infrastructure (NII) or "information superhighway" |
| November 1993 | The Health Security Act, also known as the Clinton health reform proposal, was introduced in Congress |
| 1994 | HL7 becomes an ANSI-certified Standards Development Organization and the global authority on interoperability standards |
| 1994 | Community-based HIT initiatives (e.g., CHMIS, CHINS) inspired by the Clinton health reform proposals, begin to lose momentum with the Congressional failure to pass legislation |
| August 1996 | Congress passes the Health Insurance Portability and Accountability Act (HIPAA), with administrative simplification provisions requiring development of standards for electronic exchange of health information |
| December 2000 | After a year of comments on the proposed rule, the HIPAA Privacy Rule sets national standards to protect individually identifiable personal health information used by health plans, health care clearinghouses, and health care providers (covered entities) |
| April 2001 | Institute of Medicine report "Crossing the Quality Chasm" calls for a national commitment to an electronic infrastructure to support sharing of personal health information |
| November 2001 | The National Committee on Vital and Health Statistics sets out a national strategy for health information infrastructure (NHII) |
| August 2002 | The HIPAA Privacy Rule is modified and finalized, with a compliance date of April 2003 for most entities |
| February 2003 | The HIPAA Security Rule establishes national standards to protect the confidentiality, integrity, and security of electronic personal health information |
| December 2003 | Medicare Modernization Act (MMA) requires pharmacies and health plans to follow e-prescribing standards under Medicare Part D |
| April 2004 | Presidential Executive Order creates Office of the National Coordinator for Health IT in the Office of the HHS Secretary and calls for widespread use of Health IT within 10 years |
| May 2004 | David Brailer is appointed the first National Health Information Technology Coordinator |

(continued)

| Timeline of key events in Health IT policy | |
|---|---|
| July 2004 | Markle Foundation's Connecting for Health Initiative Issues *Preliminary Roadmap for Achieving Electronic Connectivity in Health Care* |
| October 2004 | Agency for Healthcare Research and Quality (AHRQ) funds $139 million in Health IT projects |
| August 2005 | Hurricane Katrina strikes Louisiana and Hurricane Rita strikes the Gulf Coast 25 days later. Ability to provide prescription medication lists and other basic health information is limited due to destruction of paper records by the storms (Markle Foundation, 2006)[1] |
| October 2005 | Commission on Systemic Interoperability issues a report recommending a prescription medication history for every American |
| November 2005 | HHS provides support for regional electronic health record (EHR) adoption in Gulf States as part of post-Katrina response, but state legal barriers later prevent implementation[2] (HHS 2005) |
| April 2006 | A public-private collaborative funded by Markle Foundation releases Connecting for Health, a common framework to develop a networked health information environment |
| Sept 2006 | Dr. Robert Kolodner begins serving as interim National Coordinator for Health IT and is appointed to position in April 2007 |
| May 2007 | ONC releases report on the NHIN Prototype Architecture Contracts, comparing the results of four consortia to develop a "network of networks" |
| October 2007 | HHS awards $22.5 million to test implementation of nine prototype state-level health information exchanges |
| November 2007 | Federal Communications Commission provides $400 million to rural areas for broadband to promote telehealth |
| September 2008 | Government Accountability Office releases a report advising the HHS could risk losing public trust unless it creates a comprehensive privacy, confidentiality, and security strategy |
| Feb 2009 | Congress passes the Health Information Technology for Economic and Clinical Health (HITECH) as part of the American Reinvestment and Recovery Act of 2009 (ARRA), outlining a "meaningful use" incentive program for adopting electronic health records. The bill makes permanent the Office of the National Coordinator and creates the HIT Policy Committee and HIT Standards Committee to advise ONC |
| March 2009 | David Blumenthal is appointed as National Coordinator for Health IT |
| March 2010 | The Patient Protection and Affordable Care Act (ACA) is enacted |
| December 2010 | President's Council of Advisors on Science and Technology (PCAST) issues report recommending ways to accelerate Health IT adoption and reduce healthcare costs |
| April 2011 | HHS Secretary Kathleen Sebelius appoints Dr. Farzad Mostashari as National Coordinator for Health IT |
| July 2012 | The Food and Drug Administration Safety and Innovation Act (FDASIA) expands the agency's regulatory authorities in medical device innovation and launches a public debate about its authority to regulate mobile health applications |
| January 2013 | HHS releases an "omnibus" Rule that makes changes to HIPAA Privacy, Security and Enforcement Rules as required by the HITECH statute |

(continued)

[1] Patton [36].

[2] HHS Press Office [17].

(continued)

| Timeline of key events in Health IT policy | |
|---|---|
| December 2013 | Dr. Karen DeSalvo is appointed National Coordinator for Health IT, and becomes Acting Assistant Secretary of Health in October 2014 |
| April 2014 | ONC, FDA, and the Federal Communications Commission (FCC) issue a joint report mandated by FDASIA to propose a risk-based regulatory framework for Health IT, including mobile medical applications that "promotes innovation, protects patient safety, and avoids regulatory duplication" |
| January 2015 | ONC releases a draft "interoperability roadmap" to achieve interoperable Health IT infrastructure within 10 years, seeking public comments by April 2015, and also issues a 2015 Interoperability Standards Advisory to highlight specifications for interoperable clinical Health IT |

# References

1. Adler-Milstein J, et al. More than half of US hospitals are using at least a basic EHR, but Stage 2 criteria remain challenging for most. Health Affairs. 2014. http://content.healthaffairs.org/content/33/9/1664.abstract.
2. Agency for Healthcare Research and Quality (AHRQ). E-prescribing pilot projects. [Internet]. 2005. http://healthit.ahrq.gov/ahrq-funded-projects/e-prescribing-pilot-projects.
3. American Medical Association (AMA). AMA provides blueprint to improve the meaningful use program. 14 Oct 2014. http://www.ama-assn.org/ama/pub/news/news/2014/2014-10-14-1m1-blueprint-improve-meaningful-use.page.
4. Atchinson BK, Fox DM. The Politics of the Health Insurance Portability and Accountability Act (HIPAA). Health Aff. 1997;16(3):146–50. Available at http://www.library.armstrong.edu/eres/docs/eres/MHSA8635-1_CROSBY/8635_week2_HIPAA_politics.pdf. Accessed 16 Jan 2015.
5. Berwick DM. A user's manual for the IOM's 'quality chasm' report. Health Aff. 2002;21(3):80–90. doi:10.1377/hlthaff.21.3.80. http://content.healthaffairs.org/content/21/3/80.full. Accessed 20 Feb 2015.
6. Bloomrosen M et al. Anticipating and addressing the consequences of Health IT and policy: a report from the AMIA 2009 health policy meeting. 13 Sept 2011. https://www.amia.org/sites/amia.org/files/Unintended%20Consequences%20of%20HIT.pdf.
7. Bowman D. Mostashari to leave ONC. 6 Aug 2013. http://www.fiercehealthit.com/story/National-Coordinator-Health-Information-Technology-Farzad-Mostashari-resigns-onc/2013-08-06.
8. Brailer D. Remarks by David Brailer MD, National Coordinator for Health Information Technology, HIMSS. 2005. Available at http://www.providersedge.com/ehdocs/ehr_articles/DavidBrailerRemarksHIMSS2005.pdf. Accessed 28 Mar 2015.
9. Centers for Medicare and Medicaid Services (CMS). Getting started. 2015. http://www.cms.gov/Regulations-and-Guidance/Legislation/EHRIncentivePrograms/Getting_Started.html. Accessed 15 Jan 2015.
10. Commission on Systemic Interoperability. Ending the document game. 2005. http://endingthedocumentgame.gov.
11. Department of Health and Human Services (HHS). Health and Human Services (HHS) FY 2015 Budget in Brief. [Internet] Sept 2014 [cited 2015 Jan 1]. Available at http://www.hhs.gov/budget/fy2015/fy-2015-budget-in-brief.pdf.
12. DesRoches C et al. Electronic health records in ambulatory care: a national survey of physicians. N Engl J Med. 2008. http://www.nejm.org/doi/full/10.1056/NEJMsa0802005.

13. Downs S. Blue button: driving a patient-centered revolution in health care. 2011. http://www. rwjf.org/en/blogs/culture-of-health/2011/09/blue-button-driving-a-patient-centered-revolution-in-health-care.html.
14. Edmunds M, Coye MJ. America's children: health insurance and access to care. Institute of Medicine. Washington, DC: National Academies Press; 1998.
15. Fisher ES, Wennberg JE. Health care quality, geographic variations, and the challenge of supply-sensitive care. Perspect Biol Med. 2003;46(1):69–79.
16. Food and Drug Administration, Federal Communications Commission, and Office of the National Coordinator. FDASIA HIT Report. Proposed Strategy and Recommendations for a Risk-Based Framework. [Internet] Apr 2014 [cited 20 February 2015]. Available from http:// www.fda.gov/downloads/AboutFDA/CentersOffices/OfficeofMedicalProductsandTobacco/ CDRH/CDRHReports/UCM391521.pdf.
17. HHS Press Office. HHS Enters into Agreements to Support Digital Health Recovery for the Gulf Coast. 17 Nov 2005. http://archive.hhs.gov/news/press/2005pres/20051117.html. Accessed 15 Nov 2014.
18. Institute of Medicine (IOM). Crossing the quality chasm: a new health system for the 21st century. Washington, DC: National Academy Press; 2001.
19. IOM. Coverage matters: insurance and health care. Washington, DC: National Academies Press; 2001. http://www.iom.edu/reports/2001/coverage-matters-insurance-and-health-care.aspx.
20. IOM. Preventing medication errors. Washington, DC: National Academies Press; 2006. Available at https://www.iom.edu/Reports/2006/Preventing-Medication-Errors-Quality-Chasm-Series.aspx.
21. IOM. Preventing medication errors. Washington, DC: National Academies Press; 2007. http:// www.nap.edu/catalog/11623/preventing-medication-errors-quality-chasm-series.
22. IOM. Health IT and patient safety: building safer systems for patient care. National Academies Press, Nov 2011. https://www.iom.edu/Reports/2011/Health-IT-and-Patient-Safety-Building-Safer-Systems-for-Better-Care.aspx.
23. IOM. Crossing the quality chasm: the IOM health care quality initiative. 8 May 2013. http:// www.iom.edu/Global/News%20Announcements/Crossing-the-Quality-Chasm-The-IOM-Health-Care-Quality-Initiative.aspx.
24. Jha A. The final stage of meaningful use: will EHRs finally pay off? 2015. http://healthaffairs. org/blog/2015/03/25/the-final-stage-of-meaningful-use-rules-will-ehrs-finally-pay-off/.
25. Lerner B. A case that shook medicine. The Washington Post, 28 Nov 2006. http://www.wash-ingtonpost.com/wp-dyn/content/article/2006/11/24/AR2006112400985.html.
26. Lorenzi N et al. How to successfully select and implement electronic health records (EHR) in small ambulatory practice settings. BMC Med Inform Decis Mak. 2009; 9(15), http://www. biomedcentral.com/1472-6947/9/15.
27. Marbury D. IT leaders call for DeSalvo's replacement at ONC. 12 Nov 2014. http://medi-caleconomics.modernmedicine.com/medical-economics/news/it-leaders-call-desalvo-s-replacement-onc.
28. Markle Foundation. Lessons from KatrinaHealth. 2006. https://www.markle.org/ publications/894-lessons-katrinahealth/.
29. McGraw D, Leiter A. Pathways to success for multi-site clinical data research. eGEMS. 2013;1(1):1–13. Available at http://repository.academyhealth.org/egems/vol1/iss1/13/.
30. National Committee on Vital and Health Statistics (NCVHS). Information for health: a strat-egy for building the national health information infrastructure. Chapter 5. Leadership as the cornerstone of implementation. Operationalizing the Recommendations. 2001. Available at http://aspe.hhs.gov/sp/nhii/documents/NHIIReport2001/report10.htm#ops.
31. National Opinion Research Center (NORC) for AHRQ. Findings from the evaluation of e-Prescribing Pilot Sites. 2007. http://healthit.ahrq.gov/sites/default/files/docs/page/ Findings%20from%20the%20Evaluation%20of%20E-Prescribing%20Pilot%20Sites.pdf.
32. Office of the National Coordinator (ONC). Meaningful use regulations. 17 Sept 2014. http:// www.healthit.gov/policy-researchers-implementers/meaningful-use-regulations. Accessed 15 Jan 2015.

33. ONC. Connecting health and health care for the nation: a shared nationwide interoperability roadmap. Draft Version 1 10. 2015. http://www.healthit.gov/sites/default/files/nationwide-interoperability-roadmap-draft-version-1.0.pef. Accessed 10 Feb 2015.

34. ONC. Standards advisory executive summary. 30 Jan 2015. 2015. [Internet]. http://www.healthit.gov/policy-researchers-implementers/executive-summary.

35. O'Reilly K. Ways EHRs can lead to unintended safety problems. 2013. http://www.amednews.com/article/20130225/profession/130229981/4/.

36. Patton S. Health care: medical records in the wake of hurricane Katrina. 15 Nov 2005. http://www.cio.com/article/2448113/virtualization/health-care--medical-records-in-the-wake-of-hurricane-katrina.html.

37. Pennic J. AMA-led Coalition Urges ONC to Change EHR certification. 1/22/2015. 2015. http://hitconsultant.net/2015/01/22/ama-led-coalition-urges-onc-to-change-to-ehr-certification/.

38. Thune S, Alexander, Roberts, Burr, Coburn, Enzi. REBOOT: re-examining the strategies need to successfully adopt health IT. 2013. Available at http://www.thune.senate.gov/public/index.cfm?p=health-it-report-comments.

39. Stead WW, Kelly BJ, Kolodner RM. Achievable steps toward building a National Health Information Infrastructure in the United States. J Am Med Inform Assoc. 2005;12(2):113–20. doi:10.1197/jamia.M1685 http://www.ncbi.nlm.nih.gov/pmc/articles/PMC551543/.

40. Sullivan T. Senators criticize ONC's interoperability roadmap. 2015. http://www.govhealthit.com/news/senators-criticize-oncs-interoperability-roadmap.

41. Trenkle T. HHS statement by Troy Trenkle on the benefits of electronic prescribing before the judiciary committee on electronic prescribing, U.S. Senate. 2007. http://www.hhs.gov/asl/testify/2007/12/t20071204d.html. 18 June 2013.

42. U.S. Government Accountability Office (GAO). HHS strategy to address information exchange challenges lacks specific prioritized actions and milestones. GAO 14-242. 2014. http://www.gao.gov/assets/670/661846.pdf.

# Part II
# The Evolving State
# of Health IT: Reinventing Care,
# Roles and Connections

# Introduction

The second section of the book bridges the current state of health IT (Part I) to emergent information technologies and approaches that are being explored and applied in healthcare (Part III). The authors provide perspectives on how approaches, roles and tasks in information management are being reinvented and re-fitted to better meet the needs of healthcare. Collectively, these chapters capture transformation that is happening in healthcare today through enabling technologies.

- Chapter 9 by Unertl, Holden and Lorenzi (Vanderbilt Univ and Indiana Univ) and Chapter 10 by Catalina Danis (Insights-driven Wellness Services, IBM) describe how to effect usability in systems design and implementation using specific case examples from their respective organizations. Both chapters discuss the new emerging roles in clinical informatics at executive and decision making levels, and in turn, how these new roles have influenced usability and the changing healthcare delivery system.
- Chapter 11 by Mark Hagland (Healthcare Informatics) and Chapter 12 by O'Brien and Mattison (Kaiser Permanente) discuss the changing roles of Chief Medical Information Officer, CMIO, Chief Nursing Information Officer, CNIO, and Chief Knowledge Officer, CKO, and the dramatic evolution of scope and breath of responsibilities these roles entail and how they reinvent organizations by leveraging information (and other healthcare) technologies to deliver improve healthcare delivery.
- Chapter 13 by Andrew Watson (Univ Pittsburg Medical Center) continues the discussion on healthcare transformation through technology and the twenty-first century telecommunication technologies impacting options on how clinicians work, communicate and deliver care.
- Chapter 14 by Reynolds and Jones (IBM and Wake Forest Baptist Hospital) discusses the pragmatic issues surrounding financing these efforts.
- Chapter 15 by Grundy and Hodach (IBM and Phytel) provide an overview of the patient centered medical home (PCMH) model of care, its economic drivers and opportunities to link enabling technologies to improve primary care. The PCMH focus on the patient at the center of care is carried forward in Chapter 16 by Minitti and colleagues, (CarePartners Plus); and in Chapter 17 by Gibbons and Shaikh (Johns Hopkins) Both chapters focus on the use of technology to empower patients to participate in care, to enable the sharing of plans across venues and provider teams, to put the consumer, the patient into the driver's seat of care to improve the care of individuals and ultimately the health of populations.

# Chapter 9
# Usability: Making It Real from Concepts to Implementation and End-User Adoption

Kim M. Unertl, Richard J. Holden, and Nancy M. Lorenzi

**Abstract** The goal of this chapter is to explore usability, beginning with concepts and continuing through the application of these concepts to real-world health information technology implementations. Throughout the chapter, we present examples of usability concepts in practice through a case study of designing, developing, implementing, and refining an electronic health record at Vanderbilt University Medical Center. The case study presented here relates a specific implementation of a system developed in-house at an academic medical center, However, we offer the process and concepts discussed in the case as being transferable to other types of institutions and to vendor systems, as practices that extend beyond basic design principles to implementation and the outcome of usable and useful technology implementations with high rates of adoption.

**Keywords** Usability • Implementation • Human-computer interaction • Sociotechnical systems • User experience • User-centered design

K.M. Unertl, PhD, MS (✉)
Department of Biomedical Informatics, Vanderbilt University School of Medicine, Nashville, TN, USA
e-mail: kim.unertl@vanderbilt.edu

R.J. Holden, PhD
Department of BioHealth Informatics, Indiana University School of Informatics and Computing, Indianapolis, IN, USA
e-mail: rjholden@iupui.edu

N.M. Lorenzi, PhD, MA, MS
Department of Biomedical Informatics, Vanderbilt University School of Medicine and School of Nursing, Vanderbilt University, Nashville, TN, USA
e-mail: nancy.lorenzi@vanderbilt.edu

© Springer International Publishing Switzerland 2016
C.A. Weaver et al. (eds.), *Healthcare Information Management Systems: Cases, Strategies, and Solutions*, Health Informatics,
DOI 10.1007/978-3-319-20765-0_9

165

## 9.1 Introduction

Over the years of growth and development in the biomedical informatics and health information technology fields, one refrain is too often heard: "I created fantastic technology that solves a pressing problem! Why won't people use it?!?" [1, 2]. Many factors underlie success and failure of technology in healthcare settings. One component that helps set the stage for success involves planning for, integrating, and evaluating usability. The concept of usability has been defined in many different ways, drawing on multiple theories, practical experiences, and regulations [3–6].

The Food and Drug Administration in the United States has applied multiple standards from groups such as the International Organization for Standardization (ISO) and the American National Standards Institute (ANSI) in defining the role of usability in development and testing of medical devices [7]. ISO Standard IEC 62366:2015 *Medical devices: Application of usability engineering to medical devices* defines usability as "characteristic of the user interface that establishes effectiveness, efficiency, ease of user learning and user satisfaction" [8]. While these technical components of usability are crucial to establishing a standardized perspective for regulatory purposes, they omit several components beyond the technical details that are crucial to achieving overall usability, especially with respect to contextual factors (e.g., clinical setting, workflow, communication patterns, layout of space, number and type of available computers, timing of shift changes) that influence usability.

Zhang and Walji explored additional components of usability focused specifically on electronic health records in the TURF framework [9]. Dimensions included in defining usability in the TURF framework are: useful, usable, and satisfying. Each of the dimensions has multiple objective and subjective measures to evaluate overall usability. The TURF framework provides a helpful foundation for discussions about usability of health information technology, but incorporates contextual factors only in a limited fashion. Sociotechnical systems approaches towards healthcare human factors have a greater emphasis on contextual factors such as workflow and interruptions in defining and assessing usability [10–12].

**Case Study**
**Introducing a case study of a path towards usability**
Annual use statistics of the clinical systems have been maintained for years. A review of the 2013 statistics showed that the medical center had approximately 50,000 hospital discharges and 1.9 million outpatient visits. During that same period on a typical workweek day approximately 11,100 people connected into the clinical information systems. The electronic health record (EHR) system was accessed over 5.2 billion times. Users added almost 11.5 million electronic documentation notes to the EHR and a significant number of clinical items were scanned into the system in addition.

Clinicians wrote approximately 3.6 million orders through the medical center's inpatient clinical provider order entry system. In outpatient areas, physicians wrote more than 1.7 million prescriptions using the outpatient electronic prescribing system. Almost 7,000 patients logged in to the patient portal on a daily basis. Although usage statistics are not a complete indicator of usability, the growth in technology use in this case took place largely without institutional mandates requiring technology use, making usage a proxy for usability. What path did the medical center in the case study take to achieve this phenomenal technology usage rate? What were the key steps along the path?

**Back at the beginning**

Fifteen years earlier, in 1999, patient volumes at Vanderbilt University Medical Center (VUMC) began to increase dramatically. Paper-based records and processes still dominated care delivery in outpatient clinics. Leadership in both the ambulatory clinical area and the informatics operations area decided that the time to replace the paper processes with electronic processes was now, and that an assertive and concentrated effort was required.

Organizational estimates indicated that removing paper processes by implementing an EHR in outpatient areas would greatly cut costs. The institution also believed that it would have a blank slate to rework procedures, to enable maximum efficiency. The clinical and informatics leaders agreed in 2000 that they would work together to develop or purchase appropriate information systems and the E3 project (**E**lectronic by 200**3**) was launched.

The driving goal behind change became transformation of the healthcare system into a model for the future. This included both redesigning outpatient clinics and creating enabling technology tools to "**T**ransform our **O**rganization through **P**eople and **S**ystems" (TOPS). Five interconnected TOPS components constituted the transformation goals:

1. Delivering the right care and only the right care through clinical guidelines, evidence-based medicine, and reduction of process variation.
2. Delivering the right information when and where needed through information technology systems.
3. Quality patient interaction including listening to patients, meeting patient needs, and involving patients in care.
4. Supporting patient transactions through processes that minimized wait times and delays.
5. Having a culture where employees understand and model the science of improvement in their daily work.

Taken together, these five goals provided a foundation for linked organizational change and technology development.

## 9.2   Understanding the Product Design Life-Cycle

Incorporating usability principles into a software product begins far before software developers ever write the first line of code and continues well beyond the day people begin using the software. The Product Design Life-Cycle can be described as having four main phases, although the names and definitions of phases vary: Planning, Pre-design, Design and Development, and Post-design [5, 13–15]. Considering usability across all product life-cycle phases is crucial to development and implementation of a useful, usable, and satisfying technology.

The Planning Phase, illustrated in the case study segment "Back at the Beginning," is an organization and context focused phase. Understanding and modeling existing processes provides important input into design decisions [16, 17]. User-centered design and human factors engineering approaches to usability are predicated on a sociotechnical systems model, rather than viewing technology in isolation from the context of use [18, 19]. With this perspective, technology is viewed as serving the goals of the individual end users and of the organization, rather than as a neutral agent [20–22]. Technology will inevitably interact with processes, requiring fundamental choices in design about whether existing processes (a) will be supported "as is" and the technology design will be integrated into current processes or (b) will be changed in part or whole and the technology will be designed to fit into new processes [23]. Decisions made in this initial phase will fundamentally influence the direction of the overall technology design, and may result in concomitant changes to processes to ensure a usable process-technology fit.

The next phase of the Product Design Life-Cycle, the Pre-design Phase, involves approaches to gather data about the intended users, their tasks, needs, and context of use and developing conceptual models based on this data. Methodologies to gather and understand contextual data in this phase can include modeling and needs assessments. Modeling can take many different formats, including mapping of workflow, work processes, information flow, and multiple other graphical interpretations of the existing context [24, 25]. Needs assessments and development of user requirements specifications are required for a user-centered perspective on technology. Needs can be assessed and requirements developed based on multiple types of data collection, including observation of current work, interviews with stakeholders and end users, expert analysis, and focus groups. Many different disciplines can and should be involved in the process of assessing and mapping needs, including subject matter experts, human factors engineers, social scientists, engineers, and computer scientists. While there is a tendency to be overly reliant on technology expertise in needs assessment, incorporating knowledge from the social sciences and sociotechnical systems disciplines is helpful in understanding the human elements of technology usage. Usability involves multiple goals, not just user satisfaction. As the case study illustrates, these goals may include efficiency and effectiveness, but user requirements can also include other types of goals like patient engagement, improved clinical processes, and better information flow [26, 27].

The Design and Development Phase is the third phase of the Product Design Life-Cycle, and involves iterative cycles of design, Design and Development, testing, verification, and implementation. Design specifications are based on the user requirements developed in the Pre-design Phase, with the end goal of the seamless integration of user requirements into the product design. Design and Development can take many formats, including initial "mock ups" of intended technology features, to partially or fully functional interactive software versions. Continuous testing and verification of prototypes with end users continues building towards development of a usable product.

Finally, once a usable version of the software that meets the needs of end users has been developed and implemented, the product moves into the Post-design Phase. This phase involves evaluating use of the product after implementation and continuing to monitor use over time. Post-implementation surveillance of use and redesign to fit changing requirements, such as new organizational policies or shifts in responsibilities, are important parts of the user-centered design life-cycle [4, 13].

**The Early Phase of E3**

The E3 effort had three executive leaders representing three distinct groups: informatics, outpatient clinics, and nursing. The informatics leader was a physician with an extensive technology background and led the entire informatics group at the medical center. The outpatient clinic representative was the Executive Director of all outpatient clinics at the medical center, had an extensive business background, and was trained in psychology and organizational development. The nursing representative was the Chief Nursing Officer of the medical center. The individual hired to lead the E3 effort on a day-to-day basis was trained in psychology and sociology, had a doctoral degree in Organizational Behavior, and had a reputation for successfully managing large-scale change elsewhere. The strength of the leadership team for the E3 effort established credibility for the importance of the effort to the organization.

The first action in the E3 effort was to convene a Clinical Visioning Group, consisting of 12 respected clinicians from multiple disciplines. The mission of the Clinical Visioning Group was to formulate an image of information-communication needs for desired patient care in 2004. Effectively, the goal was to design what the patient care would look like in the future, with information technology support and new processes in place. Members of the group were carefully selected with the following criteria:

1. High-volume thought leaders
2. Respected quality diagnosticians
3. Experts in his/her respective areas
4. Other opinion leaders

When the Clinical Visioning Group convened, the goals of the E3 effort and the purpose of the visioning exercise were explained. The group was asked to walk through the scenario of practicing medicine 4 years in the future. Initially, the group compiled a nine-page long wish list for the future. In subsequent meetings, the group outlined priorities and established key goals from the initial list. The wish list was delivered to the informatics staff for assessment of feasibility. The top priority defined by the Clinical Visioning Group was a user-friendly front-end to unify navigation of multiple available technology products.

Concurrently, a group called the Informatics Brain Trust was created, comprised half of informatics staff and half of technology-savvy clinicians. The mission of this group was to develop an integrated picture of existing informatics tools and efforts, current opportunities, and future options – addressing the top priority defined by the Clinical Visioning Group. The group outlined a clinician-friendly front-end user interface design, and commissioned the informatics staff to design a screen layout and develop a prototype.

The new front-end user interface connected all of the existing multiple interfaces and systems. The initial prototype was distributed to seven of the clinicians on the Informatics Brain Trust. Usage grew rapidly from the initial 7 to 12–25, 75, and beyond. Suddenly over 300 people were using the prototype, without any official system rollout. At a meeting convened to name the product, the main question asked was: "What is the most significant feature of the product?" Users responded that it "assembled" all of a clinician's patients' names and information (i.e., their panel of patients), and so the StarPanel product name was created. Usage stories promoted further use of the tool. Individuals using StarPanel reported to peers that StarPanel increased the "just-in-time" information needed for patient care and made their work easier. As more and more people began using the tool, the excitement about StarPanel was palpable in the organization.

Development of a user-friendly front end was only one of the Clinical Visioning Group's priorities and goals. The group identified user requirements related to patient flow management, integrated story about the patient, actions, capturing information, internal business knowledge, and external knowledge. The long-range vision of the group also led them to specify user requirements around long-term use of informatics, recognizing that growth of information in the EHR would require robust strategies for searching through patient records for specific types of data and information.

## 9.3   Principles for Good Design and Usability

Usability must be a priority and embedded from the start, not added on as an afterthought or post-design [28, 29]. User involvement in iterative product design and development is crucial. Incorporating the perspective of intended end users into the design needs to begin before the design takes shape and needs to continue through product evaluation and usage monitoring. While physicians and other healthcare team members may not have technological skills to contribute to the design, they are the experts on the work and on the context that they work within. Finding appropriate ways for end users to contribute to the design process, such as the Clinical Visioning Group and Informatics Brain Trust in the case example, is a core usability principle. Acknowledging the expertise that end users bring to the table is a helpful strategy not just for producing usable products, but also for contributing to overall implementation success.

## 9.4 Concepts to Consider in End-User Participation in System Designs

The case study shows that several different groups contributed to the design process including clinical leaders, technology-oriented clinicians, and technology experts. Incorporating feedback from "super-users" and technology experts can push the boundaries of technology, as these individuals may be more aware of cutting-edge technology concepts than "average" users. However, working with only these types of individuals in the design process has significant implications for usability. Technology-oriented clinicians and technology experts may have different perspectives on user needs and system usability than the full range of intended end users. These individuals may make assumptions about how people will use technology based on their own experiences, which may deviate from how less technology-oriented end users will interact with the technology. By incorporating perspectives from users with a strong technology orientation and other types of users, the development process used at VUMC and illustrated in our case study helped to mitigate "designer fallacy" [1, 30]. Incorporating feedback from multiple diverse individuals (i.e., physicians, nurses, ancillary care providers) into design of a single system helped ensure that the technology was usable for different types of users. Technology intended to serve the needs of people in different roles should incorporate feedback from those different roles into the design process. For example, a system that both nurses and physicians will use should include both groups in the design process.

Furthermore, in the case, the designers and developers built on requirements specified by different types of end users and from multiple different sources of data. Design should be based on needs-assessment gathered from multiple sources [5]. Design based around the needs of highly technology-oriented end users will face significant challenges when attempts are made to implement the technology across a broader user base.

The case study also reviews how the concept of specific heuristics for usable design, e.g., Nielsen's [3] and others, were applied to the case. These heuristics promote design strategies such as grouping similar objects, reducing reliance on memory, and use of familiar metaphors – all user specifications included in the Clinical Visioning Group's prioritized feature list. The case study also demonstrated a variety of usability heuristics that comply with specific and general principles of design for usability, such as the reduction of excessive workload, combining multiple related pieces of data in a single place, putting computational burdens on machines while allowing human users to perform pattern recognition and communication functions, and avoiding the automation of decisions and action execution [3, 31–35].

Finally, in designing and developing usable systems, laboratory-based usability testing is a helpful methodology, but needs to be complemented by testing in the intended usage environment. Factors that can easily be eliminated in a laboratory setting, such as noise levels and interruptions, can have substantial impacts on the usability of technology. For example, a technology system with multiple required steps and limited ability to save work along the way may perform adequately in a laboratory setting. However, in a busy clinical environment with multiple interruptions and sources of distraction, ability to save work incrementally can be a critical feature. The sociotechnical systems approach tightly incorporates contextual factors into definitions and concepts of system usability, and stresses the importance of technology as just one element in a larger system of work. The interaction between people and technology is the key element of this perspective on usability, not just the features and functionality of the technology or the work being done by a person separately. Usability is a social process and occurs within a real-world context, not with in a closed and experimental setting.

---

**Building on Success and Moving Towards the Future**

With a successful initial prototype, the next critical step was deciding on the implementation process. There were two main implementation strategies discussed. The organization could continue with developing other components of the EHR or it could implement this panel component. The first model was referred to "an inch wide and a mile deep". The second model was referred to as "a mile wide and an inch deep." For the first model it would take much longer to develop or purchase the products requested and for the second model there would be instant benefits with practitioners using the panel component of the EHR.

The organization chose to implement the product in layers of tools and technology. The initial implementation focused on the user interface that would assemble and present a panel of patients from the underlying core electronic record. With this core functionality available, later product development cycles would focus on additional tools and functions including electronic documentation programs, electronic prescription writing, provider-patient communication support, and so on. Taken together, these various tools and functions, all united within a common user interface front-end, comprised the electronic health record technology.

A cross-functional team of individuals was assembled to manage implementation of tools across the organization. The Systems Support Team took responsibility for continuing the implementation of various features and tools across different outpatient clinics. Implementation moved rapidly through the organization. While there were setbacks and challenges along the way, the organization achieved the goal of establishing a baseline level of "Electronic by 2003" (**E3**). This marked a rapid successful expansion in the use of technology to support patient care across outpatient environments.

### Brief Overview of the Post-Implementation Years

During the 10 years from 2003 to the 2013 usage statistics, many organizational and technology changes occurred. Expansion in physical space, including a new Children's Hospital and pediatric office tower, plus the expansion to a number of off-site locations led to the continuous expansion of the EHR system. Many of the additional technology advances to support patient flow, such as an electronic outpatient whiteboard and the patient portal, were driven by the initial Clinical Visioning strategic effort.

The need to address federal Meaningful Use regulations shifted technology development to focus on achieving specific metrics, sometimes at the cost of developing responsive user-centered technology. Concurrently, the organization has integrated additional formal expertise in usability and human factors engineering, building on the original vision of organizational transformation supported by processes and technology.

## 9.5  Beyond Usability

Although this chapter has focused on usability, as the case study demonstrated, the successful design and implementation of usable systems includes multiple components beyond ensuring that technology works as needed [36]. Good project management and organizational leadership for technology design and implementation are key elements, because of the need for planning and supervision of the overall process. Planning for technology implementation through selection of appropriate strategies based on evidence is crucial. This planning needs to begin early in the design process, and needs to evolve over time and in response to specific organizational considerations. In addition, the timing of the implementation is also crucial, including building on momentum within the organization to successfully expand use. Whether the scale of the technology implementation is small or large, providing appropriate levels of support and expertise for both technology and processes can assist with achieving successful implementation. While none of these factors are explicitly usability principles, they interact with the technology design to influence the success of the technology implementation. The most perfectly designed software application with empirically proven high usability can still fail to achieve intended outcomes if these factors beyond usability are not considered. At the same time, if usability of the technology is done correctly, then the factors beyond usability will be easier to account for and can be more successfully addressed. Past success is a driver of future success. As the technology system described in our case became more embedded within an organization, demand for additional components grew and in turn adoption of the system continued to expand. If usability principles are embedded throughout all processes of system design and development, then what follows in implementation will flow more easily, with higher adoption rates and faster uptake.

We recommend a two-tiered approach to ensuring that technology is effective, efficient, easy to learn, satisfying to use, acceptable to end users, and sustainable in the organization. The first tier involves an iterative process of: field work and needs assessments to ensure that design supports users and user performance; design that follows the principles for usable interface design; and usability testing with intended end users to verify or correct the design. The second tier is an iterative process of: scanning the organizational, political, regulatory, technical, and social environments to ensure that implementation is compatible with them; creating an implementation plan that is appropriately scoped, paced, and resourced; and technology implementation that is flexible and attentive to both early wins and emerging problems. If these two processes are done in parallel and integrated so that design issues are managed during the implementation process and implementation issues are addressed through redesign, then an organization can boast both "making it real" and "really making it."

# References

1. Karsh B-T, Weinger MB, Abbott PA, et al. Health information technology: fallacies and sober realities. J Am Med Inform Assoc. 2010;17:617–23. doi:10.1136/jamia.2010.005637.
2. Bardram JE. I love the system – I just don't use it! New York: ACM Press; 1997. p. 251–60. doi:10.1145/266838.266922.
3. Nielsen J. Usability engineering. San Diego: Morgan Kaufmann; 1993.
4. Hegde V. Role of human factors/usability engineering in medical device design. Proceedings of the Annual Reliability and Maintainability Symposium (RAMS) 2013;1–5. doi:10.1109/RAMS.2013.6517650.
5. Samaras GM, Horst RL. A systems engineering perspective on the human-centered design of health information systems. J Biomed Inform. 2005;38:61–74. doi:10.1016/j.jbi.2004.11.013.
6. Holden RJ, Karsh B-T. The technology acceptance model: its past and its future in health care. J Biomed Inform. 2010;43:159–72. doi:10.1016/j.jbi.2009.07.002.
7. Weinger MB, Wiklund ME, Gardner-Bonneau DJ, editors. Handbook of human factors in medical device Design. Boca Raton: CRC Press; 2010.
8. ISO Standard IEC 62366-1:2015 Medical devices part 1: application of usability engineering to medical devices. Geneva: International Organization for Standardization; 2015.
9. Zhang J, Walji MF. TURF: toward a unified framework of EHR usability. J Biomed Inform. 2011;44:1056–67. doi:10.1016/j.jbi.2011.08.005.
10. Lindgren H. Sociotechnical systems as innovation systems in the medical and health domain. In: Editors. Context sensitive health informatics: human and sociotechnical approaches. Beuscart-Zephir M, Jaspers M, Kuziemsky C, et al., Amsterdam: IOS Press. 2013; p. 35–40.
11. Savioja P, Norros L. Systems usability framework for evaluating tools in safety–critical work. Cogn Tech Work. 2013;15:255–75. doi:10.1007/s10111-012-0224-9.

12. Carayon P, Bass E, Bellandi T, et al. Socio-technical systems analysis in health care: a research agenda. IIE Trans Healthc Syst Eng. 2011;1:145–60. doi:10.1080/19488300.2011.619158.
13. Israelski E. Testing and evaluation. In: Weinger MB, Wiklund ME, Gardner-Bonneau DJ, editors. Handbook of human factors in medical device design. Boca Raton: CRC Press; 2010. p. 201–50.
14. Toms EG. User-centered design of information system. In: Bates MJ, editor. Understanding information retrieval systems: management, types, and standards. Boca Raton: CRC Press; 2012. p. 65–76.
15. Jokela T, Iivari N, Matero J, et al. The standard of user-centered design and the standard definition of usability: analyzing ISO 13407 against ISO 9241-11. CLIHC '03 Proceedings of the Latin American conference on Human-computer interaction. ACM, New York, 2003. p. 53–60.
16. Wears RL, Berg M. Computer technology and clinical work: still waiting for Godot. JAMA. 2005;293:1261–3. doi:10.1001/jama.293.10.1261.
17. Suchman L. Making work visible. Commun ACM. 1995;38:56. doi:10.1145/223248.223263.
18. Carayon P. Human factors of complex sociotechnical systems. Appl Ergon. 2006;37:525–35. doi:10.1016/j.apergo.2006.04.011.
19. Smith SW, Koppel R. Healthcare information technology's relativity problems: a typology of how patients'physical reality, clinicians' mental models, and healthcare information technology differ. J Am Med Inform Assoc. 2014;21:117–31. doi:10.1136/amiajnl-2012-001419.
20. Forsythe DE. New bottles, old wine: hidden cultural assumptions in a computerized explanation system for migraine sufferers. Med Anthropol Q. 1996;10:551–74. doi:10.1525/maq.1996.10.4.02a00100.
21. Bullock A. Does technology help doctors to access, use and share knowledge? Med Educ. 2014;48:28–33. doi:10.1111/medu.12378.
22. Nardi BA, O'Day V. Information ecologies. Cambridge, MA: MIT Press; 1999.
23. Suchman LA. Plans and situated actions. Cambridge: Cambridge University Press; 1987.
24. Beyer H, Holtzblatt K. Contextual design. San Diego: Morgan Kaufmann; 1998.
25. Unertl KM, Weinger MB, Johnson KB, et al. Describing and modeling workflow and information flow in chronic disease care. J Am Med Inform Assoc. 2009;16:826–36. doi:10.1197/jamia.M3000.
26. Novak LL, Holden RJ, Anders SH, et al. Using a sociotechnical framework to understand adaptations in health IT implementation. Int J Med Inform. 2013;82:e331–44. doi:10.1016/j.ijmedinf.2013.01.009.
27. Holden RJ, Carayon P, Gurses AP, et al. SEIPS 2.0: a human factors framework for studying and improving the work of healthcare professionals and patients. Ergonomics. 2013;56:1669–86. doi:10.1080/00140139.2013.838643.
28. Ambler S. User interface development throughout the system development lifecycle. In: Chen Q, editor. Challenges human computer interaction: issues. Hershey: Idea Group Publishing; 2001. p. 11–28.
29. Bias RG, Mayhew DJ. Cost-justifying usability. San Francisco: Morgan Kaufmann; 2005.
30. Norman DA. The design challenge. In: Norman DA, editor. The design of everyday things. New York: Basic Books; 2002. p. 141–86.
31. Parasuraman R, Sheridan TB, Wickens CD. A model for types and levels of human interaction with automation. IEEE Trans Syst Man Cybern A. 2000;30:286–97. doi:10.1109/3468.844354.
32. Norman DA. The design of everyday things. New York: Basic Books; 2013.
33. Ben Shneiderman, Plaisant C. Designing the user interface. Boston, MA: Addison-Wesley Professional; 2010.
34. Gerhardt-Powals J. Cognitive engineering principles for enhancing human-computer performance. Int J Hum Comput Interact. 1996;8:189–211.
35. Burns CM, Hajdukiewicz J. Ecological interface design. Boca Raton: CRC Press; 2013.
36. Karsh B-T. Beyond usability: designing effective technology implementation systems to promote patient safety. Qual Saf Health Care. 2004;13:388–94. doi:10.1136/qhc.13.5.388.

# Chapter 10
# Incorporating Patient Generated Health Data into Chronic Disease Management: A Human Factors Approach

Catalina M. Danis

**Abstract** Understanding the relationships between technology design and Human Factors can help overcome barriers to incorporating patient generated health data (PGHD) into the day-to-day management of chronic disease. User Centered Design (UCD), a Human Factors approach that frames technology design in terms of users, tasks and contexts, can help developers to understand barriers to incorporating PGHD into patient and provider workflows and into electronic health record systems (EHR-S). An example of the application of UCD is presented within the context of primary care delivery for a hypothetical patient with Hypertension/Type II Diabetes Mellitus (DM2), with a focus on barriers and design issues inherent in incorporating PGHD into the EHR and into practice workflow. The results of a field trial are presented as an application of the UCD methodology in the evolution of a mobile application for collecting and using PGHD for patient disease monitoring.

**Keywords** Patient engagement • IT/information technology • Human factors • User centered design (UCD) • Stakeholders • End-users

## 10.1 Introduction

Patient generated health data (PGHD) is defined as health-related information that is "created, recorded, gathered, or inferred by or from patients or their designees" [39]. Its importance in health care has been articulated by the federal government through its projected incorporation into Stage 3 Meaningful Use criteria for certified electronic health record systems (EHR-Ss). In addition to secure messaging, health risk assessments and pre-visit questionnaires, mobile technology (smartphones) connected to EHR-Ss and data analytics hold great promise for supporting patients in chronic disease management. However, implementation and deployment of

C.M. Danis, PhD
Health Informatics Research, IBM T.J. Watson Research Center, Yorktown Heights, NY, USA
e-mail: danis@us.ibm.com

© Springer International Publishing Switzerland 2016
C.A. Weaver et al. (eds.), *Healthcare Information Management Systems: Cases, Strategies, and Solutions*, Health Informatics,
DOI 10.1007/978-3-319-20765-0_10

usable, successful and sustainable applications in healthcare present challenges for realizing the promise.

One approach to designing technology that supports the incorporation of PGHD into care lies in Human Factors. The focus of Human Factors is to understand users' (that is, patients' and providers') capabilities and needs within the contexts (day-to-day management of chronic disease) and tasks they must perform (effective management of PGHD). This approach to design and development has been shown to result in technology systems that are successful in achieving user goals and reducing costs [25, 46].

## 10.2 Patient Generated Health Data

Clinicians and policy makers have long advocated for active engagement of patients with chronic diseases in self-care [3, 4, 21, 35]. Clinical and population health research has demonstrated better outcomes when patients are engaged in at least some aspects of their own care [4, 13, 27, 28, 44, 45]. Important components of successful engagement of patients are:

- **Data collection by patients and its incorporation into ongoing care**
  When combined with traditional clinical data (physical examination, test results, etc.) and provider observations, PGHD can provide the physician a fuller picture of the day-to-day circumstances that describe patients' life situations and disease trajectories [4, 5, 41].

- **Self-awareness and learning by the patient**
  Patients attending to their health data, on their own but in the context of a patient-physician relationship, can learn how to take better care of themselves [4, 5, 41]. Evidence from the multi-year Project HealthDesign [5] has shown that patients can and do utilize their own "observations of daily living [to] draw interpretations about their daily life" and make better health and care choices.

Design of information systems to realize PGHD management has been challenging. Self-monitoring (e.g., tracking of one's behavior through journaling) has been recognized as the single most effective technique for bringing about behavior change, yet its uptake is modest. Most successful changes in patients' health behaviors are not explained by their use of existing tools, and even when urged by their health care providers to use such tools, many patients remain unable to make sustainable health behavior changes [12].

Paradoxically, healthcare providers, the principal consumers of PGHD, pose another challenge to its incorporation into care. In a recent study of physicians from 13 European countries, participants, when asked about patients' engagement in their own care, reported concerns about the potential impact of PGHD on their (the physicians') workloads [14].

On the US policy level, Stage 3 Meaningful Use (MU) criteria for certified EHR technology will focus on specific objectives for using PGHD in shared decision-making and for clinical quality measures. However, mixed success of implementing Stage 2 MU criteria [15, 43] has raised concerns and continuing debate about the feasibility of Stage 3 objectives [1, 41]. Nevertheless, interest and momentum for incorporating PGHD into care continues and is being increasingly driven by regulatory policy and insurance reimbursement decisions that impact on all stakeholders.

Given these conflicts, a fruitful approach is to examine them from a Human Factors standpoint with User-Centered Design as a tool to study, understand and mitigate the barriers and to present approaches that align stakeholders to reach the laudable and challenging goal of incorporating PGHD into chronic disease management. Beginning with definitions, the approach is applied to the primary care flow of patients with an ongoing chronic condition (Hypertension/Diabetes Mellitus, Type II).

## 10.3   A Brief Overview of the Human Factors Approach

*Human Factors* refers to a group of disciplines that share the goal of designing systems that are suited for the abilities, skills and preferences of users (i.e., people) and the task to be accomplished.

> The historical roots of Human Factors can be traced back to the early phases of industrialization. As machines replaced work previously done by humans, engineers began to consider the new relationships between man and machine. One concept was that functions could be reduced to measurable sequences of inter-related and repeatable tasks, which can be optimized and taught to workers with limited skills (known as "Taylorism") [42]. Within healthcare, productivity can be improved through systematic organization of tasks and processes and "good" design.

*Users* are humans with physical, cognitive and psychosocial capabilities that support decision-making

> The term "Human Factors and Ergonomics" originated during World War II. A major impetus that moved the discipline forward was the observation of a large number of human errors in aviation [20]. Analyses found that approximately a third of all deaths were attributable to combat, while two thirds occurred during training and normal operations [7, 9, 20]. Researchers found significant problems in training, operations and in the design of cockpit controls (which affected pilots' performance on button-pressing sequences under duress, work teams' perceptions of critical messages under noisy conditions and flight crews' work coordination during missions. [7])

*Task-analysis* has become a major methodology to understanding workflow requirements [26].

> Defined as "the study of what an operator (or team of operators) is required to do, in terms of actions and/or cognitive processes to achieve a system goal" [26], task-analysis can provide a pragmatic understanding of workers as a starting point for a better design and fit of technology [22, 24]. Techniques used in task-analysis include: activity sampling, observation, critical incident identification, and interviews. [26]

*User-centered design (UCD)* focuses on the user, the tasks and the context of work that are key factors in contributing to the overall success of system design [16, 17]. UCD stresses the importance of iterative design for evolving successful systems. In UCD, users are involved early in the design process, before any implementation, and then throughout the refinement of the system through further testing with representative intended users.

As computing has become progressively "horizontal" (general in focus) and platforms have broadened from mainframes to personal computers to mobile technologies and smartphones, the view of IT user skill sets has changed from "special expertise" (requiring training to use IT) to average knowledge (requiring little to no training). This change in user expectations has required application design and user training to be simpler, more transparent and easier to master or intuit.

*Ease of use* has become an important driver of design.

As sophisticated IT applications, enabled by personal computers and Web-based technologies, have become available to a wide range of users, there has been reduction/elimination of paper instruction/documentation and increase in common design conventions/metaphors across interfaces [6]. Guidelines for interface designs and help systems have been developed for consistency [33], with the goal of enabling average users to interact with applications with minimal training, disruption and error. Such guidelines have been embodied into standard reusable design toolkits for new applications [31] that simplify data entry and decrease other errors in data collection. As *discretionary* users (those who are not compelled/forced to use) of a given application, patients consider ease of use as a pre-requisite to using it (with the alternative being to abandon the application). This is an important factor in designing PGHD tools.

*User engagement* is important to implementing PGHD into IT-driven clinical information work.

Patients must be convinced and assured that providing accurate health data has value to them and that it provides positive return on investment (ROI), both initially and over the long-term, for management of health and chronic disease. In wellness, frequent abandonment of self-initiated usage of health tracking applications suggests that currently available tools do not provide sufficient value or ROI to the (healthy) patient over the long-term. [30]

*Coordination and collaboration* among the multiple users involved in the use of PGHD is a major area of concern for developers.

"Groupware" (collaborative) applications may fail for a number of reasons that go beyond the scope of technology [18, 19]. These include:

- *Uneven distribution of costs and benefits of the work involved in adoption.* In one example, a radiology department adopted speech recognition technology that enabled radiologists (physicians) to produce reports without the need of a human transcriptionist. The application used discrete speech recognition technology that requires users to modify their way of speaking (perceived as "unnatural") in order to be recognized by the system. Physicians were required to edit the final report (with a keyboard, something they equated with "clerical work" and not in keeping with their job role) (Danis, unpublished manuscript 1992). The department administrators strongly favored the tool because of the cost saved on transcription. The distribution of costs and benefits is more complex in the case of PGHD where both patients and providers are expected to share in the costs (and work) and would be expected to derive benefits. But, the nature of the costs and the benefits remains to be further elucidated.

- *Differential perceptions in the advantages of sharing personal information.* In an example of opposing incentives within a consultancy organization, younger consultants guarded personally-obtained information they believed gave them a competitive advantage. In contrast, senior consultants, whose positions were secure, saw advantages to the free flow of information [32]. This differential perception may be seen clinically (regarding privacy in seeking care) with adolescent patients who confide in their physicians about sensitive health issues and their parents who may wish to be alerted about by insurers whenever their teens go to the doctor. [34]

Over time, concerns for Human Factors practitioners have shifted as the nature of the machines with which humans interact has changed. Ease of use is important, but it is just one concern that potentially determines acceptance of a technology by its intended users. Increasingly, the social context in which system use is embedded has gained prominence as a factor to be considered in design. With applications that now enable multiple users, with differing roles and work incentives (such as EHR systems), social and organizational structures become an increasingly integral aspect of context. For EHR systems and other health IT, added dimensions of context and complexity are introduced by policy and regulatory constructs and constraints.

## 10.4   An Example of UCD in PGHD for Chronic Disease

We present a case of the field use of a mobile reporting application for PGHD to illustrate the iterative application of User Centered Design (UCD) to meet the challenges of designing an application and workflow for chronic disease management.

### 10.4.1   The Study

In a previously described study, a commercially available mobile reporting application tool was implemented for collecting PGHD in a primary care practice for a 6-month field trial. Seventeen patients, each of whom had a primary diagnosis of chronic hypertension (HTN) or Diabetes Mellitus, Type 2 (DM2) were enrolled [10, 11]. Data collected from use of the deployed system plus field study interviews of stakeholders provided a more realistic analysis of their needs, concerns, capabilities and limitations than possible with an experimental laboratory study. This approach also enabled a view into the important organizational and reimbursement contexts in which the application must function.

In the study, hosted by an urban, primary care practice with a largely college educated, adult patient population, the data collected included:

- Automatically logged PGHD via a mobile application.
- Pre-study interviews from a sample of participants prior to the start of PGHD collection. Patients were asked to discuss the "three most important things your physician has told you to do in regard to your primary health condition". The

interview results provided information about the challenges patients face in putting into practice the medication and lifestyle directives communicated to them by their physicians.

- Post-study interviews feedback on experiences with using the tool to accomplish the task. These provided information on patients' experiences with incorporating the task of data-generation into their daily lives, as well as with actual use of the tool.
- Questionnaire responses from physicians on attitudes and medical practices regarding their patients' self-care of their chronic medical conditions.

During the data collection period:

- Patients' tasks consisted of a "check-in" response to an automated daily request for his or her status on three health indicators. Questions were sent through a secure mobile application each morning with 24 h allotted for a response to be counted as meeting the daily requirement. The three questions were:

  1. Did you take all your prescribed medication for the day before: "Yes" or "No"?
  2. For HTN, patients were asked to measure and report their morning blood pressure. For DM2, patients were asked to measure and report their morning blood glucose level.
  3. How do you feel: Response on a 5-point scale (1–5), 5 indicating the "best"?

- Physicians' tasks was limited to an expectation that they would respond to alerts if a patient-reported blood pressure or blood glucose level exceeded threshold levels set by the medical practice. The levels selected to trigger alerts corresponded to clinically dangerous levels that normally require immediate medical intervention. The research team failed to convince the medical practice to add alerts corresponding to "high normal" (blood pressure or blood glucose) levels, which could have been used to trigger a consultation or an instruction for the patient. The medical practice defined a process whereby alerts would be sent to the on-call practice care coordinator for triaging the message according to established protocols, including one for passing the alert on to the physician if appropriate.

## 10.4.2   Initial Findings and Commentary

Results. Seventeen patients/participants generated health data for at least 4 months, some for up to 6 months. Only two participants produced daily responses for the duration of the study. The modal length of time between responses rate was every other day, with the maximum time between responses being as high as 1 week. About 80 % of patients who enrolled did not transition to the study phase (that included actively reporting data). No alerts were generated based on PGHD, so physicians were not contacted.

Patients. Patients are *discretionary* users of the application, that is, they cannot be compelled to use it. To participate in the study, patients had to have a primary diagnosis of either HTN or DM2. They were required to own a personal smartphone (iOS or Android) and to self-report as meeting a target level of proficiency with using the device for computing tasks. Observations re: lower than expected participation rates:

- Usability did not appear to be a barrier. All interview participants gave the application the top score on usability. This was not unexpected as the application used standard controls and navigation conventions for the iOS and Android systems.
- Some patients stated it was not necessary for them to respond every day to get value from using the application. Since their data did not vary significantly from day to day, they felt that reporting less often was sufficient. In addition, reporting once or twice a week was sufficient to keep them focused on their health indicators and enabled them to detect changes in their trends, if any occurred.
- A few patients reported being disappointed that "no one seemed to be paying attention" to their reports and thus they stopped replying to the daily check-in request. In fact, the physicians were largely unaware of the day-to-day progress of the study because, as we noted above, the medical practice adopted a policy that physicians were to be notified only when patient-reported levels reached thresholds that required immediate medical attention and reported levels never reached these thresholds.

Smartphones. The smartphone ownership criterion disqualified 75 % of the patients approached for participation [11]. Low penetration of smartphone ownership among this population of patients may be temporary as ownership is projected to increase rapidly over the next 5 years [40]. Smartphone ownership is inversely correlated with age, with current smartphone ownership for those aged 65+ significantly lower than younger groups [36, 37]. It is unclear if the current age related differences will be eliminated in the future due to younger users maintaining ownership of their phones as they age. Alternatively, they might abandon them due to high cost as they age, as has been reported by current seniors on fixed incomes [37].

Physicians. Physicians are *indirect* users of the application. The literature indicates a wide range of attitudes among physicians regarding patient engagement in self-care, from quite supportive to highly negative. One chief source of negative views on some types of patient engagement stems from their concerns about patients' dependence on getting medical information from untrusted sources [2, 38], requiring physician time and effort to "un-do" impressions their patients form as a result of incorrect or inapplicable information [2, 8]. Physicians in the study were found to welcome patient involvement. They believed patient involvement should include following physician directives but were less clear on the value of incorporating PGHD into care practices.

The medical practice. The practice management indicated a commitment to exploring integrating PGHD into practice, but their plans for consuming the data were constrained by the realities of their reimbursement model. Under the fee-for-service model, the practice could not afford financially to dedicate a member of their clinical team to respond solely to the incoming data (as required). Thus, they agreed to receive notifications of rare cases/reports flagged as clinically suspicious. Awareness of such events would give the medical practice a previously unavailable capability and thus it incorporated the alert-handling function into its workflow, but it was unwilling to incorporate them into the EHR system. Instead, alerts were routed to the email of a practice care coordinator at the medical practice who was responsible for handling care needs that arose outside of medical appointments.

### 10.4.3 UCD in Redesign Considerations

In considering design changes, questions from the previously described study include:

- How is it possible to satisfy patients' desire for feedback (i.e., acknowledgement that someone is paying attention, thus motivating them to continue)?
- Are there other configurations for data flow and response that are possible within the user-task-context of the practice that will satisfy the constraints (not having a full time care coordinator for managing incoming data from the application)?

An adaptive part of a possible solution is to use a worker already in the practice: the medical assistant (MA) who is paired with a physician to deliver patient care. The MA or a licensed practical nurse (LPN), already familiar with history taking, taking vital signs and blood glucose measurements, could perform the role of the care coordinator, thus providing contact to the patient, supplemented by reports generated by data analytics [23, 29]. An example of how this might play out for a hypothetical patient, John Smith:

> Mr. John Smith has had DM2 for five years. His HbA1c is at 7.0 and has trended upwards over the past year from a level of 6.0. John has agreed, at his physician's urging, to use the mobile check-in application to report his morning blood sugar level, medication adherence and "feeling good" score "a few times a week" during the three months leading up to his next regular diabetes control appointment. His reports are aggregated at a central server that logs his responses and automatically computes analytics from the data in those responses. Analyses will have been programmed to categorize glucose measurements as:

> 1. Low
> 2. Normal
> 3. Elevated but not critical
> 4. Critical

> Critical levels result in an immediate alert being communicated to the MA who follows up according to the rule-based protocols in place at the medical practice. Protocols have also been instituted to provide the MA with responses to the other new category levels, which are designed to:

> - Provide weekly feedback for Mr Smith on how he is doing
> - Identify opportunities for educating Mr Smith on elevated but not critical levels, and
> - Generate easily consumable, quarterly reports for his physician to view during the Mr Smith's next appointment.

Each of these new protocols may cover the following issues identified as barriers to use in the field study:

(a) Weekly feedback satisfies Mr Smith's need to know that someone at the practice is paying attention. If all the reported levels fell within the "normal" guidelines, he receives simple feedback noting the "normal" condition and encouragement to continue.

(b) If on occasion levels exceed normal, this would be communicated in a straightforward manner, as, for example: "Mr Smith, your blood glucose level went to 190 mg/dL once this past week. Try to keep it below 140 mg/dL each time". If a pattern of elevated levels is detected by the analytics, then an agreed upon protocol can be automatically dispatched to him. For example, perhaps elevated levels occur during the weekends but are normal for the rest of the week. The medical practice might send a message alerting the patient of the pattern, as well as directing him to take action to get more information. Perhaps something like the following: "This coming weekend, after you send in your numbers, we're going to send you a brief form for you to write in what you ate and drank the night before to see if we can figure out why you're having the higher than normal blood glucose levels. Is that OK?"

(c) If the pattern persists in spite of the dispatch of the protocol to increase awareness, then the medical practice might recommend a meeting with a diabetic educator who will be able to explore issues one-on-one with the patient.

The proposed role of automation is to detect conditions that indicate an event for which the practice wants to respond. This limits the work required by staff in consuming the new stream of data. The MA's role, when the patient comes into the office, is to review with the patient the actions taken over the past 3 months.

This scenario is a preliminary sketch of what a follow-up design might include in order to address the low participation rates by patient and physician as identified in the field trial. Targeted follow up investigations would be needed to validate each of the following components of the proposed solution, which would include:

- Will data analytics be capable of identifying patterns with the fidelity required by the medical practice to map them on to automatic response protocols?
- Will the patient accept an automated response as indication that "someone is listening"?
- How do the summary sheets have to be designed to enable the MAs to effectively and efficiently review the patient's progress during appointments?
- How can an effective summary be designed for the physician to review at the time of an appointment?

The UCD methodology provides detailed guidance for using prototypes with different degrees of fidelity (from paper sketches, through wire-frame screens, through working stand-alone systems) as a means of exploring and refining design ideas. This is particularly valuable with respect to the introduction of technologies to facilitate new processes into contexts already served by other IT systems, such as is the case with respect to technology for PGHD, and constrained by real-world conditions that create initial barriers to their adoption. Limited deployments enable all stakeholders to begin making necessary adjustments under circumstances where value is clear and to identify for themselves additional potential values from the use of the technology.

## 10.5   Conclusion

Designing an application in the area of PGHD requires understanding the context of use for the application. Using a Human Factors approach, in particular User Centered Design, provides a fruitful approach for sorting and understanding the myriad factors that embed users of an application within a clinical context. Clearly, understanding these factors does not automatically lead to an optimal design solution and good design is a continually iterative process. Such an approach (and others) will be needed to realize the vision of incorporating PGHD into EHR systems and clinical care of chronic disease as will be required in Stage 3 Meaningful Use of Certified Electronic Health Record Technology.

**Acknowledgements**   My thanks to the entire research team and the patients who participated in the field study that served as the motivating example in this chapter. I learned a great deal through the experience, particularly through a long-term interaction with the core team members: Marion Ball, Sasha Ballen, Scott Cashon, Marj Miller, and Marty Minniti. Thanks also to my colleagues Bonnie John and Tom Erickson for pointers to literature.

## References

1. Ahern D, Woods SS, Lightowler MC, et al. Promise of and potential for patient-facing technologies to enable meaningful use. Am J Prev Med. 2011;40(5S2):161–72.
2. Anderson RM, Funnell MM. Patient empowerment: myths and misconceptions. Patient Educ Couns. 2010;79(30):277–82.
3. Berwick DM. What "patient-centered" should mean: confessions of an extremist. Health Aff. 2009;28(4):555–65.
4. Bodenheimer T, Lorig K, Holman H, et al. Patient self-management of chronic disease in primary care. JAMA. 2002;288(19):2469–75. Brennan, PF. Incorporating patient-generated information to manage health HIT policy committee hearing, 8 Jun 2012. Available from http://www.healthit.gov/archive/archive_files/FACA%20Hearings/2012/2012-06-08%20 Policy%3A%20Meaningful%20Use%20WG%20Patient%20Generated%20Health%20 Data%20Hearing/patti-brennan-patient-generated-data-hearing-testimony-060812.pdf.
5. Brennan PF. Project health Design: rethinking the power and potential of personal health records. 2014. Available from http://www.rwjf.org/content/dam/farm/reports/issue_briefs/ 2014/rwjf412107.
6. Brockmann RJ. Writing better computer user documentation: from paper to online. New York: Wiley; 1986.
7. Chapanis A. The chapanis chronicles: 50 years of human factors research, education, and desing. Santa Barbara: Aegean Publishing; 1999.
8. Chase D. Patients gain information and skills to improve self-management through innovative tools. The Commonwealth Fund, Dec 2010/Jan 2011.

9. Coury BG, Ellingstad VS, Jolly JM. Transportation accident investigation: the development of human factors research and practice. Rev Hum Factors Ergon. 2013;6(1):1–33.
10. Danis CM, Ballen S, Minitti MJ, et al. Bringing patients into the loop: using technology to engage patients and improve health outcomes. J Health Inf Manag. 2014;28(1):20–7.
11. Danis CM, Minniti MJ, Ballen S, et al. Patient engagement at the point of care: technology as an enabler. In: Grando M, Rozenblum R, Bates D, editors. Information technologies for patient empowerment in healthcare. Berlin/Boston/Munich: Walter De Gruyter Inc. 2015.
12. DiMatteo MR, Haskard-Zolnierek KB, Martin LR. Improving patient adherence: a three-factor model to guide practice. Health Psychol Rev Health Psychol Rev. 2012;6:74–91.
13. DPP (The Diabetes Prevention Program Research Group at the Biostatistics Center, George Washington University). Description of lifestyle intervention. Diabetes Care. 2002;12:2165–71.
14. ECDG (European Commission Directorate General for Communication). Eurobarometer qualitative study on patient involvement. 2012. Available at: http://ec.europa.eu/public_opinion/archives/quali/ql_5937_patient_en.pdf. Accessed Nov 2013.
15. Emont S. Measuring the impact of patient portals: what the literature tells us. Oakland: California Health Care Foundation; 2011. http://www.chcf.org/~/media/MEDIA%20LIBRARY%20Files/PDF/M/PDF%20MeasuringImpactPatientPortals.pdf. Accessed 19 Apr 2015.
16. Gould JD, Lewis C. Designing for usability: key principles and what designers think. Commun ACM. 1985;28(3):300–11.
17. Gould JD. How to design usable systems. In: Helander M, editor. Handbook of human-computer interaction. Amsterdam: Elsevier Science Publishers; 1988.
18. Grudin J. Why CSCW applications fail: problems in the design and evaluation of organizational artifacts. ACM conference on computer supported cooperative work (CSCW 88); Portland; 1988. p. 362–69. p. 85–93.
19. Grudin J. Groupware ane social dynamics eight challenges for developers. Commun ACM. 1994;37(1):93–104.
20. Harris D. Improving aircraft safety. Aviat Psychol. 2014;27(2):90–5. Available from: http://www.aerotelegraph.com/sites/default/files/n238/Artikel.pdf.
21. Hibbard JH, Mahoney ER, Stock R, et al. Self-management and health care utilization: do increases in patient activation result in imposed self-management behaviors. Health Res Educ Trust. 2006. doi:10.1111/j.1475-6773.2006.00669.x.
22. Irby C, Bergsteinsson L, Moran T, et al. A methodology for user interface design. Xerox Palo Alto Research Center Internal Report. 1977.
23. James G, Witten D, Hastie T, et al. An introduction to statistical learning. New York: Springer; 2013.
24. Jones L, Danis C, Boies SJ. Avoiding the mistake of cloning: a case for user-centered design methods to reengineer documents. System sciences. 1999. HICSS-32. In: Proceedings of the 32nd annual Hawaii international conference on, Volume: Track2.
25. Karat C. Cost-justifying human factors support on development projects. Hum Factors Soc Bull. 1992;35(11):1–8.
26. Kirwan B, Ainsworth LK, editors. A guide to task analysis: the task analysis working group. Boca Raton: Taylor & Francis Group, LLC.; 1992.
27. Lorig KR, Mazonson PD, Holman HR. Evidence suggesting that health education for self-management in patients with chronic arthritis has sustained health benefits while reducing health care costs. Arthritis Rheum. 1993;36(4):439–46.
28. Lorig KR, Sobel DS, Stewart AL, et al. Evidence suggesting that a chronic disease self-management program can improve health status while reducing hospitalization. Med Care. 1999;37(1):5–14.
29. McNeill D, editor. Analytics in healthcare and the life sciences. Upper Saddle River: Pearson; 2013.
30. Michie S, Abraham C, Whittington C, et al. Effective techniques in healthy eating and physical activity interventions: a meta-regression. Health Psychol. 2009;28(6):690–701.
31. Myers B, Hudson SE, Pausch R. Past, present, and future of user interface software tools. ACM Trans Comput-Hum Interact (TOCHI) – Spec Issue Hum-Comput Interact New Millennium. 2000;7(1):3–28.

32. Orlikowslki WJ. Learning from notes: organizational issues in groupware implementation. In: Proceedings of ACM conference on computer supported cooperative work (CSCW 92). Toronto; 1992. p. 362–69.
33. Paap KR, Roske-Hofstrand RJ. The design of menus. In: Helander M, editor. Handbook of human-computer interaction. Amsterdam: Elsevier Science Publishers; 1988.
34. Paperny DMN. Privacy issues. In: Lehmann C, Kim GR, Johnson KB, editors. Pediatric informatics: computer applications in child health. New York: Springer Verlag; 2009.
35. PCPCC (Patient Centered Primary Care Collaborative). Transforming patient engagement: health IT in the patient centered medical home. 2010. Available at: http://www.pcpcc.org/guide/transforming-patient-engagement. Accessed 30 May 2014.
36. Pew Research Center. Mobile technology fact sheet. 2014. http://www.pewinternet.org/fact-sheets/mobile-technology-fact-sheet/.
37. Pew Research Center. Older adults and technology use: usage and adoption. 2014b. http://www.pewinternet.org/2014/04/03/usage-and-adoption/.
38. Schulz PJ, Nakamoto K. "Bad" literacy, the internet, and the limits of patient empowerment. AAAI Spring Symposium. 2011.
39. Shapiro M, Johnston D, Wald J, Mon D. Patient-generated health data: white paper prepared for the Office of the National Coordinator for Health IT by RTI International. Apr 2012. http://www.rti.org/pubs/patientgeneratedhealthdata.pdf.
40. Statista. Number of smartphone users in the US from 2010 to 2018. 2014. http://www.statista.com/statistics/201182/forecast-of-smartphone-users-in-the-us/.
41. Sujansky & Associates LLC. A standards-based model for the sharing of patient-generated health information with electronic health records. 2013. Available from http://www.projecthealthdesign.org/media/file/Standard-Model-For-Collecting-And-Reporting-PGHI_Sujansky_Assoc_2013-07-18.pdf.
42. Taylor F. Principles of scientific management. New York: Harper & Row; 1911. Available from https://www.marxists.org/reference/subject/economics/taylor/principles/.
43. Terry K. Meaningful use 2: a work in progress for physicians. 2014. Available from http://medicaleconomics.modernmedicine.com/medical-economics/news/meaningful-use-2-work-progress-physicians?page=full.
44. vonKorf M, Gruman J, Schaefer JK, et al. Collaborative management of chronic illness. Ann Inter Med. 1997;127:1097–102.
45. Whelton PK, Appel LJ, Espeland MA, et al. A randomized controlled trial of nonpharmacologic interventions in the elderly (TONE). JAMA. 1998;279(11):839–46. Erratum in: JAMA, 24;279(24):1954.
46. Wixon D, Jones S. Usability for fun and profit: a case study of the design of DEC RALLY version 2. Internal report, Digital Equipment Corporation. 1991.

# Chapter 11
# Transformed Roles for a Transformed Healthcare System: Where Do Clinical Informaticists Fit in Now?

**Mark Hagland**

**Abstract** Healthcare has a long history; computers being routinely used in healthcare can be traced back to the 1970s when they began to be used in the patient billing area, but clinical informaticists only go back to the 1990s. Although a short time period, they have evolved many times over. Guided by new technologies and new regulations, clinical informaticists are at the forefront of the integration of clinical medicine and information systems given a healthcare industry so dependent on data. They also work with many interdisciplinary partners whose roles themselves are evolving such as the Chief Transformation Officer and Chief Quality Officer. How will the Informaticist drive the healthcare system into the future as their roles evolve? The answer will have an impact on role of data, information technology, and information systems on an evolving healthcare delivery system.

**Keywords** Medical informatics • Informatician • Nexus leader • HITECH

When it comes to the forward evolution of clinical informatics functions and of the roles of clinical informaticists in U.S. healthcare, one need only look back two decades from the present in order to get a sense of how much has changed, and of the clear trajectory in this area going forward.

---

Mark Hagland is the Editor-in-Chief of *Healthcare Informatics* magazine, a leading publication in the healthcare IT senior leadership space. He has been a healthcare journalist for over 25 years, and is the author of two books: *Transformative Quality*: *The Emerging Revolution in Health Care Performance* (2008), and *Paradox and Imperatives*: *How Efficiency, Effectiveness, and E-Transformation Can Conquer Waste and Optimize Quality* (2007, co-authored with Jeffrey C. Bauer, Ph.D.), both published by Productivity Press/CRC Press. He is based in Chicago. Brief excerpts from *Healthcare Informatics* are provided with permission.

M. Hagland, MS Journalism
Editor-in-Chief, Healthcare Informatics Magazine, Chicago, IL, USA
e-mail: mhagland@vendomegrp.com

© Springer International Publishing Switzerland 2016                                189
C.A. Weaver et al. (eds.), *Healthcare Information Management Systems:
Cases, Strategies, and Solutions*, Health Informatics,
DOI 10.1007/978-3-319-20765-0_11

Prior to the early 1990s, only a very small percentage of hospital-based patient care organizations had implemented electronic health records (EHRs), and the percentage of physicians who had implemented EHRs in their practices was infinitesimally small. Within hospital-based organizations, most existing information systems were contained within finance departments and business, admitting, and registration offices, or scattered across completely siloed individual clinical departments and services. In "the old days" of the late 1980s and early 1990s, with a small number of exceptions, information technology professionals were largely programmers, network managers, and, at the highest levels, IT department managers. And very, very few clinicians, whether physicians, nurses, or even more rarely, pharmacists, had any involvement in information technology at all, except in relation to limited, department-specific systems, such as early-generation PACS (picture archiving and communications systems) and RIS (radiology information systems) in radiology departments, etc.

But things began to change around 1990 through 1992, and the first individuals were promoted to the title of chief information officer, or CIO, at the same time that more hospital-based organizations began to implement EHRs [3, 4].[1]

A great deal of confusion existed early on as to exactly what a CIO was or did; but over time, it became clear that a CIO needed to be more than simply a manager of information systems; she or he needed to be a strategic thinker and a high-level leader. From the early 1990s through the early 2000s, the professionalization of the CIO role evolved forward, as patient care organizations' information systems, including clinical information systems, became increasingly more comprehensive, more interconnected (if still largely not yet interoperable), and more complex.

Already by the early 2000s, most hospital-based organizations had built larger, more organized IS teams, and the vast majority had individuals with the CIO title (though some of those individuals still remained in practice high-level IT managers rather than true CIOs in the strategic sense). But widespread policy, reimbursement, and payer initiatives and mandates, along with a host of other factors, are compelling providers forward. Among those initiatives and mandates are broad pay-for-performance, outcomes measurement, and care management efforts. What's more, rapid advances in the sophistication of EHRs and the rise of numerous other IT tools such as data warehouses, data analytics tools, sophisticated infrastructure and storage capabilities, and the beginnings of real population health management and risk assessment analytics tools, as well as the growing universalization of mobile devices and the growth of telehealth capabilities, have

---

[1] HIMSS Analytics, a division of the Chicago-based Healthcare Information and Management Systems Society (HIMSS), compiles data on EHR adoption across the United States. According to its United States EMR Adoption Model, the leaders at HIMSS Analytics concluded that as of the fourth quarter of 2014, 3.6 % of U.S. hospitals had achieved Stage 7 status; 17.9 % had achieved Stage 6 status; 32.8 % had achieved Stage 5 status; 14.0 % had achieved Stage 4 status; 21.0 % had achieved Stage 3 status; 5.1 % had achieved Stage 2 status; and 2.0 % were still at Stage 1 level, according to their model of EHR adoption.

made the strategic management of IT assets essential in all but the very smallest patient care organizations.

Meanwhile, in the early 2000s, patient care organizations began the challenging work of implementing first- and second-generation EHRs and other clinical information systems. At the same time, organizations began to move into clinical transformation work, leveraging their IT systems to improve clinical performance and patient outcomes, and these trends increasingly brought clinicians into such efforts.

Fast-forward now to two watershed years in the history of healthcare informatics in the United States, 2009 and 2010. In February 2009, the U.S. Congress passed and President Barack Obama signed into law, the American Recovery and Reinvestment Act of 2009 (ARRA). The ARRA was a massive stimulus bill designed to help the U.S. economy recover from the Great Recession through job creation and other forms of stimulus, at a cost estimated to be $787 billion at the time of passage (and later revised to $831 billion). One piece of the 2009 ARRA legislation was revolutionary for healthcare and healthcare IT in the U.S., and that was the Health Information Technology for Economic and Clinical Health Act, or HITECH Act.

The purpose of the HITECH Act was to universalize EHRs and other clinical information technology across U.S. healthcare, and to channel efforts already under way to help U.S. healthcare evolve into a more connected, interoperable, patient-centered, higher-quality, and more cost-effective system. The legislation created the foundation for such development through its meaningful use (MU) program. At the time of the writing of this chapter, MU was moving forward, albeit with a number of complications and setbacks. Still, in contrast to in 2008, in which only a plurality of U.S. hospital-based organizations had fully implemented EHRs, and a very small minority of physicians in practice had done so, by the end of 2014, the vast majority of hospitals had done so, and most physicians had done so [3].

In that sense, HITECH has been a spectacular success, in its pushing providers to fully implement and significantly use core clinical and other information technology.

And then on March 23, 2010, President Obama signed, after a year-long-plus legislative saga, the Patient Protection and Affordable Care Act, widely known as the Affordable Care Act (ACA). The bulk of the ACA's provisions focused on health insurance reform, facilitating, as of the date of publication of this book, the access to affordable health insurance of well over ten million previous uninsured Americans. But while the bulk of the legislation was focused on health insurance issues, a significant portion of the legislation created new mandates and incentives for what is often referred to as "internal healthcare reform"—that is to say, incentives for hospitals, physicians, and other providers, to improve the cost-effectiveness, efficiency, quality, and patient-centeredness of healthcare for healthcare consumers/patients, families, and communities.

Indeed, mandates for hospital-based organizations to cut avoidable readmissions, and for hospitals and physicians to participate in value-based purchasing, both through the Medicare program, for the first time made clinical performance improvement mandatory as a requirement of federal law for any providers participating in the Medicare program.

What's more, provisions creating accountable care organization (ACO) development programs, and a bundled-payment program, though optional, also offered another set of channels for the potential transformation of the healthcare system.

And so, with the passage of the HITECH Act as part of the ARRA, and the passage of the ACA, U.S. hospitals and physicians were faced with a constellation of federal incentives, some required and some optional, that signaled the federal government's explicit demand for healthcare system transformation. What's more, private health insurers, which had already been moving forward with value-based purchasing, outcomes measurement, and risk-based contracting, programs, moved ahead quickly to create programs similar to the federal government's along a number of dimensions. Among those dimensions are requirements for readmissions reduction and incentives toward the development of accountable care organization development, and bundled-payment programs. In addition, payers increasingly work with provider organizations on population health initiatives. And, in relation to all of these types of programs, health insurers are demanding that providers make extensive use of EHR and other clinical information technology to improve outcomes and efficiency in healthcare.

What's more, these policy and regulatory mandates are not emerging in a vacuum. Indeed, the U.S. healthcare system appears poised to become overwhelmed by its own total cost. In October 2014, the actuaries at the federal Centers for Medicare and Medicaid Services CMS) announced that they expected total U.S. healthcare spending to increase from $3.056.6 trillion in 2014 to $3.207.3 trillion in 2015 to $4.042.5 trillion to $5.158 trillion in 2023 [7].

Furthermore, CMS projected that healthcare spending would rise as a share of the nation's gross domestic product from 17.2 % in 2012 to 19.3 % in 2023. In other words, the current cost curve of healthcare in the United States is broadly unsustainable (the authors themselves did not use the word "unsustainable," but it is obvious that the healthcare cost curve is unsustainable).

## 11.1    Clinical Informaticists as Nexus Leaders

With these policy and industry developments, and with healthcare information technology vendors moving forward to improve their products and services, U.S. patient care organizations are under pressure to transform their core patient care and operational processes as never before. And, not surprisingly, information technology, and most especially clinical information technology, is at the center of this swirl of activity and demands on the part of the purchasers and payers of healthcare (latter part unclear). Given the demands for the transformation of healthcare in the U.S. to make it more cost-effective, efficient, of higher quality, and more patient-centric, no real progress is possible without the very strong leveraging of clinical IT to create the clinical transformation needed to fundamentally change health care. Thus, cue the clinical informaticists.

## 11.2   The Rise of Clinical Informaticist Leaders

If the role of the CIO and similar executive-level IT roles (chief technology officer, or CTO, etc.) have evolved in patient care organizations in a somewhat organic, haphazard way over the years, this is doubly true for clinical informaticists. An example is CMIOs (chief medical information officers, or chief medical informatics officers; both formulations are employed in the industry). The first CMIOs evolved out of very part-time medical informatics work done "on the side" at first, as physicians who enjoyed technology (the so-called "tech-head docs") were recruited to spend a portion of their time helping to select and advise on the implementation of the first EHRs, and also systems such as PACS and RIS that at that time were very department-specific.

As information systems and the organizations and processes around them became more and more complex, intricate, and interdependent (if not actually interoperable), both physicians and nurses brought into sustained contact and collaboration with IT departments gradually moved into more extensive, and then eventually in many cases, full-time, positions as clinical informaticists, and their roles and responsibilities began to formalize to a far greater extent.

For nurses, the process was a bit more straightforward in that many nurses quickly began transitioning into full-time nurse informaticist/clinical informaticist roles. But because of the lucrative nature of physician practice and because of the unique status/stature of physicians in the health care system, the transitioning of physicians into full-time informaticist roles has been a more complicated process. Nonetheless, by the early 2000s, enough physicians and nurses had been moving into full-time or near-full-time status. In the case of physicians, even those working as informaticists 80 or more percent of their time often kept a small bit of clinical practice active, concretizing and formalizing their roles to a far greater extent. In addition, whole teams of clinical informaticists were emerging across the U.S. health care system. And, finally, some hospital pharmacists joined the physicians and nurses in their work implementing systems such as CPOE (computerized physician order entry) systems, advanced pharmacy information systems, electronic medication administration record (eMAR) systems (often incorporating barcoded meds administration elements), case and care management systems, and ultimately, population health and data analytics systems.

Now in the second decade of the twenty-first century, the U.S. health care system is encountering the full context of MU, federal healthcare reform, value-based purchasing, and population health. And as it does so, it has become readily apparent that haphazard, ad hoc, informal development of teams of clinical informaticists is no longer a viable option. Instead, we as a healthcare system are moving into the era of "clinical informaticists 2.0."

## 11.3 "Clinical Informaticists 2.0": What Does the Concept Mean?

Just what does that concept mean? Essentially, patient care organizations in the United States are transitioning from an early phase focused on the implementation of first-generation EHRs and other clinical information systems to a more mature phase involving the leveraging of those systems to improve clinical and operational performance. Increasingly, what is needed across U.S. healthcare are somewhat different skill sets and packages of experience, although a hands-on, end-user-savvy knowledge base remains important, particularly at the initial clinical informatics position levels.

Instead, however, patient care organizations need CMIOs, CNIOs (chief nursing information/informatics officers), pharmacist informaticists, and increasingly, chief health information officers (CHIOs). Occasionally, these roles are also called chief clinical information officers (CCIOs). There is a great demand for individuals to fill these positions. At the same time, the skill sets and experiences required to successfully fulfill those roles are ramping up considerably over time. What's more, these senior executives are becoming conveners, strategic planners, and leaders at higher and higher levels of activity and higher levels of position within their organizations.

This trend for chief clinical informatics officer positions with strategic skill sets is so important that we, the editors of *Healthcare Informatics* magazine, named "Health Care Informaticists 2.0" as one of the Top Ten Tech Trends of 2015 in the January–February issue of the magazine.

Among those interviewed for the article was David Levin, M.D., who served as the Cleveland Clinic Health's CMIO from 2011 to 2014. Levin explained the forward evolution of the CMIO role in particular in this way: "We as a healthcare system have been about implementation the past 5 years, getting the infrastructure into place. And we're not done, but we're well down the road." But now, he noted, the CMIO role "is starting to converge with the roles of the chief quality officer or chief medical officer, roles that are about performance management, about envisioning a better future and achieving better performance, including around concepts of the Triple Aim" [5].[2]

Dr. Levin expressed in the *Healthcare Informatics* interview the belief that what has been framed as the CMIO role has begun to morph into roles around strategy and performance management. He sees new roles, such as the chief health information officer, emerging (others have also cited the emergence of the title "chief data officer"). Dr. Levin also believes that some senior nurse informaticists will inevitably rise into CHIO roles.

Dr. Levin was part of a team led by consultant Pam Arlotto, president and CEO of the Roswell, Georgia-based Maestro Strategies consulting firm, who published a white paper entitled "From the Playing Field to the Press Box: The Emerging Role of the Chief Health Information Officer" [1, 6].

---

[2] "Triple Aim" is a set of principles being promoted by the Cambridge, Massachusetts-based Institute for Healthcare Improvement, around the improvement of patient care outcomes, the improvement of cost-effectiveness and efficiency, and the enhancement of the patient and community experience, in the U.S. healthcare system.

The essential idea of the white paper, as expressed in the white paper itself and in the *Healthcare Informatics* interview, is that patient care organizations nationwide, as they "advance" into more and more extensive levels of financial risk and into accountable care organization and population health management-based core business-organization strategies, will require senior clinical informaticists in their organizations to increasingly integrate informatics and performance and clinical quality improvement in order to satisfy the outcomes measure-based requirements of their risk-based contracts.

Operationally, this means that the integration of care and case management processes will need to be integrated into broader population health management processes, and very closely dovetailed and integrated with continuous performance improvement processes organization-wide. Such efforts will require intensified data analytics processes, very strong IT governance development, and above all, executive leadership capabilities on the part of the clinical informaticists who will need to help lead such efforts.

The challenge, as those in the trenches know, is this: how do the senior executives of patient care organizations find the physicians, nurses, pharmacists, and other clinicians who are becoming so desperately needed as clinical informaticists leaders create professional development paths and ladders for them, and move them into supported positions of leadership and influence? Increasingly, of course, in order to meet the demand for such new-generation leaders, patient care organizations will need to hire from outside their organizations, as demand is far outstripping supply. In the meantime, c-suite-level executives and even boards of directors of hospitals, large medical groups, and integrated health systems will need to identify early on those clinicians with informatics ability and skill, mentor them fully, and support their professional development into senior executive-level positions involving high-level leadership and governance activity.

Physician and nurse professional paths remain different along a number of different dimensions. As mentioned above, how to transition a physician in practice into full-time medical informatics management, and ultimately perhaps into senior executive-level organizational leadership, is a complex issue. The development of nurses with clinical informatics aptitude and interest is perhaps slightly more straightforward. What remains unknown is the extent to which the following types of positions intersect, overlap, and morph in the near future:

- Clinical informaticist, first-level
- Senior clinical informaticists
- CMIO, CNIO
- CHIO
- CIO
- Chief Data Officer
- Chief Quality Officer
- Chief Transformation Officer/similar title
- Positions involving senior care management/case management responsibilities
- Newer positions involving population health management, data analytics, and interoperability

Such overlaps and morphing among the above positions and trends are phenomena that will definitely need to be tracked. The following transformational drivers will impact the informactists' roles as they increasingly meet each other and overlap. These drivers are: evidence-based care delivery, chronic care management, avoidable readmissions reduction, continuous organizational performance improvement (such as Lean, Six Sigma, and Toyota Production System-based efforts), clinical transformation, and risk-based operational efficiency drives. To illustrate, when Health System X's leaders decide to embrace operational efficiency optimization, clinical transformation, population health management, and expanded risk contract-based operations all at once, what does the title "chief quality officer" mean? And what do the titles chief medical officer, chief nursing officer, CMIO, CNIO, CIO, CTO, and chief data officer all mean in relation to one another? And who should fill those positions?

What is clear is that different patterns are emerging in different organizations. For example, more and more clinicians are moving into CIO positions over time— both those with physician and nursing backgrounds. Indeed, some industry observers believe that, given how urgent and essential clinical transformation is to the broader policy and business imperatives facing the U.S. healthcare system, it will be inevitable that most CIOs within the next decade will have clinical backgrounds, though not everyone agrees on that point.

One particularly intriguing aspect of this discussion on executive clinical informatists' roles has to do with nurse informaticists and nurse leaders in general. What is clear is that more and more, individuals with clinical nursing and nursing informatics backgrounds will help to lead teams comprised of individuals with all types of clinical backgrounds, including medical ones. As a result, more fully blended multidisciplinary teams will increasingly emerge in leadership roles in patient care organizations nationwide. In other words, as the entire U.S. healthcare system is compelled forward towards ongoing, intensive work to improve core clinical processes and demonstrate improved patient care outcomes, efficiency, cost-effectiveness, and patient/consumer/community satisfaction, as well as to increasingly participate in risk-based contracting across all sectors (both private and public), individuals with clinical knowledge, informatics familiarity and aptitude, management skills, and leadership capabilities will become more and more prized in all forward-thinking patient care organizations.

## 11.4   How Ready Are Today's Clinical Informaticists for the New Challenges?

The question remains as to how prepared clinical informaticists are to ramp up their participation in management and leadership in their patient care organizations. Speaking specifically of the evolving CMIO role, Brian Patty, M.D., related that he is seeing shifts in dynamics taking place, and he believes that current CMIOs are totally caught up in the changes taking place.

In an interview with *Healthcare Informatics*, Dr. Patty expressed the perspective that CMIOs are increasingly becoming catalysts to action across their entire organizations, helping to lead workflow redesign, and other critical efforts. As a result, he said, the level of management, leadership, and organizational skills required is rising dramatically at the present time; and CMIOs will need to continue to advance their self-development at a pace at least equal to the demands of change [2].

As all these trends move forward, it is encouraging to note that some of the scenarios that industry observers have been predicting for years are beginning to emerge in concrete reality in U.S. healthcare. One integrated health system in which the dynamics are beginning to come together is the Falls Church, Virginia-based Inova Health, a five-hospital integrated system that serves more than two million people across the Washington, D.C. metro area and northern Virginia each year.

Ryan Bosch, M.D., Inova Health organization's vice president and CMIO, and Patricia Mook, R.N., M.S.N., its CNIO, are helping to lead their organization through its ACO and population health initiatives in a rapidly changing metro market. Helping to lead hundreds of colleagues in continuous change at their five-hospital, 16,000-employee health system, they fully embrace the "clinical informaticists 2.0" concept; indeed, Bosch claims to be one of the earliest clinical informaticists to use the phrase in public presentations.

In any case, both Bosch and Mook are living the challenges and the opportunities, as their health system dives more deeply into an expanding ACO relationship with Aetna in their market, and intensifies its population health management, population health risk assessment, readmissions reduction, and data analytics work. They and their Inova Health colleagues are exemplifying the multidisciplinary team-based leadership approach to clinical informatics work and to clinician-driven leadership in integrated health systems. And, based on their experience so far in their organization, they agree that they and their fellow CMIOs and CNIOs are going to need to ramp up their capabilities to unprecedented levels in order to meet the demands of the emerging healthcare system.

Senior clinical informaticists are going to need to "understand workflow, understand business process redesign and total quality management, in the Lean sense of the term," Bosch told me. And Mook said that, while "You need that baseline knowledge of clinical care and some informatics; and you have to understand the needs of operations, including the business side of the organization, and be able to marry the business and clinical sides."

## 11.5  Evolving Forward into the Future

In the end, while many specifics need to be worked out within patient care organizations—such as what positions and titles should be created in order to achieve their business and care delivery goals—healthcare systems will need to define who and what types of individuals need to be recruited for what roles and positions, what skill sets are needed, and how to create career paths and mentoring for internal development to meet the demand. And of course, how to support and fund all the people doing the work is a cost of doing business—the broad trendlines and imperatives are clear.

As mentioned above, the U.S. healthcare system is becoming broadly unsustainable in terms of overall cost and proportion devoted to the nation's gross domestic product. What's more, the public and private purchasers and payers of healthcare are increasingly demanding concrete results in terms of improved care quality, efficiency, cost-effectiveness, and patient-centeredness from providers. And the expert leveraging of clinical informatics will be absolutely essential to moving the needle on any of those goals.

Will clinical informaticists—and the organizations that employ them—be able to successfully "step up to the plate" to deliver the results that are not only being demanded, but that will be vital to the forward evolution of the U.S. economy and society? Only time will tell. But there is no question that the next decade will be the decade of clinical informaticists in healthcare. And that those organizations able to turn the key on transformational change will find themselves better positioned to meet the future not only with survival, but with success.

# References

1. Hagland M. CMIOs of the future: getting to the "second curve" on clinical IT governance. 2014. Healthcare Informatics http://www.healthcare-informatics.com/article/cmios-future-getting-second-curve-clinical-it-governance. Accessed 15 Apr 2015.
2. Hagland M. Top ten tech trends: "Clinical Informaticists 2.0". 2015. Healthcare Informatics http://www.healthcare-informatics.com/article/top-ten-tech-trends-clinical-informaticists-20. Accessed 15 Apr 2015.
3. HIMSS Analytics Annual study. (Capstone Database, ongoing project). http://www.himssanalytics.org/data/annualStudy.aspx. Accessed 15 Apr 2015.
4. Hsiao CJ, Hing C, Ashman J. Trends in electronic health record use among office-based physicians: United States, 2007–2012. National Health Statistics Reports No. 75. 2014. http://www.cdc.gov/nchs/data/nhsr/nhsr075.pdf. Accessed 15 Apr 2015.
5. Institute for Healthcare Improvement. A primer on defining the triple aim. 2015. http://www.ihi.org/resources/Pages/Publications/PrimerDefiningTripleAim.aspx. Accessed 15 Apr 2015.
6. Maestro Strategies. White paper—from the playing field to the pressbox: the strategic role of the Chief Health Information Officer (CHIO). 2014. http://maestrostrategies.com/from-the-playing-field-to-the-pressbox-the-strategic-role-of-the-chief-health-information-officer/. Accessed 15 Apr 2015.
7. Sisko AM, Keehan SP, Cuckler GA, et al. National health expenditure projections, 2013–23: faster growth expected with expanded coverage and improving economy. Health Aff. 2014;33(10):1841–50.

# Chapter 12
# Emerging Roles in Health and Healthcare

**Ann O'Brien and John E. Mattison**

**Abstract**  Healthcare has reached a tipping point where incremental change is not achieving the required improvements in healthcare quality, population health and affordability. The desired state of hyper-collaboration, team based, person-centered and health focused care enabled by big data and advanced analytics is described. However, gaps currently exist between the current and future states that provide opportunities for new roles both within and outside existing healthcare professions. The most significant new role will belong to informed, engaged, and activated consumers of health and healthcare pursing their desired states of health and resilience through strategies that are evidence-based, consistent with their values, goals, and preferences, and effective in their personal and social milieus. Empowered and technology savvy individuals as well as the underserved should receive the best evidence based and personalized care across the continuum of care. New team based care models require new roles and revision of existing ones to improve care and lower costs. Community Connectors, Health Coaches, Mobile Health Application Developers, Data Scientists, Informaticians and Care Experience roles are described. Virtual reality and avatars will be integrated into training and motivation of both caregivers and care receivers, and augment the health and resilience of all population segments. The roles of physicians and nurses will change in fundamental ways and become increasingly specialized and reliant on virtual care. Existing leadership roles will shift to address new values, new competencies, emerging trends and demands for consumers as co-designers of care.

**Keywords**  Hyper-collaboration • Radical personalization • Healthcare megatrends • Healthcare workforce • Emerging healthcare roles • Team-based care • Consumer-led heath • Care coordination • Informaticist roles • Person-centric care • Lay health workers

A. O'Brien, RN, MSN, CPHIMS
Information Technology and National Patient Care Services,
Kaiser Permanente, Oakland, CA, USA
e-mail: ann.o'brien@kp.org

J.E. Mattison, MD (✉)
Assistant Medical Director and Chief Medical Information Officer,
Kaiser Permanente Southern California Region, Pasadena, CA, USA
e-mail: John.E.Mattison@kp.org

© Springer International Publishing Switzerland 2016                    199
C.A. Weaver et al. (eds.), *Healthcare Information Management Systems:
Cases, Strategies, and Solutions*, Health Informatics,
DOI 10.1007/978-3-319-20765-0_12

Healthcare has reached a tipping point where incremental change is not achieving the required improvements in healthcare quality, population health and affordability. Increasingly, patients demand transparent access to their health information and autonomy to determine their health and healthcare. Decades of assertions about unsustainable escalations in healthcare costs have not driven significant changes, but we have finally arrived at the perfect storm for fundamental changes, many of which will be driven by consumers and technology. Many current professional roles must be transformed, and entirely new roles will emerge as we move from healthcare to health, shifting the focus from treating chronic disease to prevention and resilience. To understand future roles, it is helpful to briefly review the anticipated state of health and health care and the broad trends that are coalescing to create change.

## 12.1 Radical Healthcare Personalization

Since James Watson and Frances Crick unlocked the structure of DNA in 1954, it has taken many decades to begin unraveling the mystery of the genetic code and associated "omics"—a general term for a broad discipline of science and engineering that seeks to map various biological information objects (e.g., proteins and gene), identify relationships among them, and engineer the objects and their networked interactions to manipulate the mechanisms they regulate. Genetic variations reveal great diversity within common cancers—and across different clones of cancer within the same individual. Genetics also plays a significant role in chronic diseases (e.g. diabetes, hypertension, and cardiovascular disease). A complex array of genetic variations contributes to the development of these conditions and to the way individuals respond to therapies. The emerging fields of stem cell harvest, genetic alteration, and re-infusion hold wide promise for curing many genetically based diseases. These technologies will generate many new roles in the healthcare field, and which are heavily reliant on deep analytics. Finally, interplay exists between the specific genetic array of individuals and their interactions with the environment, e.g., diet, exercise, sleep, social health and responses to stress.

Genomics is the ultimate science of personalized medicine. Exponential growth across many platforms has been necessary to support the application of analytics and new knowledge to personalize care for individuals. The long-standing vision of personalized medicine is just now within grasp, due to the convergence of three factors: (1) massive amounts of data in electronic health record (EHR) repositories; (2) growing numbers of individuals whose genes have been sequenced: and (3) multinational collaborations for accelerating learning related to omics. Personalized medicine clearly supports both patient- and consumer-centric care [1]. However, what we call *radical health personalization* goes beyond personalized medicine [2, 3] to incorporate emerging concepts such as the *quantified self* in which we can know ourselves by measuring ourselves through personal data-recording devices, of which fitness monitors are an early and well-known example [4]. Another related concept is crowd-sourced *citizen science* that allows us to, for instance, get to know our own personal mix of bacteria and compare it to that of others [5].

Radical health personalization transcends patient and consumer roles to embrace the whole person—body, mind, and spirit—as he or she strives for an individually defined state of health and resilience through strategies that match his or her preferences, values, and goals and fully engage social determinants of health. Social determinants of health are the conditions in which people are born, grow, live, work, and age; they are shaped by the distribution of money, power, and resources at local, national, and global levels [6]. Unfortunately, one of the single best predictors of health is income [7], a relatively intractable factor that has relegated many social determinants of health to a neglected status within the health care system—a status that is now changing.

Over the past 8 years, the Institute for Healthcare Improvement (IHI) led the pursuit of the Triple Aim; better experience of care, better population health, and lower per capita costs [8]. Following the study of hundreds of communities globally, it is now evident that "to truly improve health requires improvement in the many determinants of health and well-being that exist outside the walls of the healthcare system" ([9], p. 2). In October 2014, IHI convened a coalition of the most forward-thinking and committed leaders in the country, representing healthcare, community health, public health, employers, policymakers, funders, patients, and community members. The coalition set an audacious shared goal of 100 million people living healthier lives by 2020. Patient advocate Cristin Lind defined health as "not the absence of disease but the addition of confidence, skills, knowledge, and connection. It is a means to an end—which is a joyful, meaningful life" ([9], p. 6).

## 12.2  Transition to Person-Centric Care

Patient engagement may be touted as the "Blockbuster drug of the 21st Century" but the operationalization of engaging and activating patients and families inside and outside the walls of the hospital is not as easy as prescribing a drug. The concept of centeredness originated from the Institute of Medicine's 2001 report, *Crossing the Quality Chasm: A New Health System for the Twenty-First Century*, in which patient-centeredness is defined as "providing care that is respectful of and responsive to individual patient preferences, needs, values, and ensuring that patient values guide all clinical decisions" (p. 6). Patient experience encompasses personal interactions, organization culture, and patient and family perceptions; it crosses the continuum of care to include clinical encounters and the edges and transition points that bind the system together [10]. Kaiser Permanente recently hosted a patient panel, *What Patient Engagement Means to You*, attended by a variety of members, from healthy members of the millennial generation to cancer survivors to spouses of patients with multiple chronic illnesses. A few broadly applicable themes emerged. First, every individual wants each health care provider or staff members from admitting clerk to nurse to anesthesiologist to *"know me when I get there"*. With the advent of EHRs, patients experience it as confusing and disheartening to be asked multiple times about allergies, preferences, or if they have an advanced directive.

Secondly, a closely related theme was "*Ask Me*". Shared decision making is emerging as a critical aspect of care as consumers want more information, options, and autonomy. Shared decision making is a collaborative process in which patients and providers make health care decisions together, weighing the medical evidence for various options against patient values and preferences. It supports the transition to a value-driven health delivery system. When patients choose what they want, many opt for less intense, less costly treatment and they report higher satisfaction in their care [11].

Our envisioned future state of person-centric care is driven by the values, preferences, and goals of individuals, draws on advanced science, technology, evidence-based medicine, and ancient wisdom, encompasses social determinants of health, and gives rise to health and resilience. As health care professionals, we support and mentor individuals as they seek higher levels of health and happiness. It is vastly different from the Newtonian cause-and-effect understanding in which a set of findings leads to a plan of care; instead, we elucidate, validate, and apply their values and objectives within their social and cultural contexts to help them achieve their health goals within their personal milieu. We must shift from aspiring to sharing decision making with our patients to enabling contextualized options for individuals and providing professional mentoring as to how they can choose among options arrayed as tradeoffs between their identified goals and values.

Our vision of radical health personalization is not immediately obvious in the current state of the health care system. Healthcare costs continue to rise in the U.S without commensurate improvements in health. Today, 75 % of healthcare costs are the direct result of lifestyle disorders, including obesity, diabetes, cardiovascular disease, cancer, and dementia [12]. The current delivery system has become increasingly unable to address prevention. Caregivers are overburdened, often with responsibilities not related to direct patient care, and the experiences of patients have deteriorated as a result. Some technologies, such as EHRs add to the work of clinicians with the burden of massive data entry [13, 14]. Many professional silos exist in healthcare and in sectors addressing social determinants of health. Care delivery systems often lack adequate coordination and communication among professionals and with patients, and social and health care systems have operated in nearly complete isolation from each other. New roles such as the Community Connector are described to rectify these issues.

## 12.3 Fully Realized Health Information Technology

Radical health personalization and the transition from healthcare to health hinges on fully realizing the power of health information technology. Tools such as voice recognition with natural language processing and natural language understanding can facilitate entering and searching EHR and PHR data. Open application programming interfaces (APIs) that allow cross vendor exchange of health data across EHR vendors will make full longitudinal health records available. Seamless and secure availability of interoperable longitudinal health data, reliable automation of identity management, and robust health information exchange will ensure that individuals' decisions are grounded in a comprehensive understanding of their health over time. Transparent data about costs and quality outcomes, including provider proficiency, will enable individuals to make sound decisions. Decision-making supports will include easily understandable graphic displays of tradeoffs between individuals' values and evidence-based options to maintain or improve health and resilience. Interactive survey tools will elicit and validate individual's preferences, values, and goals, help care providers understand individual behavioral styles and patterns, and identify ways of communication that work best for each individual, based on their preferences and evidence-based effectiveness.

Personal health records (PHRs) will engage and activate individuals on behalf of their own resilience and create a broad evidence base for understanding the influence of EHRs and PHRs on health outcomes [15]. Greater interoperability of data and services between EHRs and PHRs will lead to the realization of the value of both [16]. For instance, embedding reliable symptom checkers and motivational tools within PHRs will help realize the full potential of information technology. PHRs will include broader access to information in the EHR. Ultimately, the boundaries between untethered PHRs and EHRs must diminish in a world of shared decision making and coordination of care across professional and personal care networks. The introduction of systems such as Open Notes, in which patients view provider notes in the EHR through their PHR, will remove barriers to the flow of information between patients and caregivers [17].

Patient-provider communication through pervasive secure video services will become as frequent and fluid as current telephony-based communication is today. Attendant issues will be addressed: HIPAA compliance, platforms and processes for pre-scheduled and ad hoc video, the evidence base for video enhanced outcomes, and the elastic capacity of integrated care and other systems to absorb video-based virtual visits within diverse internal incentive models and external reimbursement protocols. Sensor technologies will offer individuals personal data, diagnostics, decision support, and therapeutic opportunities to make informed healthcare decisions more autonomously; these are currently emerging from venture-funded start-ups or competitions, such as the Qualcomm Tricorder XPrize to develop a consumer-focused diagnostic device [18]. Sensors will transmit data about markers for diseases for which individuals are at risk. Specialized digital tools will allow 'carve outs' of care for those providers who are experts in specific problems and procedures, and transparent data about provider proficiency will lead individuals toward more specific services. Robotics and visual avatars will transform how individuals interact with the health care system.

Effectively analyzing the exponentially growing body of digital data will create a learning health system that informs evidence-based approaches. Relevant data, combined with advances in Big Data analytics, and data visualization tools will generate new hypotheses that can be tested through data interrogation methods and analyses in more ontology-rich conventional databases and to help us understand how to innovate and replicate local successes globally. The combination of deep learning, fast data optimizations, heads-up displays, robotics and virtual avatars will transform how we all interact with the environment. Restorative narratives will transform new knowledge into stories that accelerate movement toward health, resilience, and happiness at the level of individuals and communities [19, 20].

## 12.4   Challenges to Fully Realized Health Information Technology

The current state of EHRs do not support data transparency and the effective and efficient communication required to effectively coordinate care for both health and disease. The most significant impediment to comprehensive personalized care is identity management. Effective digital identity management is fundamental to accurately merging records from disparate sources, without which longitudinal EHRs and PHRs are impossible. Although current initiatives exist within healthcare to create identity solutions, effective identity management is already robust in the financial sector, where identity verification for digital payments increasingly integrates physical, logical and biometric components. Technologies such as Apple Pay and bitcoin will deliver a superior method for identity management in healthcare based on logic and biometrics, such as fingerprints and voice analysis.

Currently individuals encounter unnecessary barriers to accessing personal health information and personalized advice through self-service mechanisms. Many individuals are pleading for the opportunity to become more active and involved in managing their own health and healthcare (e-Patient Dave, Regina Holliday, etc.). There is currently a backlash about the benefits of electronic health records, mobile healthcare apps, wearable sensors, genomics and big data analytics. Many researchers have become skeptical of the real value of EHRs, PHRs, and other technologies, such as mobile apps, because of slow progress toward realizing their benefits. However, full value realization requires extensive integration with workflow and coordination across technologies, and the transition over time to mature solutions can now proceed towards superior outcomes. Open Notes is a major step forward into transparent and jointly owned health records and personal health information.

Roy Amara, past president of the Institute for the Future, famously said that "futurists tend to overestimate the effect of a technology in the short run and underestimate the effect in the long run." We are firmly convinced that this aphorism applies to health information technology. These challenges will contribute to a more powerful and convenient world of sophisticated self-service supporting radical health personalization. Moreover, the inherent synergy of these complementary technologies assures acceleration toward value realization in the very near future.

Each gap between current and future states of radical health personalization and fully realized health information technology is a missed opportunity for safer, better, and less expensive pathways to health and resilience. Each gap represents a job to be done [21]. Each can be accomplished through a combination of enhanced roles for consumers, health care professionals and leaders, non-licensed health care workers, and community entities and better coordination among health care teams, health care agencies and systems, and agencies addressing social determinants of health.

## 12.5 Emerging Roles in Health and Healthcare

### 12.5.1 Consumers

Several forces create a nearly perfect storm for a consumer-led disruption in how healthcare will be delivered in the future, driving individuals to take more control of their own journeys toward health and wellness.

Patient loyalty to a personal physician has been substantially eroded. Workers may relocate regularly, resulting in transient relationships with health care professionals. Employee benefits managers seeking to contain costs for their employers may change healthcare offerings in ways that require employees to form relationships with new providers. Time pressures in ambulatory care, coupled with an epidemic of clinician 'burn-out,' may limit the ability of providers to provide mindful and empathic care.

Advances in information technology and direct-to-consumer decision support services are rapidly accumulating. Exponential growth in self-service ranges from systems allowing individuals to make informed choices without the advice or approval of a health care professional to over-the-counter medications and services that previously required physician oversight. Diagnostic services like those in development at Theranos (www.theranos.com) promise to provide cheaper and more convenient consumer access. Sensing devices that track clinically relevant metrics (e.g. glucose, blood pressure, calories burned) can provide consumers with the ability to more actively participate in managing their own care. In addition, more comprehensive and effortless PHR use will blur the boundaries separating EHRs and untethered PHRs, providing individuals with more access to their personal health information.

Increased transparency about costs and outcomes for individual providers and teams will allow patients to make value-based decisions and self-refer to providers with the highest value according to their individual preferences and goals. Similarly, transparency into the volume and risk-adjusted outcomes of procedures will help individuals self-select providers for specific procedures. Crowd-sourced assessments of providers will enhance the decision-making process for consumers.

Transparency will drive consumers to seek the right to obtain better care, even when it means crossing network boundaries of insurers, and to self-select a nearby specialist with comparable quality outcomes to avoid traveling long distances to reach an in-network provider. Increased local access to primary care, such as retail locations for healthcare services, e.g. CVS, Target and Walmart, etc., provide consumers with additional options, and medical tourism allows for off-shoring expensive US procedures, e.g. cardiac bypass, when offshore resources provide comparable quality at lower costs (primarily related to labor). Consumers will become more adept at self-service health care, more astute about evaluating cost and quality outcomes, and more informed and engaged. Together, these characteristics lead to more dynamic and meaningful interactions between individuals and members of their healthcare team.

Caregivers will need to adapt to a more engaged and informed patient with access to their complete personal health information and self-service analytics, diagnostics, prognostics, and therapeutic recommendations. The caregiver of the future must be prepared to help individuals match care options to their personal goals and values. Together, consumer and caregivers must weigh various options in terms of individual values, preferences, and goals.

### 12.5.2  Integrated Delivery Team

Healthcare leaders recognize that meeting the Triple Aim will require new leadership structures and improved team dynamics. Current work patterns of professional silos and fractured communication are primary contributors to preventable medical errors, which are now third only to heart disease and cancer as a cause of death in the United States. Although much-needed attention has been paid to the processes of care to improve safety and quality outcomes over the past 10 years, the job of improving care is far from complete.

The complexities of patient care and the challenges of information flow also require a high degree of coordination of care among all health care professionals. Care coordination is highly relational and time based. The theory of relational coordination argues that the effectiveness of coordination is determined by the quality of communication among participants in a work process, which depends on the quality of their relationships, particularly the extent to which they share goals, knowledge, and mutual respect [22]. Relational coordination is most important for achieving desired outcomes in settings that are characterized by high levels of task interdependence, uncertainty, and time constraints [23]. Improving quality outcomes with healthcare will require new ways of working together across disciplines and care settings, and new leadership structures and roles are required to foster relational coordination and improve care.

Integrated delivery networks and progressive accountable care organizations already realize that care coordination requires effective team-based care. A collaborative approach will become even more critical as care is increasingly fragmented by atomic roles of individual specialists. Ideal teams benefit from a level of stability in roles and responsibilities among team members, so the disruptive change ahead will challenge the best of teams. Effective leadership of teams requires a culture of collaboration and mutual respect, as well as team members who optimize work through coordination and allocation of tasks among themselves. As individuals become more empowered, engaged, and activated through radical health personalization and fully realized health information technology, they will become highly active team members, with implications for care coordination and leadership.

Increasing coordination across all aspects of health, mental health, nutrition, preventive medicine, and healthy behavioral approaches will result in entirely new roles. Increasingly, direct coordination with entities affecting social determinants of health in the community will become part of the fabric of achieving higher levels of health for individuals and communities. Teams achieving superior outcomes will be identified as "positive deviant teams", sought after as mentors and educators for teams addressing similar issues [24].

### 12.5.3   Community Connector

To reverse the trends of lifestyle and behavioral disorders, healthcare systems must be tightly interwoven with the communities where people live, work, learn, play, and worship. Tyler Norris, a 25-year veteran of the healthy communities movement, argues that "health cannot be understood in a silo, somehow independent of roads or jobs or education. It is best viewed as the byproduct of a community working (p. 6)" [25]. In a review of the healthy communities movement, Norris characterizes the positive changes and innovative approaches of community-based programs focused on groups at highest risk. According to Norris, "the most powerful long-term lever for ensuring affordable and equitable access to care for all is to invest first and foremost in the determinants of health and the factors that reduce health disparities. This lever is likely the ultimate contributor to cost containment" ([26], p. 7). Using systems thinking, the programs with most support and collective impact over time require partnerships and develop strategies that solve multiple problems. An example is creating safe walkable communities. Investing in simple and practical initiatives to get more people walking (www.everybodywalk.org) and more walkable communities can result in synergistic outcomes of promoting health, preventing disease, enhancing community economic development, improving community safety, and improving socially equitable access to resources such as libraries, playgrounds and healthy food. Community Health workers will require expertise in the areas of evidence based community interventions and continuous learning.

As part of the healthcare team of the future, community connectors need to be proficient at matching individuals' needs with respect to the social determinants of health with specific resources (programs, people, financial assistance, and institutions) within their local community that can help address their specific needs. Community connectors will identify the potential for system linkages and coordination and work to create them. Although linkages may be prompted by the needs of specific individuals, community connectors will establish and maintain them over time for the benefit of all patients who may need them.

## 12.5.4   Lay Health Worker

Another emerging role in the community is the lay health worker/health activator. To address health and resilience, lay health workers will link community-based organizations that address social and nonmedical needs with care coordinators associated with the healthcare delivery system. They will serve one or both of two roles: directly supporting the individual and/or directly supporting providers who care for that individual. Clear pathways for communication and documentation of this support will generate entirely new and relevant data that belongs to the individual's health record. The increasing presence of direct care delivery inside retail locations within communities may evolve into a major conduit for these community connector roles, functions, and services.

These lay health workers will need four distinct competencies gained through formal training: (1) identifying and inventorying formal and informal local resources, (2) matching resources to individual needs, (3) connecting individuals with resources, and (4) ensuring a continuous improvement cycle of the process through monitoring evidence-based benefits achieved through resource coordination.

## 12.5.5   Health Coach

Primary care is evolving to include health coaches who, by design, are not trained health care professionals. Coaches are individuals from the community who speak the language of the people they serve. These individuals may have backgrounds as diverse as exercise trainers or motivational coaches. Their essential role will be to help individuals navigate the system and proactively reach out when patients need preventive services or monitoring. They manage a set of tools and behavioral/therapeutic interventions that help achieve individual's personal objectives within their personal, social, and cultural value set. The primary skill set is listening and empathy. Health coaching is a short-term, rather than maintenance, role and is ideally orchestrated through communication and coordination with other members of individuals' personal and professional care networks.

## 12.5.6   Mobile-Health App Developer

Mobile applications have changed consumers' lives in nearly every facet of life from airline travel to uber rides. Mobile apps are increasing exponentially in healthcare to improve communication, remote physiologic monitoring, access to EHR data, outside reference materials and predictive models. Developers require knowledge of motivational science, persuasive technology science, social/gaming, and avatars, and astute insight into the varying ways that different population groups use mobile apps, as well as deep expertise in security and certification standards. Operating within highly collaborative teams will provide a collective knowledge base and foster innovation and creativity.

### 12.5.7  Clinical Informaticist

The current state of EHRs adds to the work of the clinician. Improvements in usability and knowledge at the point of care are required to decrease information gaps and improve highly reliable, best care. Near terms goals will include comprehensive biomedical device integration and IT infrastructures that support mobile smart devices for voice, secure texting, alarm management, context awareness, EHR documentation, bar coding for medication administration and patient engagement. This Clinical Informaticist role focuses on synthesizing the best evidence about care pathways with all available data including a longitudinal EHR, device and sensor data, preferences, values, and goals, in support of optimal decision-making for individuals. The intersection of big data with the quantified self requires new different constructs and approaches to quickly identify menus of treatment options for individuals that are accompanied by supporting rationales and evidence. Visualization tools, such as real time, clinician-specific graphic displays, will be essential for representing complex information in more easily comprehensible way to support clinical workflow. Rigorous training is required to develop decision support systems that encompass knowledge libraries and algorithms and specific data about individuals. Providing full transparency into how these decision support systems operate is imperative for innovation, continuous improvement, and obviation of onerous regulatory requirements. These are each very difficult tasks that require a wide array of skills that can only be represented in a team of cross-disciplinary expertise.

### 12.5.8  Physician

Physicians will be increasingly partitioned into technical proceduralists (specialty and subspecialty care) and physician partners in radical health personalization (primary care and some more general specialties; e.g., dermatology, mental health, general surgery). Licensure and privileging for specialty and subspecialty care will become increasingly restricted with more proof required for recertification and re-privileging for specific procedures. Transparency will lead to volume- and outcomes-based licensing. The net effect will be increasing fragmentation of licensure and privileging—and of care, especially in heavily populated areas. In light of the current and projected shortage of primary care physicians, an unintended consequence will be an increasing reliance on virtual care services, such as video visits and remote monitoring.

Due to its lower cost and greater convenience, virtual care will become ubiquitous as an alternative to conventional face-to-face encounters, and privileging for all forms of virtual care will develop concurrently. A new specialization in virtual care will emerge; developing over time as outcomes analyses reveal the impact of varying care models across specialties on outcomes and costs.

Increasingly, primary care providers will use digital tools to elicit and validate individual patients' values, preferences, and goals. Tools to quickly assess individual health and technical literacy will help physicians and other members of the care team best support the objectives of individual patients. Visualization tools will customize the display of diagnostic and therapeutic options to individual patients, highlighting varying preference-aligned aspects such as outcomes, risk, and required behavior changes. In this digital context, the role of partners in radical health personalization is to mentor and support patients as they choose between options. Emerging models in medical education will include more value-based, person-centric, and team-based care and become the norm. Physician training around engaging and mentoring patients using visualization tools based on individual values, preferences and goals will become standard elements.

## 12.5.9  Preventive Medicine Specialist

Health and longevity are profoundly influenced by lifestyle, so prevention will still revolve predominantly around lifestyle, healthy habits and social determinants of health [27]. However, a new subspecialty of preventive medicine will emerge, leveraging omics to provide radical health personalization as knowledge accumulates about which individuals need screening or monitoring for particular diseases. Once someone is identified as having a genetic predisposition to a disorder, early detection will include both conventional signs of disease, such as HbA1c for diabetes, and biomarkers, such as proteins in early pancreatic cancer [28]. Each individual will have a unique prescription for monitoring and prevention developed by a personalized preventive medicine specialist and implemented through an individualized combination of periodic testing and sensor use.

## 12.5.10  Chief Clinical Privacy Officer (CCPO)

While Chief Information Security Officers must focus on security and preventing breaches, there is an emerging role that must balance the needs for privacy, with the benefits of openness for optimal care, research, and connectedness. We will continue to discover the vulnerabilities to privacy and security imposed by rising connectedness and access to data, and one emerging role as a direct result of this will be the Chief Clinical Privacy Officer (CCPO), who will need to have deep understanding of the tradeoffs between technology and personal values. The virtues and mechanisms for reciprocal transparency will underpin much of the debate about personal privacy, and practical solutions. The blockchain technology will become a major facilitator of providing better security and citizen control over their own personal information.

### 12.5.11  Clinical Researcher

Personalized medicine requires segmenting the population of all patients with a condition into relevant cohorts, based on clinical, biological and outcomes data. In the emerging world of genomics and all the other—omics there will be increasing demands to publish the genomics of the cohort associated with individual outcomes. Once omics are associated with individual outcomes, a new type of meta-analysis will emerge that evaluates more coherent cohorts with more relevant outcomes. Researchers will increasingly perform meta-analyses, knowing which combination and sequence of analytic tools are best suited to answer specific questions using varying datasets.

### 12.5.12  Medical Detective

We are already witnessing the exponential growth of knowledge across numerous domains of health and disease, and we also can anticipate exponential growth in the number of people who represent "quantified selves". There are many entrepreneurs working on sophisticated clinical decision support (CDS) engines to address the mash up of knowledge with personal data, but there are still many individuals with complex undiagnosed chronic disease. As the sophistication of CDS tools rise, so will the advent of the Medical Detective. These individuals will do mostly 'virtual consults' of individuals with prolonged undiagnosed, under-diagnosed, or misdiagnosed diseases. Initially this genre will represent 'direct to consumer' business models, but eventually will migrate into the mainstream of medical care.

### 12.5.13  Information Strategist

Big data analytics hinges on large volumes of diverse data in which new knowledge can be discovered. Diverse data types include omics, current clinical data, longitudinal health data, sensor data, the quantified self, social determinants of health, and other relevant information. A new generation of information strategists is needed to lead clinical informatics teams that build analytic models to improve the care of individual patients and large populations. Valuable findings will efficiently emerge through a collaborative team of clinicians, informaticians, and data scientists; no single role can mastering both emerging analytics and visualization tools, as well as the broad disciplines constituting health and resilience and clinical domains.

### 12.5.14 Nurse

With more than three million members, the nursing profession is the largest segment of the nation's healthcare workforce. Nurses should be fully engaged with other health professionals to assume leadership roles in redesigning care. "Producing a health care system that delivers the right care—quality care that is patient centered, accessible, evidence based, and sustainable—at the right time will require transforming the work environment, scope of practice, education, and numbers of America's nurses" [29]. In reflecting on the role that HIT will play on the future of nursing, Judy Murphy wrote a seminal article stating that nurses must be supported by a health care environment that enables their knowledge-based work in nine roles [30]:

- Leaders in the effective design and use of EHR systems
- Integrators of patient information
- Full partners in decision making
- Care coordinators across disciplines
- Experts to improve quality, safety, efficiency and reduce health disparities
- Advocates for engaging patients and families
- Contributors to standardize infrastructure within the EHR
- Researchers for safe patient care
- Preparing a workforce with informatics competencies

In addition, as decision support tools become more efficient, sophisticated, and pervasive and a team-based model becomes ubiquitous in health care, advance practice nurses (APRNs) will assume more primary care and transitional care roles.

### 12.5.15 Nurse Entrepreneur

Many inner-city and rural communities have a high prevalence of uninsured, under-insured and vulnerable populations with minimal access to local, low-cost primary care. Many rural communities may not be eligible for Federally Qualified Health Clinics depending on designation as a Medically Underserved Area or proportion of the population that is medically underserved. In these communities, the community hospital emergency room is the only option for routine care. Emergency rooms are neither designed for nor capable of addressing primary care, behavioral health, disorders of lifestyle, or social determinants of health. One positive trend is the increasing numbers of Nurse Practitioner-led Community Health Clinics that manage population health in a holistic and inter-disciplinary way.

Bambi McQuade-Jones DNP, MSN, FNP-C is President and CEO of Riggs Community Health Center (CHC) in Boone County, Indiana. She brings extensive leadership expertise to Riggs CHC. Most recently, she led the expansion of the Boone County Community Clinic from a small clinic with a few hundred annual encounters to a self-sustaining medical clinic with over 4000 visits a year and significantly improved health outcomes. Nurse Practitioners with a doctorate in nursing practice (DNP) and advanced leadership and business skills are leading inter-disciplinary teams that collectively provide a wide array of medical, preventive, mental health, social, and educational services in many rural communities across the U.S. In addition to managing the health of large vulnerable populations, community clinics prevent unnecessary emergency room visits, saving millions of dollars and shifting the focus of care to total health. As virtual care becomes more widely available, specialist consultations to community clinics will become commonplace.

### 12.5.16 Primary Care Nurse Coordinator

The renewed focus on primary care and population management is requiring new models of care delivery. A comprehensive strategy to improve chronic conditions must consider the range of patients within the population. Population management tools and big data analytics can divide individuals into risk segments based on number of chronic conditions, level of health/ disease, functional status, and social needs. A lay health worker or health coach as described above can carry a large caseload of individuals in lower-risk segments, answering questions, discussing the plan, providing information, or just listening. Complex patients with multiple chronic diseases are more successfully managed by a registered nurse care coordinator. High risk patients and their families should have access to a nurse coordinator for providing education, case management, medication teaching, and team management. Shifting responsibilities require new norms, new processes and a culture change.

### 12.5.17 Chief Medical Officer (CMO)

The Chief Medical Officer role is expanding differently across settings. In care delivery organizations, the CMO will oversee the integration of strategic approaches by: (1) shaping organizational values and culture; (2) aligning incentives with the community served, e.g. for-profit vs. not-for-profit, academic vs. community medicine; (3) motivating change to adapt to market forces and trends; and (4) defining and coordinating other C-suite leadership roles (e.g., Chief Health Information Office, Chief Medical Information Officer, Chief Information Officer, and Chief Innovative Officer).

In ancillary organizations such as pharmaceutical and medical device enterprises, the CMO ensures that organizational resources focus on solving problems relevant to customers and maintains a deep understanding of the shifting landscape. He or she must have a clear vision of when to invest in new initiatives and when to move away from existing initiatives as market forces and opportunities shift. Deep experience in four areas is critical: (1) vision for future opportunities; (2) clinical landscape across many rapidly evolving domains; (3) operational imperatives of customers; and (4) the pervasive shift from provider-centric care to person-centric self-service.

In academic institutions, the most important role for the CMO will be to help define the evolving boundaries between academic research, health care professional education, and providing clinical services. As advanced analytics and decision support become ubiquitous, academic institutions will differentiate themselves from other health care services providers through a narrowed focus on sub-specialty quaternary services. The CMO must become increasingly astute at recognizing when new service differentiations need to be identified and developed.

### 12.5.18   Chief Experience Officer (CExO)

Many health care systems are recognizing that patient experience is about perception and the emotions it generates; it is central to each organization's processes and culture. It is linked to what the patient and family understand, what they remember, and how understanding and memory influence behavior and lifestyle decisions going forward. Leading a department of operational excellence, the CExO acts as a strategic partner to leaders across the health care delivery system to implement and evaluate processes monitoring patients' perceptions of their overall care experience. The CExO role embodies the recognition that every in-person or virtual interaction in health care impacts the patient's and family's perception.

### 12.5.19   Chief Health Information Officer (CHIO)

This emerging role of the CHIO resembles that of the CMO but addresses the broader scope of health, community resource integration, coordination of virtual care, and effective use of information to improve clinical outcomes and efficiency. This is perhaps the emerging role with the greatest opportunity for creative evolution and leadership. The CHIO may be a physician or non-physician executive with expertise in healthcare strategy or clinical transformation; the Chief Medical Information Officer and Chief Nursing Informatics Officer may report to or have a matrix relationship to the CHIO. This role requires strong entrepreneurial and change management skills, required to motivate change throughout large organizations that resist change and change leaders. To be effective, the CHIO must build confidence and trust among all senior organizational leadership.

### 12.5.20   Chief Medical Information Officer (CMIO)

In the past two decades, the CMIO role has flourished as digital medicine has emerged. The next step in this role is moving beyond initial implementation and support of EHRs. Next generation EHRs with open modular architectures that enable data liquidity and advanced decision support will replace existing systems but not without great struggle. New and existing products supporting data transparency, robust PHRs, and self-service tools integrated with longitudinal health records will create an urgent imperative to embrace these technologies. How well CMIOs embrace virtual care, advanced decision support tools, and radical health personalization will drive their success in this role. Their biggest challenge will be health care providers who are weary from the challenges of current generation EHRs and a generally perceived lack of control. The CMIO will need to have deep support from all senior organizational leaders to successfully drive change, but individuals who succeed in this role will shape the future of digital healthcare by providing successful exemplars of better outcomes at lower cost.

## 12.5.21 Chief Nursing Informatics Officer (CNIO)

The CNIO is a strategic leadership role that supports the clinical transformation vision of the healthcare enterprise. The CNIO partners with the Chief Nurse Executive to articulate nurses' needs and priorities for leveraging technology to improve care delivery and efficiency. Nurses are the largest users of health information technology; their role in the design, implementation and evaluation of new technology is essential. The CNIO also partners with the CMIO to lead enterprise-level initiatives, such as the development of evidence-based bundles, design of clinical decision support systems, or selection of new technology for data integration, unified communication, virtual care, or analytics. CNIO positions require knowledge of clinical practice, proficiency with health information technology and graduate education in the field of informatics with a focus on leadership [31]. This position will grow in importance over the next decade as healthcare organizations build interprofessional leadership structures that align people, processes, and technology goals.

## 12.5.22 Chief Information Officer (CIO)

Increasingly, CIOs in large institutions have become more external facing, delegating much of their former role to Chief Technology Officers (CTOs). While these roles evolve in the digital world, the necessity of greater grounding in both care delivery operations, and clinical medicine will invite individuals with clinical experience into the role of CIO.

## 12.5.23 Chief Innovation Officer (CInO)

The CInO role is perhaps the most muddled in healthcare today. To date, relatively few CnIOs have had significant impacts on their organizations because CEOs have often appointed inspired individuals who lack broad experience in all requirements

of digital innovation. Key expertise in this role includes change management, diffusion, scalability, securability, supportability, and continuous availability of digital
service. Experience in and focus on the discipline of innovation across its entire life
cycle will enhance success in this role, regardless of the professional background of
the individuals assuming it.

## 12.5.24   Conclusion

Exponential growth in knowledge and technology will enable a far-reaching expansion and revisiting of the science of health and wellness, necessitating new and
revised roles for many entities from individuals to senior leaders in health care.
Healthcare will shift from a reactive model of disease care to a proactive model of
promoting health and resilience at the level of individuals and communities.
Individuals in many roles, from community connectors and lay health workers to
bold and creative leaders with inspiring visions, will help shape the future state of
healthcare we desperately need and seek.

# References

1. Stewart M. Towards a global definition of patient centred care. BMJ. 2001;322(7284):444–5.
2. Hamburg MA, Collins FS. The path to personalized medicine. N Engl J Med. 2010;363(4):301–
   4. doi:10.1056/NEJMp1006304.
3. Weston AD, Hood L. Systems biology, proteomics, and the future of health care: toward predictive, preventative, and personalized medicine. J Proteome Res. 2004;3(2):179–96.
4. Quantified self: self knowledge through numbers. 2015. Retrieved 26 Feb 2015, from www.
   quantifiedself.com
5. uBiome. 2015. Retrieved 16 Feb 2015, from www.ubiome.com
6. World Health Organization. What are social determinants of health? 2013. Retrieved 16 Feb
   2015, from http://www.who.int/social_determinants/sdh_definition/en/
7. Marmot M. The influence of income on health: views of an epidemiologist. Health Aff
   (Millwood). 2002;21(2):31–46.
8. Institute for Healthcare Improvement. The IHI triple aim. 2015a. Retrieved 16 Feb 2015, from
   www.ihi.org/Engage/Initiatives/TripleAim/pages/default/aspx
9. Institute for Healthcare Improvement. Launch event: escape velocity to a culture of health.
   2015b. Retrieved 16 Feb 2015, from www.ihi.org/Engage/Initiatives/100MillionHealthierLi
   ves/Pages/LaunchEventEscapeVelocity.aspx
10. Wolf JA, Neiderhauser V, Marshburn D, LaVeia SL. Defining patient experience. Patient
    Experience J. 2014;1(1):7–19.
11. Butcher L. Shared decision-making: giving the patient a say. No, really. Hospitals and
    health networks. 1 May 2013. www.hhnmag.com/display/HHN-news-article-dhtml?dcrPath=
    /templatedata/HF_common/NewsArtilce/data/HHN/Magazine/2013/May/0513HHN_
    coverstory&domain=HHNMAG.
12. Committee on Quality Measures for the Healthy People Leading Health Indicators. Towards
    quality measures for population health and the leading health indicators. Washington, DC:
    National Academies Press; 2013.

13. Friedberg MW, Chen PG, Van Busum KR, Aunon F, Pham C, Caloyeras J, et al. Factors affecting physician professional satisfaction and their implications for patient care, health systems, and health policy. Santa Monica, Calif: RAND Corporation; 2013.
14. Middleton B, Bloomrosen M, Dente MA, Hashmat B, Koppel R, Overhage JM, et al. Enhancing patient safety and quality of care by improving the usability of electronic health record systems: recommendations from AMIA. J Am Med Inform Assoc. 2013;20(e1):e2–8. doi:10.1136/amiajnl-2012-001458re.
15. Kaelber DC, Jha AK, Johnston D, Middleton B, Bates DW. A research agenda for personal health records (PHRs). J Am Med Inform Assoc. 2008;15(6):729–36. doi:10.1197/jamia.M2547.
16. Studeny J, Coustasse A. Personal health records: is rapid adoption hindering interoperability? Perspect Health Inf Manag. 2014;11:1e.
17. Delbanco T, Walker J, Bell SK, Darer JD, Elmore JG, Farag N, et al. Inviting patients to read their doctors' notes: a quasi-experimental study and a look ahead. Ann Intern Med. 2012;157(7):461–70. doi:10.7326/0003-4819-157-7-201210020-00002.
18. Qualcomm Tricorder XPrize. 2014. Retrieved 16 Feb 2015, from tricorder.xprize.org/?gclid=ClSo1PHC58MCFciGfgodYkAAjQ
19. Images & Voices of Hope. Why restorative narratives are an important part of the media landscape. 2015. Retrieved 16 Feb 2015, from ivoh.org/restorative-narratives-improtant-part-media-landscape/
20. Wilson TD. Redirect: changing the stories we live by. New York: Back Bay Books; 2015.
21. Christensen CM, Anthony SD, Berstall GN, NItterhouse D. Finding the right job for your product. MIT Sloan Manag Rev. 2007;48(3):38–47.
22. Gittel J. Relational coordination: coordinating work through relationships of shared goals, shared knowledge, and mutual respect. In: Kyriakidou O, Ozbilgin O, editors. Relational perspectives in organizational studies: a research companion. Cheltenham: Edward Elgar Publishers; 2006.
23. Gittell J, Weinberg D, Pfefferle S, Bishop C. Impact of relational coordination on job satisfaction and quality outcomes: a study of nursing homes. Hum Resour Manag J. 2008;18(2):154–70.
24. Zanetti C, Bhatt J. Big data with a personal touch: the convergence of predictive analytics and positive deviance. Huffington Post; 2014. http://www.huffingtonpost.com/cole-zanetti-do/big-data-with-a-personal-_b_5206219.html. Accessed 07/30/2015.
25. Institute for Healthcare Improvement. 100 million healthier lives: an unprecedented coalition of leaders committed to improving health. Cambridge: IHI; 2014.
26. Norris T. Healthy communities at twenty five: participatory democracy and the prospect for American renewal. Natl Civic Rev. 2013;102:4–9.
27. Buettner D. The blue zones: lessong for living longer from the people who've lived the longest. Washington, DC: National Geographic; 2010.
28. Kosanam H, Prassas I, Chrystoja CC, Soleas I, Chan A, Dimitromanolakis A, et al. Laminin, gamma 2 (LAMC2): a promising new putative pancreatic cancer biomarker identified by proteomic analysis of pancreatic adenocarcinoma tissues. Mol Cell Proteomics. 2013;12(10):2820–32. doi:10.1074/mcp.M112.023507.
29. Institute of Medicine. The future of nursing: leading change, advancing health. Washington, DC: National Academies Press; 2011.
30. Murphy J. The future of nursing: how HIT fits in IOM/RWJF initiative. JHIM. 2010;24(2):8–12.
31. Sengstack P. CNIO: strategic partner for health care organizations. Voice Nurs Leadership. 2014;12(5):12–4.

# Chapter 13
# Impact of the Digital Age on Transforming Healthcare

**Andrew R. Watson**

**Abstract** Our modern society has been transformed by the arrival of the digital era – computers, communication and the impending era of cognitive computing. The roots of this digitalization transformation are deep and extensively distributed through our United States society, as well as globally. Healthcare likewise has evolved and is well launched down this digitalization journey. This chapter is written from the perspective of a practicing surgeon with over 25 years of experience, based in an academic medical center and who has also been actively engaged in EHR adoption locally as well as numerous international telehealth and EHR collaborations. The chapter reviews how our modern healthcare system has adopted six transformative core competencies – EHRs, communication, telemedicine, analytics, data/security, and the virtual point of care (healthcare takes place in the cloud). The aggregate result of these forces is immense lever forcing the transformation of healthcare far beyond economic reform as envisioned by federal policy changes. The digital era is an unstoppable and empowering driver of healthcare that will be best seen in the near future through advances in EHR functionality, streaming analytics, virtual care teams and remote monitoring. In this era of tremendous uncertainty in healthcare it is the digital evolution of our society throwing healthcare a proverbial digital lifeline of survival.

**Keywords** Mobile technologies in healthcare delivery • Virtual healthcare • Web technologies • Electronic health records • Digitization in healthcare • Cloud computing • Cognitive computing • Remote monitoring

A.R. Watson, MD, MLitt, FACS
Department of Surgery, Division of Colorectal Surgery,
University of Pittsburgh Medical Center, Pittsburgh, PA, USA
e-mail: watsar@upmc.edu

© Springer International Publishing Switzerland 2016                              219
C.A. Weaver et al. (eds.), *Healthcare Information Management Systems:*
*Cases, Strategies, and Solutions*, Health Informatics,
DOI 10.1007/978-3-319-20765-0_13

## 13.1    Introduction

The ability of the human species to evolve and adapt to environmental and technological changes over the thousands of years of man's existence is truly a defining
characteristic of our species and the societies that we create. So too is man's inventiveness and through our new technologies to impact survival, lifespan, our environment and every aspect of how we live, work and play. To illustrate, just 200 years
ago the horse was the primary form of transportation and communication relied
upon the physical delivery of paper from Point A to Point B in the form of a time
intensive and labor-intensive mail system. Contrast this picture with transportation
and communication in 2015. Today's cars are powered by electricity and higher
intelligence that can auto drive, park and warn against accidents. Electronic communication has made real-time communication possible with anyone, from anywhere and anytime through a number of social media tools, such as email, Twitter,
or Facebook. With the new technology generation cycle estimated to be 18-months
to 2 years, the rate at which we experience major new technologies that impact
every aspect of our lives feels faster today than ever before.

Early computers entered our industries by the mid-twentieth century, started to
be adapted to support healthcare in the 1970s [4] and made their way into homes in
the form of personal computers in the mid- 1980s, and by the mid-2000s web connected cell phones were in the hands of most citizens in every country [12]. As web
and computing technologies evolved and web-based telephony became ingrained in
our society, there came a Gladwellian tipping point [10] where connectivity and a
stream of electrons brought our society together and hence our patients and healthcare systems together. We saw broadband, in the forms of DSL's in the 1990s and
now we are looking at 4G and 5G LTE speeds on cellular phones with pervasive
computing and communication work as watches. For healthcare organizations and
clinicians, these profound technology changes have permeated every niche, workflow process and communication mechanism by which operations and healthcare
delivery are performed in just a short 35 years.

While we may not be able to point to a discrete start of the digital age, as of 2015,
our society is in the middle of an exponential transformation into the digital age. It
is important to recognize that over the span of this past 35 years, while we were
adapting to and shaping healthcare technologies, we have reached the point where
we are now dependent upon it [6]. The pressures for healthcare to transform our
multi-factorial are mostly financial. However, there is no doubt that the digital age
is applying as much pressure to healthcare transformation as is the economic pressure. Examples of the digital age applying pressure are seen through "electronic"
health records (EHRs) and video based "tele" medicine. These are technology
driven channels in healthcare that came from the digital evolution. Another prime
example is the imminent arrival of analytics that will take the wealth of big data (all
digital) and create streaming analytics via cognitive computing. The United States
has implemented "meaningful use" as part of healthcare reform that mandates the
use of EHRs to receive full reimbursement. In other words, there is no doubt of the
reliance of healthcare upon technology.

## 13.2    The Introduction of the Digital Age: Setting the Stage for Healthcare Transformation

As stated above, the digital age is one of the most transformative forces we have ever seen in modern society for it links all locations and all individuals and all technologies in ways we never fathomed as a society and with a potency we are still trying to understand. The two main forces that are effecting change in healthcare are computational power and communication capabilities.

The earliest computers relied upon individuals changing wires to accommodate the computation of data. It was John von Neumann who in 1946 created the concept of RAM (random access memory), and understood that one dataset could automatically act upon another dataset for desired outcome [5]. The initial computing efforts were directed at solving the complexity of the nuclear age and the ballistics. Inadvertently, but nonetheless a reality, this foundation of computing came to be applied to medicine as well. As we all have witnessed, in these intervening years, it has been developed to handle the extraordinary complexity of the human body, its organ systems, the molecules that govern and control it, and the endless variations of diseases and derangements that we as physicians and nurses and caregivers encounter. Until the late 1970s when the first personal computers began to appear in industry, computer systems took up entire rooms and there use was relegated to universities and large corporations, and were commonly depicted in science fiction films with functionality that we are just now approaching. Individuals, clinicians and patients did not associate computers with healthcare during these latter decades of the twentieth century.

Over these past six decades, computational power has increased exponentially, where by 2015 consumer-grade technology can be purchased at a local store with terabytes of storage, gigaflops of computational power, hundreds of gigabytes of RAM multiple core processors, sophisticated multidimensional graphic renderings, and come with the ability to link to high-speed communication. Arguably, the computational power necessary to extensively benefit healthcare was achieved by 2000, and now computational horsepower is essential to all aspects of life and death, in sickness and health, at home or work, and at birth and death. A hospital today is by default a digital hospital and applies to computational processing, always-present demands for security, for heating and cooling, for electronic health records (EHRs), for telemedicine, and for research.

The second component of the digital age is communication and that includes both broadband and wireless modalities that came as a direct result of computational = demands described above. The early Internet2 speeds (http://www.internet2.edu/) seen at the Argonne National Laboratory in Chicago are now commonplace at patients' and caregivers' homes, and are provided at retail prices from multiple vendors to be installed in a matter of days [1, 14]. The communication component has two parts – bandwidth and the modality. The bandwidth of communication expanded with fiber-optic communication to the homes, dark fiber paths between healthcare delivery facilities, and sophisticated wired infrastructure within healthcare settings that delivered the end result of the computational layer to the bedside or physician office. Bandwidth is critically important because health care functions and applications require the transmission of large datasets, and imaging data used in diagnostic tools, such as radiology images or digitized pathology slides [7].

Modality in communication refers to rather the tool is connected to a wired cable or line as compared to wireless, as in a SMART phone or iPad device. Since 2010, the ability of wireless communication to be reliable as well as support the necessary bandwidth has become commonplace. We no longer have to be plugged into a wall sockets, we no longer have to go to a local store or our homes to receive powerful broadband. Today, we are surrounded by high speed, powerful, reliable and capable networks that we use for almost every aspects of our lives. Even in rural America were service can be intermittent and spotty, broadband is being adopted and deployed. This commitment to extend broadband into rural America is highlighted in the 2009 Broadband Technology Opportunity Program (BTOP) that is embedded in the American Recovery and Reinvestment Act [3]. Clearly not everybody has access to broadband, but today, the vast majority of the US population has access to sufficient bandwidth.

This explosion in wireless and broadband capacity means that the endpoints of the digital era have become smaller and now fit in the pockets of patients, students, doctors, nurses, or hospital administrators. The initial cell phones were large, heavy, had limited battery life, and could dial a cell phone number. A modern smart phone will recognize your voice, a battery can last for many days, can handle video calls, can be your single source of health information, and serve as a hub for a home glucometer or pulse oximeter. In short, the endpoints are no longer single channel devices, but now pocket-sized biospheres of communication and interactions that can affect your daily health in real time.

## 13.3  Why Healthcare Is Leveraging Video, Small Endpoint and Wireless Networks

An important part of the digital age that merits special attention is the seamless delivery of video. Before video, we used speech and hearing as the staples of non-proximal communication, just closing one's eyes and communicating in this fashion gives you the perspective on how limited these two senses are. Try describing a rash or an infected wound accurately over the phone. Of the five senses, one could argue, vision is perhaps the most important and the most communicative of all. Vision can more readily substitute for speech and hearing than speech and hearing can fill in for an absence of vision. Therefore, the ability to use video around the world and as a seamless part of our everyday lives has transformed the fundamental challenge of access to healthcare. When a nurse or doctor examines a patient, there are three fundamental tenets – auscultation, palpation, and observation. Of the three, it is observation that is the most necessary and the most powerful, and now the most available at a retail level on your video-enabled phone. The availability of video has been the most important addition to healthcare arguably since the development of antibiotics or transplantation.

Healthcare is becoming addicted to the miniaturization of high-powered computers. In either an ambulatory or inpatient setting – where currently the bulk of healthcare is delivered – clinicians have at their desks or on a set of wheels a powerful computational healthcare enabler. As we examine and diagnose patients, we are looking at multidimensional, reconstructed radiology images (so called 4D imaging), we are looking at laboratory values that are accurately calculated in minutes by automated devices, and using speech to text to accelerate communication. We are using bar-code scanning to immediately document medication administration and prevent drug related medical errors. We can now offer advanced diagnostic and therapeutic modalities in our office that in the past would require a whole separate team and location. For example, portable ultrasounds that are handheld can image the ventricles of the heart, provide deep views of the portal vein, or image deep body spaces that are becoming less accessible in this era of obesity [13]. Another example is the use of robotics and procedural spaces that can refine and mature gross movements into fine-scaled arcs of a needle sewing a vein to an artery on the heart regardless of the motion of the heart or the tremor of a surgeon's hand.

The wireless or untethered endpoints means that any patient, or any employee, or any caregiver, or any administrator, can watch and interact and prescribe and predict and communicate in real time regardless of time and location and disease and state of health. The explosive arrival of tablets and cell phones that evolved with the web technologies embedded in smart phones allows us to review patient data in a true mobile and secure fashion. Pagers are being replaced by mobile devices that support secure text messaging and pictures. Providers and patients can securely and privately communicate on phones and tablets. And furthermore, the care teams and caregivers that communicated using paper in the past are making decisions in near real-time, leveraging all of the assets of the digital age that gives them immediate access to a patient's medication lists, allergies, problem lists and clinical notes. With a focus on genetics, advanced pharmaceuticals and the latest research, perhaps the greatest treatment opportunity lies in the near-term future with streaming analytics and cognitive computing. Decisions can be double-checked in real time using aggregated years of experience to ensure that high-quality care is delivered and errors or inappropriate treatment are minimized.

## 13.4 Six Core "Digital" Competencies of Healthcare Today

There are six core competencies of healthcare that exist today because of the digital transformation: EHRs, communication capabilities, telemedicine, analytics, data/security, and the virtual point of care (healthcare takes place in the cloud).

### 13.4.1  Electronic Health Records

EHRs are the most visible and simultaneously instrumental example of the digital age impacting healthcare. There are several predominant EHR vendors in the United States, with over 200 other companies aggressively positioning themselves and their products to work in this mission-critical area of healthcare. Prior to the EHR, the currency of healthcare was a combination of oral communication, a provider's memory, hands-on nursing care, and a paper chart. None of these components were linked and few were mined for analytics. Furthermore, the paper chart was siloed in multiple different physical locations, with multiple different handwriting styles, with often challenging filing requirements, and represented a physical bulk that made it difficult to carry them from location to location especially as patients got sicker and the charts became heavier.

The EHR delivered to healthcare access to information in real time, a document archive with structure, the integration of multiple clinical informatics systems, and the ability to immediately treat patients without waiting for orders to be taken off, or for a chart to be located, or a list of possible medication interactions to be investigated. ePrescribing allows for accurate, immediate and documented medication administration. Digital notes allow nurses on the floor to read what happened in the operating room only minutes before. Mediation reconciliation is a team activity between expert pharmacists and nurses in different locations across a hospital. Inpatient and outpatient records can be seamlessly tied together for all to view in offices, floors, homes, or via portals.

Despite the end-user interface and configuration critiques of EHRs, these software applications have enabled medicine to make a leap forward towards real-time and safer healthcare [2]. Asynchronous and paper based healthcare will never match the first generation of EHR functionality even with all their functionality limitations and poor usability and lack of data exchange capabilities.

### 13.4.2  Communications

Prior to our digitization era, communication between care team members, care coordination in acute care settings, and interactions with patients at home were extremely limited in features, relied upon a beeper, and were asynchronous hence frequently delaying care. Many times, nurses and doctors had to walk down the hallway or go between buildings to communicate between each other or amongst themselves. This was time-consuming, distracting, and potentially life-threatening in the setting of an emergency. During an acute change in a patient status, it is the immediacy of resources that can be assembled around the patients to save lives that is necessary. The digital age has provided the communication tools to alert and meaningfully communicate data in a number of ways. We no longer are sending a string of numbers on a disruptive loud pager without context to each other to establish communication. With cellular phones, wireless in-hospital phones, and the communication features of smart phones, we have the ability to know who to call, when to call them, and how to contact them immediately, or how to text them a critical message. Many times, we don't need to talk to a fellow care-giver or patient, we just need to get them a piece of information as an update or a reminder. Texting provides us that means and is highly appreciated widely across our society as a timelier and less distracting means to communicate information than a voice call. Therefore, the use of cellular phones and in-house phones for these different communication modes gives us the ability to reach the right provider at the right time and in a respectful and appropriate fashion.

Communication as described above has been augmented by the ability to send secure pictures and secure emails between multiple care providers at the same time. Metaphorically speaking, a picture is worth 1,000 words, and therefore sending an image of a wound or a rash immediately replaces any sophisticated attempts at describing them using words. Communication now has context, immediacy, is less distracting, can include high-resolution pictures that when seen in aggregate have revolutionized how we conduct every-day healthcare at all locations.

### 13.4.3   Telemedicine

The next significant example of the digital age impacting healthcare is the growing utilization of telemedicine. Telemedicine is a compound word, medicine being the root and is effectively unchanged. "Tele" is a reference to the telephone, but it should more appropriately be called digital medicine and not telemedicine. Using telemedicine providers, payers, and families can reach out to patients in a respectful, convenient fashion and may very well solve the challenge of access to healthcare. In the United States (US), rural telemedicine clinics link specialists to patients who may not be able to drive, may not want to drive, and may not be able to afford to drive to a clinic visit. At the University of Pittsburgh Medical Center (UPMC), we leverage rural telemedicine outreach centers with a regular sub-set of specialists and staff to conduct routine clinical work using video-communication technology. Patients are spending less money on gas, tolls, parking, child-care and no longer have to worry about driving at night on snow-covered roads. Better access to healthcare through telemedicine has significant implications on health, engagement, chronic disease management and the cost of care.

Telemedicine also functions in a pivotal role in radiology, pathology and ophthalmology. Tests are captured as images with metadata and are transmitted in a routine or urgent fashion to a specialist, who interprets the results sends them back, incorporated into the EHR. This means that specialists can be distributed across a broad landscape, making for fewer gaps in clinical service lines at hospitals, and providers do not have to waste precious caregiving time with unnecessary travel. For example, a rural hospital may have one pathologist who is not able to comfortably interpret a complex neuroendocrine tumor slide, and using digital pathology can transmit a digital slide for an expert to interpret and return a report within minutes. This enables the distribution of sub-specialty expertise, prevents wasted time with physicians driving, and helps to educate remote physicians while simultaneously treating patients.

Telemedicine has multiple implications for the health care system moving forward, and the field of remote monitoring holds tremendous potential. There is little doubt that the use of sensor-based and wearable devices at the home will give providers an early warning system to monitor longitudinal care, chronic disease management, preventative care, and well care. Importantly also, the field of remote monitoring is being driven at the level of the consumer electronics market through apps such as, biosensors, wireless scales, activity monitors, and heart-rate monitors. Remote monitoring holds promise as being the most powerful early warning system based in the home that health care will ever have.

### 13.4.4   Data Analytics

Analytics is the interpretation of data sets such as EHR structured notes or patient registries and the conversion of them into intelligence. With the growth in the computational power of healthcare and the consumer electronics market in general, the amount of data being generated within our society is exponentially increasing. In a recently published study it is estimated that 90 % of all data generated by our society in the past 2 years [16]. The era of big data is upon us, and this has been highlighted in the news and certainly in the healthcare press as well. As a result, the complexity of databases is growing, the number of databases is increasing, and this speed at which data is flowing is near real-time. These facts in isolation do not in fact improve healthcare, but in many ways hinder it due to the shear volume of data generated and its complexity. However, looking at the entirety of data sets and understanding the story they tell is critical for making healthcare become proactive and more intelligent. For example, we can look at patterns of patient healing based on locations within the hospital that may have natural light, decorated in a given décor, use music therapy or are simply quieter. We can leverage payer claims-based data to evaluate the efficacy of patient portals to see whether or not they are safe for prescribing and cost-effective for insurance companies to have to pay for them. We can look at the effect of checklists in the operating room to understand a decrease in never events, operative time, and the length of stay after a procedure. In essence, analytics makes us better understand what we have done and provides a strong context for what we need to do in the future. Winston Churchill said "history first repeats itself as a tragedy, then as a farce." Analytics gives us the tools to prevent poor decision making from happening in many ways in healthcare.

Analytics also holds tremendous potential for the field of research, in particular genomics. With the vast expanse of a genome and the environmental factors that surround it, analytics can help us understand the epigenetics, gene sequences, drug effects, and cancer mutations. For clinical outcomes, genetic-based research and pharmaceutical development, our healthcare system can become much more sophisticated through research driven by analytics of large complex data sets. We will have the opportunity to learn from our mistakes and successes.

## 13.4.5 Data Centers and Security

The next core competency of a digital health care system is the rise of data centers and security. All analytics, EHRs, telemedicine, patient communication will ride over networks and through data centers. Most of this tremendous volume of information is stored and contains sensitive personal and financial details. Healthcare systems that had terabytes of data in 2005 are looking at data-sets of over 10 petabytes in 2015. Analytics will add an additional layer of information and hence volume that needs to be store and immediately accessed as streaming analytics evolve [11].

In many ways, the storage challenges of data in healthcare is the least appealing aspect of the digital age and the least visible, but without a doubt data warehousing technologies are the most foundational element. Simple pieces of data such as where a patient is located, how old are they, what are their allergies, how many times they sent a secure email are all small fragments of data that must be stored and accessed by the application and communication layers. All caregivers and researchers and patients rely upon data and accessibility for safe patient care, for communication, for the context of their treatment, and for the quality of care. Furthermore, this information directly impacts the cost of care as knowledge of a patient's history can reduce critical expensive problems such as catastrophic drug-drug interactions or repeating unnecessary and expensive testing. How all of this information is stored and the applications virtualized have become an art form inside healthcare in the era of big data and transformative computational power. Most recently data centers have been challenged by the consumer electronics market and the "cloud" of virtualized information. Computational power and storage no longer have to reside within the healthcare campus, and can be distributed and outsourced using cloud base technologies such as those by Amazon or Microsoft. Cloud storage is fast becoming the store norm for smartphones and therefore will impact healthcare more extensively in the near future.

Data centers also have the feature of security which brings out some of the best and worst aspects of our healthcare system in the era of HIPAA (Health Insurance Portability and Accountability Act) concerns, security fraud, data breaches, and higher overall accountability. The HIPAA regulations that govern US healthcare's mandate for secured data in an expanding mobile era have never been greater nor as feared [9]. Sensitive patient information needs to be protected from unwanted intruders, healthcare providers cannot access sensitive data about a neighbor or celebrity, and patients are now entering credit cards for co-pays online. In many ways a data center in the digital age is as sophisticated as the human body in terms of its complexity, scale, and the security functions that match the human immune system.

### 13.4.6   The Digital and Virtual Point of Care

When discussing core competencies within healthcare, where healthcare actually takes place is the most important question. Is healthcare located in an office? At home? In the hospital? Or is the venue of care a combination of all the above? Today, the bulk of US healthcare still takes place in physicians' offices, ambulatory clinics or hospital settings and is driven by doctors, nurses and allied health professionals. These are the locations where a new diagnoses of diabetes is made, a new medication is prescribed, a procedure is performed or a pneumonia is treated. In the past, physicians routinely conducted home-calls and patients' care was largely home based. With the recent increase in the sophistication of medicine, the majority of care migrated to hospitals and sub-specialty care to urban settings. These areas have the most sensitive diagnostic technology, the largest collection of sub-specialists, and frequently the latest clinical trials. A standard doctor's office will have a computer, and this is as common as having a stethoscope in a provider's pocket. But the computer is also connected to the internet within the building which contains vital signs flowing from wireless thermometers, infusion pumps carrying critical rate and volumes to information systems, or telemedicine videos reaching out to a patient at home.

Technology advances in video communication, medical device monitoring and health policy that emphasize cost efficiencies are all pushing changes in point of care away from acute and ambulatory care and placing care out into the community, the primary care doctor's office and patient's home. The advent of video, broadband and smart phones has raised the potential in healthcare for care to go back to the patient at home using vehicles such as telemedicine, ePrescribing or patient portals. Using monitoring, video consultations and community based care delivery teams all raise the question of where is the "point of care"? Increasingly, the question of "where does healthcare delivery truly take place?" is found to be more virtual, more community and home based, and using communication tools that change the very nature of the provider/patient relationship.

The digital healthcare systems and the digital patients they treat are raising the real question of where should healthcare take place and can it be done virtually in the cloud? Can we afford a health care system that does not leverage the smart phone and broadband with a patient at home? Is the ambulatory setting now a hybrid of a digital home with sensor devices and the care team in a medical office building? These questions remain unanswered, but they represent the fundamental new challenge and opportunity of a virtual point of care.

## 13.5   Transformation of Healthcare

The transformation of healthcare is a byproduct of the above six digital competencies and financial reform in the United States under the Affordable Care Act that was passed during the Obama administration. The need to transform the United States healthcare system and most healthcare systems throughout the world is best recognized as economic reform. There is no doubt that the cost of healthcare in almost any country is being driven by over utilization, technology, and the perverse healthcare incentives that reward low quality and inefficient care. The current rate of growth of the United States healthcare system is not affordable, which is why "health care reform" in the United States was passed [8].

There is a much different force behind the transformation of healthcare that transcends economic reform and that is the digitalization of our society and healthcare as described above. The digital age in our society goes beyond theoretical construct and is played out in real time in the consumer electronics market every day and in all aspects of our lives. The digital era is aimed at the individual consumer and healthcare is trying to keep pace with the steep slope of innovation. The development of advanced computing is not to enable hospitals and EHRs, but rather to enable the very citizens and patients that we take care so that they have better lives, find new jobs, be more productive, and live in a smarter planet. The communication needs of smart phones and cell phones with video calls is satisfying a large gap in communication for all citizens of the world. We can video call our families when traveling in India, we can email our bosses from airplanes when going to a business meeting, and we can call a friend in trouble on a cell phone at night when not able to travel through a snowstorm to be with them. The Fortune 500 US technology companies know this trend in our society, and are making record profits from this as was recently seen by the announcement of Apple computers in January 2015 [17]. The implications for this ongoing investment in the digital marketplace is significant for healthcare, as it is for industry. Capitalism ensures that the digital trend is pushed, not healthcare methodically conducting a clinical trial or evaluating a new drug. Therefore it is concerning that healthcare is not leading the transformation of the digital age, but it is reacting to it.

There are two major trends that come out of this imbalance of evolution of healthcare versus the forward thrust of the digital age. The first trend is the expectation that patients will have of their healthcare systems and providers. As patients have real-time access to their friends and families, to data, to purchasing power, and transparency within our society, it is only a matter of time that patients hold healthcare accountable at the same level. Should healthcare tweet the latest research findings, or should doctors routinely round on Facebook patients? Currently, the economic reform of health care is placing a greater burden on patients to engage and pay for their own care; and therefore, patients will demand greater price transparency and access to care at home. This expectation will place a tremendous burden on the healthcare system to accommodate trends such remote data being securely integrated and answering video-based communications within minutes. As healthcare struggles to modernize through economic reform, it is quite possible that real pressure from the digital patients could significantly hurt or help the evolution of our care delivery systems. But it will not be an insignificant impact.

The second major trend that comes from the consumer electronics market is never ending innovation and growth. At this point in time, there is no clear end to the innovation and growth of the consumer electronics market and the money being put into innovation and marketing it to consumers. Fist sized video cameras that are waterproof to 30 m can be attached to a bicycle and controlled remotely from a smart phone. How does this impact telemedicine? If we attached an accelerometer to a patient's walker and wanted to track the progression of their movement disorder, how would you import this analyzes within a healthcare system? What if real-time, transcutaneous glucose monitoring becomes a reality? Who is responsible for that data and who will pay for the storing and interpretation? There are sensors that can be worn around your forearm that monitor the contraction of muscles and help to guide the controls of a computer or device. If the patient loses their hand from sepsis but can still remember how to use their hand that is no longer present, could this device replace the hand? The analytics surrounding communication, both voice and digital, is to the point where shopping on a website leads to predictive marketing and eventually downstream to how retail outlets stock their shelves. Could the same be said for patients searching the internet for health care problems predicting epidemics or cancer? We don't know the answer to these questions, but the power of the consumer in aggregate as witnessed by the largest technology companies in the world is threatening to push healthcare in a direction that the patients will expect and the system will be challenged to handle. But, at the same time, this same power may offer healthcare new avenues to engage patients, both sick and well, in ways that were never imagined and perhaps play a central role in solving many of the problems not just adding to complexity.

## 13.6   Discussion

It is impossible to predict the future of healthcare and it is impossible to predict the evolution of a digital society. The pressures on both go beyond any predictive capacity that we currently possess, and therefore a health care system of 2025 is beyond the scope of any reasonable confidence intervals and description. But, the digital age has taken us to the first steps of modernizing our healthcare system; and therefore we are able to see with a reasonable degree of certainty the next 5 years of our transformation.

As stated above, the health care system is under tremendous pressure to change due to the computational and communication capacity of the patients both sick and well. The devices, technologies and features that are being delivered and sold to patients are not only enabling them in terms of their daily routines, but they are simultaneously teaching our patients how to interact with the future digital healthcare system. Over the next 5 years, it is evident that four digital trends standout for their transformational impact: streaming analytics, advanced EHR functions, virtual care teams, and remote monitoring.

**Streaming analytics** is the ability for the computational layer of healthcare data centers to interpret large data-sets on the fly and understand decisions with a predictive capacity. When a patient searches Google, has a biosensor heart rate elevation, or develops a cough after an airplane ride, streaming analytics may be able to diagnose a pneumonia before it is even symptomatic. Or, streaming analytics could predict an influenza outbreak or contaminated food source. Additional examples of streaming analytics can be seen in the eICU system of VISICU whereby a multitude of patient data is interpreted in real-time and prioritized for a physician and his care team to react to. Earlier trends and sepsis can be identified, and decisions can be prioritized based on immediacy of need and capacity of the providers, not solely in a reactive fashion based on symptoms or lab values [15]. Chronic disease management, as well as cancer care, stand to make quantum leaps based on streaming analytics in the future. Ten daily biometric readings from a patient with CHF would present an impossible dataset for the human mind to interpret in real time, but streaming analytics based on cognitive computing could make sense of this. Streaming analytics will be led by IT companies such as at IBM with Watson technologies who can assemble the computational and storage capacity necessary to achieve this.

**Virtual Care Teams**: Chronic disease management is an absolute necessity for the modernization of the United States healthcare system and relies upon care teams. The cost of chronic diseases is overwhelming the payment system for healthcare, and in large part is being driven by rising obesity rates. Chronic diseases necessitate not just a nurse or doctor visit, but a team of people taking care of sick and complex patients, a different times, from different locations, and with different skills sets. There is no physical or possible way for a comprehensive care team to be with the patient in real time. The only way for a care team to holistically treat the patients and support them with a virtual care team leveraging telemedicine, EHRs, analytics, and communication. A care team must bring together the combination of asynchronous communication e.g., email or text message, real-time digital data, and the best of video telemedicine so that the patient has proactive, coordinated, communicated, and non-fragmented care. And perhaps most important, this care can now be delivered to a sick patient at or near their home as they are frequently unable to travel. The concept of a virtual care team is the aggregate of multiple features of the digital era in healthcare, and one that will require significant outcomes and patient satisfaction research moving forward.

**Advanced EHR Functions**: EHRs are still maturing in many fashions, especially in how they communicate with patients and providers, and how they communicate with each other. Market pressures and software development have left significant gaps in inter-vendor communication and the ease-of-use for end-users. However, the promise of advanced EHR functionality is starting to emerge in the marketplace. This advanced functionality includes features such as order sets, which lead to safer, more efficient, and evidence-based care to prevent medical errors. Another example is closed loop medication administration using technologies such as barcode scanners. A wireless device can identify the medication, the correct patient, the time of administration, and immediately document the transaction. The use of speech to text integrated into structured notes also means that the rise of structured text holds greater promise for more accurate diagnosis, coding, billing, and future analytics. Clinical pathways represent evidence based medicine combined with clinical decision support and are starting to bring value to healthcare through lower costs and better quality. Pathways are deployed and monitored at the provider-patient interface using EHRs. It is becoming clearer that as EHRs evolve from a data-repository and integrated billing/documentation system they will realize much greater effectiveness and capabilities within healthcare.

**Remote monitoring** has been discussed above, but its true promise is a combination of an early warning system and a lifestyle management system for healthcare delivery systems and insurance companies, respectively. Remote monitoring is the integration of sensors, information and medical peripherals wherever the patient is located. It can be as simple as an app, a text message, or rise to the complexity of multiple peripherals in a patient's home in the setting of congestive heart failure. Consumers will certainly have retail access to these devices in the near future. Regardless, these technologies will bring to bear asynchronous information reaching a caregiver who needs to understand how a patient is remaining healthy or why their healthcare status has acutely changed. A true remote monitoring system is equal to the control tower of an airport watching multiple airplanes (patients) and airlines (diseases) and locations simultaneously in real time. It helps to coordinate complexity, watch new diagnoses at home, and engage patients regardless of provider or disease or location.

## 13.7 Summary

As patients and healthcare professionals, we did not ask for the digital era. We did not ask for telemedicine, we did not want analytics to check our surgical performance, and we did not ask for electronic health records to take away the feel of writing in a patient's chart. But just because we did not ask for them, does not mean they are incorrect and not beneficial. The point is actually irrelevant because the digital era represents the natural evolution of our society and its impact on healthcare is irreversible, unstoppable and better for our society. The digital era is making health care more accessible, safer, more predictable, and also in many ways more affordable. Therefore we need to embrace, help to lead, and fully support the evolution of the health care system as it is transformed by digital era.

## References

1. Argonne National Laboratory. Whole genome analysis, STAT. Feb 19, 2014. Available at: http://www.ci.anl.gov/press-releases/whole-genome-analysis-stat. 2014. Accessed 31 Mar 2015.
2. Bell B, Thornton K. From promise to reality achieving the value of an EHR. Healthc Financ Manage. 2011;65(2):51–6.
3. BTOP. Available at: http://www2.ntia.doc.gov/. 2009. Accessed 31 Mar 2015.
4. Buchanan NS. Evolution of a hospital information system. Proc Annu Smymp Comput Appl Med Care, Nov 5. Available at: http://www.ncbi.nlm.nih.gov/pmc/articles/PMC2203735/. 1980. vol 1, p. 34–36. Accessed 31 Mar 2014.

5. Burks AW, Goldstine HH, von Neumann J. Preliminary discussion of the logical design of an electronic computing instrument. Institute for Advanced Study, 28 June 1946 (reprinted in Vol. 5 of Taub, A. H. ed. Collected Works of John von Neumann. Oxford: Pergamon Press; 1961). The Manchester copy of the report (Copy #54) is in the National Archive for the History of Computing, University of Manchester. 1946.
6. Centers for Disease Control and Prevention. Progress with electronic health record adoption among emergency and outpatient departments: United States, 2006–2001. NCHS Data Brief 187: Feb. Available at: http://www.cdc.gov/nchs/data/databriefs/db187.htm. 2015. Accessed 31 Mar 2015.
7. Costello SS, Johnston DJ. Development and evolution of the virtual pathology slide: a new tool in telepathology. J Med Internet Res. 2003;5(2):e11.
8. Emanuel E, Tanden N, Altman S, Armstrong S, Berwick D, et al. A systematic approach to containing health care spending. NEJM. 2012;367(10):929–54.
9. Feld AD. The Health Insurance Portability and Accountability Act (HIPAA): its broad effect on practice. Am J Gastroenterol. 2005;100(7):1440–3.
10. Gladwell M. The tipping point. How little things can make a big difference. New York: Little, Brown and Company; 2000. ISBN 0-316-31696-2.
11. Jamoon E, Beatty P, Bercovitz A, et al. Physician Adoption of Electronic Health Record Systems: United States, 2011. US Department of Health and Human Services. Centers for Disease Control and Prevention. National Center for Health Statistics: Hyattsville, MD. NCHS Data Brief. 2012;98:1–8. Available at: www.cdc.gov/nchs/data/databriefs/db98.pdf. Accessed July 30, 2015
12. Pew Research Center. Global publics embrace social networking: computer and cell phone usage up around the world. Dec 15. Available at: http://www.pewresearch.org/2010/12/15/global-publics-embrace-social-networking/. 2010. Accessed 31 Mar 2015.
13. Prinz C, Voigt JU. Diagnostic accuracy of a hand-held ultrasound scanner in routine patients referred for echocardiography. J Am Soc Echocardiogr. 2010;24(2):111–6.
14. Roebuck K. Presence information: high-impact strategies – what you need to know: definitions, adoptions, impact, benefits, maturity, vendors. Brisbane, QLD, Emereo Publishing; 2012.
15. Sadaka F, Palagiri A, Trottier S, et al. Telemedicine intervention improves ICU outcomes. Crit Care Res Pract 456389. Doi 10.1155/2013/456389, Epub 2013;1–5. PubMed ID: 23365729.
16. SINTEF. Big Data, for better or worse: 90% of world's data generated over last two years. Science Daily 2013. www.sciencedaily.com/releases/2013/05/130522085217.htm. Accessed 30 July 2015.
17. Wakabayashi D. 'Staggering' iPhone demand helps lift Apple's quarterly profits by 38%. WSJ July 22, 2015. Available at: http://www.wsj.com/articles/apple-earnings-boosted-by-iphone-sales-1437510647. Accessed 30 July 2015.

# Chapter 14
# Health Information Crossroad: An Opportunity to Deliver Real Measurable Outcomes for Better Health and Well Being

**Harry L. Reynolds Jr. and Christopher A. Jones**

**Abstract**  There is so much data and information in health care, but has and will it be used to truly change outcomes, cost and quality? As the focus changes to population and individual health, even more data will be needed to ensure that personalization supplants a one-size-fits-all model. Those entities that crack the code of using data for true insights and game-changing actions will reap benefits while others may fail. It is an amazing time for personal technology that can and will be used more in the future for improving individual health. The industry must undo so much in the way of process and care models now that fee-for-service is disappearing as a payment standard. This is requiring new leadership, thinking and direction unprecedented in this slow-to-change environment. As new entrants join the effort and push those who are entrenched in the past, progress is accelerating. Data and information need to play an actionable, economic and real role in changing for the better. There are more exciting examples of the new way to do it right. The future is bright and the journey is difficult. Embracing it means investing energy and courage in considerable quantities.

**Keywords**  Outcomes • Information • Insights • Data • Transformation • Consumerism • Health reform • Engagement of individuals • Convergence

## 14.1  The Current Dilemma

Health care and the models that deliver, finance and document it are undergoing dramatic change in all areas of the world. It is an industry that is made up of amazing professionals who focus on changing people's lives. The data captured by the

H.L. Reynolds Jr. (✉)
Director, Health Industry Transformation,
IBM Global Healthcare and Life Sciences Industry, Durham, NC, USA
e-mail: hreynold@us.ibm.com

C.A. Jones, MHA
Quality and Informatics, Wake Forest Baptist Hospital,
Area Health Education Center, Winston-Salem, NC, USA

© Springer International Publishing Switzerland 2016
C.A. Weaver et al. (eds.), *Healthcare Information Management Systems: Cases, Strategies, and Solutions*, Health Informatics,
DOI 10.1007/978-3-319-20765-0_14

industry has over time grown exponentially and specifically based on the entity capturing and using the data. The cost of health care has captured continuous headlines in most countries and is showing little chance of abating in the near future [1]. So many efforts are underway to change these trends and data will a dominant part of the success or failure. However, it cannot be the kinds and types of data that have always driven this industry. Instead it will need to be actionable, pragmatic, comparative, transparent, longitudinal, consumer friendly and always available.

A key filter that will be mentioned throughout this chapter is whether data and information create a landfill [2] or truly, measurably change the industry in ways not seen to date. The opportunities for data are exploding within an industry facing dramatic change and a burdensome task of creating real value before it hurts economies and individuals even further.

Every country, state, employer, payer, provider and individual are affected by current data and have a monumental hope for improvement in the future. Data is the only universal output from this industry and must become truly impactful not just be available to do processes and reporting. Everyone involved is facing dramatic and difficult decisions about healthcare and data must help not just ride along with the change.

There are pockets of the industry that are much more integrated in their organizational structures and data handling than the general industry. They are to be commended but it is difficult to extrapolate their model in most cases. However, they can share their experiences in a context that the other entities can relate to their individual pieces. Even the best fall significantly below what is needed. Neither the outcomes, costs, transparency nor engagement of individuals meet the needed levels for a successful future (Fig. 14.1).

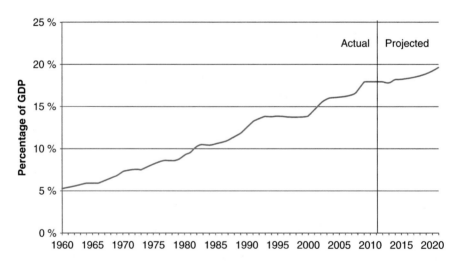

**Fig. 14.1** U.S. National Health Expenditures as a Share of GDP, 1960–2021 (Source: Centers for Medicare and Medicaid Services)

## 14.2   Data in Health and the Surrounding Industry

Each of you reading this can probably tell a compelling story about your health data, the volumes, redundancy and complexity. Most would profess that the information is important during an episode or procedure but has little use for you ongoing. Even chronically ill who live daily with issues struggle to have their data be useful, available and actionable. Care models throughout the world are made up of many processes, caregivers, systems and locations. This has helped fragment data for decades and is changing slowly [3]. Most data is kept as part of process, compliance, care documentation, and research, but does it make a real difference to changing value, quality or outcomes before, during and especially after care. Picture a beautiful quilt made from many disparate pieces of cloth into a magical and pleasing pattern. Compare that to healthcare where most entities consider their data the final product rather than making it an important part of the data about an individual who has data pieces in many caregiver and payer environments. Owning the data is a mantra of importance that many entities hold dear to their success. An admirable individual approach but will delay and actually block game-changing data sharing and usage. It is so difficult to transform data in an industry where success of individual entities is based on them being good at their piece and protecting their data. The countries and others mentioned above will be doing everything possible to redefine success factors based on value, true cost structure reduction and better population health. Only those who accept that the current world healthcare directions are not sustainable will survive the change necessary to ensure healthcare spending doesn't ruin economies, businesses and individuals seeking care.

Data standards is a subject that gets much attention and has seen progress in some countries but is not advanced at all in others. Without standards, sharing of information and real transformation will be fragmented at the very best. Countries who have not even automated basic information and its sharing.

So much is being written about the growing issue of chronic diseases such as diabetes.[1] Data and information about this disease have been available to care givers and individuals for decades but the incidence continues to rise. Devices such as glucometers, free supplies, nutrition guidelines, an internet full of information and caregivers who know how to treat the disease cannot slow its increase. The opportunities of data and information used in new ways may offer a brighter future. Such possibilities will be expanded in each of the paragraphs below to show approaches using information and process. Discussions of statistics, data, and information however can become numbing and overwhelming to the general public. As a person, who is a patient, one wants to know about themselves, in their lives and their context. So data, information and processes must matter one person at a time to show real outcomes and improve the well-being of individuals

---

[1] *Epidemiology/Health Services/Psychosocial Research*: Venkat Narayan et al. [8]

## 14.3   The New Wave of Data Sources

Smart phones, apps, social media, and wearables like fitbits etc. have changed each of your lives in an amazingly short time [4]. Monitoring patients, wherever they are, e-visits and telehealth are examples of the new data sources being embraced by the healthcare industry. More data sources whose data must be captured, stored and used. Much like you have junk mail in your inbox, what is the junk mail from these new sources? Even more importantly, what is worthwhile, to whom, for what, against real value that makes a dent in the cost, quality and outcomes so sorely needed? This data will dwarf in volume the data that has been and continues to be used in today's processes. When discussing these new sources they are considered additional to what happens now not replacements or enhancements to the old. An industry that truly needs transformation cannot just keep adding on while not replacing or making markedly significant ROI on these new sources. These new sources beg for an architecture of data for every entity that hopes to survive and thrive in this new world ahead. Just because data can be accessed doesn't help this "hoarder" industry break its habits and enhance the future.

Continuing the diabetes thread, there is an application available by smart phone for diabetics developed in Austria. You have probably heard that often, but let's dig deeper. It is an application built by individuals who have and live daily with diabetes; therefore, understanding the minute to minute life impacts. As you listen to the developers explain it's capabilities that improve their daily lives it excites you about all people's lives. Further the cost is surprisingly low and affordable, the information gathered is used to the benefit of all individuals and the application can be offered by a country to all its citizens who have diabetes. Personal to each, built by like diabetics and used differently by each person; an exciting approach for all ages, geographies and environments.

## 14.4   Data as a Conduit to Value

Just look around as you go about your normal day. What data/information are worthwhile in your life, influences your behavior and you would not want taken away. A car insurance company offers a plug-in device to evaluate your driving. It captures your driving tendencies and judges your capability. If you are good per their evaluation you get good rates! We all know that a credit score is kept on us that impacts offerings for large purchases like homes and cars. Social media has exploded with opinions about most any subject including your health, diseases and treatments. Further many people consider these opinions as valuable as those from care givers. Throw in travel sites with prices and reviews for destinations around the world, plus the new ability to schedule a taxi, track its arrival and have a set price ahead of time, people want convenience focused on them. Service, convenience and immediate access are imbedded in our daily lives. Welcome to dealing with people under their terms and conditions. How and when can the health care industry really engage in this reality of people being people and help influence their health and well-being.

Value requires changing both the existing approach to data as well as the future uses and direction. So much data exists that can be used to build baselines of performance, outcomes and cost that allow new uses of that data against new expected outcomes. Value in healthcare going forward is very difficult to define and measure as every entity tries to change or realign. It takes real leadership to accept so much change to what is successful currently. It is exciting to see governments, employers, payers, providers and individuals demanding a clearer definition of value. Watching entities adopt data models, new methods of scoring performance, and higher standards of interoperability lends so hope but too many are doing it incrementally rather than revolutionizing true value. Value in healthcare has always been based on people as patients or insurance members. Value going forward will need to think of the person as a consumer, parent, child, senior citizen, chronic, employee then patient or member. The data and its value cannot be focused on the entities in healthcare predominantly as it has in the past. Influencing individuals as they live their lives and seek wellbeing on their terms will be paramount. Value will require new sources of data that are available outside normal healthcare process [5]. Many people are asked their preferences by airlines and retail entities. That information is used to tailor value for that person. That type of engagement is almost nonexistent in healthcare so new data can be used in this manner to help value. That data however will not usually integrate well will existing systems or processes. That data used to augment value in the future will make a measurable difference. Value is look at through so many lenses in healthcare that success is dispersed. Will doctors and hospitals embrace scoring and comparisons, can the cost of healthcare be flattened, will employers demand action, and will governments dictate results.

In a European country the Minister of Health authorized the distribution of free glucometers to all diabetics in the country. The individuals are asked to bring the glucometer to each doctor visit so the doctor can actually see the readings covering the time since last visit. This data delivered by the patient to their doctor which chronicles actual readings or gaps in readings is invaluable in care. No generalities, no remembering by the patient and no uncertainty by the doctor exists. The discussion can range from controlling the disease, to daily fluctuations, to environmental effects and so on. The value is real to all involved due to the right data, personalized, accurate and shared with the doctor. An elegant approach that with good process aligned makes the data priceless. Picture further combining the application mentioned above with this capability and you have a precise data flow and information capability for each citizen that has diabetes, about them and for them.

## 14.5   Information to Change Behaviors and Affect Outcomes

Every healthcare environment is flush with data as discussed above. Turning that data into useable, actionable and continuously refreshed information is a must going forward [6]. Engaging individuals in their health and wellbeing has eluded most all healthcare arenas. Thinking of patients as people and using information accordingly is a white space yet to be captured by the industry in meaningful ways.

Unless people can really know how to engage with the information available to them everything will continue to be sporadic and episodic at best. That will ensure that 5 years from now current issues will be dramatically worse. The same issue of information is faced by all care givers and support teams in healthcare. How can each caregiver tailor the information they get, need and use to change their work flow to really impact cost, quality and outcomes? No one in the industry can escape the magnitude of data but they want to harness what they really need to fulfill their desire to make a difference every day.

Data has been for so long considered an asset itself and information hard to get that people are skeptical to transformation and weary about the journey [7].[2]

Data must be evaluated across many dimensions, uses and needs to be more than just a costly corporate asset. Data filtered by worth, usefulness, quality, is one consideration. Data across processes, procedures, patients, care givers and diseases is another consideration.

## 14.6   The End Game Expectations

True transformation discussed at length in this section requires incredibly strong leadership and foresight at so many levels, if real change is to occur. Are there enough leaders in the industry with the courage to lead toward an unscripted future. That does not just mean at the C level but throughout all levels of an organization. The experience of individuals as patients is usually clouded fractured care, unexpected costs and many insurance claims. The industry must rework itself to make that experience much easier to score from an individual's point of view. Data, information and insights must be a significant conduit to that end, but it must happen sooner not later. Embracing the journey from data to information, knowledge, insights and finally improved outcomes will take all in the industry to achieve. It will require helmets and seat belts for this difficult journey. Accepting this and leading is a true crossroad that some will take and others won't. Let's hope that the takers significantly outweigh those who do engage.

Consider a healthcare industry worldwide that delivers data and information that;

- Explains options available to caregivers and individuals needing care
- Makes everything aligned to age, health status and preferences for each user of the data

---

[2] The diabetic examples above teamed with the advancement of genomics, cognitive computing, smart phone applications and coordinated team care models paint a positive outlook for true personalized changes for individuals. Data will abound but must be turned into actionable, personal, useable and simple information that can be used by each person the masses. As health care becomes a consumer business meaning affordable capabilities, changing health status is attainable world wide.

- Educates on the transition of diseases whether one or many together
- Helps the individual get the right care in the right setting on their schedule
- Defines incentives, restrictions, cost variances and provider network alignment
- Seeks an understanding of personal compliance by patient to their care responsibilities
- Allows people to declare whether they understand their medications or diseases.
- Explains care site offerings and home monitoring that really make a difference.

This list is not exhaustive but illustrative of the future vision. Every person in the world is part of this discussion and its issues. It will take many villages to drive this transition. Shame on all of us if we don't attack these opportunities with enthusiasm, strength and vigor.

# References

1. Ginsburg P, Hughes M, Adler L, Burke S, Hoagland G W, Jennings C, Lieberman S. What is driving U.S. health care spending? In: Bipartisan policy center's health care cost containment series. 2012. http://www.rwjf.org/content/dam/farm/reports/issue_briefs/2012/rwjf401339. Accessed 19 Apr 2015.
2. Bardoliwalla N. Rescue your data from the big data landfill. 2014. CMSWire.com. http://www.cmswire.com/cms/big-data/rescue-your-data-from-the-big-data-landfill-024073.php. Accessed 20 Jan 2015.
3. Jauhar S. One patient, too many doctors: the terrible expense of overspecialization. 2014. Time. http://time.com/3138561/specialist-doctors-high-cost/. Accessed 19 Apr 2015.
4. Nield D. In corporate wellness programs, wearables take a step forward. 2014. Fortune. http://fortune.com/2014/04/15/in-corporate-wellness-programs-wearables-take-a-step-forward/. Accessed 4 Aug 2014.
5. Wharam JF, Frank MB, Rosland AM, Paasche-Orlow MK, Farber NJ, Sinsky C, Rucker L, Rask KJ, Barry MJ, Figaro MK. Pay-for-performance' as a quality improvement tool: perceptions and policy recommendations of physicians and program leaders. Qual Manag Health Care. 2011;20(3):234–45. doi:10.1097/QMH.0b013e318222c398.
6. Niland JC, Rouse L, Stahl DC. An informatics blueprint for healthcare quality information systems. J Am Med Inform Assoc. 2006;13(4):402–17. doi:10.1197/jamia.M2050
7. Bellin E, Nancy Neveloff Dubler. The Quality Improvement–Research Divide and the Need for External Oversight. Am J Public Health. 2001;91(9):1512–17.
8. Venkat Narayan KM, Boyle JP, Geiss LS, Saaddine JB, Thompson TJ. Impact of recent increase in incidence on future diabetes burden: U.S., 2005–2050. Diabetes Care. 2006;29(9):2114–6. doi:10.2337/dc06-1136.

# Chapter 15
# Health IT's Essential Role in the Patient-Centered Medical Home and Practice-Based Population Health Management

Paul H. Grundy and Richard J. Hodach

**Abstract** This chapter focuses on the IT capabilities required by patient-centered medical homes, including electronic registries and associated applications that enable care teams to automate processes and provide continuous care to their patient populations. In addition, the chapter explores new technology options, including patient portals, remote monitoring, mobile health apps, and cognitive computing. Our goal is to show how patient-centered medical homes can use automation tools, analytics, and big data to improve population health.

**Keywords** Patient centered medical home • PCMH • Population health • Healthcare transformation primary care transformation • Medical home • Primary care Health It in PCMH • Health it in population health management

## 15.1 Introduction

As chronic disease management consumes over three-quarters of US health costs [5], there is a need to redesign primary care, to change the emphasis from episodic acute care to a continuous, comprehensive preventive approach, to improve health and reduce costs [44]. The core of this redesign is the patient-centered medical home (PCMH). The PCMH model [3], a building block of Accountable Care Organizations (ACOs), organizes and optimizes care across time and medical neighborhoods (local hospitals, consultants and services) (Grundy et al. [16]), and comprises 20–25 % of US primary care practices.

P.H. Grundy, MD, MPH, IBM (✉)
IBM Industry Academy, IBM Corporation, Armonk, NY, USA

Department of Family and Preventive Medicine, University of Utah, Salt Lake City, UT, USA
e-mail: pgrundy@us.ibm.com

R.J. Hodach, MD, MPH, PhD, FACMQ
Chair, Board of Directors, American Board of Medical Quality, Tacoma Park, MD, USA

© Springer International Publishing Switzerland 2016                    243
C.A. Weaver et al. (eds.), *Healthcare Information Management Systems:*
*Cases, Strategies, and Solutions*, Health Informatics,
DOI 10.1007/978-3-319-20765-0_15

## 15.2   The Patient Centered Medical Home

The PCMH provides comprehensive primary care based on ongoing, stable relationships between patients and physician-directed integrated care teams. PCMHs charge is to enhance access, coordinate care and improve quality through the use of disease registries and health information technology [26]. The components of a PCMH [3, 27] include:

- A physician-led primary care provider/team that provides first contact and high-quality, continuous, comprehensive care for and in partnership with patients and families
- Patient-centered care with continuous (24/7) access to care providers
- Care coordination across time, settings (inpatient/ambulatory) and services
- Formal recognition: certification and reimbursement that reflects the value of these services

## 15.3   Physician-Led Care Teams

PCMHs use a physician-led, multidisciplinary (nurses, managers, health coaches, and others), team-based care model to ensure that all patients are cared for in the right place, at the right time, and in the manner most appropriate to the patient [25] to help them navigate the system and achieve agreed-upon health goals. Teams may be broadened to include professionals in the home, including specialists (especially behavioral health services), home health nurses, educators, therapists, pharmacists, social workers and increasingly, family caregivers [27, 28].

## 15.4   Patient Access

A National Committee on Quality Assurance (NCQA) recognized PCMH must provide:

- Timely appointments and enhanced access to care patients (same-day appointments, extended hours) and self-scheduling
- Access to clinical advice on a 24/7 access. Clinicians on call must have access to the EHR with phone or secure messaging

These functions may be provided through a patient portal through which patients must be able to schedule appointments, refill prescriptions, viewing lab results and access records.

## 15.5   Care Coordination

Care coordination, a PCMH requirement, is assurance of a patient's navigation through the medical neighborhood to reach specified and agreed-upon care plan goals. The assignment of roles and tasks to specific stakeholders (patient, provider, team members, consultants, service providers) helps to improve outcomes and to reduce waste and inefficiency. Care coordination extends the care team and requires the cooperation of all stakeholders in the medical neighborhood providing services to the patient. As the health status of the patient evolves, revisions in the care plan must be shared with all participants in a timely fashion.

- **Test and results tracking and follow-up**
  PCMHs must record test (laboratory, imaging, etc.) orders in an EHR and capture and store results in structured data fields. NCQA also requires tracking of and follow-up on all ordered tests, which may be supported by EHR-S alerts for missing results. Another supporting EHR-S functionality is providing patient access to results and to information about their meaning [6].

- **Referrals and follow-up**
  PCMHs must send electronic summaries of care that include the care plan and pertinent test results to other providers in more than 50 % of referrals (This is also a requirement of Stage 2 Meaningful Use). Referrals must be tracked until consultant reports are received. Some EHRs have features that allow this to be done automatically. While NCQA-recognized PCMHs meet these referral requirements, the online exchange of health information continues to be problematic.

- **Care transitions**
  PCMHs must exchange key clinical information electronically with other care providers, such as hospitals, EDs, and nursing homes, at transitions of care. They must identify patients with unplanned hospital and emergency department admissions, share clinical information with admitting hospitals and EDs and consistently obtain patient discharge summaries.
  Although, many hospitals still do not send timely discharge summaries to primary care physicians, a few institutions have modified their admission-discharge-transfer (ADT) systems to let patients' doctors know when they've been admitted and discharged (early notification system).

## 15.6   Formal Recognition

While several organizations certify patient-centered medical homes, the National Committee on Quality Assurance (NCQA) is the principal agency for PCMH recognition [13]. As of September 2014, NCQA recognized 8,112 practice sites encompassing 40,841 clinicians as PCMHs [34]. By November 2014, close to a quarter of US primary care physicians were at some stage of creating a PCMH. This growth is fueled by financial incentives from health plans that offer higher payment rates, care coordination fees, pay for performance, and shared savings [13] for recognized PCMHs. As of 2012, over 90 insurers recognized PCMHs and over four million Blue Cross Blue Shield members in 39 states were served by a PCMH [36]. A 2013 survey counted 114 payer reform initiatives for PCMHs, covering 20 million lives [13], with Medicare and Veterans Health pilots underway [36, 24].

## 15.7   Impact on Practice

Research and industry studies have demonstrated strengths and challenges in implementation of the PCMH model:

- **Strong results**
  Payers have focused on the PCMH model because it saves them more than it costs. United Healthcare, for example, recently announced that its medical home programs in four states showed average third-year net savings of 6.2 % of medical costs, resulting in a return on investment of 6:1 [49]. Similarly, a medical home pilot at the UPMC Health Plan in Pittsburgh yielded an ROI of 160 % [42]. And Geisinger Health System (which includes a health plan) estimated its net savings from its PCMH model at $3.7 million, for a return on investment of more than 2:1 [15].
  A recent peer-reviewed study found that PCMHs reduced Medicare payments by an average of $325 per patient, compared to a comparison group of non-PCMH practices. ED visits dropped by 7 % for the PCMHs, and hospitalizations of their sickest patients fell 4 %, although overall hospital admissions did not decline [33]. Much of the savings associated with the PCMH model come from avoided ED visits and hospitalizations. According to a summary of peer-reviewed PCMH studies by the Patient-Centered Primary Care Collaborative (PCPCC), 61 % of these studies reported fewer ED visits, 31 % reported fewer hospital admissions, and 13 % reported fewer readmissions [31]. The PCMH is also associated with improved access and quality. The PCPCC says that 31 % of the studies it reviewed showed improved patient access, 23 % reported higher patient satisfaction, 31 % found an increase in preventive services, and 31 % registered improvements in population health [31].

- **Areas for improvement**
  Not all PCMH studies have shown positive results. A RAND study of an early multi-payer PCMH [7] initiative in Pennsylvania found that the pilot was associated with improvement on only one of 11 quality measures and was not associated with lower ED or hospital utilization or a reduction in total costs over 3 years [14]. But a commentary by people involved in the program suggested that the results of this study might have "oversimplified" the experience of the Pennsylvania Chronic Care Initiative. The study failed to capture improvements in important intermediate outcomes such as blood pressure, LDL cholesterol and

blood sugar control in diabetic patients, the authors said. Also, they pointed out, the program had initially made a mistake by not allocating funds to hire nurse care managers for high-risk patients—an oversight that was later corrected [8].

## 15.8 Population Health Management

By emphasizing continuous proactive care and providing collective information about the ongoing health of patients they serve, PCMHs offer the opportunity to manage and improve population health. Population health is defined as "the health outcomes of a group of individuals, including the distribution of such outcomes within a group" [23].

Practice-based population health (PBPH) management uses information on specified subgroups of patients within one or a group of practices to improve the overall care and clinical outcomes of all patients within that practice ([2], 6).

Population health also depends on other factors, including health literacy, socio-economic status, geographical location, access to care, transportation, and the physical environment in which patients live [30]. Population health management (PHM) has several domains:

- Identification and characterization of subgroups of patients to stratify risk
- Guidance and support for patients and providers to assure adherence
- Measurement and feedback on practice patterns to improve performance
- Information sharing among stakeholders to assure transparency and improve quality and safety

## 15.9 Identification, Characterization and Risk Stratification

The first step in managing population health of a practice is assessment and stratification of the health risks within the practice's patient population. One method is to screen all patients proactively (health risk assessment, HRA) via questionnaires that may be distributed online at the PCMH level. If a PCMH is associated with a registry, health analytics may be able to use known indicators to identify patients at high risk [18]. Typically, 5 % of a patient population accounts for about 50 % of its health costs for a given risk [10].

## 15.10 Guidance and Support for Patients and Providers

The next step in PBPH is to identify gaps in preventive and chronic care for patients identified in population-wide registries. Analytics can identify patients that are overdue for specific services and can link them to their PCMH provider teams, customized to match the treatment preferences of patients and practices. Combined with automated messaging to patients about preventive or chronic care, analytic forecasting has been shown to increase patient adherence (Rai, et al. 2011). Combined with pre-visit prompts to providers and managers, practices can proactively assure that patients receive all appropriate, timely and up-to-date care during visits [21]. Examples of some organizations using registries today to identify patient care gaps include Group Health, Prevea and the Northeast Georgia Physicians Group.

## 15.11   Measurement and Feedback on Practice Patterns

An area of central importance in PBPH and PCMH management is ongoing measurement of practice performance, resource utilization and costs.

- **Disease-specific care quality**
  Beginning with disease-specific, risk prevalence data on populations within a registry (such as diabetes or hypertension), completion rates for clinical goals (HbA1c levels, BP measurements) and short and/or long-term health outcomes (hospitalizations, adverse events) for patients can be measured to assess performance of PCMHs and larger organizations on disease-specific targets. Registry analytics can drill down to completion of health goals and outcomes as linked to specific providers, practices or subcategories of patients and provide feedback to providers and care teams for lifelong learning and practice improvement. For long-term outcomes, PCMHs must link clinical data (HbA1c levels, BP measures) with patient-reported data (functional status, self-perceived health) and perceptions about the quality of health and the care received.

- **Utilization and Care Costs**
  Associated with performance measurement is cost management. Cost metrics are of particular importance if an organization or practice is providing care for patient populations at higher risk for high-cost care (or for other financial loss, ACO two-sided model). Economic forecasting of population care costs (how many patients will likely need expensive care) based on clinical and claims data can help guide organizations to allocate resources to meet the needs of high-cost segments and conditions within the population to anticipate and mitigate costs of Emergency Departments and hospital admissions.

## 15.12   Information Sharing Among Stakeholders

A key IT functionality needed in PBPH is timely and organized communication among stakeholders. Within the PCMH, EHR systems can facilitate internal communications and tasking, using alerts and secure messaging (via patient portals). Health information exchanges (HIEs) offer conduits for record sharing with other stakeholders in medical neighborhoods (however such HIEs and the protocols that support sharing (i.e., the Direct Protocol) are not yet widespread in the US).

Communication is essential in care transitions such as hospital admissions and discharges. Examples include:

- Hospital ADT alerts to PCMHs (Private communication: Tim Pletcher, CEO, Michigan Health Information Network) within a region to facilitate early care coordination for unexpected admissions
- Electronic messages to patients shortly after a hospital discharge to ask if they have questions about instructions or medications and to assure their connection/follow up to their PCMH [18].
- The Michigan Health Information Network (MiHIN) uses ADT feeds from hospitals to provide alerts to physicians across the state [39].

## 15.13   Health Information Technology in PHM and The PCMH

PCMH certification criteria emphasizes health IT measures related to access and electronic communication, patient tracking and registry functions, care management, patient self-management support, electronic prescribing, test tracking, referral tracking and performance reporting. NCQA Level 3 PCMH recognition is a requisite by payers for financial incentives (NCQA 2014). Recommended health information technology functionalities for achieving PHM [43] have been articulated.

## 15.14   Medical Home Technologies and PHM

- **Electronic health records, necessary but not sufficient**
  EHR systems are indispensable to providing the scope of care [19, 32] required for PCMH certification, but current systems lack complete functionalities needed for PHM. Limitations include: inability to generate population-based reports easily; problems in presenting usable alerts and reminders; inability to capture data on preventive care; and non- interoperability between different EHR systems [2]. In addition, longitudinal care plans are not used [12] and while systems may be able to alert providers about gaps in care, they do not link to relevant clinical patient data [29].

- **Automation of clerical functions, essential**
  It has been calculated that a "manual" PCMH requires 4.25 FTE staff members per FTE physician, 1.57 staffers more than the average primary care doctor uses in a non-PCMH practice. Most of this difference represents the hiring of nurse care managers [35]. At Prevea Health [37], a multispecialty group in Green Bay,

Wisconsin, automation enables managers to cover two to three times as many patients as possible with manual methods, with time savings in completion of routine tasks such as chart preparation and patient follow-up communications. Prior to deployment of the solution, managers spent an average of 188 min per high-risk patient (47 min searching the EHR for information, 2.5 patients per day). After implementation, they could process an average of 6.5 patients per day [40]. In addition to making the scope of PCMH care feasible, automated functions can make teams efficient and cost-effective [4].

- **Electronic communication, efficiency and outcomes**
  EHR system-based secure messaging and telephone calls enhance patient access and in-person visits. Patients are contacted in advance of visits to clarify concerns and expectations. Providers reviewed electronic records, including care gap alerts before each visit. A pilot study in the Seattle Group Health HMO found 6 % fewer in-person visits, 80 % more secure message threads and 5 % more telephone encounters with providers than without these tools [41]. Patient communication through email, secure messaging and access through practice portals are key components to improving PCMH outcomes.

- **Cognitive computing, great potential**
  "Cognitive computing" or harnessing the power of supercomputers to support care has great potential that is being explored and tested. One potential is as a pre-processor of current medical knowledge and literature to provide clinicians with answers and syntheses based on evidence to difficult questions. Another is to provide clinical decision support based not only on discrete data, but also unstructured information that forms about 80 % of the information stored in EHRs [1, 9, 22] to support diagnosis and management of individual patients with the potential to incorporate and integrate data from many other sources, such as geographical and income data, that have a bearing on population health, as well as the treatment of individual patients [46]. As an example, the Carilion Clinic Healthcare System in Roanoke, Va has used IBM Watson technology's [11, 20] predictive modeling power to process structured and natural language data from the EHR. From 3 years' data, Watson identified 8,500 patients at-risk for congestive heart failure, a leading source of the healthcare system's costs.

## 15.15 PHM Technologies Beyond the Medical Home

- **Patient Registries and Analytics**
  PCMH level analytics are a key enabler to help care teams manage patients effectively and efficiently [21]. By applying analytical algorithms to EHR and claims data, teams can identify and track cohorts of patients by risk, adherence and appropriate medication use. Multimodal (secure messaging, phone) automated messaging can remind patients of appointments, prescriptions and other follow ups.

One major goal of care is to reduce exacerbations of high-risk conditions that lead to ED visits or hospitalizations. Analytics can produce registry-based summaries about patient care gaps in groups, and prioritize cases re: proactive care manager interventions for high-risk patients. Depending on the PCMH's stage of technology adoption, they may conduct such programs for medium-risk and low-risk patients. Across the entire population, they endeavor to engage patients in managing their own health [21]. For example, different intervention programs might be aimed at those with Type 1 diabetes mellitus (DM), Type 2 DM, Type 2 DM plus hypertension, or poorly controlled Type 2 DM, with different educational materials and self-care recommendations sent to patients in each cohort.

Electronic registries link patient data about individuals to temporal clinical data from multiple sources (PCMH, laboratory, pharmacy, etc.) and allows for aggregation to generate knowledge about populations. In addition to helping practices identify patients at risk and to guide care and education, registries can, with appropriate analytical tools, provide practices and health care organizations with data and predictive insights for health risk stratification, identification of gaps in care, quality reporting and financial/performance evaluation. Importantly, aggregated data from multiple registries can also facilitate regional collaboration [21].

Areas where health IT has improved the efficiency of PCMH processes center on care coordination and communication tasks within a given "medical neighborhood" of a primary care based practice. Published examples of registry-enabled medical neighborhoods include the Jackson Health Network in Michigan [17] and the Northeast Georgia Physicians [38].

- **Remote patient monitoring**
This modality has been used most frequently with high-risk patients, such as those with congestive heart failure or for post-surgical home recovery, but has also been used successfully to support patients with day-to-day management of chronic disease (diabetes and hypertension, [48]). PCMH care teams may use this kind of data—which must be screened for relevance—to provide automated or live feedback to patients on their health management. In addition to tele-monitoring systems, today numerous mobile apps allow patients to self-monitor their conditions using smartphones. Increasingly, these mobile apps are being used in conjunction with portable devices such as glucometers, but integration of these patient-generated data into physicians' EHR systems is still low due to interoperability obstacles [47], as well as physicians' concerns over certification of these patient data for safety, accuracy and effectiveness.

- **Remote consultations**
No longer relegated to dedicated tele-health applications, clinician/patient remote visits are increasingly taking advantage of the availability of high-bandwidth video, well as consumer available apps on any Smart phone, such as "FaceTime" to do a "home" visit or consultation [45]. Increasingly, this form of consultation is being accepted by payers in geographic areas with low availability of specialty services, or for home visits for patients who are homebound.

## 15.16   Conclusion

The PCMH is recognized as an engine of healthcare reform. It is a building block of Accountable Care Organizations, the core of clinically integrated networks, and arguably the care delivery model that has the greatest potential to organize medical neighborhoods. PCMHs are gaining traction among primary care physicians as they cope with rising demands for services and a fast-changing reimbursement system. Information technology is an essential enabler for this transformative care delivery model as well as to achieve the Triple Aim goals in population health management. As detailed in this chapter, population health cannot be managed at an affordable cost unless providers have the needed information technology tools to apply automation to routine tasks. Moreover, the PCMH needs analytics that permit it to stratify patients by health risk, identify their care gaps, and enable care managers to intervene quickly with high-risk patients. Analytics are also essential to performance evaluation and cost management.

In conclusion, due to current lack of interoperability among EHRs and EHR systems, health IT has a long way to go before it can provide all of the support that PCMHs will need for population health management and care coordination. But, without health IT, a PCMH would have very limited capabilities. So the two trends are expected to continue evolving together.

## References

1. Agency for Healthcare Research and Quality (AHRQ). Clinical Decision Support (CDS) initiative overview. 2014. http://healthit.ahrq.gov/ahrq-funded-projects/clinical-decision-support-cds-initiative. Accessed 19 Apr 2015.
2. Agency for Healthcare Research and Quality (AHRQ). Practice-based population health: information technology to support transformation to proactive primary care. 2010. http://pcmh.ahrq.gov/sites/default/files/attachments/Information%20Technology%20to%20Support%20Transformation%20to%20Proactive%20Primary%20Care.pdf.
3. American Academy of Family Physicians (AAFP) AAoPA, American College of Physicians (ACP), American Osteopathic Association (AOA). Joint principles of the patient-centered medical home. 2007; http://www.aafp.org/dam/AAFP/documents/practice_management/pcmh/initiatives/PCMHJoint.pdf. Accessed 19 Apr 2015
4. Berner ES, Burkhardt JH, Panjamapirom A, Ray MN. Cost implications of human and automated follow-Up in ambulatory care. Am J Manage Care. 2014;20(11 Spec No. 17):SP531–40.
5. Centers for Disease Control and Prevention (CDC). Chronic diseases, the power to prevent, the call to control: at a glance. 2009. http://www.cdc.gov/chronicdisease/resources/publications/aag/chronic.htm.
6. Centers for Medicare and Medicaid Services (CMS). EHR incentive program. 2014. http://www.cms.gov/Regulations-and-Guidance/Legislation/EHRIncentivePrograms/Downloads/August2014_SummaryReport.pdf.
7. Centers for Medicare and Medicaid (CMS). Multi-payer primary care practice demonstration factsheet.2012.http://www.cms.gov/Medicare/Demonstration-Projects/DemoProjectsEvalRpts/downloads/mapcpdemo_Factsheet.pdf. Accessed 19 Apr 2015.

8. Crimm A. and Liss D. Patient-centered medical home evaluations: let's keep them all in context. Health affairs blog. 2014. http://healthaffairs.org/blog/2014/05/21/patient-centered-medical-home-evaluations-lets-keep-them-all-in-context/.
9. DataMark Inc. Unstructured Data in Electronic Health Record (EHR) systems: challenges and Solutions. white paper. http://www.datamark.net/uploads/files/unstructured_ehr_data_white_paper.pdf (Oct 2013).
10. Duncan I. Healthcare risk adjustment and predictive modeling. Winsted: ACTEX Publications; 2011.
11. Lindsey D. "Carilion Clinic Using "Watson" Technology to Identify At-Ris, Patients," Becker's Health IT and CIO Review. 2014. http://www.beckershospitalreview.com/healthcare-information-technology/carilion-clinic-using-watson-technology-to-identify-at-risk-patients.html.
12. Dykes PC, Samal L, Donahue M, Greenberg JO, Hurley AC, Hassan O, O'Malley TA, Venkatesh AK, Volk LA, Bates D. A patient-centered longitudinal care plan: vision versus reality. J Am Med Inf Assoc. doi:http://dx.doi.org/10.1136/amiajnl-2013-002454 1082-1090. First published online: 1 Nov 2014.
13. Edwards ST, Bitton A, Hong J, Landon BE. Patient-centered medical home initiatives expanded in 2009–2013: providers, patients and payment incentives increased. Health Aff. 2014;33(10):1823–31. doi:10.1377/hlthaff.2014.0351.
14. Friedberg MW, Schneider EC, Rosenthal MB, Volpp KG, Werner RM. Association between participating in a multipayer medical home intervention and changes in quality, utilization, and costs of care. JAMA. 2014;311(8):815–25. doi:10.1001/jama.2014.353.
15. Grumbach K, Bodenheimer T, Grundy P. The outcomes of implementing patient-centered medical home demonstrations: a review of the evidence on quality, access and costs from recent prospective evaluation studies Aug 2009, paper prepared for PCPCC, Washington DC.
16. Grundy P, Hagan KR, Hansen JC, Grumbach K. The multi-stakeholder movement for primary care renewal and reform. Health Aff. 2010;29(5):791–8.
17. Richard H. Population health management requires automation. Group Pract J. 2011. http://www3.phytel.com/Libraries/In-the-News-PDFs/Population-Health-Management-Requires-Automation.sflb.ashx.
18. Hodach R, Handmaker K. Population health management technologies for accountable care. Phytel white paper. 2013. 12.
19. Hsiao Chun-Ju, Hing E. Use and characteristics of electronic health record systems among office-based physician practices: United States. 2001–2013, NCHS Data Brief, No. 143. 2014. http://www.cdc.gov/nchs/data/databriefs/db143.htm.
20. IBM. Implement watson: healthcare. 2015. URL: http://www.ibm.com/smarterplanet/us/en/ibmwatson/implement-watson.html. Last Accessed 25 Mar 2015.
21. Institute for Health Technology Transformation (IHTT). Population health management: a roadmap for provider-based automation in a New Era of healthcare. 2012. http://ihealthtran.com/pdf/PHMReport.pdf.
22. Kesselheim AS, Cresswell K, Phansalkar S, Bates DW, Sheikh A. Clinical decision support systems could be modified to reduce 'Alert Fatigue' while still minimizing the risk of litigation. Health Aff. 2011;30(12):2310–7. doi:10.1377/hlthaff.2010.1111.
23. Kindig D, Stoddart G. What is population health? Am J Public Health. 2003;93:380–3.
24. Klein S. The veterans health administration: implementing patient-centered medical homes in the nation's largest integrated delivery System. 2011. The Commonwealth Fund. http://www.commonwealthfund.org/~/media/Files/Publications/Case%20Study/2011/Sep/1537_Klein_veterans_hlt_admin_case%20study.pdf. Accessed 19 Apr 2015.
25. Margolius D, Bodenheimer T. Transforming primary care: from past practice to practice of the future. Health Aff. 2010;29(5):779–84.
26. Nash D. Healthcare reform's Rx for primary care, MedPage Today, Aug. 18, 2010. Accessed at http://www.medpagetoday.com/Columns/21750.

27. NCQA. Patient-centered medical homes fact sheet. 2013. http://www.ncqa.org/Portals/0/Public%20Policy/2013%20PDFS/pcmh%202011%20fact%20sheet.pdf. Accessed 19 Apr 2015.
28. NCQA. PCMH 2011-PCMH 2014 crosswalk. (no date). http://www.ncqa.org/Programs/Recognition/Practices/PatientCenteredMedicalHomePCMH/PCMH2011PCMH2014 Crosswalk.aspx. Accessed 19 Apr 2015.
29. Nelson R. Your EHR needs a population health management system. 2013. Kevin MD. http://www.kevinmd.com/blog/2013/02/ehr-population-health-management-system.html.
30. Nguyen OK, Chan CV, Makam A, Stieglitz H, Amarasingham R. Envisioning a social-health information exchange as a platform to support a patient-centered medical neighborhood: a feasibility study. J Gen Intern Med. 2015;30(1):60–7.
31. Nielsen M. Show me the sata: do patient-centered medical homes work? PCPCC presentation, 9 June 2014.
32. Nutting PA, Crabtree BJ, Miller WL, Stange KC, Stewart E, Jaen C. Transforming physician practices to patient-centered medical homes: lessons from the national demonstration project. Health Aff. 2011;30(3):439–45.
33. O'Kane ME. Are medical homes an answer to health care's cost problem? 2014. NCQA Blog. http://blog.ncqa.org/medical-homes-answer-health-cares-cost-problem/?utm_source=SilverpopMailing&utm_medium=email&utm_campaign=Recognition%20Notes%20 1.8.14 %20(1)%20B&utm_content.
34. O'Kane ME, Barr MS, Scholle SH. Patient-centered medical homes save money and improve care. 2014. NCQA presentation. http://www.ncqa.org/Portals/0/Newsroom/PCMH%20 Research%20Slides_9-3-14_FINAL_v2.pdf.
35. Patel MS, Arron MJ, Sinsky TA, Green EH, Baker DW, Bowen JL., Day S. Estimating the staffing infrastructure for a patient-centered medical home. Am J Managed Care. 1;19:N6. 2013.Accessedathttp://www.ajmc.com/publications/issue/2013/2013-1-vol19-n6/estimating-the-staffing-infrastructure-for-a-patient-centered-medical-home/1.
36. Patient Centered Primary Care Collaborative (PCPCC). Benefits of implementing the primary care patient-centered medical home: a review of cost & quality results. 2012. http://www.pcpcc.org/sites/default/files/media/benefits_of_implementing_the_primary_care_pcmh.pdf. Accessed 19 Apr 2015.
37. Phytel. Prevea health automates population health management and improves outcomes. 2013. http://www3.phytel.com/Libraries/Case-Study-PDFs/Prevea-Health-CS-041013.sflb.ashx. Accessed 19 Apr 2015.
38. Phytel. Case study: northeast Georgia physicians group. 2012. http://cdn2.content.compendi-umblog.com/uploads/user/863cc3c6-3316-459a-a747-3323bd3b6428/4c5909e8-1708-4751-873e-4129cb2ed878/File/2eb524a34e010967789612b5ed70bd79/1392222301097.pdf.
39. Pletcher T. Changing the status quo to improve health services in Michigan: an interview with Dr. Tim Pletcher. Kanter J. 2015; 2:30–39. URL: http://www.kanterhealth.org/wp-content/uploads/Kanter-Journal-FINAL.pdf. Last accessed 24 Mar 2015.
40. Rai A, MD and Weisse JL, MS, RN. Care managers for value-based healthcare, case in point, Dorland Health Newslet. 2013;11(10). http://cdn2.content.compendiumblog.com/uploads/user/863cc3c6-3316-459a-a747-3323bd3b6428/4c5909e8-1708-4751-873e-4129cb2ed878/File/555ef563c0d60ea0c089eb2673ac8265/1391564340558.pdf.
41. Reid RJ, Coleman K, Johnson EA, Fishman PA, Hsu C, Soman MP, Trescott CE, Erikson M, Larson EB. The group health medical home at year two: cost savings, higher patient satisfaction, and less burnout for providers. Health Aff. 2010;29(5):835–43. doi:10.1377/hlthaff.2010.0158.
42. Rosenberg CN, Peele P, Keyser D, McAnallen S, Holder D. Results from a patient-centered medical home pilot at UPMC health plan hold lessons for broader adoption of the model. Health Aff. 2012;31(11):2423–31. doi:10.1377/hlthaff.2011.1002.
43. Shaljian, M., Nielsen, M. Managing populations, maximizing technology: population health management in the medical neighborhood. Patient-centered primary care collaborative. 2013. www.pcpcc.org/resource/managing-populations-maximizing-technology#sthash.P8lGuRJK.dpuf.

44. Starfield B. The future of primary care: refocusing the system. N Engl J Med. 2008;359:2087–91. doi:10.1056/NEJMp0805763.
45. Terry K. Google testing telehealth service linked to search. Medscape Med News. 2014. http://www.medscape.com/viewarticle/833823?src=rss.
46. Terry K. Mobile health tech could reduce doctor visits. InformationWeek Healthcare. 2013. http://www.informationweek.com/wireless/mobile-health-tech-could-reduce-doctor-visits/d/d-id/1112162?.
47. Terry K Is healthcare big data ready for prime time?. InformationWeek Healthcare. 2013. http://www.informationweek.com/big-data/big-data-analytics/is-healthcare-big-data-ready-for-prime-time/d/d-id/1108628?.
48. Terry K. Strategy: how mobility, Apps and BYOD will transform healthcare. InformationWeek Healthcare. 2012. http://reports.informationweek.com/abstract/105/8914/Healthcare/strategy-how-mobility-apps-and-byod-will-transform-healthcare.html.
49. UnitedHealth Center for Health Reform & Modernization. Advancing primary care delivery: practical, proven and scalable approaches. 2014. http://www.unitedhealthgroup.com/~/media/UHG/PDF/2014/UNH-Primary-Care-Report-Advancing-Primary-Care-Delivery.ashx.

# Chapter 16
# Patient-Interactive Healthcare Management, a Model for Achieving Patient Experience Excellence

**Martha Jean Minniti, Thomas R. Blue, Diane Freed, and Sasha Ballen**

**Abstract** Today technology abounds for consumers to connect in health care however, technology to date has focused primarily on the provider and claims data with little room for the patient's voice. Patient reported data comes secondhand through what providers learn as witness to patient symptoms or complaints. Unfettered access to patient reported data affords organizations and providers a pulse on performance from the patients view. Learning about individual patients' needs, problems and daily choices as the basis for improved care coordination and management provides new insights. The patient's voice makes the critical connection between care provided and continual improvement in care. In this chapter we will explore patient interactive reporting as a model for improving care and review case studies where patient feedback drove rapid cycle improvement through the use of real time feedback at the point of care (POC), exhibiting high levels of responsiveness and agility. P-IHM provides a blueprint to put more convenient, safer, higher quality healthcare into consumers' hands; the impact: improved quality at lower costs.

**Keywords** Patient experience • Patient engagement • Patient interactive reporting • Patient reported data • Rapid cycle improvement • Transformation • TQM/CQI • Adherence • Service analysis

M.J. Minniti, RN (✉)
Department of Product Development,
CarePartners Plus, Horsham, PA, USA
e-mail: mminniti@carepartnersplus.com

T.R. Blue, BS, PhD
Research, CarePartners Plus, LLC, Horsham, PA, USA

D. Freed, RN, MSN
Department of Quality, CarePartners Plus, LLC, Horsham, PA, USA

S. Ballen, MS
Vice President, Advanced Comprehensive Care Organization, LLC,
Yardley, PA, USA

© Springer International Publishing Switzerland 2016     257
C.A. Weaver et al. (eds.), *Healthcare Information Management Systems:
Cases, Strategies, and Solutions*, Health Informatics,
DOI 10.1007/978-3-319-20765-0_16

## 16.1  Introduction

I have learned what applies in manufacturing, also applies in healthcare, the better health and the higher learning of the people involved (as the products with a voice) are the real products. This is what makes P-IHM disruptive and transformative, in raising peoples voices their voices raise the quality and lower the costs of healthcare.

### 16.1.1  Health Care Costs Spiraling Out of Control

In 2006, a Public Announcement that neither Medicare nor Social Security could sustain projected long-run program costs in full under scheduled financing was made through the annual Medicare Trustees Report to Congress. For the first time in Medicare's history this meant that Medicare recipient access to care funded by Hospital Insurance (HI-Medicare Part A), entitlements that help pay for hospital, home health, skilled nursing, and hospice care for the aged and disabled, and Supplementary Medical Insurance (SMI-Medicare Part B), which help pay for physician, outpatient hospital, home health, and other services for the aged and disabled, would be curtailed. Several factors were cited for the unsustainable deficits in this report; the majority were attributed to "unnecessary" expenditures and costs. The conclusion in this Announcement was without legislative changes future beneficiaries and taxpayers would experience disruptive consequences. These would be further exacerbated and accelerated by the Recession of 2008, the greatest recession in 50 years. Combined, these events triggered an unprecedented period of international chaos. The efforts to restore health care order were eventually coined: "Health Care Transformation."

## 16.2  Background

### 16.2.1  Necessity the Mother of Invention

In 2006, preliminary aspects of the Patient-Interactive Healthcare Management (P-IHM) model were introduced through the United States Patent and Trademark Office and subsequently to several public officials appointed to protect the public interest. By 2007 the model's scope evolved into a solution to an emerging health care crisis and presented to the Office of the US Secretary of Health and Human Services for this purpose. Its scope incorporated macro and micro versions for attaining greater accountability in health care by empowering people with the ability to scrutinize quality and costs in a manner that was scalable to every individual encounter with healthcare. The ability to scrutinize billions of annual inpatient, outpatient, and home encounters and the medication and supplies that resulted would improve individual patient safety while the collective effect would decrease the Office of Management Budget's (OMB) reported $600,000,000,000 of "unnecessary" expenditures; costs significantly impairing the solvency of the Medicare Trust

Funds. According to Michael Levitt the US Secretary of Health and Human Services, "Using the patient's energy was the most forward thinking solution I have heard." Most solutions brought to him required more time and work from Physicians and staff, and this was impractical; both were at their exhaustion point and the patient's energy is unlimited. Secretary Levitt arranged for sharing the model with key staff working for the Agency of Health Research and Quality (AHRQ), the Centers for Medicare and Medicaid (CMS) and others.

By 2008 all 50 states were struggling to revive their economies due to the great recession. All 50 states number 1 priority was to get health care entitlements under control, because they were unable to balance their budgets plus meet their health-care obligations. During the next several years, the model was further introduced to administrators at state and city levels who were struggling for solutions to the ava-lanche of municipal problems caused by the great recession of 2008. For the next 7 years the national attention was focused on an electronic medical record solution while seeds for incorporating the patient's voice to complete a comprehensive national solution were slowly taking hold in the public conscience. This was vali-dated in the Patient Protection and Affordable Care Act of 2010.

## 16.2.2   Rigors and Findings

P-IHM Research and Development was initiated in earnest in 2007 and recently culminated nine demonstration projects including: three IRB clinical trials and one CMMI demonstration project. The initial span of R&D tested certain aspects of a patented series of pre-commercialized methods and electronic program codes that combined with electronic processors to provide a unique apparatus that invoked the functionality of patient-interactive healthcare management to improve healthcare. Portions of R&D concentrated on identifying and managing variations in care, effectiveness of care, patient needs, systematic deficiencies, and speed of corrective resolutions. This R&D produced substantial peer-reviewed findings that confirmed the feasibility, reliability and safety of providing of Patient-Interactive Healthcare Management to the public for consumption to improve their personal health out-comes and the healthcare systems. The model provides the overarching ability to preserve quality at a time, when healthcare cuts will continue into the unforeseeable future as indicated in the 2006 Medicare Trustees report to Congress [14] and veri-fied in the 2014 report [13]. These findings show how when health information tools P-IHMS infrastructure is implemented people will, as a regular practice, interac-tively engage which enables early warnings to be instantaneously delivered to pro-grammed users. In response, P-IHMS enables protective actions to be taken to resolve reported problems and needs at accelerated speeds, and to monitor the intended effect of these actions in real-time.

Healthcare's obsession with the electronic medical record made the scientific rigors of pioneering the reliability and economic relevance case for patient gener-ated data challenging, and all-consuming. The marketplace was pre-mobile (iphone, ipad, Android), and the Federal Government had yet to legislate a national health policy (pre-HITECH Act, Affordable Care Act, Medical Loss Ratio, ONC, Blue button, etc.) or mandate regulations for enforcement let alone promulgate compulsory patient reporting for the public good. The concept of putting decision making control at the fingertips of patients was considered radical and unreasonable by some of the status quo. It encountered significant resistance from segments that felt their market share was threatened by advancing the Patient-Centric Paradigm. Recent history shows to overcome these barriers requires a convergence of external forces: rapid changing world demographics, recession, consolidation of the banking industry, war, and the *information age*. These forces imposed their will to eclipse paradigms of generations gone by. Among these were the design, access to, delivery and monetization of healthcare. By 2009 Healthcare economics merged with *consumer information markets* and barriers broke down at unprecedented speeds. Implementing a P-IHM blueprint would quickly commercialize personalized healthcare transactions.

Part of the research activity included modeling the economic implications of P-IHM. This modeling showed how P-IHM creates an unanticipated economic spillover effect at the macro level. A prime example is Government sponsored healthcare. Because Government is the largest consumer and payer source around the world it makes Government the largest beneficiary of the unexpected dividends associated with implementing P-IHM on a macro basis. The spillover is contained in opportunities to reallocate saved, unexpended healthcare funds into public sector domains e.g. education, social services, law enforcement, environmental etc. to provide an unprecedented public benefit. The systematic configurations which enables P-IHM to scale makes achieving these economics feasible. For example at the macro level, the Federal Government adopted the P-IHM blueprint to channel information from Medicare recipients into its databases to help attack fraud and abuse. It did the same to institute a provider quality rating system; applications explained and illustrated in US Patents citing Patient-Interactive Healthcare Management [4].

This chapter is dedicated to providing a synopsis of select principles, concepts, techniques, findings and applications embodied in Patient-interactive Healthcare Management (P-IHM). It will concentrate on examining two transformational benefits enabled by Patient-interactive Healthcare Management: first, the ability to intensify the magnitude of individualized care and the corresponding outcomes in the lowest cost setting and, second, the related ability to avoid "unnecessary" costs.

## 16.3  Principles Concepts Techniques Applications

### 16.3.1  What Is It?

The P-IHM model contains configurations of Healthcare Sciences, Arts, Regulations, Standards, Financial Services, and people's one to one and contemporaneous electronic interactions with a host of stakeholders in health care aimed at instantly improving accountability, quality, effectiveness, patient safety, compliance and management, across the health care continuum. This can be accomplished from any

Point of Care (POC) where an individual resides and healthcare is rendered. At the micro level, individuals (family members) use P-IHM to intersect healthcare and improve their personal quality and cost outcomes, and because of sheer volume of annual patient encounters the macro level quality and cost outcomes also improve the system.

An example of patient-interactive health care management system provides means for healthcare services rendered to a patient to be confirmed by the patient immediately after the healthcare services are rendered. The patient is provided the ability to electronically verify the accuracy of rendered services/goods and provide an assessment of the rendered services/goods.

Healthcare is managed via patient interaction at the time the patient is visiting a health care facility to receive health care services and/or goods. As used herein, the phrase "healthcare services" refers to healthcare services and/or healthcare goods. Patient-interactive healthcare management as described herein has numerous application, including, for example, home health, skilled nursing, assisted living, hospice, teaching facilities, dental healthcare, holistic healthcare, mental healthcare, occupational healthcare, physical rehabilitation, and healthcare related encounters between patient/ consumer and a practitioner/provider.

In examples to come this contemporaneous interaction includes assessing the quality of provided health care services and verifying the accuracy of an invoice, prebill, bill, charge ticket, or the like, listing the services provided. Additionally, information can be provided to the patient to educate the patient about healthcare and about actions the patient can take to improve her/his health. The results of the patient's interaction are provided to a database for storage, to a third party responsible for delivering and managing the patients care and paying for the rendered services/goods, an agency for collecting health care information, the healthcare facility that provided the services/goods, or a combination thereof. Providing results and comparisons of the patient's interaction in this manner (e.g., feedback) can result in improvements in patient and provider behavior.

Patient-interactive healthcare management as described herein can help Federal and State governments, private practices, employers, and/or patients improve the quality and cost of healthcare. Example of patient-interactive healthcare management examples include being a web based, multimedia resource, programmed to gather useful patient and provider data using the patient's energy via surveying the patient at the end of the doctor visit. Various embodiments of patient-interactive healthcare management also can be programmed to provide periodic consumer reports to the patient. Example consumer reports include local reports, regional reports, national reports, physician office customer satisfaction reports, and statistics such as the number of procedures performed by a physician per period of time (year, month, etc.), or a combination thereof. In other examples, patient-interactive healthcare management provides patient education information, and is usable to propagate public awareness about ways to more wisely manage healthcare resources. In other examples, patient-interactive healthcare management is a consumer driven, point-of-service tool which can be placed in a healthcare facility, to empower patients to exercise normal buying behaviors When a patient sees a practitioner (e.g., physician, nurse, physician's assistant, psychologist, psychiatrist, physical therapist, or the like), patient-interactive healthcare management allows the patient/consumer to express the level of satisfaction with the quality of care received, and to verify that specific services were rendered during the visit.

"Patient-interactive health care management provides the ability for healthcare services received by a patient to be electronically confirmed by the patient, or designated person, immediately after and subsequently after the healthcare services are rendered. The patient/designated person may be provided the ability to verify the accuracy of an invoice for the rendered services/goods and may provide an assessment of the rendered services/goods. The patient/designated person may provide this information via an appropriate stationary and/or portable processor. Healthcare may be received at any appropriate location or locations. The evaluation may occur at any appropriate location or locations. An after care risk assessment may be provided to the patient/designated person to evaluate the patient's status immediately after, subsequently after, and/or in between the healthcare services rendered. Patient-interactive health care may protect the safety of patients, mitigate disparities in care, protect payers, and/or facilitate adoption of health information technology".

Because Patient-Interactive Healthcare Management empowers people with standardized health information tools and technologies to systematically and contemporaneously communicate with the healthcare system, their access to quality healthcare at lower costs can be as ubiquitous as the availability and use of electronic devices in their daily lives programmed to implement it. The breadth and scope of patient-interactive healthcare management is not limited to any single embodiment; this makes its magnitude of economic implications transformative.

### 16.3.2   Why Is P-IHM a Catalyst for Change?

Without P-IHM, systematically protecting the most susceptible aspects of health care would remain impossible. P-IHM can easily changes the way people experience healthcare for example, the ability to access healthcare the way they want, when and where they want it. Most importantly consumers will receive what they are paying for and have the ability to immediately contest if they are not. The implications and economic magnitude of its worldwide feasibility make it a catalyst for change. The findings show that when the P-IHM program code is loaded and implemented it enables immediate communications to be exchanged at both the macro and micro levels. For example, early warnings can be instantaneously delivered to programmed users, and in response, protective actions can be taken to resolve problems and needs at accelerated speeds, and the intended effect of these actions can be evaluated and monitored in real-time.

Driven by consumer engagement energy, P-IHM enables otherwise unattainable economies of scale and patient safety to be achieved through the contemporaneous communications (access, exchange, and sharing) of individual interactions, encounters and experiences – direct and indirect, clinical and non-clinical – spanning the care continuum, that comprehensively inform the health care system at unsurpassed speeds (immediacy) and accuracy (completeness). The combination of speed, completeness and standards-based real-time data driven by the interactive-patient intensifies the ability to produce an *immediacy* of quality response. The *immediacy* of quality response, is a byproduct of P-IHM. It is a critical factor in resolving patient problems, needs and preferences before situations and conditions deteriorate beyond the opportunity to take corrective actions that preserve lives, raise quality, and avoid unnecessary costs. The information derived from implementing P-IHM provides detailed costing data which organizations need to coexist in an accountable care era that expects higher quality healthcare at lower costs. While patient-interactive healthcare management allows for versatility, modifications and additions. P-IHM is not limited to any one configuration. For example, patient-interactive healthcare management may apply to any environment, whether wired or wireless, and may be applied to any number of devices connected via a network and interacting across the network.

The methods and apparatus for patient-interactive healthcare management also can be practiced via communications embodied in the form of program code that is transmitted over some transmission medium, such as over electrical wiring or cabling, through fiber optics, or via any other form of transmission, wherein, when the program code is received and loaded into and executed by a machine. While examples of P-IHM have been described in connection with various computing devices, the underlying concepts can be applied to any computing device or system capable of implementing patient-interactive healthcare management. Various techniques can be implemented in connection with hardware or software or, where appropriate, with a combination of both. Thus, the methods and apparatus for patient-interactive healthcare management, or certain aspects or portions thereof, can take the form of program code (i.e., instructions) stored in tangible media, such as diskettes, CD-ROMs, hard drives, or any other machine-readable storage medium, wherein, when the program code is loaded into and executed by a machine, such as a computer, the machine becomes an apparatus for implementing-IHM. The methods and apparatus for patient-interactive healthcare management also can be practiced via communications embodied in the form of program code that is transmitted, such as over electrical wiring or cabling, through fiber optics, or via any other form of transmission, wherein, when the program code is received and loaded into and executed by a machine, such as an EPROM, a gate array, a programmable logic device (PLD), or a client computer, the machine becomes an apparatus for patient-interactive healthcare management. When implemented on a general-purpose processor, the program code combines with the processor to provide a unique apparatus that operates to invoke the functionality of patient-interactive healthcare management. The construct of P-IHM enables many forms of electronic healthcare including but not limited to Telehealth, Telemedicine, Telemonitoring, transaction based and so on. Additionally, any storage techniques used in connection with patient-interactive healthcare management can invariably be a combination of hardware and software.

In hindsight information electronically generated from patients about their experience to identify and resolve safety, quality, clinical, administrative and financial issues before they deteriorate may seem simple or mundane. In reality engineering this technology without a national infrastructure, or guidelines, made creating Patient-interactive Healthcare Management complex, since P-IHM involves aligning databases, and IT functionality with real-time patient-interactive processes and healthcare workflows from any point in healthcare with techniques for stewards and stakeholders to contemporaneously pinpoint and protect the most vulnerable aspects and patients.

P-IHM will advance the technical fields of medical economics, health care accountability, health care management, patient adherence, engagement, safety, literacy, health care cost analysis, health care service analysis, social services, financial services and more. The versatility, improved patient outcomes and financial benefits of P-IHM constitute a specialty within health care with supported by the data suggest independent third parties credentialed and experienced in P-IHM. The chapter findings support how the functional applications of P-IHM facilitates advancements in medical, life sciences, social services and the field of healthcare management by enabling people to interactively manage their healthcare (choices, decisions, coordination and outcomes) in a structured, coordinated way while interacting with stakeholders in healthcare that sponsor, underwrite, deliver, oversee, advocate and adjudicate patient care. The patient safety and service recovery aspects alone offer unequaled economic benefits.

### 16.3.3  Conceptual Framework of Control: Who's in Control of My Healthcare?

There is a sharp contrast in how patients see their participation in health care. Some people go to the doctor to find out what's wrong with them. Others go prepared to be engaged in a shared decision making process. When it comes to a patient's outlook, perceiving their experience as internally or externally driven distinguishes health from ill-health ([15], p. 151). Patients who find their physical and mental condition "healthy" see themselves in control. Those relinquishing control to their care providers are by definition "unhealthy." As Levenson [8, 9] proposed, these two mindsets are mutually exclusive.

It is a long established principle that a change in behavior precedes a shift in values [10]. Patient-facing technology enables patients to be engaged in communicating instantaneously across the care continuum. This establishes precedence in healthcare management that significantly lowers the costs of care [6]. P-IHM enables patients to be in control of their care and "healthy." P-IHM technology enables patient engagement and its importance cannot be overemphasized.

### 16.3.4    Locus of Control

To further explain, the contrast between an internal locus of control and an external locus of control also has been long established and is shown in the Diagram below of the independent, mutually exclusive patient views of their health.

Figure 16.1 shows that with an internal locus electronic feedback and messaging aligns patient care with the standards of care. Furthermore, the under 48-h window promotes learning, avoids unnecessary costs and patient suffering, as the hallmark of patient experience excellence. The lack of success to date in verifying the accuracy and effectiveness of services rendered or in not correcting inaccuracies have been detrimental to the cost of healthcare. As the Diagram shows, higher costs and lower care quality go with the external locus of control and a window of over 48 h for the patient's standards-based report and a quality response. This 48-h window might be considered the span of the working memory [1],—the time available for a standards-based quality measure and a quality response. Elliott Jaques ([7], pp. 44 and 67) first discovered this window at Glacier Metal in London and went on to confirm it across 100 companies and 15 countries. Quality measures and quality responses within 48 h prevent unnecessary hospital admissions, readmissions or ED presentations.

### 16.3.5    Old School Methods: Eclipsed by the Information Age

Data production and analysis to date have focused primarily on provider and payer facing technologies with little room for the patient's voice. By design this excludes what happens from the patient's perspective at the Point of Care: in the hospital, the physician's office, the pharmacy, and at home. A majority of patients feel

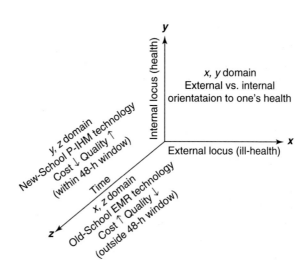

**Fig. 16.1** Independent, mutually exclusive patient views of their health

uncomfortable about openly sharing their needs and issues. They have limited tools to communicate what they need, and no system that provides a status on their requests. Even when patients are seen in the ED or the clinic, their report of symptoms and problems to clinicians can be unintentionally filtered, leaving out vital data [2] essential to care management, diagnosis and discovery. Once the patient leaves the hospital, doctor's office, or pharmacy frequently their status is not known until they experience a significant problem or emergency. A concern of prognosticators is an empowered patient may disrupt the existing order.

While information is more abundant than ever, without transforming to a comprehensive patient facing model the vital missing information necessary for achieving Patient Experience Excellence (improved outcomes) is lost. Without such information management is at a distinct disadvantage. Connecting with patients meaningfully to uncover the patient needs and status requires systematic continuous rapid cycle improvements, enabled by electronic technologies.

### 16.3.6   New School Technologies: Make for Ubiquitous Healthcare

In contrast, patient-facing technologies are incorporated into everyday electronic personal devices that can produce data direct from the source and in real-time to inform the healthcare system at speeds and accuracy levels that enable corrective actions and resolve problems, needs and preferences before a situation or condition deteriorates. The electronic industry has done a nice job of answering how to connect with consumers (e.g. smartphone, tablets, pc's etc.) Using personal devices (delivery systems) people are accustomed to providing information that may otherwise escape the health care provider. Personal devices continue to rapidly evolve. Because technologies enable unfettered access to evidence-standards based patient centered healthcare – healthcare is now readily available anywhere the patient resides. One constant is the real-time Patient-interactive element. The patient's voice transforms outdated, exclusionary practices into open, inclusive paradigms.

To put the patients at the center of their care requires empowering them with tools. Patient-interactive information then affords organizations and providers an extremely effective method for improving outcomes in the lowest cost setting. The ability to track the patient's status down to the patient – provider level is linked by the patient's voice to the standards of care. This scalable real time capability creates substantial opportunities for optimizing quality and cost outcomes.

### 16.3.7   Commercial Relevance

With P-IHM patients will have their needs and preferences met and problems resolved effortlessly and timely; out of their individual interactions, encounters and experiences – direct and indirect, clinical and non-clinical – spanning the care continuum. No more disenfranchised patients because of their inability to have their needs met or problems resolved due to the communication barriers they confront in a fractionated healthcare system. P-IHM enables consumers to raise their problems, needs and preference to have them resolved.

The commercial relevance of Patient-Interactive Healthcare Management can be seen in a series of healthcare policies and plans promulgated by the US Government that emerged in the past 5 years. For example, the HITECH Act of 2009 established the concept of "Meaningful Use" (of an electronic health record), originally promulgated for use by providers and provider organizations. MU now includes patient and family adoption of health IT. Another example is the Accountable Care Act of 2010, which broadens patient and family involvement in the electronic management of their personal care. The Medical Loss Ratio contained within the Act was devised to provide rebates to consumers. Further, national quality programs – for example, the Patient-Centered Medical Home (PCMH) model of care, and Accountable Care models are foundations upon which the Affordable Care Act is built. P-IHM provides a blueprint and methodologies for implementing the Federal Health IT goals set forth. P-IHM enables the goals specifically intended to make patient and family engagement critical to improving health outcomes and reducing costs be realized. In 2014 the Institute of Medicine (IOM) formally recommended that electronic patient management include more than the EMR and signaled the need for additional means of electronically interacting with patients. It recognized that the EMR has data appropriate for the legal medical record, but does not facilitate or provide the additional options needed for patients to self-manage their care. P-IHM enables these policies and programs to be put into practice. These policies recognize that providers can only do so much, and that patient engagement and activation produces significant savings [5]. P-IHM was introduced for precisely these reasons.

Leaders in medical informatics in the US recognize that patients are an underutilized source of missing data. 10 years ago, Dr. Charles Safran of Harvard testified to the House Ways and Means Committee of Congress as follows; "*Patients are the most underutilized resource*" in the U.S. health system. Patients "*want to be involved, and they can be involved. Their participation will lead to better medical outcomes at lower cost with dramatically higher patient and customer satisfaction*." The unanswered question was how to involve the public in a structured, productive way. New regulations intended to improve quality and reduce cost will rapidly expand now that data can be communicated directly from the patient. For example, Meaningful Use Level 3 [3], scheduled to be required by 2017, is another adoption of P-IHM, with electronic reported feedback in real time from patients about their care.

### 16.3.8   Superior Healthcare: For Everyone

To make superior patient experiences a constant requires quality data, quality responses, and patient-interactive engagement. Patient-interactive data for the purpose of producing a quality response is defined as a holistic view reported directly by the patient or their designated family member. Such reports include elements of their current health status: key data pertinent to the patient's condition, ongoing assessments of needs, lifestyle, activation levels, and barriers to care, motivation and ability to adhere to agreed plans, etc. Obtaining this data in real-time strengthens the ability to achieve superior levels of care and lower care costs. Without continuous indicators about the patient's status in real-time from the patient or family member, the best clinicians and organizations cannot transform health care.

P-IHM can be implemented from any point the patient resides and can use technology to provide information (e.g., tablets, kiosks, processors having Internet access, mobile devices, or the like), after healthcare is rendered (e.g., outpatient, physician's offices, clinics, hospitals, nursing homes, assisted living centers, home health, hospice, dental, optical offices, mental health institutions, rehab, occupational health, retail health care, or the like) wherein the services are provided. Upon completion of services provided, a patient evaluates, the pro vided services. The patient also responds to questions pertaining to the provided services. This healthcare encounter information is collected via data input devices and contemporaneously transmitted to the appropriate stakeholders (clinical, administrative, financial, family etc.).

### 16.3.9  Patient Experience Excellence: New Norm

P-IHM enables a superior level of personalized quality health care at the individual level and the ability to scale across entire populations. Patient Experience Excellence is not commonplace. It is attained from the culmination of all interactions, direct and indirect, clinical and non-clinical, spanning the care continuum. It is more wide-ranging than satisfaction. It goes beyond quality measures to include the *immediacy* of a quality response to a patient preference, need and problem through to monitoring the excellence in every patient experience. Providing the tools and technologies to institute transparent Patient Experience Excellence completes the shift from the physician-centered to patient-centered Paradigm.

### 16.3.10  Patient Experience Excellence: Misunderstood

The difficulty in attaining Patient Experience Excellence is often associated with the inadequacy of available measures, methods and tools. All too often, the measures and methods used to examine the Patient's Experience are inadequate because the tools available overlook preferences, problems and needs that patients have, and provide no way of effectively communicating them to the health care system. Thus, patient-interactive opportunities for improvement and cost avoidance are lost. Patient-interactive Health Management provides the configurations of methods and techniques that enable people to contemporaneously communicate all health care interactions and experiences spanning the care continuum, to inform the health care system at speeds and accuracy levels that enable an *immediacy* of quality response, and to resolve problems, needs and preferences before a situation or condition deteriorates.

### 16.3.11  Insights into Excellence

P-IHM provides a process for implementing Patient-Centered healthcare including patient and provider adherence. The measures capture longitudinal Patient-interactive data at the point of care and from home about direct and indirect clinical and non clinical interactions. P-IHM can be used to compare data to standards, develop profiles and improve outcomes. The act of reporting data enhances the patient experience, improves care and drives rapid cycle improvement as well as producing cultural change. Specifically, the conversation between patients and their clinician's changes when daily data is provided and the patient's unmet needs are identified. Action plans are put into place as soon as an issue is identified avoiding deterioration. Patient's data literacy also improves, making it possible for patients to connect their prior day's actions and next day results. With real -time data specific to patient conditions, providers and patients rapidly learn what works. As a result, P-IHM data allows for more personalized care plans that patients are more apt to follow.

### 16.3.12  Immediacy of a Quality Response: Golden 48

The immediacy of a quality response is core to rapid cycle improvement. The electronic real-time patient interaction needs to be followed by a quality response within 48 h ([7], pp. 44, 67). This 48-h window makes the difference between life and death. With a response within 48 h or less, acute conditions get corrected before the patient's condition deteriorates. Deteriorating health, due to responses beyond 48 h have severe consequences on patient lives and gives rise "unnecessary costs" ([12], p. 1).

### 16.3.13  Rapid Cycle Improvement: Accelerated Possible

A Rapid-cycle improvement requires real-time data to enable zero defects, continuous improvement, cost avoidance, improved care quality, and heightened patient experience excellence. In addition, electronically enabled rapid-cycle measures and responses allow care teams to break the bounds otherwise imposed by the very care delivery organizations best positioned and equipped to deliver superior care.

Rapid cycle improvements once measured in 8–12 month timeframes, get measured every 3 months or less, but need to be measured in 48 h or less. Patient-Interactive Healthcare Management. When rapid cycle improvements drop to under 48 h, they boost the quality of care, dramatically increase costs savings and patient experience improves. A kind of "boom" analogous to a sonic boom occurs [11]. The boom raises the sound of the patient's voice above the health care noise and offers clinicians even more essential data to better understand patient needs, their daily status and behaviors. With this understanding, adherence greatly improves. If "boom" is too strong a word, just picture the patient's real-time input as the catalyst—not just the catalyst for care quality and standards-based feedback, but also the source, yes the electronic source, of revenue growth and cost avoidance. Again, the shift brought about by the P-IHM transformation cannot be overemphasized.

Because P-IHMS enables the immediacy of a quality response, it accelerates the ability to perform rapid cycle improvements. In the inpatient environment, the accelerated speed and completeness of data (i.e. lab values, cardiac readings and other patient status indicators) can be dealt with rapidly, when the values or findings are out of range or indicative of a potential problem. This capability spans the entire care continuum: inpatient, outpatient and home.

### 16.3.14   Providers View

From the practice perspective, patient engagement and achieving patient experience excellence are key elements of better health, better care, and lower cost. For primary care providers, who are frequently overburdened by a malfunctioning healthcare system, effective and appropriate reporting of patient-generated data is an exciting prospect. An office visit, or a stay in an acute-care facility, produces much data about a patient – including lab results, vital signs, physician notes, diagnostic imaging, formal diagnoses, just to name a few. However, no matter the vast amount of the clinical claims data generated by an encounter with the health care system, it is still just a snapshot of the patient at a point in time. It is only with the introduction of patient reported information that the data represents the whole patient.

Managing a chronic condition is an ongoing process. If patients are not meaningfully engaged in the process, many do not maintain healthy lifestyles or adhere to their regimen of medications. However, when the patient is empowered to report their data, patterns and relationships start to emerge. When they are electronically enabled able to see the results of their choices, then they become meaningful partners in their own care.

The challenge has long been to economically provide care and guidance for patients within the confines of the US healthcare system. From the practice perspective, the P-IHM technology is an exciting prospect. Yet a flood of patient-reported data would be unmanageable. Intelligently-designed technology that surfaces the meaningful events from the patient data is a boon to providers working to identify those who would most benefit from their care team reaching out to them. These meaningful events range from patients who are improving and would benefit from support and encouragement to patients who are deteriorating and require outreach.

## 16.4 Case Studies

### 16.4.1 CHF Patient

As for the CHF patient that had multiple admissions for CHF in the past 12 months, they were given discharge instructions, the same ones they received previously. A large majority of health care organizations and payers provided a follow up call for the first few days post discharge. Home care and or nurse practitioner visit were provided for the patients with the highest likelihood of readmission. These additional services helped patients make the transition. Readmissions were avoided.

During the product development and research, the used technology and defined processes linked to evidence based standards to uncover patient needs in key areas important to achieving high quality and improving self management. This process occurred in the hospital, PCP office, pharmacy and home. Real-time data from patients was obtained through push messages, tied to standards of care, which allowed for monitoring and the elimination of variations in care. Urgent issues identified were routed to family, care coordinators and/or clinicians for assessment and intervention. Longitudinal trends were identified and analyzed as changes were made to medications and care plans. Clinical messages to patients were also tested for impact. Real time data at the POC gave providers and patients what they needed to improve care and self manage, improving the patients experience as well as improving overall efficiency and cost. Five examples are provided.

### 16.4.2 Case 1: Life or Death

This case provides an example of how P-IMH saves lives:

1. Patient if left to own devices, likely would have died
2. Patient self-medicating as a form of engagement, rather than engaging in a standards-based, evidence-based structure of patient reports on their care
3. Patient when engaged, provided vital and critical information directly applicable to her care coordinator.
4. Patient's direct engagement in her care greatly improved her safety, obviously decreased the cost of care dramatically, improved the care outcomes, and significantly improved the quality of her care.

This fist case involved mobile data from a middle age woman. Fairly new to a PCMH level 3 practices, she volunteered as a diabetic to use the technology and software to provide data about her care and daily status. The patient was given a series of questions daily on a smart phone with the responses triaged and tracked by an acting care coordinator. She reported a feeling good score with 5 as the best score and 1 as the lowest score. Using this scale, she was consistently at a 4 or 5. One day, the patient's feeling good score dropped precipitously to a 1, with a normal blood sugar. When called, she reported gaining 9 lbs in a day and a half, and she stated she was a CHF patient recently diagnosed, which was unknown to the PCP practice. She knew that she would have to go to the ED because she was so short of breath that she could not take ten steps. What she had done was to triple her daily medication by taking 240 mg of lasix in the am and pm. The patient reported diuresing profusely and felt better the next day, although weak. She was not planning to tell her cardiologist or her primary care physician of this event. The acting care coordinator encouraged the patient to see a clinician, have labs drawn and an EKG. The patient was subsequently diagnoses with a low potassium and an EKG reveled a recent MI. On review, it was determined, that without oversight and intervention the patient would have likely suffered a significant secondary event.

### 16.4.3  Case 2: Persistent Problems with Medication Related Adverse Events

This case provides an example of how P-IMH enables medication remediation across the care continuum:

1. Patient taking medication between visits, but with an out-of-range HA1C
2. Patient provided data and critical information to enable care provider to adjust medications and titrate more effectively
3. By exerting control over his healthcare, patient handled health care personally from the standpoint of a healthy person with an internal locus of control
4. The patient's report and the quality response from the clinicians made a rapid cycle improvement in the patient's quality of care and avoided unnecessary cost

A fairly well controlled diabetic with a HA1C of 8 was working to reduce his HA1C to 7 or below. He was on a new medication and an avid exerciser. During the period of medication change, the patient had fluctuations in blood sugar ranging from 150 to 70. Data provided by the patient along with additional information allowed the clinicians and patient to adjust medications and titrate more effectively. The result was a normalization of the patient's blood sugar in a shorter amount of time than usual with the patient and the clinician confident of the plan.

### 16.4.4  Case 3: Clinical Implications of Shifting to P-IHM Enabled Rapid Cycle Improvement

This case provides an example how the use of P-IHM by outpatients led to a permanent improvement in the instructions on prescriptions:

1. 42 % of patients providing input on the care provided to PCP indicated medication problem
2. Without feedback to care provider, medication problems could have persisted well beyond the 48-h window needed for rapid cycle improvement

3. With patients responding to standards-based questions, written at a sixth grade level, care providers knew of medication issues in real time through risk alerts
4. While software content came from experienced developers and administrators, independent of the clinic, the simple solution to the problem came from staff within the clinic—more fully engaging not only the patient, but also the staff in the healthcare process

Taken from post-visit data obtained at a kiosk before patients left the practice, 42 % indicated they did not feel confident to manage their medications. The practice indicated they frequently had calls on medication questions post visit, from family members managing their relative's care. The practice upon viewing the information made medication sheets for the top 10 drugs prescribed in the practice and included the instruction sheet in the patient exit paper work, circling the patient's medication information. The result was fewer phone calls regarding medications and a decrease in medication issues and an improvement in medication management scores post visit. As far as the level of patient engagement goes, patient adoption rose to 78 % when the ordering clinician asked the patient to stop at the kiosk and provide feedback prior to leaving the office [16]. What's more, a properly designed P-IHM system generates 25 times the data in one-third the time, with 30 out of 100 patients having significant undetected problems and needs.

### 16.4.5  Case 4: Economics When Clinical Pharmacists Use P-IHM to Reconcile Medication Problems

This case relates to the use of P-IHM in outpatient and pharmacy settings, related to costs potentially avoided:

1. P-IHM system enabled not only care providers to deliver services, but also for pharmacists to participate clinically in patient care
2. The interventions by the pharmacists evidenced quality responses to medication issues well within the 48-h window needed with rapid cycle responses
3. The software flagged patients reporting medication problems, thus saving the labor cost of the pharmacists combing through patient medical records
4. Patients were grateful for pharmacists intervening into potential medication complications
5. P-IHM also flagged pharmacists not delivering the needed clinical assistance

Medication safety issues were consistently high in all environments tested, patients frequently did not understand their medications, had difficulty remembering to take their medications, and had multiple questions post hospitalization on medication regimens. Pharmacists were used in conjunction with the P-IHM technology to resolve medication issues and reduce admissions and readmissions in the treated population. Avoidable costs, as verified by independent third parties, amounted to over $50 million a year. These savings did not count the reductions in costs from the improved quality of care reported by 55 % of the patients. Care

Coordinators reported being more effective, when provided risk alerts and triage list of what patients to call.

### 16.4.6   Case 5: Levels of Patient Engagement Using P-IHM

This case study shows how P-IHM aggregates data by Patient, provider, clinic, and organizational level to provide valuable data on patients and their levels of response:

1. Patient engagement correlates with health levels with control seen by the patient as in their own hands, rather than being left to their care providers
2. Patients at the higher levels of engagement reported a direct relationship between their engagement within the 48-h window and their adherence to medical advice
3. Patients at a mid-level of engagement reported greater adherence to care plans
4. Even patients at low-levels of engagement reported a sincere desire to engage more fully in their health care

In review of patient profiles patients fell into three distinct groups based on self assessments and daily patterns. The A patients, these were those who readily adapted to the technology, enjoyed providing feedback and followed their trends. They were able to correlate their daily results with the prior days or weeks choices and their adherence to medical advice. The B patients vacillated between being actively engaged and disappearing for periods of time either due to no issues or their decision to monitor less frequently. This group frequently acknowledged that medication remainders and being asked for their daily status queued them to take their blood pressure, blood sugar or to provide other relevant information. The B patients reported increased adherence to their plan of care. The C patients did not engage although they voiced the desire to engage. In many cases, their lives, by their own accounts made it too difficult to participate. In all cases, patients said they would participate more fully if they received a reward of some kind. Top of the list, as an incentive, was a deduction in copay for providing data. Patients who wanted to participate but did not have either an IPAD or Smartphone wanted to have help in obtaining a device.

## 16.5   Summary

Healthcare accountability and management are provided via patient-interactive con-temporaneous evaluation and verification of provided services.

The technical field of Patient-Interactive Healthcare Management generally relates to health care, and more specifically relates to healthcare management, health care cost analysis, financial services, and healthcare service analysis. When implemented it acts as a transformative agent of change. Patient experience excellence is key to health care transformation and provides an opportunity for new learning by adding the key stakeholder, the patient and patient reported data to the traditional picture. Accordingly, the patient is aided in adapting to changing healthcare behavior and entering into a more robust relationship with a healthcare provider. A byproduct of including the patient's voice is rapid cycle quality measures along with, enhanced care and care management. Using this transformative technology, the patient's input transforms and enlightens in a structured and manageable way, all the while improving the organizational culture and performance. The majority of the time patients' with chronic diseases and their families are on their own with few resources and disconnected from clinicians. If we want to keep chronic patients out of the hospital, we have to invest in the tools and systems to them connected. It's time to put the "me" into healthcare and how people experience it. P-IHMS provides the blueprint.

## 16.6   Appendix

### 16.6.1   Embodiments Illustrated in Patient: Interactive Health Management Patents

Figure 16.2 is a list of search results for references on Patient Interactive Healthcare Management patents history.

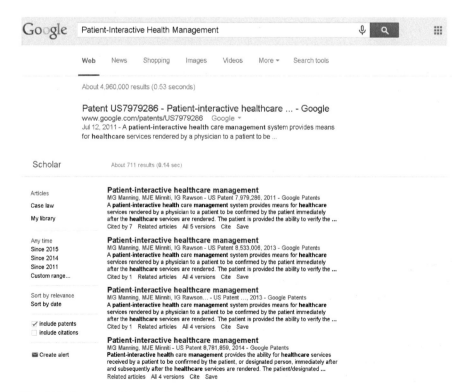

**Fig. 16.2** Search results for references on patient interactive healthcare management patents history

## *16.6.2    Figure 16.3, Adherence and Compliance Monitoring*

In this example via the data input device, the patient interacts with a user prompted interface. that collects information is an illustration (of a patient's perceptions of inter actions with a healthcare practitioner) from patients via a touch screen. A survey is conducted, using non-specialized language, about the patient's experience during the visit. The patient's perceptions pertaining to the quality of the current physician visit is gathered. Patient's perceptions of the communication of health topics in the delivery of evidence based health care during the physician visit also are collected.

Healthcare services rendered are verified by the patient immediately after treatment. This can reduce incidences of health care fraud because the information can increase accuracy as to the medical services that were actually rendered. Because the consumer/patient provides an evaluation of the office visit contemporaneously with the visit, using the consumer's energy/knowledge is a more reliable source to pinpoint and reduce billing mistakes and attempts at fraud. The patient/consumer is also the best qualified to comment on the treatment received during the office visit. Information gathered from the patient, via the information collection station, provides the ability to simplify fraud prevention activities gather physician office best practice data to reward providers for higher quality performance and to provide patient education and compliance buy-in at the time of their visit.

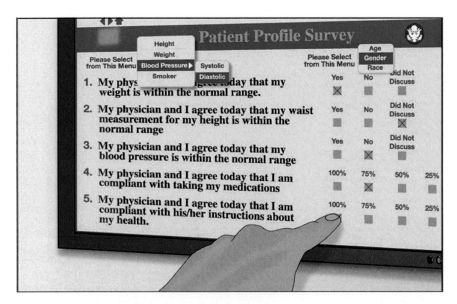

**Fig. 16.3** Illustration of patient's perceptions of interactions with a healthcare practitioner/compliance monitoring

### 16.6.3   Figure 16.4, Service Verification

In this example the patient is completing a sample verification survey. The surveys and payment information can be collected on a database or any appropriate storage means. Responses to the survey can be tabulated and provided to the physician's office (healthcare facility).

The survey offers government-pay patients (e.g., Medicare, Medicaid) the opportunity to express concerns and satisfactions with the care received from their attending health care professional (e.g., physician). The information provided by the patient can be aggregated into a database, or the like, that can be used to report a customer satisfaction score by provider, for customers and consumers accessible from a website, network, or the like. As the patient survey evolves it can yield comparative disease state management data intended to educate individuals about ways to reduce individual risk factors and achieve self-efficacy. This information can be converted into disease state management profiles that direct specific attention to various levels of analysis for the individual, the public, and the government-payer.

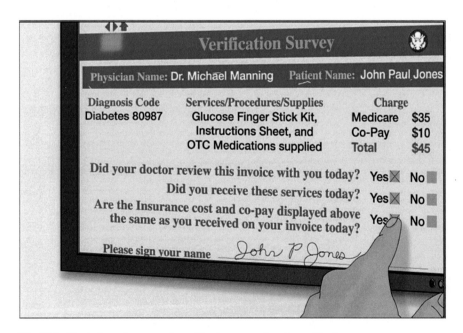

**Fig. 16.4**  Illustration of an example verification survey/service verification

### 16.6.4    Figure 16.5, Quality Transparency for Consumer Information

Is a depiction of an example provider rating report. In this example, providers are rated and the ratings are made available. The provider rating report depicted in Fig. 16.3 can be made available via the Internet, via email, via a paper report, or the like. Consumers can utilize the provider rating reports to assess practitioners before or after receiving services from the practitioner. A provider rating report can be generated from the evaluations and/or ratings of multiple patients. Information included in a provider rating report can include, for example, an assessment of the friendliness of the practitioner, the practitioner's attentiveness to patients, an assessment of the education received from the practitioner, patients' overall satisfaction with a practitioner, and an indication of patients' perception of cost and quality of rendered healthcare services/goods.

### 16.6.5    Figure 16.6, Patient/Consumer Profile

Is a depiction of an example consumer profile. The consumer profile is indicative of a patient specific healthcare report. As an example, embodiment, the patient-interactive healthcare management system stores and maintains healthcare

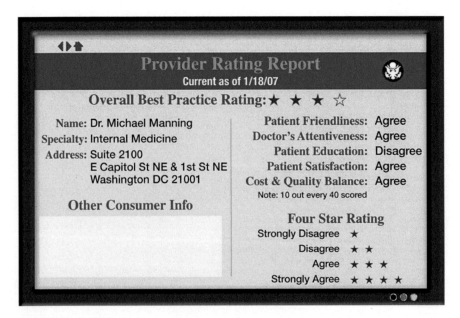

**Fig. 16.5** Depiction of an example provider rating report/quality transparency for consumer consumption

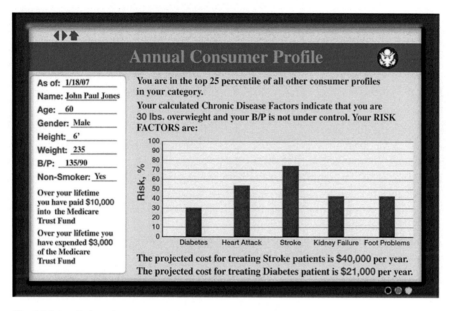

**Fig. 16.6**   Depiction of an example patient/consumer profile

information pertaining to each consumer's experiences. A consumer can access a profile containing such healthcare information. The consumer profile depicted is an annual consumer profile. However the profile can be indicative of any appropriate amount of time. The consumer profile can provide information such as the consumer's name, age, sex, and physical characteristics. The consumer profile can provide statistics pertaining to specific healthcare issues. For example, the consumer profile can provide information pertaining to chronic disease factors such as an indication as to whether the consumer is within acceptable weight boundaries and/ or whether the patient's blood pressure is under control. The consumer profile can provide information indicative of patience risk factors pertaining to various ailments such as diabetes, heart attack, stroke, kidney failure, and foot problems. Additionally, the consumer profile can run information pertaining to cost for treating specific ailments.

In this example, the patient interactive healthcare management system can be utilized as an information repository for tracking purposes. The patient-interactive healthcare management system can be utilized to track durable medical equipment or the like. For example, a patient may receive a durable medical product such as a wheelchair. At the information station, or the like, a barcode affixed to the wheelchair can be scanned into the patient interactive healthcare management system. This system will associate the wheelchair with the patient for tracking purposes. When the patient no longer needs the wheelchair, the patient can return into the practitioner, or to any appropriate location, and the location of the return wheelchair will be updated in the patient-interactive healthcare management system. The patient interactive healthcare management system also can be utilized to track prescriptions. Then, the patient interactive healthcare management system can function as a repository for tracking and maintaining a patient's medication use.

### 16.6.6   *Figure 16.7, Health Information Exchange*

Is an example illustration depicting patient-interactive healthcare management as applied to Medicare. The database comprises patient information collected via the information stations above. It provides the means for health information exchange. The database **71** can comprise, for example, information pertaining to the quality of health care provided to patients, statistics pertaining to the accuracy of invoices, information pertaining to the overall quality of healthcare services provided, or the like. The information contained in the database **71** is available to Medicare billing **75**. Medicare billing **75** can include any appropriate billing agency as the entity responsible for handling billing matters for Medicare. In an example, the information contained in database **71** is available to consumer groups **73**. Information stored in database **71** is available, via Medicare billing **75**, to the Medicare webpage **78**. Information on the Medicare webpage **78** is available to a variety of entities including, for example, a patient **80**, a healthcare provider **82**, any information seeker **84** having access to the Medicare webpage **78**, an auditor investigator **86**, the Medicare administrator **88**, and a professional association **90**.

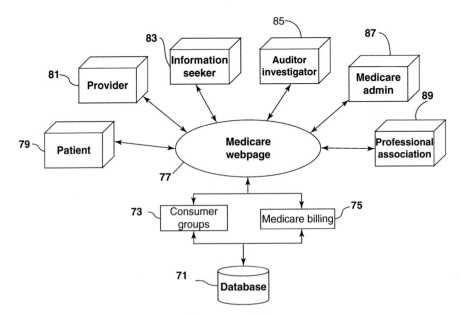

**Fig. 16.7** Diagram of an example patient-interactive healthcare management system as applied to medicare/health information exchange

# References

1. Baddeley AD, Hitch G. Working memory. In: Bower GH, editor. The psychology of learning and motivation: advances in research and theory, vol. 8. New York: Academic; 1974. p. 47–89.
2. Burgers JS, Voerman GE, Grol R, Faber MJ, Schneider EC. Quality and coordination of care for patients with multiple conditions: results from an international survey of patient experience. Eval Health Prof. 2010;33(3):343–64.
3. Dimick C. Preliminary stage 3 meaningful use recommendations released. J AHIMA. Available at http://journal.ahima.org/2014/03/11/preliminary-stage-3-meaningful-use-recommendations-released/. 2014. Accessed 26 Feb 2015.
4. Google.com. Patents. http://www.google.com/patents/US7979286. 2007. Accessed 19 Apr 2015.
5. Hibbard J, Greene J. Health affairs; new era of patient engagement- what the evidence shows about patient activation: better health outcomes and care experiences; fewer data on costs. Health Aff. 2013;32(2):207–14.
6. Hibbard JH, Greene J, Overton V. Patients with lower activation associated with higher costs; delivery systems should know their patient scores. Health Aff. 2013;32(2):216–22.
7. Jaques E. The measurement of responsibility: a study of work, payment, and individual capacity. New York: Wiley; 1972.
8. Levenson H. Multidimensional locus of control in psychiatric patients. J Consult Clin Psychol. 1973;41:397–404.
9. Levenson H. Differentiating among internality, powerful others, and chance. In: Lefcourt H, editor. Research with the locus of control construct, vol. 1. New York: Academic; 1981.
10. McGregor D. The human side of enterprise. New York: McGrawHill; 1960.
11. Ouellette J. Particle physics can help fight cancer. Discovery News, available at: http://news.discovery.com/space/particle-physics-brings-new-tool-to-110509.htm. 2011. Accessed 1 Dec 2014.
12. Pascazio S. All you ever wanted to know about the quantum zeno effect in 70 minutes. Quantum Physics, Cornell University Library, available at: http://arxiv.org/abs/1311.6645. 2013. Accessed 31 Oct 2014.
13. Social Security Administration. Status of the social security and medicare programs. A summary of the 2014 annual reports. http://www.ssa.gov/oact/trsum/. 2014. Accessed 19 Apr 2015.
14. The Boards of Trustees, Federal Hospital Insurance and Federal Supplementary Medical Insurance Trust Funds. 2006 annual report of the federal hospital insurance and federal supplementary medical insurance trust funds. https://www.cms.gov/Research-Statistics-Data-and-Systems/Statistics-Trends-and-Reports/ReportsTrustFunds/downloads/tr2006.pdf.     2006. Accessed 19 Apr 2015.
15. Wallston KA. Perceived control. In: Ayers S, Baum A, McManus C, Newman S, Wallston K, Weinman J, West R, editors. Cambridge handbook of psychology, health and medicine, Second edition. Cambridge: Cambridge University Press; 2007, p. 148–150.
16. Dirocco DN, Day SC. Obtaining patient feedback at point of service using electronic kiosks. Am J Manag Care. 2011;17(7):e270–6.

# Chapter 17
# The Patient of the Future: Participatory Medicine and Enabling Technologies

Michael Christopher Gibbons and Yahya Shaikh

**Abstract** Several forces will progressively change the current US healthcare system. First, patient factors will likely exert the greatest impact. The rapidly growing US population, a growing percentage of seniors, increasing prevalence of chronic disease, increasing racial/ethnic diversity and persisting healthcare disparities will strain an already overloaded system. Second, healthcare system factors are also contributing to challenges. Shortages in the healthcare workforce, the rising costs, complexity and chronicity of care, the burdens of caregivers as primary health providers, the failure to address social determinants of health and the emergence of retail healthcare will exacerbate that strain. This chapter discusses implications of these forces in the context of health information systems evolving to meet these healthcare challenges. We conclude with a case study of a potential future patient-centered health information system and a discussion of patient-oriented features of effective health information systems.

**Keywords** Consumer health technology • Population health • Prevention and wellness • On demand healthcare • Health innovation • Caregivers • Chronic disease self management • Populomics • Telehealth • Telemedicine

## 17.1 Changes in Patient Populations and Health Care

### 17.1.1 Introduction

A fundamental premise of this chapter is the notion that healthcare systems in the future will be very different than they are now or have been. Patients will interact with future healthcare systems in some ways that are similar to historic and current

M.C. Gibbons, MD, MPH (✉)
Medicine, Public Health and Health Informatics, Johns Hopkins University,
Baltimore, MD, USA
e-mail: mgibbon1@jhmi.edu

Y. Shaikh, MD, MPH
Department of General Preventive Medicine, Johns Hopkins University
School of Medicine, Baltimore, MD, USA

© Springer International Publishing Switzerland 2016
C.A. Weaver et al. (eds.), *Healthcare Information Management Systems:
Cases, Strategies, and Solutions*, Health Informatics,
DOI 10.1007/978-3-319-20765-0_17

practices, but undoubtedly they will need to do so in many new ways in the future. To be useful, health information systems must be responsive to current healthcare realities, and also to new and unique interactions, tasks, behaviors and needs of patients, providers and others who will engage patients, to help them achieve their personal health goals.

The chapter starts with patient and population factors which will likely exert the largest impact on healthcare, and a look at changes in healthcare itself. This is followed by a discussion on the implications of changes on health information. These factors have the potential to change many aspects of care: access, quality, costs and patients' experience and satisfaction with its delivery. Advances in information and computer technologies, especially remote clinical sensing, will facilitate the care of individuals to empower patients and to meet emerging healthcare challenges. New, more powerful health information systems will also shape the scope and practice of the healthcare processes they will support. The chapter closes with a case study of a potential health information system of the future, from the patient perspective.

## 17.1.2    The Changing US Healthcare Landscape

### 17.1.2.1    Changes in the Patient Population

*An Increasing US Population* – The US population has grown since 1950 from a base of 152 million Americans, with an additional 156 million added between 1950 and 2009 [1]. Projections suggest the number of people living in the US will increase to 400–450 million people by 2050 [1, 2]. The doubling of the US population (152 million in 1950 to 308 million in 2009) has been remarkable compared with other industrialized countries. Germany and Italy, for instance, grew by only 21 % and 30 % respectively during the same period. Several other countries particularly in Eastern Europe, have actually had reductions in population [1].

*An Aging US Population* – Since 1950, the US population has aged, with increases in the total number of seniors (those over age 65 years) and the proportion of seniors relative to the total population. In 1950, the median age of US was 30.2 years with children under the age of 5 accounting for 10.8 %. By 2000, the median age had risen to 35.3 years while children under the age of 5 accounted for only 6.8 % [1]. By 2010 the median age increased to 37.2 years with those under the age of 5 dropped to 6.5 % [3]. On the other end of the age spectrum: in 1950, seniors represented 8.1 % of the US population, increasing to 12.8 % in 2009 and projected to reach 20.2 % by 2050. By then, one in five persons or over 88 million people will be age 65 or older. Of these, 32.5 million or approximately 7.5 % of the US population are projected to be over the age of 80 [1].

*Increasing Prevalence Of Chronic Disease* – In the US, chronic diseases are the leading cause of illness, morbidity and mortality, accounting for most of health-care expenditures [4]. Half (50.9 %) of all adults in the US have at least one chronic disease and over a quarter (26 %) of all adults and more than 50 % of seniors will have two or more chronic conditions [5]. In 2011, seven of the top ten causes of death in the US were chronic conditions, including (heart disease, cancer, chronic lung diseases, stroke, Alzheimer disease, diabetes, and kidney diseases). Individuals with chronic diseases need and utilize a significant amount of health care services and resources. In addition, chronic conditions puts a tremendous burden on patients, their families and employers, among patients who stay in the workforce and those who must leave it prematurely due to disability [4].

*Increasing Racial and Ethnic Diversity* – According the Census Bureau, the US population is becoming progressively diverse, racially and ethnically. Minorities who now comprise 37 % of the population are projected to become 57 % by 2060 [2]. The non-Hispanic white population is projected to peak by 2024, at 199.6 million, and then to decrease slowly, falling by 20.6 million during 2024–2060. The overall Hispanic population is projected to more than double to 128.8 million by 2060. By 2060, nearly one in three US residents will be of Hispanic descent, up from one in six today. The Asian population is also projected also to more than double, from 15.9 million (5.1 %) in 2012 to 34.4 million (8.2 %) in 2060. The African American population is expected to increase to 61.8 million (14.7 %) over the same time period. American Indian and Alaska Native and Hawaiian and Other Pacific Islander populations are also projected to increase substantially, but will comprise about 1.5 % each of the total population over the same time frame. The number of people who identify themselves as being of two or more races is projected to more than triple, from 7.5 million to 26.7 million over the same period [2].

The cumulative effect of these changes on the total US minority population by 2060 will result in older consumers being predominately non-Hispanic white. Younger individuals will be increasingly minority and the US will become a majority-minority nation for the first time by the year 2043. At that time, the non-Hispanic white population will still be the largest single group, but no single racial group will form a majority of the total US population [2].

*Persisting Healthcare Disparities* – Racial and ethnic demographic shifts are important to consider because patients and consumers from these population groups tend to have poorer health outcomes, less access to health care, lower adoption of healthy behaviors and lower exposure to health-promoting environments. For example, non-Hispanic black adults are at least 50 % more likely to die of heart disease or stroke prematurely (i.e., before age 75 years) than their non-Hispanic white counterparts [6]. The prevalence of adult diabetes is higher among Hispanics, non-Hispanic blacks, and those of other or mixed races than among Asians and non-Hispanic whites [7]. Infant mortality is more than double the rate for non-Hispanic blacks than for non-Hispanic whites [8]. Because individuals from racial and ethnically diverse populations have and continue to experience poorer access to and quality of healthcare services than their white counterparts, they are, by definition, medically underserved and disenfranchised.

Each year since 2003, the Agency for Healthcare Research and Quality (AHRQ) has reported on the status of health care disparities in the US. The National Healthcare Disparities Report (NHDR) focuses on more than 200 health care process, outcome, and access measures, covering a wide variety of conditions and settings [9]. As in previous years, the most recent report found disparities in access to and quality of care to be common across racial and ethnic populations and that most of these are not changing [9]. A few measures of disparities have changed unevenly and inconsistently, but over time, there have been no sustained improvements [9].

The reasons for the existence and persistence of health disparities are complex and thought to be related to sociocultural, socioeconomic, behavioral and environmental factors within the context of current and historical biases and prejudices found within the healthcare system and within the larger society [10]. In addition, significant levels of mistrust and challenges in cross cultural communication have been found among many racial and ethnic minority patients and their health care providers [11–14].

### 17.1.2.2   Changes in Healthcare

*Shortages in Healthcare Manpower* – The core of US healthcare system has been historically comprised of physicians, nurses and other professionals employed within hospitals/health centers. Studies project shortages in the numbers of US healthcare providers:

- Demand for physicians continues to grow faster than supply. This will lead to a projected shortfall of between 46,100 and 90,400 physicians by 2025 [15].
- Projected shortfalls in primary care will range between 12,500 and 31,100 physicians by 2025, while demand for non-primary care physicians will range between 28,200 and 63,700 physicians [15].
- Expanded medical coverage achieved under the Affordable Care Act (ACA) once fully implemented will likely increase demand by about 16,000–17,000 physicians (2.0 %) over the increased demand resulting from changing population demographics and an aging physician workforce [15].

The greatest shortfall, percentage-wise, will be among surgical specialties (excluding obstetrics and gynecology) reflecting little projected growth in the supply of surgeons and limitations on the ability to augment staffing with other types of clinicians. While the shortfall is expected to affect everyone, it will likely be more harmful to vulnerable and underserved consumers and patients in rural or inner-city areas [16]. Some experts believe the physician shortage to be relative, a result of inadequate distribution of physicians across the country, rather than an actual overall shortage [17, 18].

Experts have also indicated that a nursing shortage exists [19]. In 2002, the shortage of registered nurses was estimated to be approximately 125,000. Primary drivers of this shortage are: an aging nursing workforce, increased demands due to population demographic shifts and expansion of government sponsored insurance. It is expected that the trend will progress over time, with a projected shortage of 400,000–808,000 RNs by 2020 [20]. Regardless of cause, whether referring to specialists, primary care providers or nurses, many patients and consumers live without adequate access to the core medical providers of our healthcare system.

*Caregivers as Providers* – The bulk of health care services to patients over the course of their lives is delivered by family members and friends, not healthcare professionals [21]. Nearly four out of ten adult Americans (39 %) report "providing care to an adult relative or friend". In addition, nearly half (47 %) of adults say that they expect to be a caregiver for an aging parent or other elderly relative at some point in their lives [21].

Caregiver activities range from providing simple assistance with routine household tasks or providing emotional support to carrying out complex medical procedures. More than half of all caregivers report having to perform medical/nursing tasks for patients with multiple chronic physical and cognitive conditions. Caregiver provided medical tasks include: managing and administering multiple medications, caring for wounds, giving injections or intravenous therapy, providing incontinence support and/or care coordination [21]. Most caregivers receive little training or support from medical professionals, having to learn to perform tasks on their own, with many reporting fear about their ability to carry out tasks properly [21]. Caregiving can be stressful and time consuming, with tremendous impacts on the physical, mental, financial and social health of caregivers. As the US population continues to age, the need for caregivers will undoubtedly continue to rise [21].

*Rising Healthcare Costs* – US health care costs have risen, largely unabated, for more than 20 years. Projections suggest that US health care spending will surpass $10,000 per person in 2015 [22] and that national health expenditures will consume more than 20 % of the US Gross Domestic Product by 2018 [23]. At the current rate, healthcare spending threatens the integrity of the Medicare and Medicaid programs and makes health care unaffordable for those with low incomes and/or without insurance. The rising rate drives employers, particularly of smaller businesses, to reduce or discontinue providing health insurance for employees because they can no longer afford premiums [23]. To help manage costs, employers and other payers are increasingly shifting costs to employees and their families by offering modest benefit packages with out-of- pocket costs. Enhanced benefits may be possible, but only at higher costs [23].

*Recognition of the Impact of Social Determinants on Health* – It has been increasingly recognized that social factors play an important role in determining morbidity, mortality, disability and health outcomes [24–32]. Growing evidence suggests that medical care, while critical to health, is not the only influence. Experts suggest that the independent influence of medical care alone on mortality may in fact be as low 10–15 % in the US [33, 34], and there is increasing acceptance of the importance of social factors in health and well-being [35, 36]. It is estimated that as many as 50 % of all deaths in the US involve behavioral causes. Health-related behaviors have been shown to be strongly shaped by social factors, including income, education, employment, isolation, social support, socioeconomic status and stress [37], and the effects of any single social factor are often contingent on a host of other factors [37].

Emerging evidence suggests that social and genetic causes of disease are not mutually exclusive and that genetic endowment is not unalterable as once thought. Gene expression may occur only when impacted by social or environmental factors. In turn, physical and social environments may be impacted by social policy [37].

*Retail Healthcare in America* – Patients and consumers can be frustrated by poor access to care, unclear or confusing health information, long wait times for physician office appointments and overcrowded emergency departments. Utilization data indicates that patients are increasingly demanding care that meets their needs [38]. Retail clinics, commercial acute care facilities that provide services evenings and weekends in convenient locations (groceries, drugstores, general retailers, etc.) have emerged as viable sources of acute and preventive care with predictable wait times, easy access, lower costs and clear, transparent patient information [38]. Growing data shows consumers satisfaction with retail clinics. In 2011, 19 % of consumers reported using a retail clinic vs 15 % in 2010 and 13 % in 2009; 30 % of consumers said that they would use a retail clinic if it considerably reduced their wait time [38]. A recent analysis of retail clinic services found they outperformed emergency departments and ambulatory care facilities in 7 measures of quality [39].

## 17.2  Implications of Change on Health Information Systems

Changes in the US population and in healthcare will affect health information systems. Systems of the future must support the needs of a rapidly expanding population of patients, caregivers and healthcare in the face of decreasing healthcare manpower. Experience with telemedicine and tele-health suggests it will be impractical, inconvenient and unnecessary for patients to see a physician for every problem.

An aging population with chronic disease will require health information systems and other information tools to support longitudinal care of increasing complexity as patients accumulate physical and cognitive limitations caused by the co-morbidities of multiple conditions over decades. Future systems will need to aggregate clinical information and data from a wide variety of sources and process as well as interpret data and provide feedback to support patients' adherence, education and health behavior changes.

Increasing racial and ethnic diversity of the population will require health information systems to facilitate and support socio-culturally and linguistically competent interactions between patients and providers. In addition to anticipating and supporting language, literacy, numeracy and health literacy needs, systems and providers will need to help patients make informed inferences, choices and decisions about their health to prevent and mitigate delays and errors in care or communication and enable truly informed consent.

The reduction of healthcare disparities presents special challenges to future health information systems and providers:

- Although patient education and training are necessary and are important means of addressing healthcare disparities, their current implementation has not resulted in discernable or sustained change or reduction. Therefore, alternatives, improvements and new techniques in teaching and training patients and their caregivers are needed if these are to have any impact on disparities.

- The assessment of social, behavioral and environmental determinants of health may require discovery and inference from new types of patient data that are currently not being collected, including those generated by patients, either actively and/or passively.
- Emerging health information systems may not reduce disparities, and in fact, may exacerbate existing and/or introduce new disparities due to differential abilities of populations to utilize and/or benefit from them.

Understanding how health information and systems, their design, implementation and deployment can impact population health to reduce disparities is a frontier in clinical and population health informatics and healthcare services research.

Health information systems of the future must support all stakeholders that comprise patient-centered care teams. As part of supporting the functions of the Patient Centered Medical Home (PCMH), systems must support the needs and activities of informal caregivers (as an integral part of care coordination). Without recognition and support in the form of (education, training and communication with the medical team), caregivers (and the patients for whom they provide services) are vulnerable to poor outcomes due to unseen, unaddressed and undocumented needs. Rather than lowering costs, this will likely increase costs because patients will continue to use expensive services emergently (i.e., emergency departments and hospitals) and unnecessarily.

Retail healthcare can provide both competition and solutions for improving support for PCMHs. Healthcare retailers have financial incentive to encourage patients to use their facilities. In the future, retail healthcare will include the deployment of information tools for patients to augment their care and deepen patient health engagement. One possible evolution is for retail clinics to become part of the medical neighborhood of a PCMH and its health information network to make all care transparent.

## 17.2.1   Patient Centered Health Information Management

The evolution of patient-centered health information management will require EHR system interoperability with a vast array of clinical, patient and consumer oriented tools, sensors and devices. Future systems must enable providers to manage these devices and their data while providing the patient culturally and linguistically appropriate just-in-time assistance and support that fits into (rather than disrupts) patient lifestyles.

Smartphones provide new opportunities for patient-centered health information support as many patients try and use personal digital health tools. It is reported that over one million "apps" are available through Android, Google and Apple [40], with 40,000 health apps being available on the iTunes (Apple) store alone! [41]. In addition, while consumers are increasingly turning to online resources for first-line health information and support, possibly because access is easier than for providers

[42]. Many patients also engage in online communities of care (i.e. Patients like me, Cure Together) that connect patients with similar illnesses and/or problems.

Consumer-targeted health information technologies [43, 44] help patients manage their own care and decisions and can be beneficial in improving health [43–45]:

- Web-based interventions have been shown to improve depression, anxiety or stress [46].
- Mobile messaging supports chronic disease self-management [47] with a variety of tools aimed at helping patients to control asthma [48].
- Social media and/or video-based digital health tools also augment in-person interactions with peers and health professionals as patients navigate their conditions and search for support.
- Social media is also challenging fundamental notions of medical research:

  – Electronic recruitment of geographically dispersed or sparse cohorts can occur quickly.
  – "Citizen science" (patient originated and conducted "studies") conducted in online communities (Patients like me, Cure Together, Association of Cancer Online Registries, Smart Patients) may ignore traditional constraints of research: evidence-based hypotheses, theory-based intervention design, peer review and even informed consent. Many patients, caregivers and consumers view the ability to conceive and conduct these "studies", independent of formal research communities, as empowering and able to challenge traditional research processes. "Citizen science" does not wait for the approval of the scientific community and may provide the patient's voice in hypothesis generation.

The rapid growth of the use of these platforms and innovations suggests that these trends will continue for the foreseeable future and that future health information systems could benefit by incorporating these technologies into care to better engage and empower patients [49–51], and to meet the IHI "Triple Aim" of (a) improving the patient experience of care (including quality and satisfaction), (b) improving the health of populations and (c) reducing the per capita cost of health care [52].

## 17.3   The Patient of the Future: Care, Self-Care and Technology

Understanding how patients, consumers, providers and organizations located in different places may work together in an integrated and coordinated fashion may be facilitated by an "ecosystem" organizational perspective. Serbanati defines a healthcare ecosystem as a collaborative, multidisciplinary and cross-organizational medical and social care delivery network, with the patient or consumer at the center. Using an Internet-based broadband infrastructure, participants share electronic information, use e-services and collaborate as needed and as directed by the patient to address health concerns [53]. Marschollek [54] refers to such systems as sensor enabled Health Information Systems, highlighting the need for such systems to support decentralized, patient-centered and personalized care while seamlessly interfacing with the many sources of information in a person's environment.

At least three types of benefits will be realized by patients using these systems:

*First: Patients will be in constant connection with digital sensors and tools.* These tools will provide real time decision support, enhance patient engagement in health and enable them to stay in contact with the people, information and resources they need to become healthy and stay well. Patients will live in constant contact with medical, social and behavioral supports to reach their health goals. These virtual "health and care" ecosystems will be accessible by patients "on demand", anytime, anywhere they need them. Providers will be able to manage patient-generated health data using emerging big data techniques to study the health of populations for care and research.

*Second: Patients will benefit when data from multiple sources are integrated to yield new insights ("smart" environments).* For example, it may be useful to know an asthmatic patient's respiratory rate heart rate and blood pressure during exercise. A clinician (using an algorithmically generated display) can calculate the patient's work of breathing. This information can enable real time predictions for the likelihood of an impending asthma attack.

*Third: "Smart" environments will be able to respond to real-time patient sensor data and adjust to benefit the patient.* To illustrate this point, imagine that our asthma patient lives in a "smart" home (a residence equipped with technology that facilitates monitoring of residents aiming to improve health, quality of life and promote independence) [55]. Mobile sensor and wireless network technologies can extend monitoring beyond the "smart" home into external activities. Such ubiquitous computing provides the basis for "ambient" assisted living technologies [55]. The "smart" home can be networked to a broader "health and care" ecosystem to become part of the patient's personal ecosystem in which clinical algorithms detect when the patient's work of breathing is consistent with an impending asthma attack and can assess measures of contributory factors such as temperature, medication utilization and patient activity to determine the need for an intervention such as raising the humidity of the home environment, delivering a dose of rescue medication and/or alerting an on-call nurse to the potential of an emerging asthma attack.

This "network of networks" of wireless body sensors, "smart" home, "ambient" assisted living environment and the broader "health and care" network (medical and social information, services and providers) can (using big data and cloud technologies) allow processing of immense amounts of data [56] and integration of that data from a wide variety of sources (i.e., all asthmatic patients within a geographic region) in real time [56]. Over time, these "health and care" ecosystems will be able to "learn and predict" patient behaviors, needs and outcomes, and automatically respond in ways to prevent acute events or to optimize health outcomes based on aggregated patient data.

## 17.4   Case Study: The "Interactive Remote Lifestyle Assistant" (Irla)

To illustrate these benefits, we present a case study of a hypothetical sensor- enabled health information system for supporting chronic disease management:

*Ruby C. is a 76 year old Hispanic patient with congestive heart failure (CHF). She lives alone in a semi-urban mid-western state. Her husband died of a heart attack three years ago. Their three adult children have done well for themselves, but now live in other states with their own families. For many years Ruby struggled, requiring at least 3 hospitalizations a year. Even though she was doing her best, Ruby and her children constantly lived in fear of the worst. But now, things are much better. Ruby's new bathroom carpet automatically records her weight, just before she gets in the shower each day and the information is automatically sent to her health information system and appropriate information forwarded to her electronic medical record. As Ruby tells it:*

> *Whenever I gain 5 pounds or more, this "magic" carpet contacts IRLA. IRLA (the Interactive Remote Lifestyle Assistant) analyzes my eating patterns over the last week. Depending on the results, IRLA will suggest simple ways I can adjust my diet or cooking. IRLA also is able to contact the local grocery store and order foods I like and need and have them delivered right to my door or make a reservation for me at the neighborhood YMCA so I can get the exercise I need. Whenever my kids want to know how I am doing, IRLA keeps track of everything and can tell them anything they want to know. Whenever I need her or just want to talk, all I have to do is turn on the TV and press this button on one of my grandson's game boxes and there she is. We talk and chat for as short or as long as I would like, day or night! If IRLA gets real worried, she will actually call my children to let them know what is going on, set up an appointment with my doctor and arrange for my church van to pick me up and bring me home after the visit.*

*In addition to CHF, Ruby also has asthma. Her doctor recently gave her a new digital asthma inhaler that automatically records the temporal and geospatial context of each use then sends the data back to Ruby's smartphone, IRLA and other connected devices within the network. IRLA automatically integrates this information with data from these data streams are then utilized by an algorithm to identify patterns highly related to an asthma exacerbation. IRLA then activates connected devices such as humidifiers, air filters and heaters in Ruby's home to optimize her environment and decrease the likelihood of an asthma attack.*

*Over time IRLA "learned" that Ruby's asthma triggers include, among other things, the spicy foods that she loves so much. Using this information, IRLA suggested flavorful recipes and foods that Ruby could cook, without the spicy ingredients that lead to asthma attacks, based on what was already in her refrigerator and kitchen cabinets. In addition, IRLA noticed that Ruby usually ate out at a restaurant once a month, usually between the 1st and 5th of the month. Using this information, IRLA provided Ruby, on the last week of each month, with local restaurant and menu suggestions that avoided the spicy foods that often triggered her asthma attacks.*

In this example, IRLA is the convenient, culturally and linguistically appropriate and competent, patient-facing interface to a sensor enabled health information system. IRLA is managed by Ruby's providers but under her control. IRLA is more than a database that collects and transmits data. IRLA relys on data from Ruby's total environment:

- Ruby's medical history, encoded in her electronic health record
- Data from multiple sensors and sources including:
  - Weight scale in the Bluetooth-enabled bathroom mat that wirelessly and automatically transmits weight data to a "cloud" repository
  - Radio frequency identification (RFID) tags embedded in food labels and bottle caps of the food items she buys to help monitor sodium and nutritional intake
  - Continuously indoor and outdoor atmospheric pollution sensors
  - Humidity and temperature sensors
  - Local traffic conditions (for diesel exhaust fumes) and weather patterns
  - Direct input from Ruby
  - Information from her internist
  - The Bluetooth enabled peak flow meter attached to her asthma inhaler to monitor potential airway obstruction
  - Ruby's activity and appointment calendar and diet tracker
  - Food databases from her favorite restaurant and grocer

IRLA helps coordinate Ruby's health and social care activities and provides culturally appropriate behavioral feedback to motivate long term behavior change. With data streams from Ruby's ecosystem of devices and doctor, IRLA can then use machine learning and artificial intelligence, initiate certain actions autonomously and automatically record these actions in Ruby's electronic health record for viewing by caregivers to whom Ruby has granted access (her physician, her pastor and her adult children).

Prior to IRLA, Ruby and her children always worried about keeping up with everything the doctor told them the last time they saw him. It was difficult because he always had to rush and the paperwork was always confusing. IRLA simplifies the paperwork Ruby receives from her doctor and provides verbal reinforcement to help Ruby to become and stay healthy. Ruby's children no longer worry about not knowing what is going on because they can obtain understandable online summaries of her activities, eating patterns or doctor's instructions at any time without having to take off valuable time from work and loose income.

Finally, IRLA provides Ruby with suggestions and regular behavioral feedback. Timely practical feedback and instruction is a powerful form of reinforcement based on the data from recent patient actions. Regular behavior feedback has been shown to be critical to initiating and sustaining behavior change and has been found to be a key component of successful consumer health informatics tools. This form of teaching has its roots in so-called "edutainment" and "health gaming". Time and rigorous evaluation will be needed to determine the superiority of these approaches to traditional methods (which have not worked).

## 17.5   Conclusions

As healthcare systems evolve, so too must health information systems and tools to meet the changing needs of patients and healthcare systems. The story of IRLA is hypothetical but the described technologies are currently possible or being developed. Their implementation into publicly or commercially available connected health information ecosystems is only a matter of time as industry and federal efforts are underway to lay the foundation for realizing these possibilities.

Health information systems of the future must provide much more than just a mechanism for health information exchange with a provider or health system. Robust health information systems of the future will likely share the following characteristics:

- Systems will consist of distributed networked devices, tools, sensors and technologies, working together to provide alignment of decision support, behavioral motivation, education and health task support, while maintaining awareness of patient activity, response and needs. They will need to automate pre-programmable tasks where and when possible within patient home environments, in response to real time aggregated data.
- Systems must be interoperable with any patient's health information ecosystem. They will need to receive and share data with a variety of clinical and nonclinical sources (including patient generated health data), based on patient preferences, information needs and tools (apps, consumer devices, fitness trackers and other emerging technology), in human accessible/readable forms.
- Systems must put patients at the center of care. They must:
  - Integrate and incorporate tele-health and remote technologies to make healthcare accessible, usable and convenient for patients
  - They must facilitate communication and other interactions among all stakeholders in a patient's care
  - They must summarize data and present it in forms that meet the literacy, numeracy and health literacy needs of patients at all levels in a culturally acceptable fashion.

It is challenging to conceive how healthcare services will be delivered to meet the needs of all Americans, but the evolving US patient population will require evolving ways of managing health information. Networked, sensor-enhanced, patient-centered health information systems hold great promise to facilitate this evolution, to empower patients and to make the work of providers care teams and families more efficient, more cost-effective and more responsive to patient needs to help the nation achieve its national health goals.

# References

1. Shrestha LB, Heisler EJ. The changing demographic profile of the United States. Washington, DC: Congressional Research Service; 2011. Report No.: 7-5700.
2. U.S.Census Bureau. Projections show a slower growing, older, more diverse nation a half century from now. https://www.census.gov/newsroom/releases/archives/population/cb12-243.html. 2012.
3. Howden LM, Meyer JA. Age and sex composition 2010: 2010 Census brief # C2010BR-03. https://www.census.gov/prod/cen2010/briefs/c2010br-03.pdf. 2011.
4. Bauer UE, Briss PA, Goodman RA, Bowman BA. Prevention of chronic disease in the 21st century: elimination of the leading preventable causes of premature death and disability in the USA. Lancet. 2014;384(9937):45–52.
5. Ward BW, Schiller JS. Prevalence of multiple chronic conditions among US adults: estimates from the National Health Interview Survey, 2010. Prev Chronic Dis. 2013;10, E65.
6. Gillespie CD, Wigington C, Hong Y. Coronary heart disease and stroke deaths – United States, 2009. MMWR Surveill Summ. 2013;62 Suppl 3:157–60.
7. Beckles GL, Chou CF. Diabetes – United States, 2006 and 2010. MMWR Surveill Summ. 2013;62 Suppl 3:99–104.
8. MacDorman MF, Mathews TJ. Infant deaths – United States, 2005–2008. MMWR Surveill Summ. 2013;62 Suppl 3:171–5.
9. Agency for Healthcare Research and Quality. National healthcare disparities report 2013. Washington, DC: AHRQ; 2014.
10. Institute of Medicine. Unequal treatment: understanding racial and ethnic disparities in health care. Washington, DC: National Academies Press; 2002.
11. Boulware LE, Cooper LA, Ratner LE, LaVeist TA, Powe NR. Race and trust in the health care system. Public Health Rep. 2003;118(4):358–65.
12. Casagrande SS, Gary TL, LaVeist TA, Gaskin DJ, Cooper LA. Perceived discrimination and adherence to medical care in a racially integrated community. J Gen Intern Med. 2007;22(3):389–95.
13. LaVeist TA, Isaac LA, Williams KP. Mistrust of health care organizations is associated with underutilization of health services. Health Serv Res. 2009;44(6):2093–105.
14. LaVeist TA, Nickerson KJ, Bowie JV. Attitudes about racism, medical mistrust, and satisfaction with care among African American and white cardiac patients. Med Care Res Rev. 2000;57 Suppl 1:146–61.
15. Dall T, West T, Chakrabarti R, Iacobucci W. The complexities of physician supply and demand: projections from 2013 to 2025. Washington, DC: IHS; 2015.
16. Association of American Medical Colleges. Physician shortages to worsen without increases in residency training. https://www.aamc.org/download/153160/data/physician_shortages_to_worsen_without_increases_in_residency_tr.pdf. 2010.
17. Council on Graduate Medical Education. Physician distribution and health care challenges in rural and inner-city areas. Washington, DC: HRSA; 1998. Report No.: 10th.
18. Petterson SM, Liaw WR, Phillips Jr RL, Rabin DL, Meyers DS, Bazemore AW. Projecting US primary care physician workforce needs: 2010–2025. Ann Fam Med. 2012;10(6):503–9.
19. Goodin HJ. The nursing shortage in the United States of America: an integrative review of the literature. J Adv Nurs. 2003;43(4):335–50.

20. Keenan P. The nursing workforce shortage: causes, consequences, proposed solutions. The Commonwealth Fund; Report No.: Issue Brief #619. 2003.
21. Adler R, Mehta R. Catalyzing technology to support family caregiving. Washington, DC: National Alliane for Caregiving; 2014.
22. Centers for Medicare & Medicaid Services. National health expenditure fact sheet. http://www.cms.gov/Research-Statistics-Data-and-Systems/Statistics-Trends-and-Reports/NationalHealthExpendData/NHE-Fact-Sheet.html. 2014.
23. Battani J, Zywiak W. US healthcare in the year 2015. Falls Church: Computer Sciences Corporation; 2015.
24. Ferrie JE, Shipley MJ, Davey SG, Stansfeld SA, Marmot MG. Change in health inequalities among British civil servants: the Whitehall II study. J Epidemiol Community Health. 2002;56(12):922–6.
25. Marmot M. Income inequality, social environment, and inequalities in health. J Policy Anal Manage. 2001;20(1):156–9.
26. Marmot MG, Smith GD, Stansfeld S, et al. Health inequalities among British civil servants: the Whitehall II study. Lancet. 1991;337(8754):1387–93.
27. Kawachi I, Kennedy BP, Wilkinson RG. Crime: social disorganization and relative deprivation. Soc Sci Med. 1999;48(6):719–31.
28. Pickett KE, Wilkinson RG. Income inequality and health: a causal review. Soc Sci Med. 2015;128:316–26.
29. Wilkinson RG, Pickett KE. Income inequality and population health: a review and explanation of the evidence. Soc Sci Med. 2006;62(7):1768–84.
30. Wilkinson RG. Income inequality and population health. Soc Sci Med. 1998;47(3):411–2.
31. Braveman P, Egerter S, Williams DR. The social determinants of health: coming of age. Annu Rev Public Health. 2011;32:381–98.
32. Williams DR, Sternthal M. Understanding racial-ethnic disparities in health: sociological contributions. J Health Soc Behav. 2010;51(Suppl):S15–27.
33. McGinnis JM, Foege WH. Actual causes of death in the United States. JAMA. 1993;270(18):2207–12.
34. McGinnis JM, Williams-Russo P, Knickman JR. The case for more active policy attention to health promotion. Health Aff (Millwood). 2002;21(2):78–93.
35. Mackenbach JP. The contribution of medical care to mortality decline: McKeown revisited. J Clin Epidemiol. 1996;49(11):1207–13.
36. Mackenbach JP, Stronks K, Kunst AE. The contribution of medical care to inequalities in health: differences between socio-economic groups in decline of mortality from conditions amenable to medical intervention. Soc Sci Med. 1989;29(3):369–76.
37. Braveman P, Gottlieb L. The social determinants of health: it's time to consider the causes of the causes. Public Health Rep. 2014;129 Suppl 2:19–31.
38. Kaissi A, Charland T. The evolution of retail clinics in the United States, 2006–2012. Health Care Manag (Frederick). 2013;32(4):336–42.
39. Shrank WH, Krumme AA, Tong AY, et al. Quality of care at retail clinics for 3 common conditions. Am J Manag Care. 2014;20(10):794–801.
40. Freierman S. One million apps and counting at a fast pace. New York Times. 2011 Dec 12 pB3.
41. Aitken M, Gauntlet C. Patient apps for improved healthcare: from novelty to mainstream. Parsippany: IMS Institute for Healthcare Informatics; 2013.
42. Cybercitizen Health v8.0. New York: Manhattan Research; 2008.
43. Gibbons MC. Personal health and consumer informatics. The impact of health oriented social media applications on health outcomes. Yearb Med Inform. 2013;8(1):159–61.
44. Gibbons MC, Wilson RF, Samal L, et al. Impact of consumer health informatics applications. Evid Rep Technol Assess (Full Rep). 2009;(188):1–546. AHRQ Publication No. 09(10)-E019
45. Gibbons MC, Wilson RF, Samal L, et al. Consumer health informatics: results of a systematic evidence review and evidence based recommendations. Transl Behav Med. 2011;1(1):72–82.
46. Davies EB, Morriss R, Glazebrook C. Computer-delivered and web-based interventions to improve depression, anxiety, and psychological well-being of university students: a systematic review and meta-analysis. J Med Internet Res. 2014;16(5), e130.

47. de Jongh T, Gurol-Urganci I, Vodopivec-Jamsek V, Car J, Atun R. Mobile phone messaging for facilitating self-management of long-term illnesses. Cochrane Database Syst Rev 2012;(12):CD007459.
48. Morrison D, Wyke S, Agur K, et al. Digital asthma self-management interventions: a systematic review. J Med Internet Res. 2014;16(2), e51.
49. Househ M, Borycki E, Kushniruk A. Empowering patients through social media: the benefits and challenges. Health Informatics J. 2014;20(1):50–8.
50. Winbush GB, McDougle L, Labranche L, Khan S, Tolliver S. Health empowerment technologies (HET): building a web-based tool to empower older African American patient-doctor relationships. J Health Care Poor Underserved. 2013;24(4 Suppl):106–17.
51. Calvillo J, Roman I, Roa LM. How technology is empowering patients? A literature review. Health Expect. 2013. doi:10.1111/hex.12089.
52. Dahl D, Reisetter JA, Zismann N. People, technology, and process meet the triple aim. Nurs Adm Q. 2014;38(1):13–21.
53. Serbanati LD, Ricci FL, Mercurio G, Vasilateanu A. Steps towards a digital health ecosystem. J Biomed Inform. 2011;44(4):621–36.
54. Marschollek M. Recent progress in sensor-enhanced health information systems - slowly but sustainably. Inform Health Soc Care. 2009;34(4):225–30.
55. Demiris G, Thompson H. Smart homes and ambient assisted living applications: from data to knowledge-empowering or overwhelming older adults? Contribution of the IMIA Smart Homes and Ambiant Assisted Living Working Group. Yearb Med Inform. 2011;6(1):51–7.
56. Bryant R, Katz RH, Lazowska ED. Big data computing: creating revolutionary breakthroughs in commerce, Science and Society. Washington, DC: Computing Research Association; 2008.

# Part III
# Looking Forward: Near Future Initiatives to Make Things Better

## Introduction

The eight chapters in this section explore new areas in the science of patient safety; new virtual training environments for healthcare professionals and students; standards, architecture and infrastructure needed to support a viable and usable Personal Health Record; and the new emerging technologies and care delivery models that they enable that support person-centric care and consumers choice in care utilization. Part III's chapters report on current innovative initiatives in the early conceptual stages of development and testing that are directed at key areas of transformative change.

- In Chapter 18, Michael Rosen and his group of authors from the Armstrong Institute lay out a number of in-process, data-driven patient safety pilot programs being conducted under their Emerge Project.
- Dev Parvati, in Chapter 19, addresses the potential of virtual, clinical simulation laboratories and their underlying technologies that present medical and nursing students the opportunity to learn clinical skills and critical thinking in the medium of medical devices and electronic record technologies that are often not available in actual clinical settings.
- As we address the efforts to date to engage patients in models of patient centered care and self-management, the thorny area of Personal Health Records (PHR) continues to be an elusive reality. In Chapter 20, William Yasnoff offers a vision for achieving a usable and effective PHR by addressing the interdependent issues of information architecture, business models, and standards needed.
- In Chapter 21, Hsueh, Chang and Ramakrishnan takes us into the world of new emerging technologies that offer the promise of broader consumer involvement in their daily health; while Zhu and Cahan explore the "wearable revolution", telehealth and mobile devices as enabling technologies that fundamentally change the way healthcare is delivered in support of patient-centered care in Chapter 22.
- And just as methods of care delivery are changing at lightning speed, so too is the way care is being reimbursed with the opportunity for consumers to be more engaged in their choices of insurance and care utilization (Yuen-Reed and Mojsilović – Chapter 23); coded for payor reimbursement, quality and cost effectiveness big data analysis (David Meyers – Chapter 24) and managed as data inside organizations to address the ever more demanding requirements for data security from internal and external threats (Kiel et al. – Chapter 25).

# Chapter 18
# Data Driven Patient Safety and Clinical Information Technology

Michael A. Rosen, Grace Tran, Howard Carolan, Mark Romig,
Cynthia Dwyer, Aaron S. Dietz, George R. Kim, Alan Ravitz,
Adam Sapirstein, and Peter J. Pronovost

M.A. Rosen, PhD (✉)
Armstrong Institute for Patient Safety and Quality, Johns Hopkins University School
of Medicine, Baltimore, MD, USA

Bloomberg School of Public Health, Johns Hopkins University,
Baltimore, MD, USA
e-mail: mrosen44@jhmi.edu

M. Romig, MD • A.S. Dietz, PhD
Armstrong Institute for Patient Safety and Quality, Johns Hopkins University
School of Medicine, Baltimore, MD, USA

G. Tran, MS
Applied Physics Laboratory, Human Factors/Systems Integration, Johns Hopkins University,
Laurel, MD, USA

H. Carolan, MBA, MHA
Armstrong Institute for Patient Safety and Quality, Johns Hopkins University
School of Medicine, Baltimore, MD, USA

C. Dwyer, RN
Surgical Intensive Care Unit/Intermediate Care Unit, The Johns Hopkins Hospital,
Baltimore, MD, USA

Armstrong Institute for Patient Safety and Quality, Johns Hopkins University
School of Medicine, Baltimore, MD, USA

G.R. Kim, MD
Division of Health Sciences Informatics and Armstrong Institute for Patient Safety
and Quality, Johns Hopkins University School of Medicine, Baltimore, MD, USA
e-mail: gkim9@jhmi.edu

A. Ravitz, MS
Healthcare, Research and Exploratory Development and Human
Factors/Systems Integration, Applied Physics Laboratory,
Johns Hopkins University, Laurel, MD, USA

© Springer International Publishing Switzerland 2016                    301
C.A. Weaver et al. (eds.), *Healthcare Information Management Systems:
Cases, Strategies, and Solutions*, Health Informatics,
DOI 10.1007/978-3-319-20765-0_18

A. Sapirstein, MD
Armstrong Institute for Patient Safety and Quality, Johns Hopkins University School of
Medicine, Baltimore, MD, USA

Division of Adult Critical Care Medicine, The Johns Hopkins University School of Medicine,
Baltimore, MD, USA

P.J. Pronovost, MD, PhD
Director, Armstrong Institute for Patient Safety and Quality, Johns Hopkins University
School of Medicine, Baltimore, MD, USA

Professor, Department of Anesthesiology and Critical Care Medicine, Johns Hopkins
University School of Medicine, Joint Appointment in the School of Nursing, School of
Medicine, Baltimore, MD, USA

Senior Vice-President for Patient Safety and Quality, Johns Hopkins Medicine,
Baltimore, MD, USA

**Abstract** Healthcare information technology has improved the business of health-care with mixed results for its impact on the delivery of care itself. As industry and regulatory pressures to improve the quality and safety of care through the reduction of preventable harms, it becomes imperative to align information systems to (a) collect real-time clinical data with patient care workflows and (b) provide quality and patient safety teams (and other stakeholders) easy access to meaningful process and outcomes data. To accomplish this, hospitals and other healthcare organizations must adopt emerging practices from the science of high reliability organizations (HROs). In addition, they must employ and adapt clinical IT systems to facilitate real-time collection, analysis and feedback of performance (on multiple levels) with data directly from care. An example, Project Emerge, from the Johns Hopkins Hospital, is presented.

**Keywords** Patient safety • Care quality • Intensive care unit • Critical care • Surgical critical care • High reliability organizations • Real-time patient monitoring • Data reuse • Armstrong Institute for Patient Safety and Quality • Johns Hopkins Hospital • Project Emerge (safety) • Ventilator associated events (VAE) • Patient/family engagement in care

## 18.1   Introduction

Modern day healthcare organizations are inefficient and wasteful [3], unsafe [14], and frequently fail to deliver care consistent with either evidence-based practices [13] or the values and preferences of patients and their loved ones [1]. Converging pressure from regulatory agencies, public and private payers, as well as the general population create conditions requiring transformative, disruptive, and radical change to the status quo. Healthcare organizations need new ways of managing and providing care. Information technology has been a critical driver of efficiency and reliability on other industries, and is heralded as one key solution to the current challenges in healthcare [20]. However, the current health information technology (HIT) infrastructure in most healthcare organizations fails to support the needs of those charged with improving safety and quality.

HIT has contributed improvements in care delivery [11], but the record has been mixed [9]. Much remains to be done if the true promise of better information technology is to be realized. HIT shortcomings manifest in multiple ways within healthcare organizations. For example, quality and safety improvement teams frequently lack accessible and meaningful process and outcome data needed to drive projects; clinicians must use information tools that do not fit their workflows, adding complexity, workload and opportunities for error; patients and their loved ones must manage an increasingly complex care process with very few information tools designed with them in mind. These shortcomings can be traced back to the origins of HIT as billing systems and a failure to adopt systems engineering and human factors design principles that are common to other safety critical domains [16].

HIT can and must better support healthcare organizations as they strive to meet the mounting industry pressure to increase the quality and value of care through the reduction of preventable harms. To that end, we pursue three goals in this chapter. First, by drawing from the science of High Reliability Organizations (HROs) and emerging practices in healthcare, we outline management functions that HIT must provide to better support patient safety and care quality processes. Second, we discuss data collection, analysis, and feedback functions that HIT currently has and will need to have to support safety and quality improvement. Third, as a Case Study to illustrate the possibilities of the rigorous application of systems engineering and human factors approaches to the development of HIT in the interest of patient safety and care quality, we describe Project Emerge, a project in critical care at the Johns Hopkins Hospital.

## 18.2 Information Technology to Enable Patient Safety: Implications of an Evidence-Based Approach to Managing Safety

In order to build a better HIT infrastructure for safety and quality, system designers need a detailed understanding of the requirements: What tasks and functions will HIT need to support? We explore this question below, first by summarizing implications of the science of High-Reliability Organizations with respect to HIT; and second by examining emerging organizational management practices for safety and quality in healthcare.

### 18.2.1 Principles of High-Reliability Organizations

High-Reliability Organizations (HROs) has emerged as a topic of inquiry from a group of researchers at the University of California, Berkeley. This group was studying how organizations within highly hazardous industries (e.g., nuclear power generation, military and civil aviation) were able to perform with rates of accidents far below what could be expected [12]. Their discovered principles of HROs have informed current visions of a safe and high quality healthcare system [5, 15, 22].

The definition of an HRO is: an organization with the potential for reaching catastrophic outcomes due to mistakes, but that actually achieves high levels of relatively error-free performance over the long term [4]. Research on HROs has led to an understanding of how these organizations achieve this remarkable level of performance.

Individuals within HROs possess a common set of core values relating to risk, errors and safety [21]. These are:

- *Preoccupation with failure.* This manifests in two key ways:

  - First, they scrutinize any deviation from expected outcomes or standard practice. When things do not go as planned, it is treated as an opportunity to learn more about how the system works and how to more effectively manage operations in the future.
  - Second, even when operations are within normal and safe boundaries, members of HROs dedicate significant effort towards anticipating how things may go wrong. This proactive approach to identifying potential threats to safe operations leads to a continual effort at improving when actual errors or deviations become very infrequent.

- *Extreme reluctance to simplify.* HRO members do not accept easy answers to complex problems and understand that seemingly insignificant events can produce dire consequences. Superficial explanations are not tolerated and true underlying causes are pursued.
- *Acute sensitivity to operations.* Members of the organization actively seek a clear understanding of how the organization is currently performing in terms of outcomes as well as deviation from standard operating procedures.
- *Unwavering commitment to resilience.* HRO members adopt a learning-oriented perspective and react to problems and failures as opportunities to improve. This mindset helps them respond to unanticipated situations rapidly and effectively.
- *Deference to expertise* when solving problems. They do not use status (e.g., rank, title, or tenure) to determine who is qualified to address a given task or situation. They seek to recognize expertise in others and adjust their response to make sure the best ideas and interpretations of situations are used in decision making regardless of where (or who) those ideas come from.
- *High levels of competence.* Expertise is prized highly and developed continually, both as individuals and as collective units. There are formal (e.g., continuing professional development) and informal (e.g., mentoring and peer review) processes to ensure that people have the opportunity to continue to grow professionally.

### 18.2.2  Emerging Safety and Quality Management Structures in Healthcare

HROs achieve high levels of performance by creating mechanisms to enact the values described above. Healthcare is attempting to transition to the levels of performance characteristic of HROs, but currently is far from being a member of this class. However, healthcare organizations are developing new forms of management capable of operationalizing HRO principles that are feasible given the unique constrains of the industry.

The fractal-based quality management infrastructure [17] is one such approach. In general, fractals are repeating structures at different levels of analysis. This approach is important for managing safety and quality due to the complexity of healthcare organizations. The fractal-based management structure is currently being implemented within the Johns Hopkins Health System and articulates core functions of managing safety that can be replicated in different ways across levels of the organization. These functions include:

- *A centralized improvement core of experts in a broad array of improvement and safety related disciplines* such as information technology and analytics, organizational science, and human factors engineering. This core works to coordinate efforts across the system and to ensure that the best evidence and practices around safety and quality improvement are included used in the organizations efforts.
- *Sufficient resources, including training and salary support for physician and nurse safety and quality improvement professionals at each level of the organization.* This is critical for managing safety at the local level and both identifying and mitigating risks that may be uniquely present in one area as well as serving as an effective change mechanism for system wide interventions.
- *A system of clear goal setting using standardized measurement, transparent reporting, and assigned accountability.* These goals must be aligned across levels of the organization.
- *Horizontal learning structures cut across traditional boundaries to ensure that lessons learned are spread throughout the organization.* Many problems are local in nature, but there is great value in sharing solutions to safety problems throughout the organization. Some can be adopted organization-wide, while others can serves as models to spur further innovation.
- *Inclusion and involvement of patient representatives in safety and quality improvement work* in different ways including both advisory committees as well as seats on improvement teams at different levels.

This framework articulates the fundamental infrastructure necessary for managing safety and quality. The development of HIT can be informed by these functions, as most, if not all, safety management functions can be enabled by better HIT tools. Clearly, setting goals using standardized metrics and ensuring transparent reporting is tightly coupled with HIT implementation. Using current data streams (e.g., EMRs) to track progress and provide needed process and outcome data is critical to scaling this function. HIT needs to be flexible enough to adapt to changing data needs for safety and quality improvement projects. Currently HIT can serve as a valuable tool for standardization (e.g., creating common order sets). However, the challenge is avoiding the potential pitfall of rigidity. For example, when the entire organization uses one standardized workflow or order set, changing that component of HIT can become highly bureaucratic involving approval and sign off from numerous committees. Similarly, healthcare leaders need to consider and plan for the HIT resources needed at different levels of the organization, specifically, which HIT resources are centralized and distributed (e.g., developed within clinical departments, or contained within in HIT department). These decisions will impact how effectively safety and quality improvement teams are able to make use of the HIT infrastructure.

## 18.3   The Use and Re-use of Data for Quality and Safety

In 1966, Avedis Donabedian proposed the model of healthcare quality as measurements linked to structures, processes and outcomes of care [6]. Since then, progress toward creating, computing and using databases of process-based measures to demonstrate impact on outcomes has leveraged the power of information technology to incorporate active clinical data. With the enactment of the Patient Safety and Quality Improvement Act of 2005 (Public Law 109-41), the Federal Government formally committed to foster patient safety through the definition and creation of Patient Safety Organizations (PSOs) to collect, aggregate, and analyze confidential information reported by health care providers.

Mandates to measure the quality of federally-funded care have produced a corpus of data for use in research, quality improvement and innovation from the Centers for Medicare and Medicaid and the Agency for Healthcare Research and Quality. Databases and data collection/reporting systems related to drug safety and adverse events have been established by the Food and Drug Administration for safety and adverse events reporting for drugs and biologics (including post-market surveillance) and by then Centers for Disease Control and Prevention for public and population health (including vaccine safety). The federal government has also made these data resources available to the public along with tools needed to manipulate them.

These advancements in measurement have not yet resulted in large scale improvements in safety or quality. As an industry, healthcare is currently in the process of re-discovering hard won knowledge from the organizational sciences. While measurement practices continue to progress, there is a striking failure to put that data to use in many cases. For example, the American College of Surgeon's National Surgical Quality Improvement Program (NSQIP®) is the most comprehensive and trusted database of surgical process and outcome data available. However, several recent articles have been unable to detect a significant difference in patient outcomes between NSQIP® participating and non-participating facilities [2, 8]. In essence, the improvement infrastructure, like that detail in the fractal model above, has not matured enough to make effective use of the growing data resources.

There are of course gaps in the data collection mechanisms. Not everything that is measured is important, and not everything important is measured. For example, studies have indicated that current quality measurement systems only capture about 50 % of the reasons patients are readmitted [7]. Additionally, moves towards transparency and financially incentivizing performance based on these still developing data sources has the potential to skew improvement efforts. For example, systems used to assess the value of care based on patient's presenting symptoms (i.e., those present and indicated before the clinician has arrived at a diagnosis) can skew measures of value [10].

In sum, three trends would seem to dominate data for safety and quality in healthcare: more data (of increasing quality), more transparency, and more account-ability. While there are still many challenges for developing good measurement systems for safety and quality, the state of the art and science is progressing. More people now have access to this data, both internally within healthcare organizations via the proliferation of data dashboards, and externally through regulators. Public accountability for these data requires organizations invest in generating and using high quality data. The following section details a case example of how better sys-tems engineering and human factors design processes can lead to more effective HIT for safety and quality.

## 18.4   Case Study: Project Emerge

The current state of the health information technology infrastructure in critical care environments does not incorporate the level of good user-center design needed to support high quality, safe, efficient and patient centered care. Rather, current inten-sive care technology, workflows, and culture have incrementally evolved over time into a disintegrated set of system components. The Armstrong Institute for Patient Safety and Quality at the Johns Hopkins University School of Medicine in collabo-ration with the Johns Hopkins University Applied Physics Laboratory are currently leading a significant HIT initiative with the aim of redressing these issues through the application of systems engineering and human factors design and evaluation principles and methods. Project Emerge is an example of how this approach can be applied to develop more effective HIT and ultimately to improve the quality, safety, and patient-centeredness of care delivery systems [19]. We describe the aims, over-view and current state of Project Emerge and discuss challenges associated with implementation, and future goals based on the lessons learned.

### 18.4.1   Project Aims

Project Emerge is focused on balancing three core aims related to improving value: (1) improve the safety and quality of care by eliminating preventable harm and ensuring patients receive care consistent with evidence-based guidelines, (2) elimi-nate waste, and (3) support respect and dignity for patients and their loved ones. To achieve these aims, Project Emerge seeks to demonstrate the potential of a patient-centered, systems engineering approach beginning in ICU environments and expanding over time to include the full continuum of care. The project is guided by three fundamental assumptions. First, the process of care in the ICU is complex, dynamic, and the array of clinicians in the ICU and hospital is not optimally config-ured to deliver consistent high-quality, safe, efficient care. Second, the delivery of care can be perceived as disrespectful and indifferent to the needs and values of the patients and family members despite the key roles that they can play in their own care. Third, accountability and learning mechanisms (e.g., timely and actionable data, transparency of performance and non-performance; feedback loops to correct and prevent mistakes, etc.) are critical for ensuring high-reliability of healthcare services, but currently are immature, absent, or insufficient.

With the overall goal of developing an integrated ICU to enhance the safety, quality, and patient-centeredness of care delivery, the initial phases of Project Emerge targeted five clinical harms: Central Line Associated Blood Stream Infections, Venous Thromboembolism, Delirium, ICU Acquired Weakness, and Ventilator Associated Events. These clinical harms where chosen because the represent a significant portion of preventable harms in the ICU, and relatively well developed evidence-based protocols exist to reduce risk. Additionally, two non-clinical harms were targeted: the loss or diminution of respect and dignity of patients and families, and failure to align care with patient goals. Previous approaches to managing risks associated with these harms have functioned independently. Project Emerge approached the problem from a different perspective. The historical lack of integration and appropriate prioritization has fueled errors and inefficiencies. Project Emerge started by building an integrated model that accounted for (1) technical interoperability, (2) the workflows and tasks of stakeholders including clinicians, patients, and their families, and (3) the culture of healthcare and the local culture where the system is being implemented.

Project Emerge included a diverse set of team members including software engineers, clinicians, human factors, patient safety and bioethics experts, biostatisticians, and patient/family advocates. The Project Emerge team is arguably the first demonstration of a trans-disciplinary engineering effort in clinical medicine. This broad team was necessary to address the multiple issues involved in addressing the aims stated above.

## 18.4.2   Overview of the Project Emerge System

The Project Emerge system is an open architecture with a front-end of interactive displays facilitating situations awareness, risk perception, decision support, and communication. The system functions as a middle-layer architecture for translating disparate information into an integrated presentation format for end users of the system. Currently, the lack of interoperability between data sources in the ICU (e.g., electronic medical records, infusion pumps, ventilators, monitors, environmental sensors) creates hazards and complicates the process of building and maintaining shared situational awareness of patient status, trajectory, and risks. From the earliest phases of the project, there was a heavy emphasis on connecting data to analytics. A key belief among the project team is that real-time data and analytics are crucial to driving meaningful change. A human factors working group was convened to develop design concepts for representing the data pulled from various data streams with the goal of enabling safe and efficient work processes. Human factors work included conducting user needs analyses with patient, family, and clinician stakeholder groups to develop and refine design requirements and prototype displays, iterating and redesigning prototypes based on user feedback. While systems integration is a central concept for Project Emerge, creating better information tools is necessary to capitalize on the integrated infrastructure. The user-centered approach taken in this project produced innovative displays (see Fig. 18.1) to support the work of clinicians as well as the engagement and activation of patients and their loved ones.

Initial iterations of two major components of the Emerge System are described in the following sections: the Care Team Portal (CTP), and the Patient and Family Portal (PFP). These portals target unique information needs of clinicians and patients and their families, but they are interconnected. They serve to facilitate critical interactions between clinicians, patients, and their loved ones. The portals do not replace existing communication channels, but attempt to improve the quality of those interactions.

### 18.4.3   The Care Team Portal

The Care Team Portal (CTP) was designed to promote harm prevention and humanization of patients. Existing information systems display patient data as lines or numbers on spreadsheets or graphical displays and rely on clinicians to digest and integrate the data into actionable information themselves. In contrast, the CTP currently imports data from the EMR and patient/family tablet to display risks at the unit and patient-level in relation to the seven harms presented earlier.

Figure 18.1 depicts several key CTP displays. There are three main levels to displays of clinical information: the unit-view, patient-view, and condition specific displays. These are all designed to support real-time situational awareness of patients' risks for harm, and each is described in detail below. In addition, there are components of the displays designed to support patient and family engagement.

On first logging in to the system, clinicians view a unit-level overview of the status of each patient along with a simple indicator of risk. At the unit-level, if a patient is at risk for a specific harm, but does not have all evidence-based protocols in place, a red X is displayed next to that patient's picture along with a link to alerts associated with that patient (i.e., the number of preventative measures that should, but are not currently in place for that patient). If a patient is currently receiving all preventative measures for the relevant and targeted harms, a green check-mark is displayed. Clinicians can select a patient on the unit-level display by touching that patient's picture. This will provide a deeper dive on the patient view.

The patient view displays each of the seven harms as a segment of a wheel. If a patient is at risk for a specific harm, that segment of the wheel will be red. If all required therapies and interventions are in place for a given harm, that segment of the week will appear green icon. If the harm is not applicable to the patient (e.g., due to a contraindication), that segment of the wheel will be grey. Clinicians can then dive deeper by touching one of the wheel segments. This will bring them to the Condition-Specific Display (CSD).

CSDs provide fine-grained access to all details surrounding prevention strategies for a specific targeted harm. For example, a clinician may notice that the Ventilator

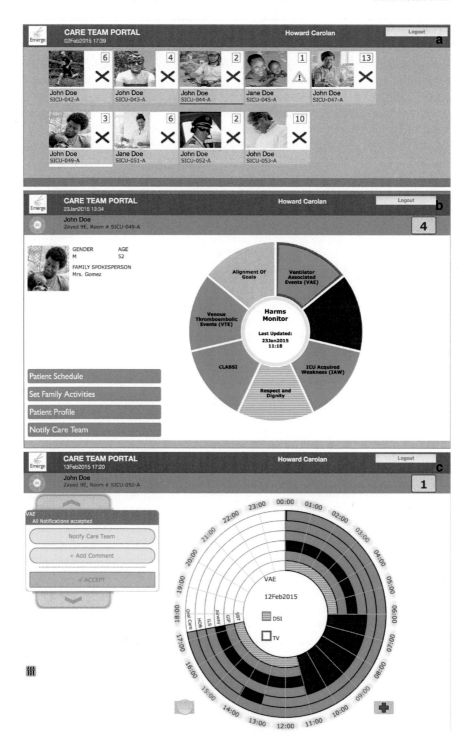

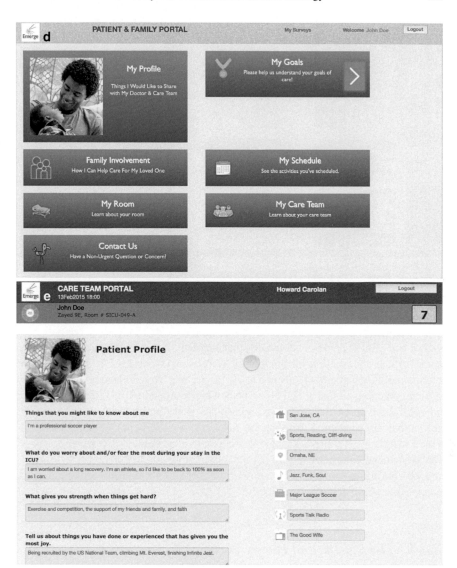

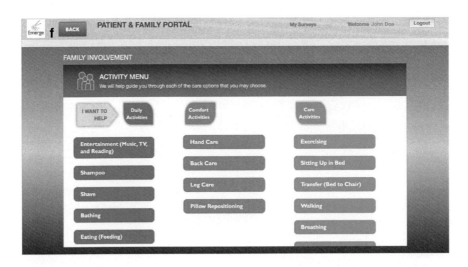

Associated Event (VAE) harm is out of parameter (i.e., a red wheel segment on the patient view). They can identify the underlying cause by clicking on the VAE wheel segment. Here, there is a visualization of each element of preventative strategies for VAE, and whether or not they are within parameter. For example, if the patient's head of bed (HOB) angle is below 30°, that segment of the VAE wheel will be red, as one critical intervention for preventing Ventilator Associated Pneumonia (VAP) is to maintain the patient's HOB bed at 30° or greater. To help ensure adherence to best care practices in this area, patient beds were equipped with HOB sensors. The Emerge system can access this data and use it to drive both visualizations and real time support for managing patient harm risks as described here and analytics. Prior to the Emerge system, there was no mechanism to alert clinicians whether this protocol was out of parameter (e.g., a team member adjusting the bed for a test/procedure and failing to return it to the proper height) and clinicians were required to calculate the angle of the bed manually.

### 18.4.4   The Patient and Family Portal

The Patient and Family Portal (PFP) focuses on enhancing patient and family member engagement in care. To do so, the PFP includes training and education materials, two way communication tools for expressing care priorities, tools for sharing information about themselves and asking questions as well as information about the care team and schedule of events. Several of these functions are detailed below.

The PFP supports several basic information functions designed to familiarize patients and families with the ICU environment. These include information about the patient room, frequently asked questions about ICU care, identification of types of care team members, and ICU visitor policies. Additionally, the PFP provides journaling and image upload features for the exclusive use of the patient and their family members as well as an "about me" section that the patients can use to describe themselves as a person to the care team. The PFP also integrates a Family Involvement Menu (FIM; [24]). This is a truly novel feature designed to support the role of patients and families as *members* of the care team and not just passive recipients of care [23]. Specifically, the FIM allows family members to learn about certain care activities in which they can participate. These activities range from basic (e.g., assisting with comfort related tasks such as pillow positioning, managing the entertainment system) to more advanced (e.g., oral care, wound care, physical therapy). After learning about these specific activities, the family member can use the PFP interface to indicate a desire to participate in this care activity. This information is displayed on the CTP to alert care team members that there is interest in participation. This integration facilitates better scheduling and coordination to include family members in patient care activities. The FIM is not designed to replace existing interactions encouraging involvement in care, but as mechanism to increase the likelihood family members will understand the opportunities available and express desire to participate.

Another important feature of the PFP is the ability for patients and their loved ones to ask questions directly to care team members and for the organization to solicit real time feedback regarding the quality of their care experience. The PFP includes tools for ensuring patient's goals of care are aligned with those of the care team to this end. The PFP allows patients and family members to indicate their care goals while in the ICU. These responses are then compared to those of the attending physician. On the CTP, the harms monitor and CSD for the alignment of care with patient goals indicates with a color code if the goals are adequately aligned. While many patient-family tools are commercially marketed, they are rarely integrated with health information systems. As a result, they are unlikely to drive improved communications or process of care.

### 18.4.5  Implementation Challenges

EMERGE has transitioned from a concept to being implemented in an ICU at Johns Hopkins Hospital as well as a second site at the University of California, San Francisco. While the speed of this process is encouraging, there have been challenges. Chief among these challenges are issues relating to the quality of information available in current electronic medical records and system stability. The first challenge concerned the timeliness of data. In the earliest phases of the project, security and concerns from network administrators over bandwidth usage precluded automated feeds from the hospital servers to the CTP. Initially, data from the EHR required manual entry, beginning at a rate of once a day and progressing to three times a day. Data at this frequency undermined the utility of using the CTP. The Emerge system now extracts data from the Johns Hopkins Hospital EHR every hour, but the ultimate goal is for data to be presented in real-time. Another factor involves the quality of the data itself. The quality of data presented on the CTP is dependent on the data that are available for it to access. For example, data may be missing from the EHR entirely. If a pain or RASS (i.e., delirium) goal is not entered into the EHR, assessments of pain and delirium throughout the day cannot be displayed on the CTP. Issues such as these limit the adoption of any real time situational awareness and decision support tool such as Project Emerge. People will not (and should not) make decisions based on old or inaccurate data. These data quality issues are rooted in current use of EHRs. However, by building visualization displays and more sophisticated analytics for EHR data, these gaps in data quality become more apparent. Short term solutions involve interventions to improve documentation. Longer term solutions involve developing automated data feeds to remove documentation burden from staff and improve overall data quality.

We are also only at the beginning stages of engaging patients and family members with the PFP tablets. Challenges in this area include the absence of family members visiting the ICU, mental status of patients that precludes their use of the tablet, and a rather lengthy, detailed research consent process for participation. A key strength of the PFP is its integration with the CTP, but this integration requires the CTP to be functioning optimally to support information that may be entered by patients in the PFP. Improvements in the consenting process, such as simplification of the script for participation as well as remote (e.g., telephone-based) consenting of family members should improve the level of participation and better engage patients and families as the project advances.

### 18.4.6    Future Goals

Project Emerge seeks to advance the state of Healthcare IT and address the critical goals of improving safety and quality, reducing waste, and supporting patient and family member activation in the care process. As described above, novel aspects of Project Emerge include the (1) application of a systems approach, (2) delineation and reduction of preventable harms that include not only avoidable clinical complications, but also loss of dignity and respect for patients-families by the care delivery system, and (3) creation and implementation of a model that reinforces learning and accountability at the individual, team, and unit levels. Project Emerge is a new system for preventing harm that has been created by a multidisciplinary team focused on improving the technology, workflow, and culture in the ICU. The initial versions of the CTP and PFP have been developed and implemented and iterative improvement is ongoing.

Future research will not only be dedicated to making system improvements, but also focused on outcomes analysis. Improvements in clinical processes and outcomes will be targeted and tracked for patients admitted to the units where the Emerge system is currently being implemented. Additional metrics, such as time saved by providers using the Emerge system to complete patient safety assessments, as well as improvements in providers' situational awareness and accuracy of information for decision making will be important to study and quantify.

The Project Emerge team has created a platform into which important clinical safety data can be imported from a hospital EHR and environmental sensors and ultimately used for improving care in real time and over time with better data quality and analytics. Yet an overwhelming amount of additional clinical and safety data lives in medical devices, the majority of which function as closed systems that do not allow for easy extraction of relevant medical information. A major effort to extract information from medical devices as well as to motivate vendors to open their systems to the Emerge platform will be key to achieving the full potential of an integrated ICU. Over time, the inclusion of a growing number of automated data streams will enable better real time management of patients as well as the care team itself [18].

## 18.5   Conclusion

The opportunities to improve healthcare safety, quality, patient activation, and overall value with better information technology are significant. These range from real time monitoring and decision support to guide care, to more sophisticated analytics to drive learning and accountability mechanisms in a safety management system, to tools to help manage population health. As the industry moves forward, it will be important to ensure that the data infrastructure evolves to meet the needs of different stakeholders, and ultimately to keep patients safe.

## References

1. Barry MJ, Edgman-Levitan S. Shared decision making—the pinnacle of patient-centered care. N Engl J Med. 2012;366(9):780–1.
2. Berwick DM. Measuring surgical outcomes for improvement: was Codman wrong? JAMA. 2015;313(5):469–70.
3. Berwick DM, Hackbarth AD. Eliminating waste in US health care. JAMA. 2012;307(14): 1513–6.
4. Bourrier M. The contribution of organizational design to safety. Eur Manag J. 2005; 23(1):98–104.
5. Chassin MR, Loeb JM. The ongoing quality improvement journey: next stop, high reliability. Health Aff. 2011;30(4):559–68.
6. Donabedian A. Evaluating the quality of medical care. Milbank Memorial Fund Q. 1966;44(3): 166–206.
7. Dimick JB, Ghaferi AA. Hospital readmission as a quality measure in surgery. JAMA, 2015;313(5):512–13.
8. Etzioni DA, Wasif N, Dueck AC, Cima RR, Hohmann SF, Naessens JM, Mathur AK, Habermann EB. Association of hospital participation in a surgical outcomes monitoring program with inpatient complications and mortality. JAMA. 2015;313(5):505–11.
9. Harrison MI, Koppel R, Bar-Lev S. Unintended consequences of information technologies in health care—an interactive sociotechnical analysis. J Am Med Inform Assoc. 2007;14(5): 542–9.

10. Kanzaria HK, Mattke S, Detz AA, Brook RH. Quality measures based on presenting signs and symptoms of patients. JAMA. 2015;313(5):520–2.
11. Kaushal R, Jha AK, Franz C, Glaser J, Shetty KD, Jaggi T, Middleton B, Kuperman GJ, Khorasani R, Tanasijevic M, Bates DW, Brigham and Women's Hospital CPOE Working Group. Return on investment for a computerized physician order entry system. J Am Med Inform Assoc. 2006;13(3):261–66.
12. LaPorte TR, Consolini PM. Working in practice but not in theory: theoretical challenges of " high-reliability organizations". J Public Admin Res Theory. 1991;1:19–48.
13. McGlynn EA, Asch SM, Adams J, Keesey J, Hicks J, DeCristofaro A, Kerr EA. The quality of health care delivered to adults in the United States. N Engl J Med., 2003;348(26):2635–45.
14. Pham JC, Aswani MS, Rosen M, Lee H, Huddle M, Weeks K, Pronovost PJ. Reducing medical errors and adverse events. Annu Rev Med. 2012;63:447–63.
15. Pronovost PJ, Berenholtz SM, Goeschel CA, Needham DM, Sexton JB, Thompson DA, Lubomski LH, Marsteller JA, Makary MA, Hunt E. Creating high reliability in health care organizations. Health Serv Res. 2006;41(4p2):1599–617.
16. Pronovost PJ, Bo-Linn GW. Preventing patient harms through systems of care. JAMA. 2012;308(8):769–70.
17. Pronovost PJ, Marsteller JA. Creating a fractal-based quality management infrastructure. J Health Organ Manag. 2014;28(4):576–86.
18. Rosen MA, Dietz AS, Yang T, Priebe CE, Pronovost PJ. An integrative framework for sensor-based measurement of teamwork in healthcare. J Am Med Inform Assoc. 2014. amiajnl-2013.
19. Tropello SP, Ravitz AD, Romig M, Pronovost PJ, Sapirstein A. Enhancing the quality of care in the intensive care unit: a systems engineering approach. Crit Care Clin. 2013;29(1): 113–24.
20. Williams C, Mostashari F, Mertz K, Hogin E, Atwal P. From the Office of the National Coordinator: the strategy for advancing the exchange of health information. Health Aff. 2012;31(3):527–36.
21. Weick KE, Sutcliffe KM. Managing the unexpected: resilient performance in an age of uncertainty, vol. 8. San Francisco: Wiley; 2011.
22. Wilson KA, Burke CS, Priest HA, Salas E. Promoting health care safety through training high reliability teams. Qual Saf Health Care. 2005;14(4):303–9.
23. Wyskiel RM, Chang BH, Alday AA, Thompson DA, Rosen MA, Dietz AS, Marsteller JA. Towards expanding the acute care team: learning how to involve families in care processes. 2015.
24. Wyskiel RM, Weeks K, Marsteller JA. Inviting families to participate in care: a family involvement menu. Jt Comm J Qual Patient Saf. 2015;41(1):43–6.

# Chapter 19
# Simulation: A View into the Future of Education

Parvati Dev

**Abstract** With the growth of the research enterprise, and its increasing emphasis on laboratory research and the molecular basis of medicine, the education process has changed from an apprentice-based approach to one with intensive classroom learning and an unfortunate reduction in hands-on practice. Further, any clinical experience has become highly supervised, with learners being allowed very little responsibility for patient care and, consequently, not having the opportunity to develop the experience and skill needed to practice autonomously. Medical, nursing, and other healthcare students graduate without the confidence or practical knowledge that would allow them to be independent practicing professionals. Simulated clinical experience has been proposed as a solution to the urgent need to provide early and frequent clinical experience to healthcare learners. While no simulation can entirely replace actual clinical practice, there is much that can be taught about procedures, process, critical thinking, and decision making in an environment that supports practice and reflection, without the pressure of clinical responsibility. In this chapter, we review this new direction in education, and present examples of the many ways in which simulation will enrich the learning process in healthcare.

**Keywords** Healthcare education • Nursing education • Medical education • Simulation • Simulated patient • Simulation • Online learning • E-learning

## 19.1 Introduction

### 19.1.1 Status

Modern healthcare education is based on the Flexner model of learning, the scientific basis of medicine, which postulated that learners should be taught the science behind the functioning of the human body, and that such learning should be

P. Dev, PhD
President, Innovation in Learning, Inc, Los Altos Hills, CA, USA
e-mail: Parvati@parvatidev.org

© Springer International Publishing Switzerland 2016
C.A. Weaver et al. (eds.), *Healthcare Information Management Systems: Cases, Strategies, and Solutions*, Health Informatics,
DOI 10.1007/978-3-319-20765-0_19

mastered through its application in clinical practice [11]. This was an advance on the earlier approach of medicine and nursing as a craft, without a scientific basis, and learnt through on-the-job apprenticeship. Typically, in medical school, the Flexner approach was implemented as 2 years of lecture and laboratory-based learning followed by 2 years of rotations through various clinical departments. Nursing, dental, and other healthcare disciplines followed a similar approach of didactic learning and bedside practice.

What was not anticipated was how significantly the nature of academic medicine would change. With the growth of the research enterprise, and its increasing emphasis on laboratory research and the molecular basis of medicine, "research has outstripped teaching in importance", with ever fewer teachers bringing a depth of clinical knowledge to the classroom [6]. At the same time, healthcare has become increasingly commercialized, with in-hospital teachers being forced to prioritize clinical productivity over clinical teaching. As a consequence, medical, nursing, and other healthcare students experience an ever-diminishing access to actual hands-on clinical practice, and they graduate without the confidence or practical knowledge that would allow them to be independent practicing professionals.

## 19.1.2 Problem

Today's students graduate without the necessary knowledge, practical skills, and professional values that they need to be contributing partners in the healthcare enterprise. As nursing and medicine evolved from being crafts to becoming professional practices with a scientific basis, the education process also changed from an apprentice-based approach to one with intensive classroom learning and an unfortunate reduction in hands-on practice. Further, this clinical experience became highly supervised, with learners being allowed very little responsibility for patient care and, consequently, not having the opportunity to develop the experience and skill needed to practice autonomously.

The current system, with time-stressed clinician-teachers, and significantly reduced hands-on clinical practice hours, is not expected to change in the near future. Medical graduates without any specialty experience are finding it increasingly difficult to find a position to practice as physicians. Nursing graduates who, upon graduation, used to move into hospital positions as licensed nursing professionals, find that current programs in nursing schools simply cannot provide them enough clinical exposure to qualify for hospital-based nursing positions.

Therefore, medical students must expect to spend 4–10 years beyond graduation from medical school before they are board certified to practice any medical specialty. Nursing students are usually required to undergo an additional residency year to learn the necessary clinical skills before they are considered for hospital positions.

Therefore, a significant and increasing problem is access to adequate, high quality clinical training, with the necessary clinical guidance and feedback essential to mastery learning.

### 19.1.3 Proposed Solution

Simulated clinical experience has been proposed as a solution to the urgent need to provide early and frequent clinical experience to healthcare learners [17]. While no simulation can entirely replace actual clinical practice, there is much that can be taught about procedures, process, critical thinking, and decision making in an environment that supports practice and reflection, without the pressure of clinical responsibility. Current issues of patient safety and quality of care can be addressed and practiced in a simulated environment till competence, and then mastery, are achieved.

In a recent seminal study, Hayden et al. [16] presented the premise that, "with high-fidelity simulation, educators can replicate many patient situations, and students can develop and practice their nursing skills (cognitive, motor, and critical thinking) in an environment that does not endanger patients". They showed that, in "students who had 50 % of their traditional clinical hours replaced by simulation", "at the end of the nursing program, there were no statistically significant differences in clinical competency as assessed by clinical preceptors and instructors". With this, and other, evidence to support its learning efficacy, simulation is likely to see explosive growth as a learning tool.

In this chapter, we will review the many types of simulators, some existing and upcoming methods of using simulation, the place of simulation-based learning in current theories of learning, and the need to provide realistic and usable clinical experience to healthcare learners at all levels of their profession.

## 19.2 What Is Simulation

When a teenager plays an auto racing video game on the computer, the appearance and the underlying physical behavior of the computerized car is a very satisfactory representation, or "simulation", of the appearance and behavior of a real car. Simulations have also been used extensively in fields other than healthcare. Pilot training through flight simulation is a well-known example. Nuclear reactor technicians practice crisis management in simulations because such practice is simply not possible in real life. Businesses train sales people in customer response using simulated encounters with virtual customers. Similarly, the opportunities for simulation-based training in healthcare are enormous.

Gaba [14] points out that "simulation is a technique—not a technology—to replace or amplify real experiences with guided experiences that evoke or replicate substantial aspects of the real world in a fully interactive manner." With this view-point, it is clear that numerous methods and technologies fall within the realm of simulation, though some may be in greater use than others. Further, the simulation may be solely of the patient or a part of the patient, or it may encompass the environment within which the patient is situated, along with equipment, people, policies, and other aspects of a healthcare event.

Clinical learning in healthcare is usually opportunistic, and dependent on the cases that arrive at the hospital or clinic. Simulation provides the opportunity for scheduled, constructed clinical learning sessions, targeted to the learner's need and readiness, and scaling with the learner's ability to absorb the knowledge. Simulation can provide learning opportunities that may never be available in real life, such as a mass casualty or a pandemic. It can also support learning ranging from routine processes to rare but critical situations to dangerous events that can be practiced safely in a simulation.

## 19.3 The Place of Simulation in Current Learning Theory

### 19.3.1 Current Theories of Learning

Current theories of learning emphasize a *constructive* approach, where the learner controls their learning process, and builds their knowledge through exploration and interaction with content and with other learners [4]. The *role of the teacher* is elevated from being a source of knowledge to being a *coach* who applies different pedagogic approaches, such as questions, hints, requests for clarification, and guidance, adapting the pedagogic approach to the learner's gaps in knowledge.

*Flow theory* maintains that optimal learning occurs when the learning activity is both demanding but achievable, leading to a state of satisfaction where the learner continues the tasks because of the pleasure derived from the process of learning [7].

To achieve expertise or mastery in a skill, extended practice is necessary. Ericsson et al. [10] show that a skilled practitioner, such as a world class violinist or football player, will have spent over 10,000 hours of practice to achieve their expert performance. Further, simple repetitive practice is not enough. This must be *deliberate practice*, or practice that is focused on improving specific areas of lack of performance, through learning tasks usually designed by a teacher [9].

Kolb's [18] influential work identified *experiential learning* as being the most effective driver of learning, and he described a cycle of learning where reflection and abstraction from concrete experiences lead to a new level of understanding, and an ability to experiment with the new knowledge and to identify the next areas of concrete learning.

## 19.3.2 Learning in Simulation

Working in a simulated environment allows learners to experience a realistic work situation, to explore information and action options, and to receive feedback from the environment and the virtual patient as they work. If the simulation includes other learners, together they can practice collaboration and team interaction, studying and improving their interpersonal interaction, their ability to lead or be a supporting member of a team, and to resolve problems such as conflicts or information transmission up a hierarchy.

Kolb's model of experiential learning closely fits the learning process ongoing in the simulation experience. Feedback or debrief provides the opportunity for reflection and abstraction that consolidates the learning, leading to a new level of understanding and the readiness to accept the next level of knowledge.

Simulation, by its nature, is best used with the teacher acting as a facilitator or guide. The learner constructs their own learning through a process of experimentation and feedback within the simulation.

A well-structured curriculum of simulation can implement Czikszentmihalyi's flow theory, balancing challenge and the learner's ability, to keep the learner engaged while they learn. In practice, simulation experiences are not made available in a structured and graded fashion, thus losing a significant opportunity for high quality learning. As more simulation content becomes available, it is possible that flow theory will become one of the guiding principles in simulation-based learning.

Because simulation is still not a large component of the curriculum, it also cannot satisfy Ericsson's definition of deliberate practice as a requirement for mastery learning. This failing also may be rectified in the future, as more curricular time and curriculum content becomes available for healthcare learners.

## 19.4  Simulators

### 19.4.1  Tissue Surrogates for Skills Training

Healthcare students have a long list of psychomotor skills that they are expected to acquire as undergraduates. For nursing students, these may include moving or lifting the patient, acquiring cultures using swabs, puncturing the skin for vessel access or injections, or inserting or removing a urinary catheter [1]. For medical students, routine technical procedures may include venipuncture, inserting an intravenous catheter, arterial puncture, thoracentesis, lumbar puncture, inserting a nasogastric tube, inserting a urinary catheter, and suturing lacerations [2].

Psychomotor skills have always been practiced on objects that are obtained easily, such as an orange, to simulate human skin for an injection, a chicken breast for

**Fig. 19.1** Multi-layered soft tissue pad for the practice of intradermal, subcutaneous, and intramuscular tissue injection techniques (Image from website of Limbs and Things)

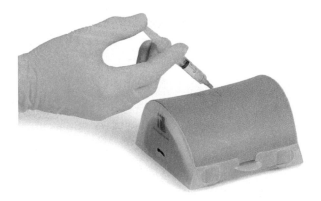

biopsy, or a pig's foot with skin, to practice layered suturing. Students also practice on each other, conducting a physical examination, or learning venipuncture. However, some skills, such as inserting a urinary catheter, or conducting a female pelvic examination, cannot easily be practiced on fellow students because of issues such as ethics or physical discomfort.

Synthetic models that simulate human tissue are available from many manufacturers. Plastic tissue models visually represent wounds or pressure ulcers, and are used to teach recognition of these problems. Other models may include internal anomalies, representing tumors, such as synthetic models of the breast that support palpation to learn breast examination. Still other models may include embedded tubes with fluids, to teach catheterization or central line insertion (see Fig. 19.1).

## 19.4.2 Digital/Physical Part-Task Trainers, Surgical Skill Trainers

Hybrid digital and physical simulators significantly increase the training capability of these simulators. Known as part-task, or surgical skill simulators, these simulators include realistic visualization and haptics (the sense of touch, feel and kinesthesis), as well as the ability to track performance automatically and provide feedback.

The female pelvic examination simulator embeds the uterus and surrounding related organs within a model of the female pelvis. After inserting the fingers into the vagina, the learner can palpate the uterus and the ovaries, using correct palpation technique. Pressure sensors embedded in the synthetic uterus measure the location and pressure of the palpation, and display details of the action on a computer screen. The enormous value of this visual feedback can be understood when one realizes that there is no comparable way to visualize one's actions when palpating within a real human. Studies by Pugh and Youngblood [21] demonstrated that students trained using the simulator showed more confidence and less errors, when conducting a real pelvic exam, than students trained only with text, graphics and a video

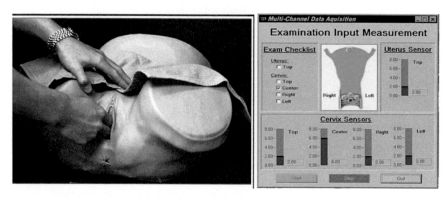

**Fig. 19.2** The pelvic exam trainer combines a physical pelvic model with digital pressure sensors to measure the positioning and applied pressure as the learner practices examining the female pelvis (Images courtesy Carla Pugh, MD, PhD)

(Fig. 19.2). Further, tissue anomalies, such as a cyst or tumor, may be placed within the synthetic uterine tissue, and the learner is then required to detect the presence and size of the pathology. Similar training simulators have been developed for the breast exam, the rectal exam, and the prostate exam.

### 19.4.3   Role Playing, Actors, Standardized Patients

Role play is widely used as a method for learning communication. A learner is asked to assume the role of a character, such as a patient, and to respond to questions from the other learners as though he or she were a real patient. The exercise provides a realistic representation of a patient encounter, particularly if the simulated patient has a script for expected responses. Nextel and Tierney [19] show that role playing is very effective in providing opportunities for rehearsal and for discussion about the encounter.

Alternatively the role of the patient is played by a "standardized patient", a paid actor, who is trained to follow a conversation script. This simulation can be carried further, into the space of physical examination, where the learner practices the skill of inspection, palpation, auscultation and percussion on the real human.

### 19.4.4   Digital Patients, Virtual Patients

Digital or virtual patients are an alternative to human standardized patients. There is a high cost of hiring and training actors, as well as significant turnover of actors. It is also difficult for different actors to present a consistent and uniform, standardized patient. Virtual standardized patients provide immense opportunity to create experiences that teach critical thinking, diagnostic reasoning and even communication [5, 23]. Figure 19.3 shows an example of a virtual patient in a simulated clinic.

Accurate and useful virtual patients require upfront effort to develop, but they are particularly easy to deploy, both on desktops and on mobile phones and tablets. Many virtual patient programs have been developed for general purpose simulation of any disorder. However, because of the potential for rich interaction, virtual patients are also being developed for a variety of niche learning applications. University of Southern California's SimCoach, for patients with post-traumatic stress disorder, emphasizes dialog with a sympathetic and non-judgmental coach. Shadow Health's nursing mentor also uses free text dialog to teach nurse-patient encounter communication. DecisionSim focuses on practicing decision making, with each virtual patient's state modeled as a detailed branching tree of decisions. Prognosis uses simple text interaction, on mobile phones, to teach clinical reasoning.

Virtual patient simulations will become widely available and easy to use. As they become embedded in curriculum and in textbooks or e-books, they will become the accepted approach to assess a learner's understanding of clinical concepts, as well as their ability to reason and act on clinical information.

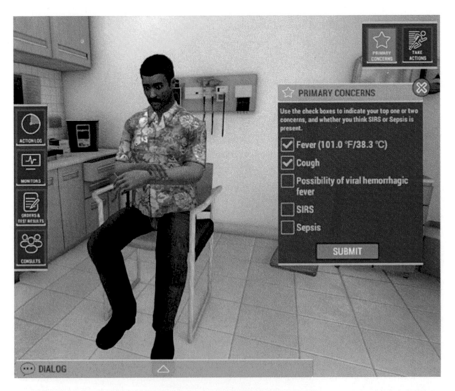

**Fig. 19.3** An example of a virtual patient in a simulated clinic. The learner can obtain information through a dialog interface or by using clinic equipment. They must demonstrate their critical thinking process by choosing their top concerns and their selected actions (Image courtesy of SimTabs, LLC, 2015)

### 19.4.5   Digitally Controlled Physical Manikins/Simulated Physical Environments

The first digitally controlled manikin-based patient simulator was introduced in 1967 [3]. It was a full size lifelike manikin, with a heartbeat and a pulse, and the ability to respond to selected intravenous drugs and anesthetic gases. A similar manikin, focused on teaching cardiovascular events, was developed a year later, and is still in use today in most academic centers [15]. Additional simulators were developed that improved on the simulated physiology and behavioral realism presented by the manikin [13], and today there are a large range of lifelike, computer-controlled, physical simulators for applications across much of healthcare, including obstetrics, trauma, and pediatrics. Figure 19.4 shows an adult manikin in a simulation center.

Computer-controlled manikins, with realistic physiologic responses, are usually used in clinical scenarios, usually preceded by a didactic briefing session, and followed by a debrief and reflection session. During the scenario, the learners are required to work as if in a real clinical environment, acquiring information from the patient and the monitoring devices, making decisions, consulting with teammates, and managing the consequences of their clinical decisions. The real learning occurs after the scenario, when all participants gather to debrief about the events and actions, with the guidance of a facilitator. This is Kolb's approach of experiential learning, with learning occurring through the process of reflection and discussion.

The wide availability of manikin-based simulators has led to the development of a considerable number of scenarios and curricula. Some sites integrate this content

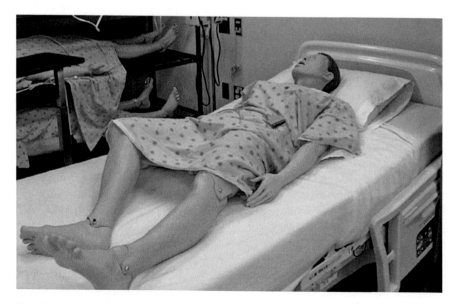

**Fig. 19.4** An adult manikin in a simulation center at Samuel Merritt University, Oakland, California (Image courtesy of P. Dev)

with the curricular learning objectives of entire programs, such as the curriculum for a Bachelor of Sciences in Nursing (BSN). However, in many other academic settings, not enough time or budget is allocated to manikin-based simulation, and learners do not get enough simulation experience to learn more than a selected few topics.

### 19.4.6  Virtual Worlds, Immersive Virtual Reality

Virtual world simulations, and immersive virtual reality, move beyond simulations using virtual patients in that they also simulate the working environment in which the patient is situated. Consequently, they provide increased realism, and they also create additional learning opportunities with regard to the team settings and the systems within which healthcare is practiced [12].

A typical virtual world represents a view, on the computer screen, of a clinical space such as an acute care ward, with a nurses' station, a waiting area, and private rooms for patients (Fig. 19.5). Students log into the virtual world on their personal laptops, choose their 'avatar' or character, such as a nurse, physician or administrator. Through the use of a headset and microphone, they are heard by others in the world, and participate in a conversation. The virtual patient in the room is computer-controlled or is controlled by one of the participants. Learners click on items in the environment to read vital signs, conduct a physical examination, review the electronic medical record, or give medications. The virtual patient's vital signs and other physiological parameters change dynamically based on the learners' actions. All actions are tracked and used for feedback [8].

The greatest advantage of virtual world systems is that, since they are not physical, there is very little cost, beyond the software license, to scale up to a large number of learners. They do not require additional building space and, since they are not physical electro-mechanical objects as manikins are, they do not require maintenance by skilled technical personnel. A second advantage is that, since software can be updated with relative ease, changes in healthcare procedures or policy are easily introduced into the software. A third, and fortuitous, advantage is that today's learners are digital natives who have grown up with the Internet and with online video games. To them online virtual worlds are a natural follow-on to their prior online experience, and acceptance of the technology is rarely a problem.

Because of the cost and lack of accessibility of physical simulators such as manikins, most academic programs cannot provide the breadth of experience to truly provide a significant amount of meaningful clinical experience. Virtual world simulations have the potential to fill this gap, and to provide simulation experiences that can range well beyond what is easily possible within the physical confines of a simulation space.

As compared to laptop screen-based virtual worlds, *immersive* virtual reality systems project the image of the world on goggles worn by the learner, such that, when the learner turns their head, they see other parts of the world. This differs from the screen-based view of the virtual world where, to look around, the learner must use the arrow key or a joystick to change the view on the screen. The sense of being able

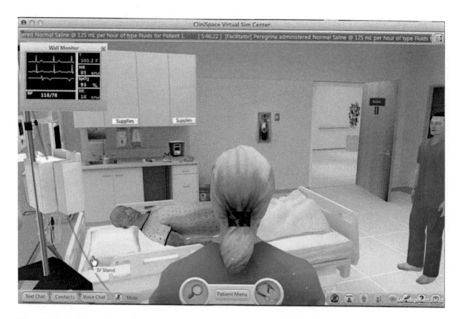

**Fig. 19.5** A three-dimensional clinical environment where learners can move between rooms to care for patients and collaborate with co-workers (Image of CliniSpace environment, courtesy of Innovation in Learning, Inc)

to turn one's head to look around corresponds so closely to natural action that these systems are legitimately described as immersive. Some immersive systems also include a view of the learner's hands in the virtual world, interacting with virtual objects. Immersive medical virtual reality systems are still in their infancy but we can expect to see a sharp increase in the next 2 years.

## 19.5   A Virtual Hospital?

It is possible to conceive of a virtual hospital, similar to an actual hospital, populated by staff, patients, and family, in which learners enter (log in) and leave according to their learning schedule. The learner can request a mix of cases suited to their learning objectives, or they work on their assigned cases. Tasks within the virtual hospital can range from shadowing to care giving to managing entire departments. Learning to communicate with patients and other caregivers becomes a natural outcome of working in the virtual hospital.

Besides the cases themselves, perhaps even more important is the opportunity to use patient cases to work with the range and complexity of the systems that support actual clinical care. These include information systems, such as the electronic medical record, the safety policies, from hand washing to catheter care, and interpersonal interaction, such as team work, mentoring and practicing empathetic encounters with family members.

Linking virtual and physical simulations brings the practice of psychomotor actions, such as a working with a manikin or a surgical simulator, into the larger context of the clinical scenario within a virtual hospital. While the surgeon learner works on the simulated patient with the surgical simulator, the nursing team sees and speaks with the surgeon and the virtual patient within the virtual operating room, and practices the actions and decisions around the surgical procedure. The concept has been extended in the Wide Area Virtual Environment [24] where room-size screens simulate the environment of war while soldiers and medics conduct a rescue mission with numerous manikins representing injured soldiers.

The use of the virtual hospital need not be restricted to a constructed set of systems and patient cases for use by learners. It can also be used to improve healthcare operations. Simulation of an actual department, with a mix of real or representative cases, can be used to identify problems with allocation of space or staff. Adding a financial overlay, allows simulation of business options. Researchers have created a virtual representation of the waiting area and triage rooms of the emergency department at Erie County Medical Center, and have simulated all expected triage actions, including the time needed to perform each action. With this simulation, they are studying the potential impact of different types of extreme events, such as a pandemic or a mass casualty.

Simulation of large-scale environments has long been recognized as material of science fiction. Niven and Barnes [20] developed the idea of virtual theme parks where players could safely experience the beauty and dangers of travel in remote lands. Stephenson [22] conceived of an entire world for recreational purposes. The technology for large-scale simulation is here today. Constructing such a world, and giving it a learning purpose, is within our means, and virtual hospitals in virtual neighborhoods may well be in the future of our educational approach.

## 19.6 Conclusion

Achieving competence in a healthcare profession requires knowledge of the scientific foundations of healthcare, as well as extensive and deliberate practice in the craft of healthcare. Simulation, in its many manifestations, will provide the opportunity for this practice, and we can expect its use to expand rapidly in the near future. As simulations become the standard-of-practice in education, we will even see them become required learning before the student is ready to work with the real patient.

## References

1. AACN. Essentials of baccalaureate education for professional nursing practice. Washington, DC: Association of American Colleges and Universities; 2008.
2. AAMC. Report I: learning objectives for medical student education-guidelines for medical schools. Washington, DC: Association of American Medical Colleges; 1998.

3. Abrahamson S, Denson JS. A computer-based patient simulator for training anesthesiologists. Educ Technol. 1969;9(10):55–9.
4. Bransford JD, Brown AL, Cocking RR, editors. How people learn: mind, brain, experience and school. Washington, DC: National Academy Press; 2000.
5. Cook DA, Triola MM. Virtual patients: a critical literature review and proposed next steps. Med Educ. 2009;43(4):303–11.
6. Cooke M, Irby DM, Sullivan W, Ludmerer KM. American medical education 100 years after the Flexner report. N Engl J Med. 2006;355:1339–44.
7. Csikszentmihalyi M. Flow: the psychology of optimal experience. New York: Harper Perennial Modern Classics; 2008.
8. Dev P, Heinrichs WL, Youngblood P. CliniSpace: a multiperson 3D online immersive training environment accessible through a browser. Stud Health Technol Inform. 2011;163:173–9.
9. Ericsson KA. Deliberate practice and the acquisition and maintenance of expert performance in medicine and related domains. Invited address. Acad Med. 2004;79(10):S70–81. October supplement.
10. Ericsson KA, Krampe R, Tesch-Römer C. The role of deliberate practice in the acquisition of expert performance. Psychol Rev. 1993;100:363–406.
11. Flexner A. Medical education in the United States and Canada. Bulletin No. 4. New York: Carnegie Foundation for the Advancement of Teaching; 1910. http://archive.carnegiefounda-tion.org/pdfs/elibrary/Carnegie_Flexner_Report.pdf. Accessed 22 Dec 2014. For a brief, lay summary, see: Flexner A. Medical education in America. The Atlantic. 1910. http://www.the-atlantic.com/magazine/archive/1910/06/medical-education-in-america/306088/. Accessed 22 Dec 2014.
12. Foronda C, Gattamorta K, Snowden K, Bauman EB. Use of virtual clinical simulation to improve communication skills of baccalaureate nursing students: a pilot study. Nurse Educ Today. 2014;34(6):e53–7.
13. Gaba D, DeAnda A. A comprehensive anesthesia simulation environment: re-creating the operating room for research and training. Anesthesiology. 1988;69:387–94.
14. Gaba DM. The future vision of simulation in health care. Qual Saf Health Care. 2004;13 Suppl 1:i2–10.
15. Gordon MS, Ewy GA, Felner JM, Forker AD, Gessner I, McGuire C, et al. Teaching bedside cardiologic examination skills using "Harvey", the cardiology patient simulator. Med Clin N Am. 1980;64(2):305–13.
16. Hayden JK, Smiley RA, Alexander M, Kardong-Edgren S, Jeffries PR. The NCSBN national simulation study: a longitudinal, randomized, controlled study replacing clinical hours with simulation in prelicensure nursing education. J Nurs Regul. 2014;5(2):S3–64. Supplement.
17. Institute of Medicine. The future of nursing: leading change, advancing health. Washington, DC: The National Academies Press; 2011.
18. Kolb DA. Experiential learning: experience as the source of learning and development. Englewood Cliffs: Prentice-Hall; 1984.
19. Nextel D, Tierney T. Role-play for medical students learning about communication: guidelines for maximising benefits. BMC Med Educ. 2007;7:3.
20. Niven L, Barnes S. Dream park. New York: Ace Books; 1981.
21. Pugh CM, Youngblood P. Development and validation of assessment measures for a newly developed physical examination simulator. J Am Med Inform Assoc. 2002;9:448–60.
22. Stephenson N. Snow crash. New York: Bantam Books; 1992. 480 pp.
23. Talbot T, Sagae K, John BS, Rizzo A. Sorting out the virtual patient: how to exploit artificial intelligence. Game technology and sound educational practices to create engaging role-playing simulations. Int J Gaming Comput Mediated Simul. 2012;4(3):1–19.
24. WAVE. Wide area virtual environment. 2014. http://simcen.usuhs.edu/facility/virtual/Pages/wave.aspx. Accessed 27 Dec 2014.

# Chapter 20
# The Health Record Banking Model for Health Information Infrastructure

William A. Yasnoff

**Abstract** The goal of health information infrastructure (HII) is to assure the availability of comprehensive electronic patient records when and where needed. An effective HII must overcome the challenges of privacy, stakeholder cooperation, incomplete information, and financial sustainability. The recent increased adoption of electronic health records by providers has created a real opportunity for HII implementation. Attempts to implement HII with systems that attempt real-time aggregation of institution-centric records stored in multiple locations for each person has been unsuccessful. The high implementation costs, incomplete data that inevitably results from lack of availability of all relevant information sources, and the difficulty of assuring ongoing stakeholder cooperation are key factors. A network of health record banks, community repositories of electronic health records with access controlled by patients, can address the key HII challenges. Privacy is protected by patient control, allowing each individual to establish and maintain their own privacy policy. Stakeholder cooperation can be accomplished by having individuals request their own data, invoking the legal requirement for providers to supply digital copies of their records on patient request. To achieve interoperability, ongoing financial incentives to providers can ensure that data supplied uses acceptable standardized formats. Financial sustainability can be achieved through new value created by the information itself when utilized for innovative applications for both patients and other health care stakeholders that are only possible when comprehensive records of individuals are available. Health record banking can therefore unlock the potential of HII to simultaneously lower costs and improve the quality of care.

**Keywords** Health information infrastructure • Health record bank • Electronic health records • Privacy • Interoperability • Financial sustainability

W.A. Yasnoff, MD, PhD, FACMI
Founder and Managing Partner, NHII Advisors, Arlington, VA, USA
e-mail: william.yasnoff@nhiiadvisors.com

© Springer International Publishing Switzerland 2016    331
C.A. Weaver et al. (eds.), *Healthcare Information Management Systems:
Cases, Strategies, and Solutions*, Health Informatics,
DOI 10.1007/978-3-319-20765-0_20

## 20.1   Introduction

Longitudinal patient data of individuals has great value for medical care and prevention as well as public health and research. Accessing such information is currently impossible, since the records for any given patient are fragmented over multiple locations, providers and formats (i.e., paper/electronic). The goal of universal access to comprehensive and lifetime patient data requires an electronic record and data model that (a) can aggregate all data for an individual in a usable, efficient and timely fashion, (b) maintains information assurance (confidentiality, integrity, availability), (c) aligns the interests of all stakeholders, and (d) is financially sustainable.

Design of an infrastructure to successfully support this vision requires consideration of the interdependent issues of information architectures, business models and standards that can overcome the flaws in current approaches. In addition to these considerations are the pragmatic issues of policy and governance (and modifications required to realize the vision) as well as the identification and monitoring of metrics to accurately assess progress in achieving a working health information infrastructure.

## 20.2   Need for Longitudinal, Patient-Centric Health Information Infrastructure (HII)

Healthcare data from individual patients is essential for medical care, the management and improvement of population health, and research. At present, longitudinal, lifetime health records of individuals are effectively unavailable. An additional challenge comes from the increasing use of personal monitoring devices, such as glucometers and pedometers that produce growing amounts of individual health data that have no natural "home" and are not easily combined with other health data to produce actionable information. The need to include genomic and other types of data (e.g. patient location data over time to assess environmental exposures) adds further complexity.

As a consequence, health care providers routinely utilize unpredictably incomplete patient information resulting in varying combinations of undertreatment, overtreatment, and inappropriate treatment producing both adverse outcomes and unnecessary costs [1]. A health information infrastructure (HII) that ensures the availability of comprehensive electronic patient information when and where needed could effectively address these issues.

Further exacerbating the problem of incomplete information is the complexity of current medical practice, which depends upon the "clinical decision-making capacity and reliability of autonomous practitioners for classes of problems that routinely exceed the bounds of unaided human cognition" [2]. Electronic health information systems could help address this problem with decision support to alert practitioners about recommended actions at the point of care. Many research studies have shown that such reminders improve safety and reduce costs [3, 4]. One study showed that medication errors could be reduced by 55 % [5]. A widely cited study by the Rand Corporation found that only 55 % of U.S. adults were receiving recommended care [6]. The same decision support methods used to reduce medical errors with electronic health information systems can also help ensure that needed care is provided. The importance of this grows as the population ages and the prevalence of chronic diseases increases.

HII has the potential to reduce the costs of healthcare. Inefficiencies as well as duplication in today's healthcare system are well documented and common. One estimate of anticipated nationwide savings from implementing advanced computerized physician order entry (CPOE) systems in the outpatient environment is $44 billion per year, [7] while another study [8] predicted $78 billion in additional savings from health information exchange (HIE) (for a total of $112 billion per year). Growing use of electronic prescribing has decreased the administrative costs of outpatient paper prescriptions and reduced transcription errors. More savings are possible in the inpatient setting – many hospitals have documented large net cost reductions from implementation of EHRs. A widely cited study anticipated that the patient safety and efficiency cost reductions from HII would be from $142 to 371 billion each year [9], and a literature survey found predominantly positive benefits from HII [10]. Of course, much of the predicted savings requires not only the widespread adoption of EHRs, but the effective electronic exchange of EHR data to ensure that comprehensive, lifetime medical records for every patient are readily available regardless of care setting.

### 20.2.1 Key Applications of HII

#### 20.2.1.1 Decision Support

Guidelines and reminders also can accelerate the dissemination and routine adoption of new research results. At present, it is estimated that widespread clinical use of new research findings takes an average of 17 years [11]. Decision support that generates reminders about new research results at the point of care could substantially accelerate this process.

#### 20.2.1.2 Research

An effective HII could also improve the efficiency of clinical trials. Today, most large clinical trials are supported by their own custom-built information infrastructure to ensure protocol compliance and collect research data. Comprehensive longitudinal records from an HII would allow clinical trials to be deployed via the dissemination of decision support guidelines that encoded the research protocol. Data collection could then occur automatically in the course of care, reducing time and costs. In addition, an HII would be able to support the analysis of de-identified aggregate patient care data to evaluate the outcomes of various treatments, as well as monitor the health of the population.

### 20.2.1.3 Public Health Surveillance

HII is also a valuable tool for early detection of disease patterns, especially outbreaks of newly virulent microorganisms or even bioterrorism. Our current system of disease surveillance, based on alert clinicians diagnosing and manually reporting unusual conditions, is both unreliable and slow. An example is the delayed detection of the anthrax attacks in the Fall of 2001, when seven cases of cutaneous anthrax in the New York City area that occurred 2 weeks before the "index" case in Florida were not reported to public health authorities [12]. Since all of these patients were seen by different providers, the overall pattern would not have been evident even if they had each been correctly diagnosed. Effective surveillance systems must have immediate electronic reporting to ensure early detection [13].

## 20.2.2   Increasing EHR Adoption Provides a Key Opportunity to Move Towards HII

The substantial increase in EHR adoption over the past few years creates a real opportunity for the information they contain to be used to compile more timely and complete longitudinal records for individuals as well as population health information. In 2013, over 50 % of health care providers were using EHRs, according to the Office of the National Coordinator for Health Information Technology (ONC) [14]. While this is very positive, much more progress is needed before we have a fully electronic health information system that can effectively monitor population health in real-time. EHRs alone are not sufficient for this purpose – mechanisms are needed to aggregate the information for each person into a longitudinal record and search those records across the entire population. So far, efforts to develop and deploy such "health information exchanges" (HIEs) have been problematic, with just a few partial successes [15].

It is clear that an HII providing anywhere, anytime comprehensive electronic patient records can simultaneously accomplish the goals of reduced costs, improved care, more effective population health, and more efficient research. Each individual's longitudinal record needs to be accessible for health care encounters, and must also be available for searching to perform population monitoring and customized preventive interventions.

## 20.3   Health Information Infrastructure Challenges

Establishing an effective HII has proven to be a challenging problem. At least four key obstacles have been identified: (1) *privacy* – the privacy of each individual's medical records must be protected; (2) *incomplete information* – all the records must be electronic in order to facilitate organizing and delivering comprehensive records for each patient; (3) *stakeholder cooperation* – physicians, hospitals, laboratories, pharmacies, imaging centers, etc., must all contribute their patient records; and (4) *financial sustainability* – operational funding must be available on an ongoing basis [16]. A recent study found that 75 % of HII projects in the U.S. have yet to achieve financial sustainability [17].

In considering HII, the critical questions are how such a system would operate and how it can be built. One promising vision that has been proposed is a network of health record banks (HRBs), community repositories of health records with access controlled by patients. Storing health records for each person in one place (but not everyone's health records in the same place) and letting patients control access provides a potentially effective approach for solving the complex, interrelated problems of privacy, stakeholder cooperation, incomplete information, and financial sustainability [16]. In this section, we will discuss the HRB approach in more detail in the context of the first two major HII challenges. The other two challenges will be addressed in the following section on Architecture.

### 20.3.1   Privacy

*Privacy* has been defined as the right of individuals to hold information about themselves in secret, free from the knowledge of others [18]. This definition implies that private information has not been disclosed to any third party. *Confidentiality* is the assurance that information about identifiable persons, the release of which would constitute an invasion of privacy for any individual, will not be disclosed without consent (except as allowed by law) [18]. The exception for release of confidential data without consent when allowed by law may at first seem objectionable. However, this exception may be more comfortably interpreted as "community" consent through elected representatives who have determined that this information must be available for the good of all. Confidential data should never be released without consent – but community consent implies that the consent has been codified legally through the legislative process.

It is clear from these definitions that concerns about the release of medical information typically relate to confidentiality rather than privacy, since "privacy" strictly refers to prevention of information release while confidentiality covers the appropriate use of sensitive information after it is released. However, we will adopt the common (although arguably somewhat inaccurate) use of the term privacy to refer to concerns about release of sensitive information.

From the perspective of consumer acceptance, privacy is the most important and overriding requirement of HII. While other aspects of information assurance, such as integrity and availability of information, are also essential to an effective HII, consumers generally focus their concerns on privacy. Clearly, health records comprise a very sensitive – perhaps the most sensitive – type of personal information. Disclosure of medical information can be frankly embarrassing and can even lead to employment (or other) discrimination. Perhaps more importantly, failing to assure the privacy of medical records will make patients much less willing to divulge critical personal details to their providers – and perhaps even avoid seeking medical care at all. Besides the actual contents of the records, the very existence of some records (e.g., a visit to a clinic for sexually transmitted diseases) is sensitive even if no other information is available. Clearly, any HII system must rigorously prevent unauthorized disclosure and use of medical records.

In the U.S., the HIPAA Privacy Rule [19] that governs the release of medical information generally requires patient consent for medical record disclosure and use. However, consent is waived for sharing of records for the purpose of treatment, payment, and healthcare operations. These "TPO" exceptions have, over time, allowed healthcare organizations to utilize medical records extensively without patient consent. An organization that collects and stores medical information has full discretion to decide whether a proposed disclosure is or is not eligible for one of the TPO exceptions. Until recently, there was no requirement for such TPO disclosures to be recorded, thereby effectively eliminating the possibility of audits to determine the existence of improper disclosures. While the 2009 HITECH legislation requires an audit trail of TPO disclosures, such disclosure records are not readily available to patients. As a result, individuals both lack control over the dissemination of their medical records, and are not informed when they are disclosed beyond the provider site (or other location) where they were created.

Overriding individual consent as allowed in the HIPAA privacy rule can be problematic. Most people understand that improving the availability of electronic patient records for appropriate and well-justified purposes simultaneously means they will be more accessible for undesirable uses. Additional efforts to prevent the latter with more stringent protections of the information are therefore needed to avoid (or at least minimize) abuses. Allowing anyone other than patients themselves to approve disclosure of personal medical records inherently erodes trust. By doing this, the message to patients is, in essence, "other people are going to determine who should be able to see your medical records because they understand what's in your interest better than you do." It is inherently difficult for patients to understand why, if a given disclosure is in their interest, their consent should not be obtained. Not seeking patient consent clearly leads to suspicion that the disclosure is in fact not in the interest of the patient, but rather benefits whoever is deciding that records will be shared.

These concerns about medical record privacy are not theoretical. Surveys have shown that 13–17 % of consumers already use "information hiding" behaviors to prevent access to their medical records [20, 21]. Examples of this include using an alias for laboratory testing or seeking treatment in another state. This substantial minority of consumers would certainly refuse to participate in an electronic medical information system unless it provided them with the opportunity to fully control access to their own records. Furthermore, these surveys likely underestimate the proportion of the population with concerns about these privacy issues because of the natural reluctance of respondents to admit to such behaviors. In addition to opting out of a system that did not provide individuals with control over their records, it is likely that these concerned consumers would organize and apply political pressure to prevent the development and operation of such a system. An example of this occurred in response to the original HIPAA legislation that called for a unique medical identifier for all U.S. residents. An extremely small percentage of concerned citizens, citing the threat to privacy, successfully lobbied Congress to defund these unique identifier provisions shortly after their enactment, effectively preventing any implementation activities.

In view of these considerations, a strong case can be made that decisions about access to patient records should be entrusted to the patients themselves (except in rare cases such as mental incompetence) [22]. It is also clear that these access control issues are especially important for enabling HII, because success depends on patients trusting that their records will only be used for their benefit. While there are legitimate concerns that some patients may not be sufficiently informed to make such decisions and could make access choices that may be harmful, delegating this decision-making to anyone other than the patient will likely have a much larger (and more certain) negative impact. As an analogy, we as a society agree that individuals should retain the right to decide how their financial resources are allocated, even though this clearly leads to negative consequences when consumers act unwisely. Indeed, prior to the 2002 HIPAA Privacy Rule establishing the TPO exceptions, patient consent had always been required for access to medical records.

In a system where patients control access to their own medical information, education and assistance related to decisions about sharing that information would clearly be needed. Managing access to personal information is a new concept for most people, so some confusion about this new responsibility is inevitable. Similar to current policies for patient consent to treatment, rules and guidelines need to be established for delegating information access decisions when patients are unwilling or unable to decide for themselves.

While the need for consumer education about decisions relating to release of medical records is clear, medical information privacy policy issues are both important and urgent in the context of the enhanced trust necessary to implement an effective and widely accepted HII. In particular, we will see in the following sections that a key advantage of an HII comprised of health record banks is that privacy is protected through individual control of access to each individual's own records. Each person is therefore able to establish and maintain his/her own custom-tailored privacy policy. As a practical political matter, such a system of individually determined (and easily modifiable) privacy policies is much more likely to engender widespread support than any specific, uniform policy that does not provide for individual choices.

## 20.3.2    Availability of Electronic Records

To ensure the availability of comprehensive patient information, every medical record from all healthcare providers must be electronic and available for immediate use. With respect to the latter issue, it would be ideal if stakeholder cooperation in supplying these records were voluntary. However, assuring long-term collaboration of competing healthcare stakeholders to make electronic records readily available is extremely difficult. In practice, only a very few communities have been successful in developing an organization with the active participation of the majority of health-care providers. Even in these rare communities, the arbitrary withdrawal of one or more participants is an ongoing risk, and would be disruptive to the system. The experience in most communities is that healthcare stakeholders, fearing loss of competitive advantage, are quite reluctant to share patient records. Because of this, legally mandated sharing of records is necessary.

Clearly, the electronic exchange of health information requires the information itself to be in electronic form. Although laboratory results and prescription medication information are nearly all electronic already, patient records, particularly in the outpatient domain, are not. While estimates vary, it is clear that a major fraction of office-based physicians have not yet adopted comprehensive EHR systems, even though there have been substantial government incentives to do so for the past several years. In addition, many physicians who do use electronic records have systems with limited capabilities [23].

### 20.3.2.1    Cost as an Obstacle to EHR Adoption

The biggest cost-related challenge for physician EHR adoption is that most of the benefits of outpatient EHRs accrue not to the physician, but to other stakeholders. One study reported that physicians derive only 11 % of the economic benefit, with the remaining benefits attributed to other stakeholders [24]. It is not surprising that physicians are reluctant to assume 100 % of the cost of systems for which they receive a small fraction of the benefits.

While the substantial EHR subsidies in the 2009 HITECH Act ($44,000–$63,750 over 5 years) have greatly increased EHR usage over the past several years, they only partially cover the costs of physician EHR systems. In particular, conversion costs related to reduced revenue from lost productivity during the transition from paper to electronic records are quite substantial. Furthermore, while the costs of EHRs continue indefinitely for physicians, the HITECH subsidies are temporary. In view of this, it is clear that providing ongoing reimbursement and/or other offsetting benefits for EHRs would better allow physicians to recoup their costs and promote higher levels of EHR adoption. This is important in building a sustainable HII since its effectiveness depends on all the records being electronic.

Hospitals, on the other hand, have a more substantial economic incentive for EHRs, since reducing costs will improve their financial performance under the diagnosis-related groups (DRG) reimbursement system that pays fixed amounts for specific conditions. In addition, it appears that the large HITECH incentives for hospitals have been sufficient to induce widespread EHR adoption. Even so, coordinating patient records during a hospital admission is largely an internal problem that does not benefit from an HII (although having an HII is very helpful prior to and at the time of admission, and can even help prevent unnecessary hospitalizations). But the vast majority of healthcare encounters do not involve hospitals, so HII efforts have the greatest potential for benefit in the outpatient environment.

While universal EHR adoption is necessary for an effective HII, it is not sufficient. In essence, each individual EHR system converts a "silo" of paper-based information into electronic form. EHRs are therefore capable of managing each individual provider's information about each patient, but, with rare exceptions, do not contain *all* the information for each patient. To ensure availability of comprehensive patient information, it is necessary to have a cost-effective and efficient mechanism that compiles and combines the records of each patient that are currently scattered among all their providers. It is these truly comprehensive records that can improve quality and reduce costs, e.g., through elimination of duplicate tests and procedures.

## 20.4   Health Information Infrastructure Architecture

### 20.4.1   Institution-Centric Architecture

Most existing HII systems utilize an institution-centric approach to data storage that leaves patient records stored wherever they are created (Fig. 20.1). To efficiently retrieve the records when needed, it is necessary to establish and maintain

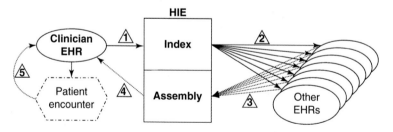

**Fig. 20.1** Institution-centric HII architecture. *1*. The clinician EHR requests prior patient records from the health information exchange (HIE); this clinician's EHR is added to the index for future queries for this patient (if not already present). *2*. Queries are sent to EHRs at all sites of prior care recorded in the HIE Index. *3*. EHRs at each prior site of care return records for that patient to the HIE; the HIE must wait for all responses. *4*. The returned records are assembled and sent to the clinician EHR; any inconsistencies or incompatibilities between records must be resolved in real time. *5*. After the care episode, the new information is stored in the clinician EHR only. (Used with permission of the Health Record Banking Alliance [25])

a central index of the locations of information for each patient. If such an index were not available, finding all the information for a given patient would be impractical, requiring queries to every possible source of medical information worldwide. When a patient's record is requested, the index determines which locations are queried to retrieve the needed information. The results of queries to those locations are then combined (in real time) to retrieve and compile the patient's complete record. After the patient encounter is complete, any new data that was generated is entered into the clinician's EHR system. The index is then updated with a pointer to that system (if not already present) so that it will be queried (in addition to all the other prior locations) when that patient's record is subsequently requested.

Healthcare stakeholders like this architecture because it allows them to "control" the records they generate. However, it does not allow efficient searching, is complex and expensive to operate, and does not scale. With this approach, searching the data, e.g., to find all patients with an elevated HbA1c (hemoglobin A1c, an important indicator of blood sugar control in diabetics), requires each patient's records to be assembled from their various locations and checked one at a time. In contrast to routine computer searching techniques that use a pre-computed index (much like using an index of a book to find the location of a word of interest), this is a slow sequential search.[1] This is a huge computing and communications burden that both increases the cost of EHR operation (since the EHR must be able to perform the additional processing associated with queries) as well as reducing security because of the risk of interception of information which is transmitted in full for each query. Standard database systems pre-index the contents of their records to greatly reduce search times. In this architecture, pre-indexing would effectively create a central repository of indices that could be used to reconstruct most of the original data, creating the same security vulnerabilities as a central database itself (which would defeat the purpose of this approach to avoid such a central repository).

To address this problem of slow sequential searching, it has been proposed that queries in an institution-centric architecture could be distributed to each provider system and the results aggregated. However, this approach cannot reliably produce correct output because individual patient records in each system are incomplete. As a result, queries that request multiple patient data items (e.g., patients with diabetes who have taken a certain medication in the past 6 months), will produce anomalous results unless all the relevant data for a given patient happen to be stored in a single provider system (i.e., if one system finds a patient with diabetes, but with no record of the medication of interest [which is in a different system], that patient will not be counted as satisfying the query). In addition, if multiple systems have all the data

---

[1] The completion time of such a sequential search increases linearly with the number of records being examined. For example, in a modest-sized community with 500,000 patients, with retrieval and processing time of each patient's records of just 2 s (a low estimate), such a search would take at least 12 days (1 million seconds). Even worse, every search requires that each connected EHR retrieve and transmit all its information.

needed about a specific patient for a given query, that person may be counted twice or more as meeting the specified conditions. Therefore, queries across multiple institution-centric data sources produce unpredictable numbers of undercounts, overcounts, or both.

Besides searching issues, response times for assembling a patient record can also be problematic. To assemble a given patient record, the locations where the patient has available records are determined by the central index. Then, each location where patient records are available is queried to obtain the patient's information. After all the systems have responded, the results are then integrated into a comprehensive record to be sent to the requestor. While the queries can all be done in parallel, the final integration cannot be completed until the last response has been received. As the number of queried systems increases, so does the likelihood of a slow (or missing) response from one of them. Also, more queried systems require more processing time to integrate all the information into a single record. As a result, the response time grows as the number of queried systems increases.

The institution-centric architecture is also operationally complex. To ensure complete patient records, all the systems that contain information about each patient must be available. Assuring this requires a $24 \times 7$ network operations center (NOC) that constantly monitors the operational status of every medical information system. This NOC must be staffed with senior IT personnel to rapidly troubleshoot and correct any problems that are detected. Even with highly reliable systems (e.g., with failure rates of one per thousand), an institution-centric system with thousands of EHR information sources will frequently have systems that are unresponsive to patient record queries that need immediate expert repair. The cost for such a NOC is very substantial, since least five full-time staff would be needed to assure round-the-clock coverage 7 days a week.

Adding to the cost of the NOC, each EHR in an institution-centric system must have the built-in capacity to respond to $24 \times 7$ queries in real-time. This means that every EHR would require additional hardware, software, and communications capacity so that it can both serve its local users efficiently and simultaneously respond to outside queries for records. The volume of such outside queries would be substantial, since each patient's records will at a minimum be queried whenever they receive care at any location. This is in contrast to a central repository model (such as health record banking, discussed below), where information from each care episode is transmitted once to the repository and no further queries to the source system are ever needed. A recent simulation study demonstrated clearly that both the transaction volume and probability of incomplete records (because information was not retrieved from a malfunctioning network node) increase dramatically with the average number of sites where each patient's data is stored in an institution-centric architecture [26].

## 20.4.2  Person-Centric Architecture (Health Record Banking)

Health record banks represent a person-centric approach to community HII that can overcome the challenges faced by current efforts while meeting all the necessary functional requirements [27]. A health record bank (HRB) is defined as "an independent organization that provides a secure electronic repository for storing and maintaining an individual's lifetime health and medical records from multiple sources and assuring that the individual always has complete control over who accesses their information" [28].

### 20.4.2.1  Overview

The operation of an HRB is much simpler than an institution-centric architecture (Fig. 20.2). Upon enrollment or prior to a care episode (except an emergency), the patient's consent for the provider to access his/her HRB records (either all or part) is captured and stored. The caregiver then accesses (and/or downloads) the records through a secure Internet site. When the encounter is complete, the provider uploads the newly generated information to the HRB, which is added to the account-holder's lifetime health record. The updated record is then immediately available for further use.

Storing health records for each person in one place (but not everyone's health records in the same place) and letting patients control access allows the complex, interrelated problems of privacy, stakeholder cooperation, incomplete information, and financial sustainability to all be successfully addressed. In contrast to the

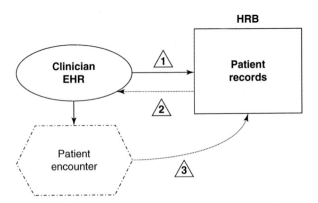

**Fig. 20.2** Person-centric HII architecture. *1*. The clinician EHR requests prior patient records from the HRB. *2*. The prior patient records are immediately sent to the clinician EHR. *3*. After the care episode, the new information is stored in the clinician EHR and sent to the HRB; any inconsistencies or incompatibilities with prior records in the HRB need to be resolved before that patient's records are requested again (but not in real time). (Used with permission of the Health Record Banking Alliance [25])

frequently used institution-centric architecture for managing electronic health records, where each patient's records are stored where they are created and only assembled when needed (in real time), the centralized HRB approach has been demonstrated in simulations to be considerably more efficient and less subject to retrieval errors [26]. It can also support efficient searching of health records for research and policy purposes, with patient consent.

### 20.4.2.2  History

The person-centric health record banking architecture was first described by Szolovits [29]. Several years later, it was called a "health information bank" in the U.K. [30], and was subsequently termed the "bank of health" [31]. The legal aspects of a "health record trust" were described in 2002 [32], and the "health record bank" architecture was highlighted by Dyson in 2005 [33]. In 2006, a policy paper from the Heritage Foundation recommended health record banking [34], other authors provided details of their HRB vision [35, 36], and the non-profit Health Record Banking Alliance (HRBA) was organized [37]. That same year, Washington State recommended HRB implementation after a 16-month health information infrastructure study [38] and the non-profit Dossia consortium of several large employers was started to develop an HRB for their employees [39]. The following year, the Information Technology and Innovation Foundation endorsed the health record banking approach for the U.S. HII [40], and Gold and Ball termed the architecture an "imperative" [41]. Also in 2007, both Google and Microsoft introduced their own patient-controlled medical record repository products designed for general consumer use. In 2009, an HRB pilot was started in Rotterdam, Netherlands,[2] three more pilot HRBs received initial grants from the State of Washington, and the privacy protection benefits of HRBs were described [42]. The HRBA has released white papers describing HRB architecture [25], business models [43], and policy recommendations showing how HRBs can promote and achieve interoperability [44]. Another recent article describes the practical implementation experiences of a community-wide HRB startup in 2010 [45]. The person-centric, patient-controlled architecture of HRBs continues to be regularly referenced in articles discussing the need for comprehensive EHRs [46–50, 15, 51].

### 20.4.2.3  Security

One security concern about the health record banking approach to HII relates to the misguided belief that information security is weaker in a central database than if the information is physically dispersed. However, it is well known that a properly protected repository is really more secure than the equivalent distributed system [52]. First, the protocol for immediately locating and retrieving each patient's records in

---

[2] http://webwereld.nl/nieuws/54340/rotterdam-start-eigen-versie-elektronisch-patiDOUBLEHY-PHENntendossier.html. Posted January 14, 2009 (Accessed 26 December 2014).

a distributed system is just as vulnerable as retrieval from a central data repository. Second, when data is aggregated from distributed locations, the risk of interception doubles since data are transmitted twice for each use: once between the storage site and the aggregation point, then again from the aggregation point to the end user. Third, data in a central system are more easily protected because it is "much easier to enforce strict security access controls when there are fewer doors or when the entry points are centralized" [53]. Fourth, double encryption of the data can prevent unauthorized "total access" to the entire database, with one key held by the patient and the other by the HRB. Finally, the use of multiple community-based HRBs limits the quantity of data in any single system, establishing an upper limit on the potential consequences of a breach. Overall, HRB security is objectively superior to an equivalent distributed system.

### 20.4.2.4 Financial Sustainability

Long-term financial sustainability for HII can be achieved with three general mechanisms either individually or in combination: (1) taxation; (2) redirecting healthcare cost savings; or (3) leveraging new value created by the HII. Advocates of public funding through taxation assert, with some justification, that an effective HII is a public good with universal benefit, analogous to other important infrastructure such as roads. However, new taxes are generally unpopular and therefore politically challenging to enact. Also, there are examples of other critical infrastructure, such as public utilities and the Internet that, although regulated, are supported with user fees rather than taxation. Nevertheless, there are at least two states, Maryland and Vermont, that are using public funds to at least partially support their HII systems.

Redirecting health care savings to pay for HII is the most common sustainability approach. The justification for this is sound, relying on the large evidence base indicating that higher quality and lower cost care can be achieved with the availability of more comprehensive electronic patient records [10, 54]. Examples include several large, generally closed healthcare systems such as Group Health, the Veterans Administration, and Kaiser Permanente, where the widespread adoption and use of electronic medical records has resulted in better care at lower cost. While the evidence that HII can reduce healthcare costs is persuasive, the timing and distribution of the savings cannot reliably be predicted. Also, one healthcare stakeholder's cost savings is another's revenue loss. The organization losing income will of course find this result very undesirable, and as a result will strongly oppose any initiatives that even *appear* to have the possibility of this outcome. In addition, the distribution of savings is not known in advance, making all organizations unable to make specific financial commitments with the confidence that a positive return on their investment will be forthcoming.

The third approach to financial sustainability of HII, utilizing the new value created by the availability of comprehensive electronic information, has generally not been explored. Although there is widespread agreement that HII information will have substantial value for many important and worthy purposes, minimal attention has been devoted to specific methods for capturing this value to create a viable business model. One example of such new value that has been recognized in a few communities is reducing the cost of delivering laboratory results to ordering physicians. A unitary community infrastructure providing electronic lab result delivery to physicians is much more efficient than current duplicative systems. Another example of potential value is the use of medical information for research – both for research queries and to find eligible subjects for clinical trials. Even though the use of the medical information for research can produce revenues that cover a substantial part of the costs of HII, the required supporting mechanisms for both searching data and recording and maintaining patient consent have not typically been implemented in today's HII systems.

Innovative applications that deliver compelling value to consumers and other healthcare stakeholders based on the underlying information are potentially one of the largest and most promising sources of HII revenue [45]. These include timely and accurate reminders and alerts to patients (and their families) for preventive services, medication refills, and other medically related events of immediate interest. Another example is applications that assist consumers to more easily manage their chronic diseases. Such an "application ecosystem" was described as a key element of the business model to support Microsoft's HealthVault™ personal health record system [55]. Utilizing the new value of medical information to sustain HII avoids the allocation, timing, and prediction issues inherent in leveraging anticipated healthcare cost savings, with the added benefit that with this model any such savings accrue to the stakeholder that achieves them.

Finally, the person-centric health record bank approach facilities revenue generation from advertising to consumers (who are more likely to engage with their comprehensive records), including sponsorship of specific patient groups by interested healthcare stakeholders.

### 20.4.2.5 Interoperability

Interoperability requires the use of standards so that information transferred from one medical information system to another can be understood and interpreted correctly, retaining the same meaning. Ultimately, standards compliance must be mandatory to ensure universal adoption. Such mandates can take the form of regulations, payment incentives, or both. To be effective, compliance must also be monitored continuously.

The HRB approach can incentivize the use of standards to ensure interoperability. If, as has been proposed [45], cloud-based EHRs are provided at no charge to outpatient physicians by an HRB, the HRB will only select those systems that can transmit information back to the HRB in a standard format. For physicians who currently have EHRs, an HRB may provide payments for data deposits from those systems that would be conditioned on the consistent use standards-based transactions. Over time, additional encoding and structuring of medical information can be required with gradually more stringent data deposit requirements (with sufficient lead time to allow systems to be upgraded). Overall, compliance with standards can be consistently assured through the direct relationship to ongoing payments.


#### 20.4.2.6    Challenges

Although the HRB approach can successfully address the key obstacles to a successful HII, as of this writing there are no large-scale operational examples in communities. The most obvious reason has been lack of funding. ONC did not allow any of the $564 million allocated to the states for HIEs over the past several years to be used to build HRBs, even for those few states bold enough to propose this. To some extent, this is because the healthcare stakeholders (and the general public) have been very wary of centralized repositories because of the perceived vulnerability to loss of all the data in a single security breach. As discussed in the Security section above, despite the fact that state-of-the-art computer security requires sensitive information to be segregated in one place so that it can be effectively protected, the fear of the "database in the sky" has permeated HII discussions. A requirement to avoid centralization has been a consistent "precondition" to nearly all such efforts. For HRBs to gain traction, it may be necessary to find an alternative architecture that can store each person's records in one place (with patient control of access) while still allowing efficient searching across records without the need for a central repository or index.

In addition, while HRBs do have a feasible business model, a large critical mass of subscribers are needed to generate sufficient revenue to offset the substantial fixed costs, particularly for the first implementation. The cost of achieving the necessary scale (perhaps $10 million) represents a one-time obstacle that must be overcome to provide an initial successful HRB demonstration project. While these funds could logically be provided by one or more of the many current initiatives promoting innovation in health care, such an investment has yet to occur.

Finally, healthcare stakeholders have been reluctant to cooperate in the creation of HRBs in their communities, fearing loss of competitive advantage when comprehensive information for each patient is readily available. However, the increasing focus on population health, incentivized by the Affordable Care Act, makes HRBs an important potential asset. Population health activities require comprehensive information on each patient, which is not otherwise accessible to Accountable Care Organizations (ACOs) created to promote health and reduce the need for medical care with effective prevention. Hopefully, the recognition that HRBs can solve this problem will accelerate their adoption.


## 20.5    Policy Issues in Health Information Infrastructure

The trust problems inherent in the current HIPAA policy framework, as modified by HITECH, were described above in the Privacy section. An alternative, and arguably more effective, policy approach would be to require patient consent for any and all use of personal health information. This would reinstate the policy in place prior to the 2002 HIPAA Privacy Rule that created the "treatment, payment, and operations" exceptions to patient consent for medical record disclosure. Such a policy change would be an important first step toward transferring ownership of the medical records to the patient. Today, providers own patients' medical records, with patients entitled to a copy on request. Reversing this would be very helpful in ensuring privacy since the provider's copy of the records would then be available only for the provider's own use. Provider disclosure of records to other parties without patient consent would be prohibited.

However, to avoid disruption of current systems of care, such a major policy change in handling medical information would need to be implemented gradually. One potential first step of such a process could be a large-scale demonstration showing that patient ownership and control of records is practical, can be readily implemented with today's HIT technology, and can facilitate both better health care for both individuals and the population. After a successful initial project, a plan for gradual transition could be developed and executed in an orderly fashion over several years, allowing sufficient time to implement needed changes in provider health record systems.

## 20.5.1   Necessary Exceptions to Patient Control of Access to Their Information

Despite patients' ownership and control of their medical information, there are justifiable cases for overriding individual consent for the good of the community. For example, reporting communicable diseases to public health authorities has historically been done without individual consent since it is necessary to protect the general population. Availability of controlled substance prescription information to providers is another case where consent must be balanced with community needs. It would not make sense to enable fraudulent multiple prescriptions for narcotic painkillers by letting individuals deny consent for providers to access their medication information. However, limitations on individual consent for access to information should be as minimal as necessary to address the specific problems identified. In the case of patients denying providers access to their controlled substance prescription records, for example, any provider treating the patient and accessing their medical records might receive a message indicating that some medication information has been withheld (without actual information being displayed). Providers would thus be alerted to a potential problem, while patients would still have some ability to protect their information. With medical information access controlled by patients, it seems likely that a limited number of additional public policies, such as access control policies for minors, will be needed to ensure that, when it is appropriate, essential community interests supersede individual rights.

Another commonly cited need for an exception to patient control of access to medical information is "break the glass" functionality in an emergency. This would allow emergency providers to access patient records regardless of consent. However, this can easily be addressed by asking patients to agree to such emergency access in advance. If patients indicate that they do not want emergency providers to have access to their records, they would be clearly informed of the potentially lethal consequences of such a decision. Should a patient insist despite this warning, it is difficult to argue that their request should be overridden. Of course, to make such a system of emergency access effective, all providers would need to be aware that abusing the system (i.e., by fraudulently accessing patient records claiming a nonexistent emergency) would immediately and consistently result in serious sanctions.

## 20.5.2   Current U.S. Government Programs

Under the HITECH Act, the Meaningful Use regulations provide substantial financial subsidies for physicians and hospitals adopting and using EHR systems. This has resulted in a substantial increase in EHR usage. For the Stage 1 Meaningful Use criteria, it has been reported that over 50 % of physician offices [56] and 42 % of hospitals [57] are using qualifying EHR systems. However, even if all eligible physicians and hospitals met all Stages of the Meaningful Use criteria, the availability of comprehensive electronic patient records when and where needed would not be assured. To accomplish this, an effective HII that can aggregate each person's individual records from all sources is also necessary. As recognized in the HITECH legislation, which provided $564 million of HII funding to the states distinct from the Meaningful Use incentives, this aggregation requires additional infrastructure and cannot be accomplished solely by individual providers.

The view, download, and transmit (VDT) requirement included in Meaningful Use Stage 2 (effective October, 2013, for hospitals and January, 2014, for office-based providers) has the potential to be very helpful in facilitating HII. VDT mandates that all providers must give patients the capability to access and electronically transmit their records to any destination they choose using standard coding and formats. To fully qualify, providers must also demonstrate that at least 5 % of their patients are taking advantage of this service. VDT compliance is also required for EHR technology certification, so EHR vendors are adding this capability to their systems. The resultant widespread implementation of VDT will allow patients to routinely direct that their electronic medical records be transmitted to a destination of their choice. This will enable patient-selected third parties (such as health record banks) to compile comprehensive person-centric records over time and make them available to subsequent providers at the direction of each patient.

A related messaging standard, the ONC Direct protocol,[3] is designed to enable transmission of medical record information from one point to another using standards. Although Direct was initially designed to be a "provider to provider"

---

[3] http://wiki.directproject.org/file/view/DirectProjectOverview.pdf (Accessed 26 December 2014).

communication capability, it can also effectively transmit patient information as required by VDT. This could, for example, involve sending patient data to a health record bank where it can be integrated with prior information for that patient and stored as a longitudinal record. Therefore, the Direct protocol also has the potential to be very helpful in facilitating HII development.

### 20.5.3   Opportunities for Innovation and Discovery

The availability of population data from an HII can enable greater health policy flexibility and experimentation. Today, it typically takes years before information is available to assess the impact of a health policy intervention. Naturally, this makes policymakers very reluctant to make changes without compelling justification of the anticipated positive benefits. But if near real-time population data were available for analysis, policy changes would be much less risky because unanticipated negative consequences could be ascertained rapidly. If needed, a new policy that was not working as expected could be reversed before its negative impact was widespread.

Timely availability and appropriate use of population health data can also inform other policy domains at federal, state, and local levels that impact health, such as education, housing, the environment, and criminal justice. An effective HII can provide aggregated personal health data to guide government policy decisions, greatly improving our ability to understand and address critical citizen needs and promote a healthier society.

In addition, population health data would facilitate our discovery and understanding of unanticipated relationships between activities and events, e.g., emergency room visits and air quality. Today, investigating such correlations often requires expensive and time-consuming clinical trials. Readily available data allows these correlations to be found more quickly and easily, and also can facilitate the analysis of complex interactions.

### 20.5.4   The Information Economy

There is growing value in aggregating many types of personal information, not merely health records. Our progress in extracting this value will be accelerated by replacing our current "whoever has it can use it" approach to the management of highly valuable personal information with a policy of personal ownership and control by declaring each individual's personal information as their property, only to be used by others with permission. Not only is this approach inherently fair and protective of privacy, but persuasive arguments have been made that "permission-based" use of personal information would create huge new markets and economic activity [58]. A recent example of this is the $60 million Genentech agreement with 23andMe for access to the health and genetic information of thousands of patients (with their permission) [59]. Regardless of how policy evolves, it is clear that individual health records have tremendous value for both individuals and the whole community. The policy challenge is to move rapidly to extract those benefits for the good of all, while simultaneously minimizing potential harm.

## 20.6 Measuring Progress

Metrics that can quantify our progress toward an effective HII have largely been neglected. Several desirable features of such HII progress measures have been described [60]. First, they should be sensitive enough to reflect changes over reasonable time periods, for example, 1 year. A progress measure that remains unchanged over many years despite real advances toward the goals would not be helpful. Second, the measures should be comprehensive so that they incorporate the activities and outcomes that are important to the key stakeholders. A measurement system that ignores a key element that must be present in an effective HII would be suboptimal. Third, the measures should be meaningful to policymakers. If the metrics are overly technical or otherwise difficult to understand, they will not be useful in guiding priorities and resource allocation. Fourth, the measures should be easy to determine (or estimate) so that the evaluation process does not divert substantial resources from the actual work. Finally, when the target values for all the measures are attained, the original goals of a complete and fully functional HII should have been reached.

Based on these criteria, currently used metrics are largely ineffective. For example, measuring whether or not health information is being exchanged at all or how many "exchange messages" occur has little value. The number of messages that need to be exchanged in order to assure the availability of comprehensive information for each patient is unknown (and unpredictable). Therefore, monitoring the message count over time does not indicate whether or not the goal of comprehensive information for all patients is close to being met. Although an increasing number of "exchange messages" would show progress, it does not allow assessment of how much more needs to be accomplished.

Using the above measurement criteria as a guide, Labkoff and Yasnoff identified and validated a combination of four measures for the quantitative evaluation of HII progress in communities: (1) completeness of information, (2) degree of usage, (3) types of usage, and (4) financial sustainability [61]. Using this assessment method, four of the most advanced community HII projects in the U.S. at that time earned scores of 60–78 (on a 0–100 scale), indicating that substantial additional work was required before their community HIIs could be viewed as complete.

However, one critical dimension of progress not covered in the Labkoff and Yasnoff evaluation framework is the extent of semantic encoding of electronic health records. Clearly, the electronic exchange of images or pdfs of clinical documents, where the content is not readily machine-interpretable and can only be read by an end user, will not enable the record integration, analysis, and decision support that an HII must ultimately provide. The end goal is fully standardized and encoded electronic health records so that all the information is computable. A progress measure that would capture the degree to which this standardized encoding has been accomplished would be an important and valuable addition to the evaluation process.

## 20.7   Conclusion

Health information of individuals is critical to medical care, research, and population health. Clearly, the timely availability of this information can contribute significantly to the overall health of our society. However, in order to successfully implement an effective health information infrastructure (HII), the complex and interrelated problems of privacy, stakeholder cooperation, incomplete information, and financial sustainability must all be addressed. One proposed approach to HII that can overcome these problems and appears to provide a feasible path toward an effective HII is health record banking. This or a similarly effective alternative approach is likely to be the basis of HII implementation over the next few years. Regardless of how it is architected, an HII comprised of both EHRs and mechanisms to aggregate records from them for each person will be a key ongoing data source for monitoring and improving both individual health and the health of our communities in the years ahead.

## References

1. Institute of Medicine. Committee on quality of health care in America. To err is human: building a safer health care system. Washington, DC: National Academy Press; 1999.
2. Masys DR. Effects of current and future information technologies on the health care workforce. Health Aff. 2002;21(5):33–41.
3. Bates DW. Using information technology to reduce rates of medication errors in hospitals. BMJ. 2000;320:788–91.
4. Kass, B. Reducing and preventing adverse drug events to decrease hospital costs. Research in action, Issue 1. 2001. AHRQ Publication Number 01-0020. Available at http://archive.ahrq. gov/research/findings/factsheets/errors-safety/aderia/ade.html. Accessed 26 Dec 2014.
5. Bates DW, Leape LL, Cullen DJ, et al. Effect of computerized physician order entry and a team intervention on prevention of serious medication errors. JAMA. 1998;280(15):1311–6.
6. McGlynn EA, Asch SM, Adams J, et al. The quality of health care delivered to adults in the United States. NEJM. 2003;348:2635–45.
7. Johnston D, Pan E, Walker J, Bates DW, Middleton B. The value of computerized provider order entry in ambulatory settings. Boston: Center for Information Technology Leadership, Partners Healthcare; 2003.
8. Walker J, Pan E, Johnston D, Adler-Milstein J, Bates DW, Middleton B. The value of healthcare information exchange and interoperability. Boston: Center for Information Technology Leadership, Partners Healthcare; 2004.
9. Hillestad R, Bigelow J, Bower A, Girosi F, Meili R, Scoville R, Taylor R. Can electronic medical record systems transform health care? Potential health benefits, savings, and costs. Health Aff. 2005;24:1103–17.

10. Buntin MB, Burke MF, Hoaglin MC, Blumenthal D. The benefits of health information technology: a review of the recent literature shows predominantly positive results. Health Aff. 2011;3:464–71.
11. Balas EA, Boren SA. Managing clinical knowledge for health care improvement. In: Yearbook of medical informatics 2000: patient-centered systems. Stuttgart: Schattauer; 2000. p. 65–70.
12. Lipton E, Johnson K. The anthrax trail; tracking bioterror's tangled course. New York Times, Section A, p. 1, 26 Dec 2001.
13. Wagner MM, Dato V, Dowling JN, Allswede M. Representative threats for research in public health surveillance. J Biomed Inform. 2003;36(3):177–88.
14. U.S. Department of Health and Human Services. Update on the adoption of health information technology and related efforts to facilitate the electronic use and exchange of health information. A report to congress. HHS Office of the National Coordinator for Health Information Technology. 2013.
15. Yasnoff WA, Sweeney L, Shortliffe EH. Putting health IT on the path to success. J Am Med Assoc. 2013;309(10):989–90.
16. Yasnoff WA. Health information infrastructure. In: Shortliffe EH, Cimino JJ, editors. Biomedical informatics: computer applications in healthcare and medicine. 4th ed. New York: Springer; 2014. p. 423–41.
17. Adler-Milstein J, Bates DW, Jha AK. Operational health information exchanges show substantial growth, but long-term funding remains a concern. Health Aff (Millwood). 2013;32(8):1486–92.
18. Yasnoff WA. Privacy, confidentiality, and security. In: Magnuson JA, FU PC Jr., editors. Public health informatics and information systems. 2nd ed. New York: Springer-Verlag; 2014. p. 155–72.
19. U.S. Department of Health and Human Services. The HIPAA privacy rule. Available at: http://www.hhs.gov/ocr/privacy/hipaa/administrative/privacyrule/index.html. Accessed 12 Jan 2015.
20. California Health Care Foundation. National consumer health privacy survey. 2005. Available at: http://www.chcf.org/publications/2005/11/national-consumer-health-privacy-survey-2005. Accessed 26 Dec 2014.
21. Harris Interactive. Many U.S. adults are satisfied with use of their personal health records. 2007. Available at: http://www.harrisinteractive.com/vault/Harris-Interactive-Poll-Research-Health-Privacy-2007-03.pdf. Accessed 26 Dec 2014.
22. Blumenthal D, Squires D. Giving patients control of their EHR data. J Gen Intern Med. 2015;30 Suppl 1:S42–3.
23. DesRoches CM, et al. Electronic health records in ambulatory care – a national survey of physicians. N Engl J Med. 2008;359:50–60.
24. Hersh W. Healthcare information technology: progress and barriers. JAMA. 2004; 292:2273–4.
25. Health Record Banking Alliance. A proposed national infrastructure for HIE using personally controlled records. 2013. Available at: http://www.healthbanking.org/docs/HRBA Architecture White Paper Jan 2013.pdf. Accessed 26 Dec 2014.
26. Lapsia V, Lamb K, Yasnoff WA. Where should electronic records for patients be stored? Int J Med Inform. 2012;81(12):821–7.
27. Yasnoff. Health record banking: a practical approach to the national health information infrastructure. 2006. Available at http://williamyasnoff.com/?p=26 Accessed 26 Dec 2014.
28. Health Record Banking Alliance. Principles and fact sheet. 2008. Available at http://www.healthbanking.org/docs/HRBA Principles & Fact Sheet 2008 FINAL.pdf. Accessed 26 Dec 2014.
29. Szolovits P, Doyle J, Long WJ, Kohane I, Pauker SG. Guardian angel: patient-centered health information systems. 1994 Technical report MIT/LCS/TR-604, Massachusetts Institute of Technology Laboratory for Computer Science.
30. Dodd B. An independent "health information bank" could solve health data security issues. Br J Healthc Comput Inf Manag. 1997;14(8):2.

31. Ramsaroop P, Ball M. The "bank of health": a model for more useful patient health records. MD Comput. 2000;17:45–8.
32. Kostyack P. The emergence of the healthcare information trust. Matrix J Law Med. 2002;12(393).
33. Dyson, E. Personal health information: data comes alive! 2005. Release 1.0 24,1 (Sep).
34. Haislmaier EF. Health care information technology: getting the policy right. 2006. Available at http://www.heritage.org/Research/Reports/2006/06/Health-Care-Information-Technology-Getting-the-Policy-Right. Accessed 26 Dec 2014.
35. Ball M, Gold J. Banking on health: personal records and information exchange. J Healthc Inf Manag. 2006;20(2):71–83.
36. Shabo A. A global socio-economic-medico-legal model for the sustainability of longitudinal health records. Methods Inf Med. 2006;45:240–5 (Part 1), 498–505 (Part 2).
37. Health Record Banking Alliance. 2006. http://www.healthbanking.org. Accessed 26 Dec 2014.
38. State of Washington Health Care Authority. Washington state health information infrastructure: final report and roadmap for state action. 2006. Available at http://www.providersedge.com/ehdocs/ehr_articles/Washington_State_Health_Information_Infrastructure-Final_Report_and_Roadmap_for_State_Action.pdf. Accessed 26 Dec 2014.
39. Dossia Consortium. 2006. http://www.dossia.org. Accessed 26 Dec 2014.
40. Castro D. Improving health care: why a dose of IT may be just what the doctor ordered. Information Technology and Innovation Foundation. 2007. Available at http://www.itif.org/publications/improving-health-care-why-dose-it-may-be-just-what-doctor-ordered. Accessed 26 Dec 2014.
41. Gold JD, Ball MJ. The health record banking imperative: a conceptual model. IBM Syst J. 2007;46(1):43–55.
42. Kendall DB. Protecting patient privacy through health record trusts. Health Aff. 2009;28(2):444–6.
43. Health Record Banking Alliance. Health record banking: a foundation for myriad health information sharing models. 2012. Available at http://www.healthbanking.org/docs/HRBA Business Model White Paper Dec 2012.pdf. Accessed 26 Dec 2014.
44. Health Record Banking Alliance. Comments on: advancing interoperability and health information exchange (CMS- 0038-NC). 2013b. Available at http://healthbanking.org/pdf/HRBA Response to CMS-ONC RFI FINAL.pdf. Accessed 26 Dec 2014.
45. Yasnoff WA, Shortliffe EH. Lessons learned from a health record bank start-up. Methods Inf Med. 2014;53(2):66–72.
46. Steinbrook R. Personally controlled online health data – the next big thing in medical care? N Engl J Med. 2008;358(16):1653–6.
47. Mandl KD, Kohane IS. Tectonic shifts in the health information economy. N Engl J Med. 2008;358(16):1732–7.
48. Kidd MR. Personal electronic health records: MySpace or HealthSpace? Br Med J. 2008;336:1029–30.
49. Miller H, Yasnoff WA, Burde H. Personal health records: the essential missing element in twenty-first century healthcare. Chicago: Health Information and Management Systems Society; 2009.
50. Krist AH, Woolf SH. A vision for patient-centered health information systems. JAMA. 2011;305(3):300–1.
51. Yasnoff WA, Shortliffe EH, Shortell SM. A proposal for financially sustainable population health organizations. Popul Health Manag. 2014;17(5):255–6.
52. Turn R, Shapiro NZ, Juncosa ML. Privacy and security in centralized vs. decentralized database systems. Policy Sci. 1976;7:17–29.
53. Evaristo JR, Desouza KC, Hollister K. Centralization momentum: the pendulum swings back again. Commun ACM. 2005;48(2):66–71.
54. Agency for Healthcare Research and Quality. Costs and benefits of health information technology. Evidence report/technology assessment 132, publication 06-E006. 2006. Available at http://www.ahrq.gov/research/findings/evidence-based-reports/hitsys.pdf. Accessed 26 Dec 2014.

55. Microsoft. 2012. http://msdn.microsoft.com/en-us/healthvault/hh922966. Accessed 26 Dec 2014.
56. Hsiao CJ, Jha AK, King J, Patel V, Furukawa MF, Mostashari F. Office-based physicians are responding to incentives and assistance by adopting and using electronic health records. Health Aff (Millwood). 2013;32:1470–7.
57. Desroches CM, Charles D, Furukawa MF, et al. Adoption of electronic health records grows rapidly, but fewer than half of US hospitals had at least a basic system in 2012. Health Aff (Millwood). 2013;32:1478–85.
58. Laudon K. Markets and privacy. Commun ACM. 1996;39(9):92–104.
59. Herper M. Surprise! With $60 million genentech deal, 23andme has a business plan. Forbes, January 6, 2015. Available at: http://www.forbes.com/sites/matthewherper/2015/01/06/surprise-with-60-million-genentech-deal-23andme-has-a-business-plan/. Accessed 18 Jan 2015.
60. Yasnoff WA, O'Carroll PW, Freide A. Public health informatics and the health information infrastructure. In: Shortliffe EH, Cimino JJ, editors. Biomedical informatics: computer applications in healthcare and medicine. 3rd ed. New York: Springer-Verlag; 2006. p. 537–63.
61. Labkoff SE, Yasnoff WA. A framework for systematic evaluation of health information infrastructure progress in communities. J Biomed Inform. 2007;40(2):100–5.

# Chapter 21
# Next Generation Wellness: A Technology Model for Personalizing Healthcare

Pei-Yun Sabrina Hsueh, Henry Chang, and Sreeram Ramakrishnan

**Abstract** Personalization or individualization of care is essential to the behavioral modifications and lifestyle changes that result in patient wellness (for good health or chronic disease management). The implementation of effective personalized care is hampered by the lack of reliable means to collect and process real-time data on individual contexts (preferences, constraints) and on adherence to care protocols and mechanisms to provide timely, customized cognitive coaching that is structured, consistent and informative to users.

The advent of personal embedded biosensors is creating an accumulation of patient-generated data from numerous "touch points" (data interfaces and exchanges between patient and healthcare services before, during and after traditional clinical encounters). A major technical challenge is the establishment of a patient-centered infrastructure that can:

- Provide the customized, timely, evidence/knowledge-driven messaging based on data from multiple touch points for continuous feedback to individual patients
- Support this functionality within an information infrastructure of multiple service providers to provide access to unified views of patients' data across touch points and time for multiple users (patients, providers, administrators, researchers)

We propose the implementation of a cloud-based platform to support the analytics and other services to implement this infrastructure. From an IT perspective, we explore

- Modeling of patient contexts (preferences, behaviors) within a risk-based framework

P.-Y.S. Hsueh, PhD (✉) • H. Chang, PhD
Healthcare Informatics Group, IBM T.J. Watson Research Center,
Yorktown Heights, NY, USA
e-mail: phsueh@us.ibm.com

S. Ramakrishnan, PhD (Industrial Engineering)
Wellness Ecosystems and Analytics, Taiwan Colloboratory, IBM T.J. Watson Research,
Hawthorne, NY, USA

© Springer International Publishing Switzerland 2016
C.A. Weaver et al. (eds.), *Healthcare Information Management Systems:
Cases, Strategies, and Solutions*, Health Informatics,
DOI 10.1007/978-3-319-20765-0_21

- Calibration of individualized, evidence-based recommendations based on patient-generated data
- Deployment of analytics functionalities within the platform model

**Keywords** Personalized healthcare • Patient centered-care • Data Analytics • Precision Medicine • Personalization Analytics • Watson mobile applications • Knowledge coupling with data

## 21.1   Introduction

### 21.1.1   Personalized Health and Care

Personalized healthcare [4, 17, 35], highlighted by President Barack Obama's 2015 initiative on "precision medicine", can be defined as "[disease] prevention and treatment strategies that take individual variability into account" [20]. System biologists have extended this concept as "P4 Medicine" (personalized, predictive, preventive, and participatory) [46] to incorporate personalized healthcare that actively engages patients, since it is estimated that more than 60 % of "health" is based on patient contexts, that is: behavioral patterns, social circumstances and environmental exposures [64, 80].

As populations age, the prevalence of chronic and pre-morbid conditions (such as obesity) rises, and with them the overall cost of healthcare. In Japan, seniors (those over 65 years) represent 21 % of the population and in the United States (US), the ratio of seniors to non-seniors is projected to increase by 80 % in coming decades [12]. According to the Agency for Healthcare Research and Quality [6], more than 84 % of US healthcare costs go to chronic care, with its annual cost amounting to $1.65 trillion (or 15 % of the gross domestic product (GDP)) [18].

Longitudinal studies have shown that tailoring lifestyle interventions can reduce the burden of chronic disease, through primary prevention (e.g., Finnish Diabetes Prevention Study (FIN-D2D) [75], US Diabetes Prevention Program (DPP) [27, 28], China Da Qing IGT and Diabetes study [66]) and secondary prevention via targeted screening (e.g., the US Diabetes Control and Complications Trial/ Epidemiology of Diabetes Interventions and Complications Study (DCCT/EDIC) [23] and the UK Prospective Diabetes Study (UK PDS) [85]). Quantification of the benefits of such tailored interventions has demonstrated a 42 % risk reduction (RR) for all cardiovascular disease events, 57 % RR for nonfatal heart attacks, strokes or death from other cardiovascular causes [93] and 58 % RR for Type 2 Diabetes Mellitus for patients with impaired glucose tolerance [84].

Despite this, personalized healthcare has not gained traction as might be expected for wellness, prevention and chronic disease management. Patient-Centered Medical Home (PCMH) models [68] have faced challenges in transforming current encounter-based practice into truly patient-centered care. Improving case management guidelines [19] for coordination of care alone does not appear to solve the problem.

There is need to engage and empower patients in their own care, using strategies that incorporate individual variability and that gives patients incentives and access to evidence and data to assert themselves in crucial healthcare discussions and decisions.

## 21.1.2   Challenges in Achieving Personalized Health and Care

Existing care delivery is structured on applying evidence-based guidelines to the care of individuals at risk. Guidelines are population-based, that is, they are designed to serve average patients, with the assumption that one guideline "fits all". An example of this is the standard JNC7 high blood pressure guideline [16] which uses a single rule, i.e., whether a patient's systolic blood pressure (SBP) is higher than 135 mmHg, to determine the prescription of anti-hypertensive therapy, which may not be optimal for diabetic patients (for whom a lower SBP threshold may be more appropriate). Studies have shown that overall, at least 45 % of patients do not receive recommended care and that there is large variation in guideline implementation [36, 60].

Measuring patient variability is difficult as there are few standard proxy measures to assess different contexts. This difficulty extends into assessing baseline and adaptive contexts (abilities and preferences) in individual responses to specific interventions (that include habit formation, non-adherence, aversion, etc.). Thus, patients frequently make "free-style" decisions, without adequate guidance, resulting in low adherence rates (estimated to be less than 50 %, with one example being a report of 20–30 % of prescriptions left unfilled [8, 24, 43]).

The financial potential is compelling. The estimated worldwide cost of non-adherence is $30–$594 billion dollars annually [55]. In the European Union alone, non-adherence accounts for 194,500 deaths and adds 125 billion euros to the costs per year [71]. In the United States, non-adherence has been estimated to account for 69 % of hospital admissions, adding $100 billion and $290 billion annually in terms of excessive hospitalization and avoidable medical spending respectively [49]. Stakeholders in healthcare spending, such as self-insured employers, have taken interest and action.

## 21.1.3   Personalized Healthcare, Patient Empowerment and Technology

To overcome challenges inherent in realizing personalized healthcare:

(a) **Physicians and healthcare systems must recognize patients as full partners in the dialogue of evidence-based care**. In this dialogue, the patient is a source of continual, reliable, time-specific data (ongoing reports of point-of-care measurement: serial blood glucose, blood pressure, etc.) and physicians and systems provide tools to facilitate active and ongoing two-way communication.

(b) **Patients must be actively engaged as full partners in their individualized care**. Patients and families must use education and support to their best ability to make empowered decisions (with support from their providers) about their health and care. Patients must also generate information that prime analytics tools to identify "teachable" moments, to personalize messages according to patient contexts/challenges [42] and to mediate/mitigate non-adherence risk by tracking and optimizing the effectiveness of incentives [82].

To support this vision of an active ongoing health dialogue between patient and care team with a bi-directional real-time flow of information to and from the patient, wearable biosensor and cloud technologies are providing new opportunities and possible solutions for exploration.

### 21.1.3.1    Mobile Phones

The ubiquity of mobile phones provides an open terrain for communication and engagement, with the worldwide mobile health market expected to grow to $49 billion by 2020, with a projected annual growth rate of 49.7 % in monitoring services.

One report revealed that 27 % of mobile phone users "would like a personalized plan to help guide them through their journey to better health" [13].

### 21.1.3.2    Wearable Biosensors and Cloud Platforms

Wearable patient monitoring devices are being developed to monitor asthma [61] and chronic obstructive pulmonary disease (COPD) [67] by tracking physical parameters (movement, heart/respiratory rates) via accelerometers and physiologic sensors. Sensors are also being developed to detect biochemical changes in sweat [44] and to quantify changes in body movement in patients with Parkinson Disease [57]. Non-invasive sensors have been deployed into smoking cessation programs to monitor a patient's smoking habits by monitoring breathing and hand-to-mouth gestures [54].

The market of "connected health and wellness devices" is expected to reach $8 billion by 2018. As the Internet of Things (IoT) and Machine to Machine (M2M) technologies and infrastructures mature, 20–50 billion connected devices are predicted to emerge around the world by 2020 [2, 48]. The progressive integration of mobile sensors and cloud technologies is making possible "smart" and "connected" personal health networks that are raising awareness of healthcare and health [38]. As of 2014, the accumulation of patient-generated health data at finer levels of granularity has stimulated understanding of patient contexts (i.e., disease states, self-management capabilities, and preferences).

### 21.1.4 Personalized Healthcare Recommendations as a Platform-Based Service

The vision of transforming episodic office-based practice into continuous data-driven patient-centered care requires a paradigm shift to unify care and information transactions (patient-generated data, information and recommendations about care) across "touchpoints" (i.e., all contacts between a patient and healthcare services across time, providers and settings (within and beyond face-to-face encounters)). One possibility, which we are exploring, is the use of a platform, that is, a data-brokering mechanism that connects consumers/patients to services/providers in real-time. In this service model, information can be exchanged wirelessly to provide real-time feedback loops of patient data, assessment and guidance that encourage participatory decision-making.

Cloud-based services are an intrinsic part of the platform approach, but they do not solve the problem entirely. Analytics tools must be available to process incoming health data from multiple sensors into meaningful outputs for interpretation and decision support by users (patients and providers). A major challenge with analytics has been the specification of functionalities to map clinical guideline-based recommendations to personalized care in a safe, effective and sustainable way. As such, healthcare has been slow to implement analytics [22] and thus, progress has been limited.

Other barriers to platform implementation have been:

- *Uncertainties in the regulation of medical devices and health information assurance*: As mobile and personal health information technologies mature, the definition of "medical device" becomes less clear. In previous years, the US Food and Drug Administration (FDA) cleared more than 100 medical mobile applications (MMA) as its 510(k) medical devices, but it has also prioritized safety. The FDA further released the two guidelines on MMA [32] and its associated medical data storage systems (MDDS) [33]. In addition, non-alignment of business interests and the ever-changing regulatory environment for information assurance and security complicate data sharing among federated entities.
- *Data capacity and costs*: The sheer size of data has posed challenges to service providers, incurring the need to hire subject matter experts and IT support personnel to handle the quantity and formats of data. The high staffing expense in turn creates barriers to small- and mid-sized providers who do not have enough data volume to justify the costs of analytics and/or cloud services that may be needed.

## 21.2 A Personalization Framework

Our research investigates the feasibility of a sustainable wearable sensor-driven cloud-based analytics platform for providing evidence-based feedback based on patient-generated data. We introduce a technical framework for healthcare information personalization, and we begin by asking three questions:

1. How can patient contexts (abilities, preferences, choices, etc.) be modeled within personalized healthcare?
2. How can personalized recommendations be chosen/generated in response to patient data and contexts?
3. What is a vision for implementing these on a service platform?


## 21.2.1   Individualized Risk Stratification

One model of patient contexts (abilities, preferences, choices, etc.) poses such attributes in terms of the outcomes risk they confer upon a patient within diseases and treatments. The stratification of risk has been studied with regard to ICD-9 codes and claims data [77] and in relation to patients' self-reported data on their chronic diseases to produce numerical scores [15, 31, 56]. Using this model, analytics techniques have been used with electronic health record (EHR) data to:

- Detect abnormalities in healthcare delivery quality [51, 77]
- Identify significant associations between medication use and disease outcomes (Ex. heart attack risk and use of a specific drug, subsequently removed from the market) [78].
- Identify risk factors for cardiovascular diseases for prediction [21].
- Correlate health outcomes of patients with environmental data to analyze behavioral risk factors at the community level [47, 79]

Similarly, "big data" analytics techniques have been used with genetic biomarkers from genomic databases to capture signals of risk-conferral:

- Disease-indicative genetic variations have been discovered by cross-examining individual genetic profiles [83] with genome-wide association studies [62].
- Correlations between gene expressions and exogenous data, such as physical activity and nutrition intake, have been proposed but not been studied extensively [81]. Complex diseases, such as obesity and metabolic syndrome may be associated with variable expression of thousands of genes across functional categories.
- High-throughput screening techniques have been applied to identify "dietary signatures" (i.e., sets of distinctive patterns in nutrients, non-nutritive food components and nutritional regimes that can influence the protein expression and regulate the progression of metabolic syndrome) [65, 74].
- Molecular analyses (e.g., differences in genes, gene expression, protein expression, and metabolites) are used to assess the relationship between clinical outcomes and individual variations. Such analyses can support individualized interventions based on individual genetic differences in addition to physical activity and other lifestyle choices on chronic disease management for better outcomes [63].

The term "sub-health" has been defined by the World Health Organization as a state between health and disease where standard tests may be normal, but in which a patient is in distress or at risk for ailments. This is the conceptual basis for modeling contexts as contributors to a patient's sub-health or risk status [53].

## 21.2.2   Individualized Guidelines for Wellness Management

An individualized guideline is an ideal that provides patient-specific feedback and recommendations with respect to the patient's contexts and data for optimal wellness management for chronic disease and prevention. As part of individualization, such guidelines (or programs) must include contingencies for acute illness (i.e., "sick" day management), for changes in patient responses over time, for different life circumstances (i.e., home vs work vs vacation vs school) and for their impact on patient contexts (i.e., stress) and management. An individualized guideline should also predict, prevent and overcome treatment resistance and failure.

As an example, the medical management of "diabetes mellitus" (DM) must be individualized:

- Type and severity of disease (Type I DM vs Type II DM) determine pharmacologic approaches. Type I DM typically requires insulin early in the course of the disease, whereas Type II may require it later
- Diabetic patients may be at higher cardiovascular risk (for heart attack and stroke), more so as they age
- Some therapies can increase insulin resistance in some individuals [92]
- Exogenous insulin may increase cardiovascular risk, but better glucose control 240 over time has decreased risk (U.S. Diabetes Control and Complications Trial [23] and UK Prospective Diabetes Study (UKPDS) [85, 86])
- Some patients with Type I DM may lose their ability to respond to hypoglycemia (low blood glucose) over time.

In this case, individualization of guidelines helps optimize medical care (drug choices depend on specifics of the illness), risk reduction (cardiovascular disease prevention depends on a number of factors, including diabetic management), wellness (day-to-day management depends on diet, exercise, weight management, medication adherence and other factors) and contingencies ("sick" days) to balance physiologic and individual needs as the condition evolves [3]. In addition, measures of patients' self-efficacy and literacy may be useful in selecting and developing appropriate educational approaches and partnerships (such as with diabetic educators) [76].

Failure to accommodate individual needs may result in mixed effects on different individuals. In many cases, patient-generated health data (including self-reports and monitoring data) can provide important feedback on tailoring and customizing clinical recommendations to individuals. The importance of patient-generated health data in diabetes has been demonstrated in a study at the Juvenile Diabetes Research Foundation (JDRF), which shows that continuous glucose monitoring and individualized insulin adjustment significantly decrease hypoglycemic episodes [50].

### 21.2.3 Coupling Information to Wellness Best Practices

#### 21.2.3.1 Data

Mobile and wearable health devices can provide "real-time" patient data (vital signs, exercise, intake and exposure, surveys/assessments, etc.). PricewaterhouseCoopers' Health Research Initiative (HRI) [70] report on "wearables" has demonstrated that 21 % of Americans are already using personalized technology (wristband/watches to record physical activity, sleep patterns, etc.) to measure and record biometric data. For example, the Apple HealthKit [7] supports many observations: date of birth, height, weight, body mass, BMI, body fat percentage, blood pressure, heart rate, RR interval, respiratory rate, body temperature, oxygen saturation, spirometry, peripheral perfusion index, blood glucose, blood alcohol content, dietary intake – carbohydrates, fat, sugar, vitamins, number of times fallen, regular steps, distance, flights climbed, workout information, etc. that may impact on an individual's health. In addition to providing opportunities for health improvement and health IT development, these technologies provide a potential foundation for health and health informatics research, with great opportunities for investigators to develop and explore questions and hypotheses on wellness, interventions, diagnosis, and interventions, with new sensor features providing the potential for a wide array of data on populations (using "big data" techniques).

#### 21.2.3.2 Knowledge

Knowledge on wellness and prevention that meets the needs and preferences of individuals can be divided into three dimensions:

(a) Lifestyle programs that include regimens for managing nutrition, exercise, weight loss, relaxation, pain and stress (Example: customized daily cardiovascular fitness regimens)
(b) Messaging tools that deliver timely, contextual messages to users to inform and encourage them at the right time and place (Example: a smartphone reminder about portion control prior to a scheduled social event)
(c) Health state analysis and prediction tools that answer patient health questions from the literature and predict outcomes of recommended actions from published guidelines (Example: a patient-friendly summary of the relevant information from the Framingham heart study based on his/her cholesterol level).

In one commercial venture, IBM Watson (artificial intelligence/question answering system) and its capability to process natural language materials is being leveraged to help answer personal health questions from consumers [90]. Through a mobile interface connected to evidence-based knowledge sources, pre-processed by Watson, patients/users can participate more actively in the clinician-prescribed management plans. One challenge to widespread diffusion of this tool and approach is the need to meet the literacy/health literacy needs of patients/users, and its current principal market is employer-based health plans; patients must qualify for self-care (inferring a baseline literacy level for users). One possible vision is that such a tool can provide a focal point for social networking in health condition-related communities (e.g., patientslikeme) to extend patient engagement and empowerment in lifestyle interventions as a part of consumer-driven healthcare (Fig. 21.1).

## 21.3   Platform Support

We now explore system design requirements for a cloud-based platform that incorporates the personalization framework and support the necessary analytics. The personalization framework consists of four components that fit into clinical information workflow:

- Guideline-based personalized treatment plan: A clinical diagnosis triggers initiation of a condition-specific wellness management plan according to high-level guidelines with constraints. For example, for a diagnosis of "dyslipidemia" the recommended diet constraints are: "carbohydrates 50–60 %; protein 10–20 %; fat $\leq 30$ %; total cholesterol $\leq 300$ mg; and fiber 25–35 mg" (e.g., National NCEP/ATP III guideline for blood lipid control [37])
- Analytics-driven individualized guideline refinement: Analytics stratify an individual patient's risk factors according to the patient's longitudinal record in comparison to a cohort (patients of a similar age, gender and weight, etc.) for disease and risk mitigation strategies according to guidelines, patient/provider preferences and the patient's needs (according to existing data). For example, a patient with a diagnosis of dyslipidemia with an extremely high fasting cholesterol level may be referred for genetic testing and intensive dietary and medical management.
- In-context outcome-driven personalized recommendation: A user profile specifies guideline recommendations for specific contexts (user preferences and abilities, day-to-day activities, vacation modifications) and filters and ranks them based on the patient's current context (time of day, event). For example, reminders on diet and portion control may be scheduled prior to dinner at a restaurant (as noted in a patient's personal calendar).
- Personalized feedback generation and service plan adaptation: Given an incoming data stream by a user, real-time messages provide feedback on adherence/compliance levels in response to defined abnormalities. For example, an unusually high blood pressure measurement may deliver a prompt to a patient for symptoms, inquire about medication adherence and suggest the blood pressure to be re-checked, with an accumulation of high blood pressure events over time.

We define service flow as a sequence of information operations in which some action (knowledge delivery, analytical calculation, mapping to a specific guideline) is invoked by data or other output. Within the personalization framework, the operations of the service flow require inputs from the patient (electronic record data,

**Fig. 21.1** "Ask Watson"
mobile application, source
IBM.

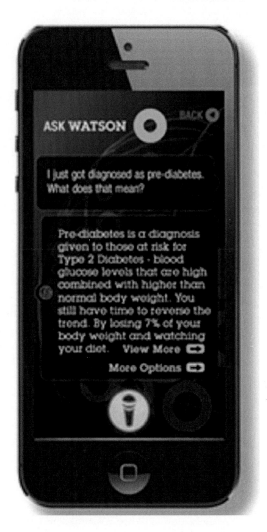

contexts, sensor data, etc.) and from systematic risk/benefit calculations of specific healthcare interventions (general guidelines) for the patient. These inputs are then mapped to individualized recommendations/guidelines (service plans) that are delivered as specific interventions (services) to the patient for wellness and disease management.

Our cloud platform consists of three layers that use HL7 CDA [26] messaging to interoperate with other health information technology systems for care coordination:

(a) The **information service layer** provides analytics utilities connected to other platform components via messaging protocols
(b) The **living service layer** orchestrates information services to offer personalization functionalities with application programming interfaces (APIs) that enable

programmers to generate personalized information services that can be consumed and delivered

(c) The **care solution layer** allows clinical case managers to "jumpstart" personalized care service offerings with simple configuration tools to specify user interactions and interfaces (Fig. 21.2).

We now focus on analytics (information service layer functions) for three components/tasks of the personalization framework individualized guideline refinement, in-context outcome-driven recommendation and personalized feedback generation (The selection of a guideline-based personalized treatment plan, being triggered principally by diagnosis, requires no analytics within this framework).

### 21.3.1 Support for Analytics-Driven Individualized Guideline Refinement

To initiate an active personalization cycle (i.e., design and implement an individualized guideline), the platform must absorb patient-centric information from multiple sources and identify predisposing risk factors. The platform must interact with a care provider to allow:

1. Profiling of the patient's personal wellness and health risks

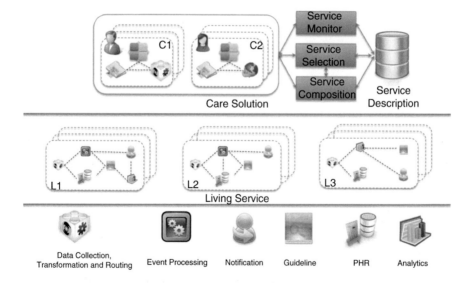

**Fig. 21.2** Platform support for personalized care application development

2. Design of effective and interactive presentations of interventions with regard to the profile and contexts
3. Individualizing patient interaction with service options with regard to risk mitigation

To start, clinical and patient-generated data repositories are stored in a patient wellness record (PWR) on the platform [40]. For each disease or condition, individual risk stratification is performed based on the importance of patient contexts and data in relation to what is known about similar patients and/or what is specified by the care provider. Once the conferral of risks with regard to patient contexts (risk profile) has been performed, specific service plans (recommendations/interventions) are chosen and linked to visual objects/widgets to be presented to the patient for discussion and testing for acceptance and usability.

Therefore, one property that a platform must support is interactive guideline refinement for participatory decision-making [59, 88], by which clinicians and patients can jointly make health management decisions that fit the patients' contexts (preferences, abilities, constraints, etc.). Once patients have navigated through service plan options with regard to specified constraints and preferences, guidelines can be refined according to perceived importance to generate personalized service plans ready for patient use.

## 21.3.2   Support for In-Context Outcome-Driven Personalized Recommendation

To complete an active personalization cycle (i.e., implement an individualized guideline), the platform must match services/recommendations according to a patient's contextualized needs. It must provide support for services/ recommendations that are reactive to what the patient does, situated in context and proactive to future steps in care.

To accomplish this, our platform provides:

(i) Pre-screening (contextual factor analysis) uses analytics utilities that use low-frequency variations across specific risk factors [72] to identify risk or susceptibility in complex conditions. For personalized wellness management (in health and chronic disease), these include variations in: nutrition intake, physical activity, social network lifestyle, compliance behavior, and many other external environment factors such as air pollution. This yields a set of contextual risk factors.

(ii) Modeling (context-driven personalized query) uses identified contextual risk factors to create context-aware queries as the input to the framework to search for suitable personalized service plans/recommendations.

(iii) Post-screening (context-driven user model solicitation) uses filtering utilities to tailor model-generated recommendations with respect to patients' current contexts.

The product of these two components/tasks is a user-centered, context-aware disease management program, which is coupled with adherence monitoring, instant feedback and location-based recommendations.

### 21.3.3   Support for Personalized Feedback Generation

To sustain the personalized healthcare design framework, the platform must assess incoming data streams for changes, generate interactive feedback and trigger individualized risk mitigation services/recommendation in a reliable and timely fashion. Therefore, two properties that the platform must support are: the detection and reliable identification of significant dynamic changes in incoming data and the ability to monitor for projected changes in incoming signals based on a user's health and wellness status.

## 21.4   Discussion and Conclusion

### 21.4.1   The Place of Analytics in Personalized Healthcare

Although existing patient education and participatory decision support approaches that require in-person sessions have been shown as effective in initiating behavioral changes [9, 89], they yielded mixed effects in sustaining behavioral changes. This is largely due to the lack of reinforcement and reinforcement based on patient-generated data. The analytics and platform framework to provide this that we have described can help to sustain behavioral change.

The recent acceleration of mobile and sensor development has increased demand for context-aware recommendations systems [1, 5, 87] with experimentation to better capture contextual factors that matter for personalized recommendation [91]. The rising trend of context awareness and intelligence opens up many new possibilities in the wellness domain (user-centered, context-aware disease management by instant compliance checking and location-based recommendations).

### 21.4.2   Data Quality

An important issue in deployment of the system we describe is assurance of data quality and integrity. This is especially important for service platform when the data originates from multiple stakeholders (including the patient), more so because of the impact of the service provided (health recommendations to patients at risk).

One approach we have taken is to create a data quality monitor to determine whether an identified risk group is sufficiently representative to be used for predicting risk [39]. Specifically, the monitor follows possible sources of prediction errors in three major categories: risk group noise, case ambiguity, and noise-adjusted case ambiguity.

- Risk group noise quantifies deviations of the predicted and assigned risk from each risk group identified
- Case ambiguity quantifies average deviation of all predictions yielded on one single case, based on all relevant risk groups
- Noise-adjusted case ambiguity modifies case ambiguity scores reweighted with respect to the noise level of each risk group involved in case ambiguity determination

With the aid of the data quality monitor, developers can implement proactive learning programs to determine which data source to ask for future cases to analyze. When analysis results do not appear to be reliable, the monitor can also help filter cases that are ambiguous.

### 21.4.3  Health Risk Appraisals

Health risk appraisals (HRA) are used by health plans and employer wellness promotion programs. These have also been used to drive treatment for targeted populations. For example, KP Care Management Institute's clinical trial in Hawaii [29] showed that the treatments driven by individualized guidelines could prevent 6,000 myocardial infarctions (MIs) and strokes annually if applied throughout KP. The results can be translated into 43 % of improvement over the JNC7 guideline for the same cost.

Despite the successful trials and pilots of HRAs in screening, diagnosis and prognosis, their use in computer-supportive personalized wellness management remains conceptual. Previously, government-sponsored trial programs such as Finnish diabetes prevention study group (Finland D2D) and U.S. Diabetes Prevention Program (DPP) have attempted to provide individualized wellness management by having health professionals manually analyze individual risk and send out personal reminders. However, such a labor-intensive operation is difficult to scale.

The movement to use innovative approaches to make care more patient-centered and accountable and coordinated, such as direct payment model [69] and collaborative care model [10], would benefit from a personalization framework and system design on a service platform that are easily accessible, scalable and elastic.

### 21.4.4  Innovative Models for "Open Wellness"

Wellness management involves multiple business partners handling different healthcare and wellness issues, including physical examination and screening, physical activity coaching and nutrition regimens, etc. for chronic disease management.

Many of these services can be transformed with better understanding of the target users. A service platform business ecosystem can allow health service providers in partnership to provide personalized services based on the shared knowledge of patients' current status and the level of their individual needs [14]. This will help providers tailor patients' personal intervention plans accordingly in the context of their service provisioning.

Emerging opportunities for value-added services such as healthcare data brokering of patient-generated health data for exploratory and comparative effectiveness research, benchmarking for identifying useful attributes for quantifying patient populations of risk and provisioning and repurposing of analytics tools and methods are compelling. The resulting networks of providers could serve to further increase the business ecosystem efficiency and performance of personalization prediction and maintain a competitive edge of the participating service providers.

A major challenge of the ecosystem-based business model is sharing the burden of data protection [41, 45]. In addition to assuring the privacy and security of data within the system, there must consideration of governance regarding proper use and reuse of data and analytics products.

Another major challenge comes from the questions regarding how to systematically characterize patient-specific properties previously unobservable without cross-layer data integration support. For example, evidence has emerged for the importance of personal social network factors on wellness outcome [11]; however, it remains unclear how to integrate data streams from social network to characterize individual differences in factors such as psychosocial stressors and self-esteem [52, 58].

An industry vertical solution is thus expected to fill in the space and provide sustainable system support to the service providers who would like to add a layer of personalization analytics in their own service delivery systems. The development of cloud services that encompass a common personalization analytics component can provide use cases beyond utility computing.

Many new business opportunities, as a result, will emerge from an industry vertical solution that focuses on the ease of employing data-driven analytics approaches that are seemingly too sophisticated in the past and deploying data processing capabilities to handle a large amount of data on an incoming basis.

### 21.4.5   Future Work

In addition to the questions outlined in this chapter, our further explorations will involve cognitive modeling to provide insights into the causes of non-compliance and how to devise counter-strategies [25, 30, 34, 73]. It is important to tie personalization technology to behavioral medicine regimens that focus on sustaining change.

**Acknowledgments**   Many thanks to our colleagues at the IBM T.J. Watson Center and Taiwan Collaboratory who developed the earlier prototypes of the system described here.

# References

1. Abbar S, Bouzeghoub M, Lopez S. Context-aware recommender systems: a service-oriented approach. In: Proceedings of the 3rd VLDB international workshop on personalized access, profile management, and context awareness in databases (VLDB PersDB Workshop, IBM Almaden, San Jose). 2009.
2. ABI Research. More than 30 billion devices will wirelessly connect to the internet of everything. 2013. Available at: https://www.abiresearch.com/press/more-than-30-billion-devices-will-wirelessly-conne.
3. Abrahamson M, et al. Insulin-treated type 2 diabetes: balancing physiologic and individual needs. Medscape Educ. 2006. http://www.medscape.org/viewprogram/5955 [last accessed 30 July 2015].
4. Adams J, Mounib E, Shabo A. IT-enabled personalized healthcare. IBM Institute for Business Value Report, Somers, NY. 2010.
5. Adomavicius G, Tuzhilin A. Context-aware recommender systems. In: Proceedings of the ACM conference on Recommender systems RecSys '08, Lausanne. 2008.
6. AHRQ. Medical expenditure panel survey. Rockville: Agency for Healthcare Research and Quality; 2014.
7. Apple Inc. HealthKit. 2015. URL: https://developer.apple.com/healthkit/. Last accessed 22 Apr 2015.
8. Bardel A, Wallander MA, Svärdsudd K. Factors associated with adherence to drug therapy: a population-based study. Eur J Clin Pharmacol. 2007;63:307–14.
9. Brown LL, Lustralia MLA, Rankins J. A review of web-assisted interventions for diabetes management: maximizing the potential for improving health outcomes. J Diabetes Sci Technol. 2007;1(6):164–74.
10. Butler M, Kane RL, McAlpine D, Kathol, RG, Fu SS, Hagedorn H, Wilt TJ. Integration of mental health/substance abuse and primary care no. 173 AHRQ Publication No. 09-E003, Agency for Healthcare Research and Quality. 2008.
11. Carrell SE, Hoekstra M, West JE. Is poor fitness contagious? Evidence from randomly assigned friends. National Bureau of Economic Research Working Paper No. 16518. 2010. https://www.google.com/url?sa=t&rct=j&q=&esrc=s&source=web&cd=1&cad=rja&uact=8&ved=0CB4QFjAA&url=http%3A%2F%2Fciteseerx.ist.psu.edu%2Fviewdoc%2Fdownload%3Fdoi%3D10.1.1.378.6489%26rep%3Drep1%26type%3Dpdf&ei=ZHE7Va6jEMnEgwTPyICwBw&usg=AFQjCNEWKhLPdSb1CevCMynelpPOS_q2xg&sig2=ilFnsgN3-YHAHLg0d7dvqg.
12. Census Bureau. 2012 national population projections. Washington (DC): Census Bureau. Available from: http://www.census.gov/population/projections/data/national/2012/summary-tables.html.
13. Consumer Electronics Association (CEA) report. The Connected Health and Wellness Market. Online available at: http://www.ce.org/News/News-Releases/Press-Releases/2013-Press-Releases/CEA-Releases-Report-on-Dramatic-Rise-of-Connected.aspx. Last Access 24 Apr 2015.
14. Chang H, Chou PB, Ramakrishnan S. An ecosystem approach for healthcare services cloud. IEEE international conference on e-business engineering. (ICEBE '09, Macau, China). 2009.
15. Charlson ME, Pompei P, Ales KL, Mackenzie CR. A new method of classifying prognostic comorbidity in longitudinal studies: development and validation. J Chronic Dis. 1987;40(5):373–83.
16. Chobanian AV, et al. The seventh report of the joint national committee on prevention, detection, evaluation, and treatment of high blood pressure. JAMA. 2003;289(19):2560–71.
17. Christensen C, Grossman J, Hwang J. The innovator's prescription: a disruptive solution for health care. New York: McGraw-Hill; 2008.
18. CMS, Office of the Actuary, National Health Statistics Group. National health expenditures by type of sponsor: calendar years 1987–2012. Baltimore: Centers for Medicare and Medicaid Services; 2012. Available at http://www.cms.gov/Research-Statistics-Data-and-Systems/Statistics-Trends-and-Reports/NationalHealthExpendData/Downloads/tables.pdf.

19. CMSA (Case Management Society of America). The case management adherence guidelines (CMAG-1). 2004. Retrieved 16 Oct 2004, from http://www.cmsa.org/cmag/[Context Link].
20. Collins FS, Varmus H. A new initiative on precision medicine. N Engl J Med. 2015;372:793–5.
21. Sr D'agostino RB, Vasan RS, Pencina MJ, Wolf PA, Cobain M, Massaro JM, Kannel WB. General cardiovascular risk profile for use in primary care: the Framingham Heart Study. Circulation. 2008;117(6):743–53.
22. Davenport JG, Harris TH. Competing on analytics: the new science of winning. Boston: Harvard Business School Press; 2007.
23. DCCT/EDIC (The Diabetes Control and Complications Trial/Epidemiology of Diabetes Interventions and Complications Study Research Group). Intensive diabetes treatment and cardiovascular disease in patients with type 1 diabetes. N Engl J Med. 2005;353:2643–53.
24. DiMatteo MR. Variations in patients' adherence to medical recommendations: a quantitative review of 50 years of research. Med Care. 2004;42(3):200–9.
25. De Vries H, Kremers S, Smeets T, Brug J, Eijmael K. The effectiveness of tailored feedback and action plans in an intervention addressing multiple health behaviors. Am J Health Promot. 2008;22(6):417–25.
26. Dolin RH, Alschuler L, Boyer B, Beebe C, Behlen FM, Biron PV, Shabo A. HL7 clinical document architecture, release 2. J Am Med Inform Assoc. 2006;13(1):30–9.
27. The Diabetes Prevention Program (DPP) Research Group. The Diabetes Prevention Program (DPP): description of lifestyle intervention. Diabetes Care. 2002;25(12):2165–71.
28. DPP (Diabetes Prevention Program). NIH Publication No. 09–5099, 2008, US Department of Health and Human Services. 2008.
29. Eddy D, et al. Individualized guidelines: the potential for increasing quality and reducing costs. Ann Intern Med. 2011;154:627–34.
30. Elder P, Ayala G, Harris S. Theories and intervention approaches to health-behavior change in primary care. Am J Prev Med. 1999;17(4):275–84.
31. Elixhauser A, Steiner C, Harris R, Coffey R. Comorbidity measures for use with administrative data. Med Care. 1998;36(1):8–27.
32. FDA report. Mobile medication applications: guidance for industry and food and drug administration staff. 2015a. http://www.fda.gov/downloads/MedicalDevices/DeviceRegulationand Guidance/GuidanceDocuments/UCM263366.pdf.
33. FDA report. Medical device data systems, medical image storage devices, and medical image communications devices: guidance for industry and food and drug administration staff. 2015b. http://www.fda.gov/ucm/groups/fdagov-public/@fdagov-meddev-gen/documents/document/ucm401996.pdf.
34. Gonzalez V, Goeppinger J, Lorig K. Four psychosocial theories and their application to patient education and clinical practice. Arthritis Care Res. 1990;3:132–43.
35. Goodman C. Comparative effectiveness research and personalized medicine: from contradiction to synergy. In: Lewin Group Report prepared for the conference of comparative effectiveness research and personalized medicine: Policy, Science, and Business, National Pharmaceutical Council and Personalized Medicine Coalition, Falls Church, VA. 2009.
36. Grol R. Improving the quality of medical care. JAMA. 2001;286(20):2578–85.
37. Grundy SM, et al. Detection, evaluation, and treatment of high blood cholesterol in adults (adult treatment panel III). In: The Third Report of the National Cholesterol Education Program (NCEP) expert panel. Circulation. 2002:17;106(25):3143–421.
38. Hirst W. Connected health and the rise of the patient-consumer. Health Aff. 2014;33(2):191–3.
39. Hsueh P, Lin R, Hsiao J, Zeng L, Ramakrishnan S, Chang H. Cloud-based platform for personalization in a wellness management ecosystem: why, what, and how. IEEE international conference of collaborative computing. Chicago, IL, 201.
40. Hsueh P, Lan C, Deng V, Zhu X. From clinical requirement to personalized wellness decision support: a data-driven framework for computer-supported guideline refinement. Proceedings of the 24th European Medical Informatics Conference (MIE 2012). 2012a.

41. Hsueh P, Grandison T, Zhu X, Pai H, Chang H. Challenges and requirements on privacy in enabling evidence use service on wellness cloud, frontiers in service conference. 2012b.
42. Hsueh PS, Marschollek M, Peres Y, von Cavallar S, Martin Sanchez FJ. Gap analysis of insight-driven personalized health services through patient-controlled devices. MIE 2014 Workshop, Istanbul.
43. Ho PM, Bryson LC, Rumsfeld SJ. Medication adherence: its importance in cardiovascular outcomes. Circulation. 2009;119:3028–35.
44. Huang X, Liu Y, Chen K, Shin WJ, Lu CJ, Kong GW, Patnaik D, Lee SH, Cortes JF, Rogers JA. Stretchable, wireless sensors and functional substrates for epidermal characterization of sweat. Small. 2014;10(15):3083–90.
45. Grandison T, Hsueh P, Zeng L, Chang H. Privacy protection issues for healthcare wellness clouds. Chapter 10. In Privacy Protection Measures and Technologies in Business Organizations (Ed. GOM Yee), IGI Global, Hershey, PA, 2011.
46. Hood L, Friend SH. Predictive, personalized, preventive, participatory (P4) cancer medicine. Nat Rev Clin Oncol. 2011;8:184–7.
47. Irigaray P, et al. Lifestyle-related factors and environmental agents causing cancer: an overview. Biomed Pharmacother. 2007;61(10):640–58.
48. IMS Institute for health care Informatics. 2012. Press Releases. Available at: http://www.ims-research.com/news-events/presstemplate.php?pr_id=2743.
49. IMS Institute for health care Informatics. Avoidable costs in U.S. health care: the $200 billion opportunity from using medicines more responsibly. 2013. Available at: http://www.imshealth.com/deployedfiles/imshealth/Global/Content/Corporate/IMS%20Institute/RUOM-2013/IHII_Responsible_Use_Medicines_2013.pdf. Accessed 10 Oct 2014.
50. JDRF (The Juvenile Diabetes Research Foundation Continuous Glucose Monitoring Study Group). Continuous glucose monitoring and intensive treatment of type 1 diabetes. N Engl J Med. 2008;359:1–13.
51. Kansagara D, Englander H, Salanitro A, Kagen D, Theobald C, Freeman M, Kripalani S. Risk prediction models for hospital readmission: a systematic review. JAMA. 2011:19;306(15):1688–98.
52. Kuper H, Marmot M. Job strain, job demands, decision latitude, and risk of coronary heart disease within the Whitehall II study. J Epidemiol Community Health. 2003;57(2):147–53.
53. Lloyd-Jones DM, et al. Cardiovascular risk prediction: basic concepts, current status, and future directions. Circulation. 2010;121:1768–77.
54. Lopez-Meyer P, Tiffancy S, Patil Y, Sazonov E. Monitoring of cigarette smoking using wearable sensors and support vector machines. IEEE Trans Biomed Eng. 2013;60(7):1867–72.
55. Luga AO, McGuire MJ. Adherence and health care costs. Risk Manag Healthc Policy. 2014;7:35–44.
56. Macknight C, Rockwood K. Use of the chronic disease score to measure comorbidity in the Canadian Study of Health and Aging. Int Psychogeriatr. 2001;13(Supp 1):137–42.
57. Maetzlera W, Domingosc J, Srulijesa K, Ferreirac JJ, Bloemd BR. Quantitative wearable sensors for objective assessment of PD. Mov Disord. 2013;28(12):1628–37.
58. Marmot MG, Rose G, Shipley M, Hamilton PJ. Employment grade and coronary heart disease in British civil servants. J Epidemiol Community Health. 1978;32(4):244–9.
59. Mayo Clinics Shared Decision Making resource center. Available at http://shareddecisions.mayoclinic.org/resources/general-resources/.
60. Mcglynn EA, Asch SM, Kerr EA. Quality of health care delivered to adults in the United States – Reply. N Engl J Med. 2003;349:1867–8.
61. Misra V, Bhansali S, Muth J, Jackson T, Lach J. NSF Nanosystems Engineering Research Center for Advanced Self-Powered Systems of Integrated Sensors and Technologies (ASSIST). Available at: http://www.nsf.gov/awardsearch/showAward?AWD_ID=1160483&HistoricalAwards=false.

62. Moore JH, Asselbergs FW, Williams SM. Bioinformatics challenges for genome-wide association studies. Bioinformatics. 2010;26(4):445–55.
63. Mori M, et al. Genetic basis of inter-individual variability in the effects of exercise on the alleviation of lifestyle-related diseases. J Physiol. 2009;587(23):5577–84.
64. Mcginnis JM, Williams-Russo P, Knickman JR. The case for more active policy attention to health promotion. Health Aff. 2002;21(2):78–93.
65. Müller M, Kersten S. Nutrigenomics: goals and perspectives. Nat Rev Genet. 2003;4:315–22.
66. Pan XR, et al. Effects of diet and exercise in preventing NIDDM in people with impaired glucose tolerance. The Da Qing IGT and Diabetes Study. Diabetes Care. 1997;20(4):537–44.
67. Patel S, Mancinelli C, Bonato P, Healey J, Moy M. Using wearable sensors to monitor physical activities of patients with COPD: a comparison of classifier performance. IEEE workshop on wearable and implantable body sensor networks. 2009, Berkeley, CA. p. 234–39.
68. Peikes D, Zutshi A, Genevro J, Smith K, Parchman M, Meyers D. Early evidence on the patient-centered medical home. Final report (prepared by Mathematica Policy Research, under Contract Nos. HHSA290200900019I/HHSA29032002T and HHSA290200900019I/HHSA29032005T). AHRQ Publication No. 12-0020-EF. Rockville: Agency for Healthcare Research and Quality; 2012.
69. Pierre Y. The healthcare imperative: lowering costs and improving outcomes: workshop series summary. Washington DC: The National Academies Press; 2010. p. 141–74.
70. PricewaterhouseCooper report. Consumer intelligence series: the wearable future. Online available at: http://www.pwc.com/us/en/industry/entertainment-media/publications/consumer-intelligence-series/. Last access 24 Apr 2015.
71. Pharmaceutical Group of the EU Staff. Targeting adherence: improving patient outcomes in Europe through community pharmacists' intervention adherence. PGEU policy statement on adherence to medicines. 2008.
72. Pritchard JK. Are rare variants responsible for susceptibility to complex diseases? Am J Hum Genet. 2001;69(1):124–37.
73. Prochaska JO, Diclemente CC, Norcross JC. In search of how people change. Am Psychol. 1992;47(9):1102–14.
74. Roche HM. Nutrigenomics—new approaches for human nutrition research. J Sci Food Agric. 2006;86(8):1156–63.
75. Saaristo T, Peltonen M, Keinanen-Kiukaanniemi S, Vanhala M, Saltevo J, Niskanen L, Oksa H, Korpi-Hyovalti E, Tuomilehto J. National type 2 diabetes prevention programme in Finland: FIN-D2D. Int J Circumpolar Health. 2007;66:101–12.
76. Burke SD, Sherr D, Lipman RD. Partnering with diabetes educators to improve patient outcomes. Diabetes Metab Syndr Obes. 2014;7:45–53.
77. Sloan KL, et al. Construction and characteristics of the RxRisk-V: a VA-adapted pharmacy-based case-mix instrument. Med Care. 2003;41(6):761–74.
78. Solomon DH, Schneeweiss S, Glynn RJ, Kiyota Y, Levin R, Mogun H, Avorn J. Relationship between selective cyclooxygenase-2 inhibitors and acute myocardial infarction in older adults. Circulation. 2004;109(17):2068–73.
79. Schaefer C, et al. The Kaiser permanente research program on genes, environment and health: a resource for genetic epidemiology in adult health and aging. In: Proceedings of 17th annual HMO research network conference, Boston, 2011.
80. Schroeder SA. We can do better — improving the health of the American people. N Engl J Med. 2007;357(12):1221–8.
81. Scott CT, Caulfield T, Borgelt E, Illes J. Personal medicine—the new banking crisis. Nat Biotechnol. 2012;30:141–7.
82. Sherman BW, Chris B. Beyond incentives: the impact of health care reform on employer population health management strategies. Popul Health Manag. 2014;17(2):67–70.
83. Thorisson GA, Smith AV, Krishnan L, Stein LD. The international HapMap project web site. Genome Res. 2005;15(11):1592–3.

84. Tuomilehto J, et al. Prevention of type II diabetes mellitus by changes in lifestyle among subjects with impaired glucose tolerance. N Engl J Med. 2001;344(18):1343–50.
85. Turner RC, et al. Risk factors for coronary artery disease in non-insulin dependent diabetes mellitus: United Kingdom prospective diabetes study. Br Med J. 1998;316:823.
86. UKPDS Group. Intensive blood-glucose control with sulphonylureas or insulin compared with conventional treatment and risk of complications in patients with type 2 diabetes (UKPDS 33). UK Prospective Diabetes Study (UKPDS) Group. Lancet. 1998;352:837–53.
87. van Setten M, Pokraev S, Koolwaaij J. Context-aware recommendations in the mobile tourist application COMPASS. In: Nejdl W, De Bra P, editors. Lecture notes of computer science, vol 3137. Springer, Eindhoven, The Netherlands, 2004. p. 235–44.
88. Volk RJ, Llewellyn-Thomas H, Stacey D, Elwyn G. Ten years of the International Patient Decision Aid Standards Collaboration: evolution of the core dimensions for assessing the quality of patient decision aids. BMC Med Inform Decis Making. 2013;13 Suppl 2:S1.
89. Webb TL, Joseph J, Yardley L, Michie S. Using the internet to promote health behavior change: a systematic review and meta-analysis of the impact of theoretical basis, use of behavior change techniques, and mode of delivery on efficacy. J Med Internet Res. 2010;12(1):e4. doi:10.2196/jmir.1376.
90. Welltok caféwell concierge introduction. 2015. Available at: http://welltok.com/solutions/cafewell-concierge.html.
91. Zimmermann A, Specht M, Lorenz A. Personalization and context management. User Model User-Adap Inter. 2006;15(3–4):275–302.
92. Wilcox G. Insulin and insulin resistance. Clin Biochem Rev. 2005;26(2):19–39.
93. Stampfer MJ, Hu FB, Manson JE, RimmEB, Willett WC. Primary prevention of coronary heart disease in women through diet and lifestyle. N Engl J Med 2000;343:16-22.

# Chapter 22
# Wearable Technologies and Telehealth in Care Management for Chronic Illness

**Xinxin Zhu and Amos Cahan**

**Abstract** Telehealth is the use of technology for remote patient monitoring and care. Wearables are small electronic devices that can seamlessly collect data about a patient for prolonged periods of time and support the implementation of telemedicine in the patient's natural environment. In a reality where patients are becoming older and sicker, medicine is becoming more and more a multidisciplinary team work and healthcare resources are limited, telehealth holds promise as a way to improve patient care while cutting on costs. It may improve coordination between care providers, allow for bringing top notch expertise to remote, rural settings, provide a more complete picture of the patient's condition and support independent living of the elderly and patients with chronic diseases. In this chapter, we review some of the related technology and application and portrait how they may be integrated in the near future in the healthcare delivery system.

**Keywords** Wearable • Sensor • Telehealth • Chronic condition • Care management

## 22.1 Outline

After presenting the medical, technological and financial context for the rise of telehealth in Sect. 22.2, we will introduce the (sometimes ambiguous or overlapping) main terms and concepts in this domain in Sect. 22.3. Section 22.4 will explore the roles of telehealth in delivering healthcare and the potential held by wearable devices in facilitating telehealth use. In Sect. 22.5 we illustrate the use of telehealth

X. Zhu, MD, PhD (✉)
Department of Healthcare Informatics, IBM T.J. Watson Research Center,
Yorktown Heights, NY, USA
e-mail: zhux@us.ibm.com

A. Cahan, MD
Research Staff, IBM T.J. Watson Research Center, Yorktown Heights, NY, USA
e-mail: acahan@us.ibm.com

technologies in a few real-world applications. Section 22.6 elaborates on challenges that implementation of telehealth faces, and Sect. 22.7 offers a glimpse into the near future of wearables. We conclude this chapter in Sect. 22.8.

## 22.2 Introduction

### 22.2.1 Wearables Revolutionize the Capture of Clinical Data

Traditionally, medicine was practiced at the presence of the physician, either at the patient's home, in the clinic or hospital. This was because the tools used for diagnosis and treatment were sparse, expensive and manually-operated. With the advent of technology, some diagnostic and therapeutic procedures could be performed automatically or by other professionals (e.g., lab technicians). These allowed for the concept of patient monitoring to develop.

Yet, even today, most of the clinical data is collected in the clinic- be it the physician's office or an inpatient ward. Enormous amounts of patient-related data such as temperature, heart rate, blood pressure and blood oxygen saturation are captured and stored. These data may be used for secondary analysis, to leverage insights on disease characterization and progression, improving prediction of future events and supporting individualized care. However, the data captured in the clinic settings does not necessarily reflect the patient's condition in other setting such as at home or at work. For example, a patient's blood pressure measured at the physician's office may systematically differ from that taken outside the clinic. Moreover, clinical (diagnostic and therapeutic) decision points are limited to times when new data is available. Since data is collected on a periodic basis, often with long intervals between observations, opportunities to react to changes in a patient's condition are limited.

Indeed, several monitoring devices are widely available for home use. These include blood pressure monitors, simple EKG devices and pulse oximeters, to mention some. However, continuous monitoring using such devices is impractical and rarely done. A few monitoring systems that allow for continuous outpatient data collection are available (e.g. Holter test, ambulatory blood pressure monitoring) but these are cumbersome, expensive and are used for short, infrequent monitoring sessions. Moreover, interpretation of the data collected by such devices requires expertise and is not commonly done in real time.

Recent years have brought about the ubiquitous use of smartphones and wireless connectivity (e.g., WiFi and Bluetooth technologies). Enabling this revolution in part was the development of various small and cheap sensors and transmitters. As computers have become closely intertwined with our daily life, it was only natural for gadgets based on such technology to be introduced, that can be carried around continuously and interact with computers and with one another. Wearable technology has emerged and it is growing fast.

For the most, commercially available wearables target the wellness market. Heart rate sensors continuously monitor pulse, whereas motion sensors and accelerometers are used to count steps and minutes of sleep. Wearables are frequently integrated with smartphone and personal computer applications that allow for review of the recorded data as well as for capturing of other types of data (e.g., caloric intake). Such applications often provide recommendations related to wellness maintenance including diet and exercise.

Strict regulations enforced by the FDA and other governmental agencies, higher development costs and liability concerns have kept medical wearables lagging behind. Yet the healthcare ecosystem is undergoing tremendous changes which are likely to turn wearables into an integral and important component of patient care in the next few years.

## 22.2.2 Medical, Economic and Social Factors Are Driving the Development of Telehealth and Wearable Systems

### 22.2.2.1 Chronic Patients Are Increasing in Number and Require Costly Care

Healthcare costs are constantly rising. Sophisticated imaging techniques and advanced therapeutics offer hope to patients whose diseases have previously been beyond cure. The successes of modern medicine in prolonging life are leading to more and more patients living with chronic conditions for many years. The population is aging, and Baby Boomers are gradually entering the eighth decade of life, further increasing the burden on the healthcare system. As medicine is growing in knowledge and expertise, patients are becoming more complex. The traditional model of a "village doctor" has been replaced by a multidisciplinary team of care providers, including physicians of various specialties, nurses, physical therapists, psychologists, social workers, pharmacists, nutrition consultants and others. Their coordinated actions are essential in achieving therapeutic goals.

Chronic patients consume a large volume of medical services. The United States alone spent \$2.8 trillion on health care in 2012 [12], with more than 75 % of these expenditures directed toward the treatment of patients with chronic diseases [45]. Chronic diseases—such as diabetes, cardiovascular disease, chronic obstructive pulmonary disease, and cancer—are persistent or recurring, and frequently debilitating conditions that require prolonged care. Due to their fluctuating nature, effective management of chronic diseases requires frequent follow up and treatment adjustments. Good control of chronic conditions may reduce morbidity and mortality. Adherence issues play a major part in achieving good control over chronic conditions, as patients have to be active monitoring measures such as blood glucose or weight and persistent in taking their medications. Patients are required to keep a log of their home measurements, to help their doctor have a better understanding of their day to day condition, but keeping such records is very demanding and many of them fail to do this.

### 22.2.2.2  Technologic Solutions Are Part of the Attempt to Contain Healthcare Costs

In light of the increasing burden of healthcare costs, ways to provide good medical care at reduced costs are vigorously sought. The understanding that better coordination between healthcare agencies and practitioners is required has contributed to the Meaningful Use Act, which drives the computation of health records and information communication between providers. Adaptation of a "pay by performance" model is increasing the incentives for stakeholders to prevent diseases rather than perform procedures. Attempts are made to shorten hospitalizations and reduce readmission rates. As it turns, this new model aligns medical and financial incentives.

Telehealth and wearable technology offer tools that are a natural fit to the new healthcare model demands. Sensors used to continuously capture and record patient data provide a more complete, real-time understanding of the patient's condition. Combining such sensors systems with advanced analytic tools and audiovisual communication may turn the collected data to actionable knowledge to enable better care at reduced costs while maintaining independent living and improved quality of life to the elderly and to patients with chronic diseases. With telehealth, care providers can utilize communication technologies to provide education, assess patients, supervise procedures, and monitor patients with chronic conditions at home. Telehealth for patients with chronic disease can not only improve symptom management, but also provides an avenue to assess and improve compliance and adherence to prescribed regimens of care.

### 22.2.2.3  Cost Effectiveness of Telehealth

Expansive promises have been made about the potential role of telehealth in reducing healthcare expenditure. For example, Cusack et al. [16] modeled cost savings of $4.3 billion a year if telehealth were implemented to facilitate consultations between healthcare providers in the USA, and this is without considering savings associated with the provision of care direct to the patient. However, demonstrating the effect of telehealth on costs in real world settings is challenging, and in fact, no valid answer exists. This is due to the marked and multidimensional variability between studied applications, the continuous and rapid progress in the field as well as methodological flaws in published studies. Recently, Bergmo [6] reviewed the quality of economic evaluations in telemedicine, reporting highly diverse evaluations, many of which did not adhere to standard economic evaluation techniques. Specifically, statistical, sensitivity, and marginal analyses, and information on the perspective of the studies were often lacking. Whereas this review pointed out methodological deficiencies, it did not aim to draw conclusions about the cost-effectiveness of telemedicine.

Here we bring a few examples of cost effectiveness studies summarized by Wade et al. [49] to illustrate their strengths and limitations. A review of tele-health provision of accident and emergency support to primary care found several studies with utility analysis, all indicating cost-effectiveness; however it concluded that the case was far from proven [10]. Two reviews of telepsychiatry concluded that cost-effectiveness could not be demonstrated because the volume of consulting was too low [34, 37], while a third review reported conflicting evidence of both increased and decreased costs [19]. A review of the use of tele-health in intensive care units found two clinical trials reporting cost savings [15]. Paré et al. [40] conducted a number of reviews on home care for chronic disease and reported that very few detailed economic analyses had been done, leading to no confirmation of economic viability. Applied to heart failure patients, home monitoring reduced costs of hospital admissions [31] in one study, and in another, despite initial excess costs, substantial long term cost savings were found [47].

## 22.3 Definitions

### 22.3.1 Telehealth

The Health Resources Services Administration defines telehealth as the use of electronic information and telecommunications technologies to support long-distance clinical health care, patient and professional health-related education (e.g., continuing medical education), and public health and health administration [21]. Through telehealth technology, medical practitioners are able to evaluate and diagnose patients remotely, prescribe treatment, e-prescribe medications, and quickly detect fluctuations in the patient's medical condition at home, to be able to alter therapy or medications accordingly. Under the general scope of telehealth are include *telemedicine*, i.e., remote doctor-patient consultations, and *telecare*, referring to the remote monitoring of vital signs and other health condition metrics, and patient assessment (Fig. 22.1). Telehealth technologies include videoconferencing, the internet, store-and-forward imaging, streaming media, and terrestrial and wireless communications. Based on timing of communication, two types of telehealth systems are defined:

- Real-Time Interactive Systems (Synchronous) telehealth: requires the presence of both parties at the same time and a communication link between them that allows a real-time interaction to take place. Video-conferencing equipment is one of the most common forms of technologies used in synchronous telehealth. There are also peripheral devices that can be attached to computers or the video-conferencing equipment which can aid in an interactive examination.

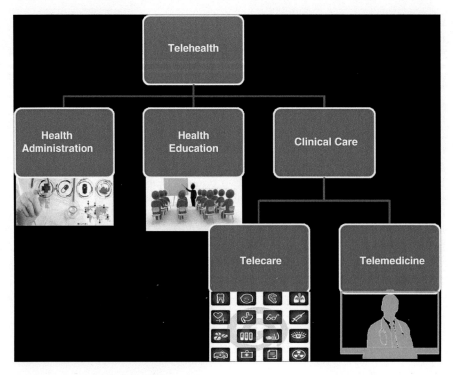

**Fig. 22.1** Components of telehealth

- Store-and-Forward (Asynchronous) telehealth: involves acquiring medical data (like medical images, biosignals, voice recordings, etc.) and then transmitting this data to a doctor or medical specialist at a convenient time for assessment offline. It does not require both parties to be available at the same time

## 22.3.2 Telecare

Telecare uses remote monitoring of patients to receive alerts about real-time emergencies and to track lifestyle changes over time. Telecare is managed through the use of telecommunications technology including telephones, computers and mobile monitoring devices such as warden alarms, automatic gas shut-off devices and home entry videophones. Telecare allows patients to stay safe and independent in their own homes. The concept of remote patient monitoring (RPM) relates to medical applications of telecare, utilizing information and communication technology (ICT) to deliver health services at a distance. RPM includes the collection of disease-specific metrics from biomedical devices used by patients in their homes or other settings outside of a clinical facility. RPM systems typically collect patient readings and then transmit them to a remote server for storage and later examination by healthcare professionals. Once available on the server, the readings can be used in numerous ways by home health agencies, clinicians, and informal care providers.

### 22.3.3 Telemedicine

Telemedicine is a subtype of telehealth defined as the use of electronic communications and information technologies to provide clinical services to patients in locations and times other than where the care provider is present. While telehealth can refer to remote non-clinical services, telemedicine refers specifically to the provision of health care services and education over a distance through the use of telecommunications technology. Examples of telemedicine include video consultations with specialists, remote medical evaluations and diagnoses and the digital transmission of medical imaging.

### 22.3.4 Mobile Health, Wearable Technologies

Broadly and somewhat loosely viewed, a wearable sensor is typically a small electronic device located in proximity to, or implanted within, the body of a user, which can transduce information related to the user or their ambient environment. Wearable sensors (commonly referred to as "wearables") use various technologies to capture physical or chemical signals [42].

Some wearable sensors have been used for decades. These include home blood pressure monitors, glucose sensors and pulse oximeters (measuring blood oxygen saturation). Most of these are stand-alone devices that perform on-demand measurements. Some of the newer ones can keep a log of results or communicate them to a personal computer application. Event-triggered devices include, for example, implantable cardiac pacemakers equipped with loop recorders to capture episodes of arrhythmia, or home apnea monitors for infants.

However, the wearable technology revolution now offers much more sophisticated designs. These rely on miniaturized sensors, with some at the micro- and even nano- scale being developed. For instance, off-the-shelf millimeter-scale products with a triaxial accelerometer, a gyroscope and magnetometer are currently commercially available and widely used in gadgets [42].

Wearables use sensors that transduce various types of signals to electric impulses. They can be classified by their location, the technology they use or the determinants they monitor (Table 22.1). A general distinction can be made between physical and chemical sensors. Physical sensors measure vital signs such as heart rate, blood pressure and temperature, but also activity (e.g., movement, and location). Chemical sensors monitor the concentration of substances in or on our body (known

**Table 22.1** A classification of parameters associated with wearable systems features and capabilities

| Determinant | Type [examples] |
|---|---|
| Location | External (Apple Watch (Apple Inc.), Samsung Gear (Samsung Inc), fitbit bracelet (Fitbit Inc.), tattoos) |
| | Implanted- usually embedded in another implantable medical device [cardiac pacemaker, Implantable cardioverter-defibrillator, cardiac resynchronization therapy] |
| Sensing type | Physical (heart rate, blood pressure, respiratory rate, peak-flow, oxygen saturation, body movement, speech, pupil diameter, electrodermal activity, speech) |
| | Chemical (glucose, sodium, potassium, lactate, pH) |
| Power supply | Battery- rechargeable (including wireless charging) or replaceable |
| | Energy scavenging/harvesting (using mechanical movement, vibration or heat) |
| Configuration | Stand alone |
| | Coupled with an external device (smartphone, laptop) |
| Data storage | Store on device memory and/or transmit to other devices for storage |
| Transmission technology | Wired (uncommon) |
| | Wireless (radio frequency, bluetooth) |
| Transmission frequency | Continuous |
| | Scheduled: at predetermined intervals |
| | On-demand: user activated |
| | Triggered: such as by signals from other sensors |
| Data analysis | Local- integral (within the device) |
| | Local-external (e.g. on a smartphone) |
| | Remote (on the cloud) |
| Data clients | User |
| | Care provider |
| | Hotline |
| Notification- content and scope | All data collected |
| | Interpretation of raw data, such as in the form of outstanding values, summaries or alerts |
| Guidance/advice | None |
| | Local- relying on an adjunct device such as a smartphone |
| | Remote- web-dependent |
| Therapy administration | User supervised/facilitated (patient-controlled analgesia) |
| | Autonomous-closed loop (bionic pancreas) |

as biosensors). This is commonly done using an electrochemical sensor. The measured substance (analyte) attaches to a receptor (e.g. an antibody) and a physico-chemical transducer then generates an electric signal that is proportionate to the substance concentration. While attractive, this approach faces some challenges, including low sensitivity at low substance concentration and limited long term resilience [4]. Other technologies, particularly using spectroscopy are being adapted to wearable devices and avoid the need for using a receptor.

Smart fabrics are made with conductive material which allows for sensors to be embedded in textile (e-textile). These provide convenience of use while performing continuous monitoring, facilitated by a wide contact area with the body.

Body area networks (BAN) are formed by an array of sensors that measure various physiological parameters [17]. BAN's, aka Smart Wearable Systems (SWS) [27] use wireless technology such as radio frequency (RFID) or Bluetooth for communicating captured data. Data collected can be stored and transmitted to a local microprocessor (in a smartphone or personal computer) or to a distant server for analysis. Information can then be made available to the user or a care provider (Fig. 22.2). If a need for immediate action is detected by the system, the user and/or a care provider may be alerted, and interim advice may be provided independently by the system. Coupling sensing with decision rules or artificial intelligence may be used to autonomously control the administration of therapeutics in closed loop systems. Many concerns are associated with this idea, however a working Bionic Pancreas, coupling continuous glucose sensing and insulin administration has been recently evaluated in patients with type-1 diabetes in a clinical trial [44]. SWS are most commonly noninvasive, although implantable systems are also being developed. Novel ways to power such devices, including miniature batteries, wireless charging using induction, and ways to use energy harvested from the sensor's environment are explored [32]. Table 22.1 lists the different levels of capabilities offered by wearables.

## 22.4   Impact of Telehealth and Wearables

### 22.4.1   Telehealth Supports a Healthier Healthcare System

The advantages offered by telehealth are multifold, and all of the healthcare system stakeholders may benefit from its use:

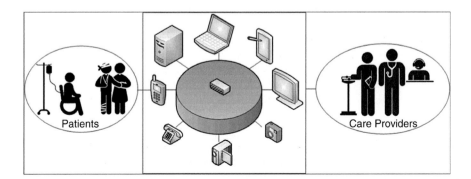

**Fig. 22.2** Communication networking of mobile telehealth systems

- **Patients** may achieve better access through telehealth to specialists who can apply higher standards of care associated with their clinical discipline, avoiding long distance travel. With the ability to better manage their health situations at home using remote monitoring, patients can remain closer to the support network of family and friends to avoid unnecessary admissions or delay readmissions.
- In **outreach clinics**, telehealth services enable clinical staff to better cope with challenging diagnostic and therapeutic questions arising during patient care by having real time access to specialist support networks. Easy access and geographical convenience offered by widespread outreach clinics can help attract clients, as well as improve patients' adherence to appointments and treatment. The ability of outreach clinics to retain patients rather than transfer them to another facility or possibly out of their health system altogether has the potential to improve care continuity and coordination.
- **Consulting physicians** may extend their clinical reach to a wider range of patients who can benefit from their expertise. They can save the time lost traveling between facilities to see patients, and increase their productivity.
- **Payers** may reduce expenditures by optimizing the use of specialist resources. For example, remote consultation may save unnecessary transfers, admissions or readmissions, and reduce length of stay. In addition, timely access to physicians with right expertise may help optimize care and reduce the risk for costly complications.
- Telehealth can be beneficial to the **healthcare system** as a whole by providing tools to cope with the growing shortage of physicians, delaying the need to provide nursing home services to elderly and chronic patients, and shortening the lifecycle needed for new practices and guidelines to be implemented in the community setting. Overall costs can be reduced by telehealth through more comprehensive preventive and early stage care rather than having to face patients with conditions complicated by delayed medical intervention.

### 22.4.2   Wearables Power the Widespread Use of Telehealth Services

Wearable systems provide better data on patients. Quantitatively, they can capture much more data; a sensor is used on a single patient and does not have to be shared with others, so it can be used to monitor the patient continuously for prolonged periods of time. Moreover, data is collected in the patient's natural environment, not only in a designated point in time and space. As such, it is of higher clinical quality or utility since it better reflects the patient's true condition.

Improved data collection means not only better understanding of a single patient's disease characteristics and course, but also, in the aggregate, better understanding of conditions at the population level. Coupled with advanced analytics, data capture by wearable devices may generate insights that could transform the way in which diseases are diagnosed and managed.

### 22.4.2.1 Diagnosis

Widespread use of sensor systems among healthy individuals offers a potential to diagnose conditions before patients actively seek medical advice and even before they are symptomatic. Take for instance silent cardiac ischemia, a condition wherein impaired blood supply to the heart is not accompanied by chest pain. This condition is easily missed unless specifically sought. ECG changes consistent with ischemia may be captured by wellness wearable devices during physical exercise and prompt performing additional tests to exclude or establish ischemic heart disease.

Wearables may be useful in diagnosing other conditions as well. Continuous home monitoring of blood pressure could more efficiently identify conditions such as white coat hypertension (abnormally high clinic blood pressure with normal out-of-clinic readings) and masked hypertension (normal readings in the clinic that mask hypertension in other settings).

Importantly, wearables can provide useful data in real time. A commonly performed test in traditional medicine is the Holter test, which is used to capture episodes of arrhythmia (abnormal heart rhythm) by continuously monitoring ECG in the outpatient setting for 24–48 h. The ECG is recorded and stored in the memory of the device. When the test is completed, the device is returned to the clinic and a physician reviews the data stored on it. If there is an episode of arrhythmia during the test, it would only be detected days or even weeks after it had occurred. In some cases, immediate intervention to control potentially fatal (and sometimes asymptomatic) arrhythmia may be indicated, and so real time detection of abnormalities may be life-saving. Smart Wearable Systems offer the ability to capture and transmit data from monitors in real-time, as has been used in Remote-ICU (intensive care unit) programs [11].

Sensors can be used in the patient environment to collect data without even touching the body. Although not truly wearables, wall-mounted motion detectors installed in a patient's home may be used to detect changes in patients' behavioral patterns potentially indicative of an arising or aggravating health problem.

### 22.4.2.2 Management

SWS engage patients in managing their own conditions by making them aware of their state without requiring them to invest time in measuring and documenting the monitored attributes. They allow care providers to be kept updated about their patients' condition, giving them the opportunity to follow up on their recommendations in a fast and flexible way, and facilitate effective communication between patients and providers. Close home monitoring may allow for earlier hospital discharge, as well as for timely measures to be taken to avoid readmission. Monitoring can provide reassurance to elderly persons living alone and their families. Their input can be used to optimize a treatment protocol to achieve better disease control, so as to anticipate events and address them preemptively. As part of an integrative outpatient care program framework, better patient data can be used to prioritize interventions. Moreover, ongoing monitoring of patients, dynamic evaluation of their needs and flexible allocation of resources to meet them may enable healthcare systems to cope with increasing needs and ever-limited funding. Such enhanced monitoring capabilities utilized in advanced care models may be able to delay the need for institutionalization and improve the quality of life of persons living independently.

## 22.5  Real-World Applications on Telehealth and Smart Wearable Systems

There is an almost infinite number of potential applications for telemedicine using SWS. In this section, we bring a few examples of solutions that have been developed and clinically evaluated.

### 22.5.1  At-Home Monitoring of Patients with Heart Failure

Patients with heart failure tend to be complex, commonly having comorbidities and taking multiple medications. In the course of heart failure, exacerbations may manifest as fatigue and shortness of breath, sometimes severe enough to lead to respiratory failure. Patients with heart failure are required to maintain a strict diet and monitor their weight frequently as a marker of fluid retention. Sensors embedded in implantable devices such as cardiac pacemakers and implantable cardioverter-defibrillators have been developed, that can measure heart rate and heart rate variability, EKG, patient mobility and intra-thoracic impedance. Their use has been demonstrated to improve the prediction of heart failure decompensation at home, which may allow for preventive measures to be taken. A trial in which a pressure sensor was implanted in the left atrium of the heart of patients with severe heart failure and used to support patient self-management by titration of medications reported a reduced risk of acute decompensation or death compared to the control group reviewed in [14].

### 22.5.2  Early Detection and Management of Atrial Fibrillation

A program in which EKG streams were transmitted by cardiac pacemakers routinely to a medical team showed improved early detection of arrhythmia (atrial fibrillation) that affected patient management [43]. The European Union-funded MobiGuide project developed an intelligent decision-support system for patients with chronic illnesses, including atrial fibrillation. Wearable sensors monitor heart rate and blood pressure and transmit data wirelessly to the patient's smartphone, and through it to a back-end server. A decision support framework that can access the patient's medical records analyzes the data streams and uses clinical practice guidelines adapted to be computer-interpretable to reach management recommendation. The system can interact with the patient to collect additional information and prompt alerts to the patient and to caregivers. Advice is personalized to meet the patient's circumstances (e.g. living alone). A limited set of off-line decision support tools is also available through the mobile device [33].

### 22.5.3 Automatic Detection of Fall Among the Elderly

Falls occur yearly in one third of adults older than 65. Apart from potentially serious injuries inflicted by falls, fear of fall is common and adversely affects quality of life [25]. Half of the patients falling are unable to get up, resulting sometimes in a "prolonged lie", which carries medical and psychological consequences. Patients with impaired cognitive function are at increased risk of fall and may not even be able to activate a user-operated wearable panic alarm device [7]. Wearable sensor-based applications to detect falls are usually based on accelerometers. Real life evidence for their effectiveness is limited, perhaps due to the low frequency of falls, and reported performance measurements based on simulated falls may be overly optimistic [3]. A comprehensive review on automatic fall detection has been recently published [39].

### 22.5.4 Mental Health Monitoring Applications

Assessing the level of stress is commonly done using markers of increased tone of the autonomic sympathetic nervous system (e.g., heart rate, heart rate variability, and electrodermal activity). Attempts to capture electroencephalogram (EEG) streams to assess cognitive and mental function are also made. Speech analysis, using semantics or on patterns of speech flow have been able to detect thought disturbances [35]. The European PSYCHE project couples e-textile and smartphones in the outpatient mental patient environment for long-term (day and night) recording of physiological and clinical parameters, including voice recording. It aims to detect and eventually predict mood changes in those patients, directing preemptive interventions to be carried out [23].

## 22.6 Challenges

### 22.6.1 Information Challenges in Telehealth Applications

The amount of health data collected from patients is growing rapidly and the volume of which can be overwhelming. A telehealth system using biomedical devices or video conference tools to generate, collect, and transfer patients' health data presents challenging requirements in the area of content management and system capacity.

- **Scalability**: Millions of patients suffering from chronic conditions are the potential clients of telehealth systems. Such systems are required to scale to support large numbers of patients and their associated care providers while adhering to proper identity matching when managing patients and their associated devices and data streams.
- **Interoperability**: to ensure effective and efficient delivery of health care and maintain transparency regarding care quality and pricing, any new telehealth system development or acquisition faces the challenge of using a wide range of health information exchange standards and protocols, to the greatest extent possible. Interoperability and certification standards are important but take time to develop and are constantly evolving. Among many efforts, one notable initiative is the eHealth Exchange, formerly known as the Nationwide Health Information Network (NwHIN), developed under the auspices of the U.S. Office of the National Coordinator for Health Information Technology (ONC), and now managed by a non-profit industry coalition called HealtheWay [38].
- **Reliability**: As the complexity of telehealth function increases, there is a higher demand on network bandwidth and reliability. While patient access to online electronic medical record or Web-based health information requires lower bandwidth, clinical video conferencing or image streaming can pose a greater challenge in terms of system infrastructure support. Patients may be at home or travel to places where network connectivity is poor. Even in the face of network failures, the system should collect, cache, or store patient data for later transmission to the back-end system to avoid data loss.
- **Privacy and security**: The U.S. Congress has passed the Health Insurance Portability and Accountability Act (HIPAA) [18] to improve the efficiency of electronic health record systems while protecting patients' rights by reducing instances of information fraud and abuse. Medical privacy and confidentiality issues involved in the telehealth industry may be extremely complex. When communicating with patients through telehealth, there are risks that the telehealth encounter itself would result in a privacy or security law violations. Because these interactions, by definition, involve communications with patients who are not physically present, there is a heightened risk of disclosing information to the wrong person, which would likely be an unauthorized disclosure under the HIPAA Privacy Rule. Telehealth encounters may also be vulnerable to third party interference, signal errors, or transmission outages. These types of incidents can result in data loss, interrupted communications, or the alteration of important clinical information, which, in addition to other liability risks, could be considered HIPAA privacy and security violations. In certain cases, transmission outages or the loss of important clinical data during transmission could be seen as a failure to adequately maintain the integrity or availability of protected health information (PHI) as required under the HIPAA security regulations. In addition, electronic transmission of information can be susceptible to hackers and other

breaches of security. Telehealth networks often require technical teams to run the systems, independent of medical staff, which means more people have potential access to patient records. This is associated with higher risks of undue exposure to private patient data. The HIPAA privacy rules provide a framework for securing protected health information held by covered entities and specify patients' rights with respect to that information. Under HIPAA, telemedicine clinicians have the same responsibility to protect patients' medical records and keep information regarding their treatments confidential. Electronic files, such as images or audio/video recordings, must be stored with the same precaution and care as paper documents. Telehealth providers should have in place reliable methods for verifying and authenticating the identities of the patient and practitioner(s) at the beginning of each telehealth encounter. Patients and clinicians should communicate via phone, text, emails through a secure portal to protect PHI.

### 22.6.2 Regulation and Licensure

Licensure is a major concern facing telehealth, especially in the United States. The US has federal standards for medical training and testing, however licensure is on a state-by-state basis with each state having its own licensing board. Providing telehealth services across state lines therefore creates licensure and insurance challenges. Most states require not only that physicians providing tele-consultation services be licensed to practice in their original state, but also in the state where the patient is located [20].

Another factor that has been limiting the acceptance and growth of telehealth is reimbursement. Today, not all telehealth costs are reimbursed. The Centers for Medicare and Medicaid Services (CMS) views telehealth as a cost-effective alternative to traditional medical care, but the decision to reimburse for telehealth services is at the discretion of each state [13]. Indeed, most states have chosen to reimburse for Medicaid telehealth services, and some also require that such services be covered by private medical insurance plans. Medicare reimburses for telehealth services when the originating site (where the patient is) is in a Health Professional Shortage Area (HPSA) or in a county that is outside of any Metropolitan Statistical Area (MSA), defined by HRSA [22] and the Census Bureau respectively. This originating site must be a medical facility and not the patient's home. Medical facilities include practitioners' offices, hospital, and rural health clinics. This reimbursement is not affected by the location from which the telehealth services are being delivered (the "distant" site). Medicare will only pay for synchronous, "face-to-face" interactive video consultation services wherein the patient is present. In most states, asynchronous "store-and-forward" applications such as teleradiology, telepathology and remote EKG are not reimbursable.

There is no single widely-accepted standard for telehealth adoption and reimbursement by private payers. Some insurance companies value the benefits of telehealth and will reimburse a wide variety of services [1]. Others have yet to develop comprehensive reimbursement policies, and so payment for telehealth may require prior approval. Likewise, different states have various standards by which their Medicaid programs will reimburse for telehealth expenses [36].

The American Telemedicine Association publishes standards and practice guidelines for delivering telehealth care in different clinical domains, including but not limited to telemental health, teledermatology, teleICU, telerehabilitation and telepathology [2].

### 22.6.3   Technical Support and Informatic Training on Telehealth Services

#### 22.6.3.1   Physician Information Overload

Because telehealth aims to leverage scarce care resources and improve care efficiency, medical practitioners may treat more patients in a telehealth environment than in the traditional face-to-face medical settings. As clinicians are already overwhelmed by information, more electronic data in the form of numbers, images, or messages may be too much to handle. Proper use of technology is a key factor in the long-term success of telehealth programs, and this entails finding ways to avoid dumping of information on physician.

#### 22.6.3.2   Patient and Clinician Technical Skills

Operation of sophisticated telehealth devices and wearable technologies can be challenging for clinicians and patients alike. Comprehensive training programs will be needed, particularly in the early stages of implementation, to overcome the lack of familiarity with new technologies, or an initial reluctance to rely on telehealth technologies to make diagnosis and treatment decisions. For example, properly using fiber optic scopes (e.g., dermascope and naso-pharyngoscope, remote otoscope, telephonic stethoscope) by a patient during video conferencing, and correct interpretation of this information by a remote physician without operating them require coordinated interaction achieved by experience and practice by both parties. A telehealth program should not underscore the importance of training to achieve increased utilization of the system, improved data collection capabilities, and greater confidence in diagnosis when relying on data collected through telehealth technologies.

### 22.6.4   Challenges to Utilizing Wearable Technologies

Noninvasive sensing involves considerable "noise" generated by various factors. Assuring an acceptable signal to noise ratio, as well as maintaining sensor resilience under real-life conditions is therefore not trivial. The more data is collected about patients, the higher the chances of detecting abnormal patterns. Whereas this serves the goal of early diagnosis and close follow up on patients, some abnormal patterns may generate false alarms, which are counter-productive. Ways to minimize false alarms should be sought, and the use of collateral data captured by different sensors to validate the readings of one another may be beneficial in this regard. All systems require energy to power data capture, storage and especially transmission. Providing power supply for prolonged periods of time is mandatory in the case of implanted sensors, the replacement of which requires invasive interventions. Solutions using energy scavenged from the body or environment are sought but are not yet ripe.

The volume of data generated by continuous monitoring is another challenge. It has been estimated, for example, that a single multifunctional sensor may generate over 150 MB of data per day [42]. The amount of data that has to be saved and transmitted may be reduced by filtering or processing of captured data at the sensor level. Reducing unnecessary data transmission may also be used to prolong battery life. Analyzing the enormous amounts of data collected by multiple sensors over time carries the promise of leveraging new insights, but requires sophisticated expertise and expensive technical resources.

As of yet, there is no agreed method for standardization of data measurements, storage and transmissions that supports integration of inputs from various sources. Even if there were such standardization protocols, the patterns identified in the data from a particular patient may not be characteristic of those of another patient. Between- subject variability increases the complexity of analysis and limits the generalizability of its results. On the other hand, using patients as self-controls by comparing data from multiple time points may help reduce the noise and improve the prediction of future events based on past trends. Moreover, uncommon patterns or signal features shared by a subset of the population may be discovered using the power of so called Big Data.

In the development of SWSs, special attention should be given to the discomfort and inconvenience of use, societal stigma and privacy considerations [42]. A wearable device should have minimal impact on the user's daily life. A small device which may be discretely carried is more likely to be accepted by patients than a visible, bulky one, especially when wearing it implies a disease (this does not apply to fashionable gadgets used for wellness management). Privacy considerations arise from the transmission of data from sensors to other devices such as cell phones, which may be intercepted. As with other personal medical information, measures to assure that only those approved by the user could access data collected by SWS should be taken.

## 22.7 Future Directions

Telehealth and wearable technologies are gaining increasing attention from healthcare organizations across the globe, and the body of evidence supporting telehealth and wearable technologies and their outcomes continues to grow. Telehealth promises immense potential on cost savings. Improved communication between doctor and patient telehealth facilitates will inevitably make remote medical services and telemedicine technologies an integral part of many healthcare organizations. The following are some of the most prominent emerging telehealth trends:

## 22.7.1 Emerging Telehealth Trends

### 22.7.1.1 Patient-Centered Home Telehealth

The ability to record and capture vital patient and environmental information makes telehealth a powerful assessment service for home care. Vendors are focusing on home-based healthcare solutions that give patients more control over their own care, especially for patients suffering from one or multiple chronic conditions. In this environment, telehealth technologies assist home care nurses to monitor a patient's vital signs, capture images and video of wounds or perform stroke assessments at home and share it with other health care professionals. These applications also enable nurses to identify changing trends in the patient's physiological state from a distance. The home care team can discuss next steps of management and attach the information to the client's record. This type of technology can also assist with medication compliance and decrease the need for in-home care or office visits.

### 22.7.1.2 Health and Wellness

Health and wellness programs, including diet and exercise routines and consultations with life and wellness coaches, are being implemented to provide disease prevention or to improve post-discharge care to reduce complications and avoid costly readmissions. Many chronic conditions can be improved or prevented through lifestyle management.

### 22.7.1.3 Long-Term Care Facilities

Often long-term care facilities do not have physicians on premise and health concerns can be beyond an onsite care giver's scope. In these situations, traditional telehealth technology is not sufficient. Patients are typically transported by ambulance to an acute care facility, which is resource and labor intensive and also stressful for patients. The mobility of a telehealth kit can be used in these situations to bring a physician or specialist right to the resident's bedside to make a proper assessment of the situation and decide on appropriate follow-on actions.

### 22.7.1.4 Remote Nursing Stations

Remote nursing stations can benefit from many of the use case applications described above. Nurses can engage medical specialists to provide enhanced quality of care while saving money on transportation costs and logistics. Connectivity options for remote nursing stations can be accomplished through terrestrial internet options or cellular and satellite communications if available.

### 22.7.1.5 Telesurgery

Remote robot-assisted surgery has recently been made feasible through Asynchronous Transfer Mode (ATM) technology, which was designed for the high-speed transfer of voice, video, and data through public and private networks [29, 30]. Telementoring, a subset of telemedicine, allows a surgeon at a remote site to offer intraoperative guidance via telecommunication networks. As robotic surgery continues to evolve, telementoring will become a viable alternative to traditional on-site surgical proctoring, particularly minimally invasive surgery (MIS). Newcomers to MIS need the guidance of more experienced, 'high volume' mentors to achieve the superior outcomes promised by MIS over conventional techniques [46]. As the cost of surgical systems decreases and reliable data networks become more available, barriers preventing the routine use of telesurgery may fall, allowing a more broad involvement in future surgical practice. Teletransmission of active surgical manipulations will continue demonstrating the potential to ensure availability of surgical expertise in remote locations for difficult or rare operations, and to improve surgical training worldwide.

### 22.7.1.6 Teleradiology

Teleradiology is the practice of transferring medical images electronically through the internet from a primary system to a remote location for the diagnosis or treatment of patients. Today teleradiology has many purposes worldwide ranging from services for expert or second opinions to international commercial diagnostic reading services. Not only does teleradiology improve the accessibility of radiologists but it also improves the quality of the interpretations for the patients [5]. Although teleradiology has become a reality for several years to date, its existence still has not been freed from all obstacles. Over years, the main issues have shifted from image quality, transmission speed and image compression to clinical governance, legal concerns and quality assessment. The increasing use of teleradiology reflects the changing world of clinical practice, service delivery and technology. With the widespread availability of fast connectivity, adoption of picture archiving and communication systems (PACS) and other advanced technologies, the sharing of medical imaging between physicians will become more commonplace in the foreseeable future [9].

### 22.7.1.7 Social Networking

Social networks are being recognized for their potential in helping people maintain healthier lifestyles. Keeping people accountable to family and friends can be much more effective than mandates from physicians, especially for patients with chronic conditions. Convergence of wearable, mobile technologies, telehealth and social networking is leading to a new healthcare delivery model. Patients can not only connect with other patients with similar medical conditions, they can also track and compare health data to better understand their bodies and contribute data to research. Telehealth and mobile health markets are anticipated to reach $2.9 billion and $1.5 trillion by 2019 due to the use of billions of smart phones and connected tablet devices all over the world [50]. Without a doubt, telehealth and mobile health markets are poised for tremendous growth and one could predict that these markets collaborate and innovate for devising healthcare delivery models in the coming years.

Over recent years, telehealth has increasingly demonstrated its value in supporting the delivery of healthcare. From teletriage services as a portal into healthcare through to telemonitoring of patients with chronic conditions, technology is already increasing the ability of practitioners to provide care remotely, empowers patients and improves clinical outcomes. In the future, telehealth services have the potential to have an even greater impact on the provision of healthcare. Embedding telehealth services into mainstream medical care, the development of more sophisticated devices and the utilization of technology in a wider range of clinical contexts will help to accelerate the adoption of telehealth throughout healthcare. In the fast-growing telehealth and wearable technology fields, new and valuable trends and telehealth technology solutions will continue to emerge and be adopted. Making use, or at least being aware of these trends will benefit providers, practitioners and patients as the market advances.

### 22.7.2   The Near Future of Wearables

A vibrant research and development environment exists, in which technological advancements are being explored to overcome some of the challenges of widespread use of SWS and to address more clinical needs. Technologies and projects are too numerous to cover here, and this section does not aim to be comprehensive but only to give a taste of this evolving industry through examples.

Energy harvesting methods may eliminate the need for battery charging or replacement [32]. Wireless-enabled garments with sensor-embedded textile (e-textile) are already appearing in the market to capture multiple signals simultaneously and continuously in a seamless manner [27]. Some systems incorporate electro-chemical sensors that can measure electrolyte concentration, pH, lactate, ammonium, glucose and other substances in saliva, sweat or tear fluid [4]. Noninvasive glucose monitoring is one of the most sought after applications. Various technologies have been attempted to achieve reliable glucose readings. The GlucoWatch® wristwatch-mounted glucose sensing device used an electric current to extract interstitial fluid through the skin and determined glucose concentration by reverse ionophoresis. The device has been withdrawn from the market following reports on skin irritation. Occlusive spectroscopy is used in the approved for marketing in Europe finger-mounted NBM-200G (OrSense Ltd., Israel) device for glucose, hemoglobin and oxygen saturation monitoring. For a comprehensive review on noninvasive glucose sensing, the reader is referred to [48]. Micro- and nanotechnology is making its way towards clinical use [26] with demonstrated ability of a tattoo-like flexible printed electrochemical biosensor to measure lactate in sweat [24]. Aids for the visually impaired include electronically augmented walking sticks [28], wearable systems [41] and even (at a prototype phase), a bionic contact lens which transforms images captured by a front facing camera to tactile stimulation of the densely innervated cornea [8].

## 22.8  Conclusions

Advancements in medicine, technology and the need to find more efficient ways to sustain the heavily burdened health system are strong forces driving the development and implementation of telehealth solutions. The evolving telehealth market will soon have a dramatic impact on the way healthcare services are provided.

## References

1. Antoniotti NM, Drude KP, Rowe N. Private payer telehealth reimbursement in the United States. Telemed J E-Health Off J Am Telemed Assoc. 2014;20(6):539–43. doi:10.1089/tmj.2013.0256.
2. ATA. American Telemedicine Association standards & guidelines. American Telemedicine Association; 2012. Retrieved from http://www.americantelemed.org/resources/standards/ata-standards-guidelines#.VHM4T2P-HGA.
3. Bagalà F, Becker C, Cappello A, Chiari L, Aminian K, Hausdorff JM, Klenk J. Evaluation of accelerometer-based fall detection algorithms on real-world falls. PLoS One. 2012;7(5):e37062. doi:10.1371/journal.pone.0037062.
4. Bandodkar AJ, Wang J. Non-invasive wearable electrochemical sensors: a review. Trends Biotechnol. 2014;32(7):363–71. doi:10.1016/j.tibtech.2014.04.005.
5. Barneveld Binkhuysen FH, Ranschaert ER. Teleradiology: evolution and concepts. Eur J Radiol. 2011;78(2):205–9. doi:10.1016/j.ejrad.2010.08.027.
6. Bergmo TS. Can economic evaluation in telemedicine be trusted? A systematic review of the literature. Cost Eff Res Allocat C/E. 2009;7:18. doi:10.1186/1478-7547-7-18.
7. Bianchi F, Redmond SJ, Narayanan MR, Cerutti S, Lovell NH. Barometric pressure and tri-axial accelerometry-based falls event detection. IEEE Trans Neural Syst Rehabil Eng Publ IEEE Eng Med Biol Soc. 2010;18(6):619–27. doi:10.1109/TNSRE.2010.2070807.
8. Bionic contact lens. (n.d.). Retrieved from http://www.digitaljournal.com/article/351212.
9. Bradley WG. Teleradiology. Neuroimaging Clin N Am. 2012;22(3):511–7. doi:10.1016/j.nic.2012.05.001.
10. Brebner JA, Brebner EM, Ruddick-Bracken H. Accident and emergency teleconsultation for primary care – a systematic review of technical feasibility, clinical effectiveness, cost effectiveness and level of local management. J Telemed Telecare. 2006;12 Suppl 1:5–8. doi:10.1258/135763306777978542.

11. Breslow MJ. Remote ICU care programs: current status. J Crit Care. 2007;22(1):66–76. doi:10.1016/j.jcrc.2007.01.006.
12. CMS. National health expenditure projections 2012–2022. Centers for Medicare and Medicaid Services; 2012. Retrieved from http://www.cms.gov/Research-Statistics-Data-and-Systems/Statistics-Trends-and-Reports/NationalHealthExpendData/downloads/proj2012.pdf.
13. CMS. Reimbursement for Telemedicine. Centers for Medicare & Medicaid Services; 2014. Retrieved from http://www.medicaid.gov/Medicaid-CHIP-Program-Information/By-Topics/Delivery-Systems/Telemedicine.html.
14. Cruz J, Brooks D, Marques A. Home telemonitoring in COPD: a systematic review of methodologies and patients' adherence. Int J Med Inform. 2014;83(4):249–63. doi:10.1016/j.ijmedinf.2014.01.008.
15. Cummings J, Krsek C, Vermoch K, Matuszewski K. Intensive care unit telemedicine: review and consensus recommendations. Am J Med Qual Off J Am Coll Med Qual. 2007;22(4):239–50. doi:10.1177/1062860607302777.
16. Cusack CM, Pan E, Hook JM, Vincent A, Kaelber DC, Middleton B. The value proposition in the widespread use of telehealth. J Telemed Telecare. 2008;14(4):167–8. doi:10.1258/jtt.2007.007043.
17. Custodio V, Herrera FJ, López G, Moreno JI. A review on architectures and communications technologies for wearable health-monitoring systems. Sensors (Basel, Switzerland). 2012;12(10):13907–46. doi:10.3390/s121013907.
18. HHS. The Health Insurance Portability and Accountability Act of 1996 (HIPAA) privacy, security and breach notification rules; 1996. Retrieved from http://www.hhs.gov/ocr/privacy/.
19. Hilty DM, Marks SL, Urness D, Yellowlees PM, Nesbitt TS. Clinical and educational telepsychiatry applications: a review. Can J Psychiatry Rev Can Psychiatr. 2004;49(1):12–23.
20. HRSA. Telehealth licensure report. Health Resources and Services Administration; 2010. Retrieved from http://www.hrsa.gov/healthit/telehealth/licenserpt10.pdf.
21. HRSA. Telehealth. Health Resources and Services Administration; 2014. Retrieved from http://www.hrsa.gov/ruralhealth/about/telehealth/.
22. HRSA. What are the reimbursement issues for telehealth? Health Resources and Services Administration; 2014. Retrieved from http://www.hrsa.gov/healthit/toolbox/RuralHealthITtoolbox/Telehealth/whatarethereimbursement.html.
23. Javelot H, Spadazzi A, Weiner L, Garcia S, Gentili C, Kosel M, Bertschy G. Telemonitoring with respect to mood disorders and information and communication technologies: overview and presentation of the PSYCHE project. BioMed Res Int. 2014;2014:104658. doi:10.1155/2014/104658.
24. Jia W, Bandodkar AJ, Valdés-Ramírez G, Windmiller JR, Yang Z, Ramírez J, Chan G, Wang J. Electrochemical tattoo biosensors for real-time noninvasive lactate monitoring in human perspiration. Anal Chem. 2013;85(14):6553–60. doi:10.1021/ac401573r.
25. Ludwig W, Wolf K-H, Duwenkamp C, Gusew N, Hellrung N, Marschollek M, Wagner M, Haux R. Health-enabling technologies for the elderly – an overview of services based on a literature review. Comput Methods Prog Biomed. 2012;106(2):70–8. doi:10.1016/j.cmpb.2011.11.001.
26. Lymberis A. The era of micro and nano systems in the biomedical area: bridging the research and innovation gap. In: Conference proceedings: … annual international conference of the IEEE engineering in medicine and biology society. IEEE Engineering in Medicine and Biology Society. Annual Conference, 2011; 2011. p. 1548–51. doi:10.1109/IEMBS.2011.6090451.
27. Lymberis A. Wearable smart systems: from technologies to integrated systems. Conference proceedings: … annual international conference of the IEEE Engineering in Medicine and Biology Society. IEEE Engineering in Medicine and Biology Society. Annual conference, 2011; 2011. p. 3503–6. doi:10.1109/IEMBS.2011.6090946.
28. Maidenbaum S, Hanassy S, Abboud S, Buchs G, Chebat D-R, Levy-Tzedek S, Amedi A. The "EyeCane", a new electronic travel aid for the blind: technology, behavior & swift learning. Restor Neurol Neurosci. 2014. doi:10.3233/RNN-130351.

29. Marescaux J, Leroy J, Rubino F, Smith M, Vix M, Simone M, Mutter D. Transcontinental robot-assisted remote telesurgery: feasibility and potential applications. Ann Surg. 2002;235(4):487–92.
30. Marescaux J, Rubino F. Robot-assisted remote surgery: technological advances, potential complications, and solutions. Surg Technol Int. 2004;12:23–6.
31. Martínez A, Everss E, Rojo-Alvarez JL, Figal DP, García-Alberola A. A systematic review of the literature on home monitoring for patients with heart failure. J Telemed Telecare. 2006;12(5):234–41. doi:10.1258/135763306777889109.
32. Mitcheson PD. Energy harvesting for human wearable and implantable bio-sensors. Conference proceedings: annual international conference of the IEEE Engineering in Medicine and Biology Society. IEEE Engineering in Medicine and Biology Society. Annual conference, 2010; 2010. p. 3432–6. doi:10.1109/IEMBS.2010.5627952.
33. Mobiguide- guiding patients anytime everywhere. (n.d.). Retrieved from http://mobiguide-project.eu/.
34. Monnier J, Knapp RG, Frueh BC. Recent advances in telepsychiatry: an updated review. Psychiatr Serv (Wash, DC). 2003;54(12):1604–9.
35. Mota NB, Vasconcelos NAP, Lemos N, Pieretti AC, Kinouchi O, Cecchi GA, Copelli M, Ribeiro S. Speech graphs provide a quantitative measure of thought disorder in psychosis. PLoS One. 2012;7(4):e34928. doi:10.1371/journal.pone.0034928.
36. NCSL. State coverage for Telehealth services. National Conference of State Legislatures; 2014. Retrieved from http://www.ncsl.org/research/health/state-coverage-for-telehealth-services.aspx.
37. Norman S. The use of telemedicine in psychiatry. J Psychiatr Ment Health Nurs. 2006;13(6):771–7. doi:10.1111/j.1365-2850.2006.01033.x.
38. ONC. Nationwide Health Information Network. Office of the National Coordinator for Health Information Technology (US); 2011. Retrieved from http://www.healthit.gov/policy-researchers-implementers/nationwide-health-information-network-nwhin.
39. Pannurat N, Thiemjarus S, Nantajeewarawat E. Automatic fall monitoring: a review. Sensors (Basel, Switzerland). 2014;14(7):12900–36. doi:10.3390/s140712900.
40. Paré G, Jaana M, Sicotte C. Systematic review of home telemonitoring for chronic diseases: the evidence base. J Am Med Inf Assoc JAMIA. 2007;14(3):269–77. doi:10.1197/jamia.M2270.
41. Pradeep V, Medioni G, Weiland J. A wearable system for the visually impaired. Conference proceedings: … annual international conference of the IEEE Engineering in Medicine and Biology Society. IEEE Engineering in Medicine and Biology Society. Annual conference, 2010; 2010. p. 6233–6. doi:10.1109/IEMBS.2010.5627715.
42. Redmond SJ, Lovell NH, Yang GZ, Horsch A, Lukowicz P, Murrugarra L, Marschollek M. What does big data mean for wearable sensor systems? Contribution of the IMIA wearable sensors in healthcare WG. Yearb Med Inform. 2014;9(1):135–42. doi:10.15265/IY-2014-0019.
43. Ricci RP, Morichelli L, Santini M. Remote control of implanted devices through home monitoring technology improves detection and clinical management of atrial fibrillation. Europace Eur Pacing Arrhythmias Card Electrophysiol J Work Group Card Pacing, Arrhythmias Card Cell Electrophysiol Eur Soc Cardiol. 2009;11(1):54–61. doi:10.1093/europace/eun303.
44. Russell SJ, El-Khatib FH, Sinha M, Magyar KL, McKeon K, Goergen LG, Balliro C, Hillard MA, Nathan DM, Damiano ER. Outpatient glycemic control with a bionic pancreas in type 1 diabetes. N Engl J Med. 2014;371(4):313–25. doi:10.1056/NEJMoa1314474.
45. RWJ. Chronic care: making the case for ongoing care. Princeton: Robert Wood Johnson Foundation; 2010. Retrieved from http://www.rwjf.org/content/dam/farm/reports/reports/2010/rwjf54583.
46. Santomauro M, Reina GA, Stroup SP, L'Esperance JO. Telementoring in robotic surgery. Curr Opin Urol. 2013;23(2):141–5. doi:10.1097/MOU.0b013e32835d4cc2.

47. Seto E. Cost comparison between telemonitoring and usual care of heart failure: a systematic review. Telemed J E-Health Off J Am Telemed Assoc. 2008;14(7):679–86. doi:10.1089/tmj.2007.0114.
48. Vashist SK. Non-invasive glucose monitoring technology in diabetes management: a review. Anal Chim Acta. 2012;750:16–27. doi:10.1016/j.aca.2012.03.043.
49. Wade VA, Karnon J, Elshaug AG, Hiller JE. A systematic review of economic analyses of telehealth services using real time video communication. BMC Health Serv Res. 2010;10:233. doi:10.1186/1472-6963-10-233.
50. WGR. Telemedicine and M-Health Convergence: market shares, strategies, and forecasts, worldwide, 2013 to 2019. Winter Green Research; 2013. Retrieved from http://www.research-moz.us/telemedicine-and-m-health-convergence-market-shares-strategies-and-forecasts-worldwide-2013-to-2019-report.html.

# Chapter 23
# The Role of Big Data and Analytics in Health Payer Transformation to Consumer-Centricity

Gigi Yuen-Reed and Aleksandra Mojsilović

**Abstract** Historically, information management for payers has been focused on enabling efficient operations, such as claims administration and group management. Recently, with the rise of individual insurance and increasing pressure to reduce cost through better health management, healthcare payers are transforming its business to be increasingly consumer-centric. In the healthcare payer setting, consumer-centricity means to put individual consumer at the focus of payer operations. It is to understand and engage individual consumer throughout the insurance lifecycle, from assisting prospects to choose the most suitable product, engaging new enrollees in wellness, to assisting members navigate the healthcare system. In this chapter, we discuss the implications of consumer-centricity and external data explosion on payer information management, ranging from data management, analytics applications and use cases, to the analytics delivery platform. We also discuss how consumer data and open data support this transformation, shedding insights into range of business processes, and expanding the role of informatics in the payer organization.

**Keywords** Consumerism • Retailization • Health insurance • Managed care • Predictive analytics • Data platform

## 23.1 Introduction

Healthcare is following a similar transformation the financial and travel industries experienced over the last several years. The shift to consumer-driven health is evolving rapidly. Healthcare payers need to transform their operations, processes and culture to retain their members, stay relevant and manage costs. Consumer-centric healthcare is a way to approach, design and deliver healthcare by placing the customer experience and value above other priorities. The consumer

G. Yuen-Reed, PhD (✉) • A. Mojsilović, PhD, EE
Data Science, IBM T.J. Watson Research Center, Yorktown Heights, NY, USA
e-mail: gigi.yuen@us.ibm.com; aleksand@us.ibm.com

© Springer International Publishing Switzerland 2016                         399
C.A. Weaver et al. (eds.), *Healthcare Information Management Systems:
Cases, Strategies, and Solutions*, Health Informatics,
DOI 10.1007/978-3-319-20765-0_23

experience includes the traditional patient experience, but expands across the continuum of care. Because consumers will be making the buying decisions, providers must increasingly think like retailers, whether it is in formulating marketing, pricing and risk management strategies, or in establishing new billing and payment practices.

Considering the consumer is important not only for the sake of improving the consumer experience – this strategy is critical to healthcare payers' financial and operational decisions and their ability to manage costs more effectively, grow their business and transition to outcome-driven organizations.

The rise of consumer-centricity in healthcare has been investigated from different perspectives. The work described in [3] discusses the consumer-centricity from the point of view of building trusted relationships and useful interactions between healthcare payers and their members; [11] discusses the implications of consumer-centricity in healthcare to finance functions, and highlights many of the ways payers and providers – including their treasury functions – will need to respond to prosper in this new environment. As payers begin to consider direct-to-consumer relationships, they will also have to address the automation and reengineering of their back-office processes and the underlying IT infrastructure. The need to understand the individuals better brings in new IT requirements and a need for far more detailed insights and information tailored to the individuals. As a result, Big Data and advanced analytics capabilities will become a key enabler in the success of the consumer-centric transformation in healthcare.

In this work, we provide an overview of the role of Big Data and analytics in this consumer-centric transformation. In Sect. 23.2, we discuss the background of healthcare payer function and driving forces of consumer-centric transformation. In Sect. 23.3, we address the implications of consumer-centricity in healthcare to payer processes and operations. We also provide several analytics use cases central to consumer-centric business processes and supporting data-driven applications. In Sect. 23.4, we address the information management strategy and roadmap needed to enable such transformation, from data management, analytics platform to API enabled shared services. In Sect. 23.5, we offer concluding remarks and future directions.

## 23.2 Background and Industry Trends

### 23.2.1 The Evolution of the Role of Healthcare Payer in the US

Health insurance in the United States has roots in the Civil War period and has grown and evolved with market need over times.

One of the first group policies giving comprehensive health benefits was offered in 1847 by Massachusetts Health Insurance of Boston. In 1929, the first modern group health insurance plan was formed. A group of teachers in Dallas, Texas, contracted with Baylor Hospital for room, board, and medical services in exchange for a monthly fee. As the popularity of health insurance increased, several large life insurance companies entered the health insurance field in the 1930s and 1940s. In 1932, nonprofit organizations called Blue Cross or Blue Shield first offered group health plans. Blue Cross and Blue Shield Plans were successful with discounted contracts negotiated with doctors and hospitals.

In return for promises of increased volume and prompt payment, providers gave discounts to the Blue Cross and Shield plans. Employee benefit plans proliferated in the 1940s and 1950s, as influential unions bargained for better benefit packages and tax-free, employer-sponsored health insurance. During the World War II (1939–1945) wage freezes imposed by the government accelerated the spread of group health care. Prevented by law to attract workers by paying more, employers instead improved their benefit packages, adding health care. Government programs to cover health care costs began to expand during the 1950s and 1960s. Disability benefits were included in social security coverage for the first time in 1954. When the government created Medicare and Medicaid programs in 1965, private sources still paid 75 % of all of the health care costs. By 1995, individuals and companies only paid for about half of the health care, with the government responsible for the other half. During the 1980s and 1990s, the cost of health care rose rapidly and the majority of employer-sponsored group insurance plans switched from "fee-for-service" plans to the cheaper "managed care plans." As a result, most Americans with health insurance were enrolled in managed care plans by the mid-1990s. For more details in US health insurance history, see [15].

Through growing market adoption and consolidations, many of the early third party payer systems evolved and matured to today's healthcare payers. As of 2013, about 87 % of the US population is covered by health insurance offered by public or private health payers [24]. Amongst the insured population, about 55 % are covered by employer-based insurance, 38 % are covered by government-sponsored plans like Medicare and Medicaid, and less than 7 % are covered by non-group-based insurance.

Traditionally, healthcare payers focused their operations on providing support to their members through transactional processes and managing their risk through underwriting. Transactions included tasks such as looking up benefits, submitting claims, and searching for providers. Improving the efficiency of the transactions, especially claims processing, was the key lever behind running a successful healthcare payer organization. As a result, claims operations centers focused on the speed and accuracy of processing and paying healthcare claims, ensuring that providers were reimbursed in a timely manner, and that members received proper coverage, as prescribed in their health plans. Another critical focus area of payer operations was risk management. Risk management centers were established to ensure financial soundness of the insured portfolios, such that premium collected was sufficient to support the claims and administrative expenses and risk adjustment payments are properly accounted for. Given these priorities of the traditional healthcare payer role, the organizational structure and underlying Information Technology (IT) and Information Management (IM) strategies was centered on maximizing operational efficiencies and ensuring financial soundness. Typical performance measures included claim cost per member per month and claims adjudication speed. Consequently, technology investments amongst healthcare payers typically focused on supporting group management, risk management and achieving operational efficiency.

## 23.2.2   The Affordable Care Act and Changing Landscape of Health Insurance

The passage of Affordable Care Act (ACA) in 2009 had significant impact on the US health insurance environment. With the overarching goal to expand access to insurance coverage, the ACA legislation directly impacts many of the foundational tenants of the healthcare system.

ACA requires most US citizens and legal residents to obtain health insurance; failure to compile results in penalties. ACA provided for the creation of public health insurance exchanges in all states. These exchanges, also known as "marketplaces," offer a set of government-defined and standardized healthcare plans from which individuals may purchase health insurance and be eligible for federal subsidies, thereby creating a boost in commercial individual insurance market. Individual insurance targets individuals who do not currently qualify for government-sponsored insurance and group-sponsored insurance, mostly the self-employed, employees of small businesses and unemployed. Enrollment in the healthcare exchanges began in October 2013. During the first open enrollment period of public health exchanges in 2013–2014, around eight (8) million Americans enrolled and the number is expected to increase to 25 million in 2017 and subsequent years [6]. Many Americans are expected to obtain healthcare insurance through privately administered health insurance exchanges, to which their employers are directing them. Published reports indicate that Fortune 500 companies such as Time Warner, IBM, Caterpillar and DuPont are among the companies using private exchanges for retirees or for certain groups of employees as a way to move toward a defined contribution model of healthcare benefits. In such setting, employers create a set of health insurance plan options through a private exchange, and their employees can choose a plan from participating payers. For employers, one advantage is they can continue to offer the company subsidy and some level of employee healthcare benefits in the form of pre-tax premiums, while controlling their costs.

As a result, the individual insurance increased from around 14 million members in 2011 to 20 million in 2014 [24]. The growth is expected to continue, reaching 26–73 million by 2020, corresponding to 8–22 % of the commercial insurance market [5]. Unlike group insurance, purchasing decisions are made by individuals (or families) and hence, require a consumer-based marketing, sales and retention approach.

In addition to creating the boost for the commercial individual market, ACA also introduced requirements that are altering how payers manage risk. For example,

ACA prohibits the maximum lifetime limits on individual and group health plans. It also requires the payers to provide essential benefits coverage, without the ability to differentiate premium pricing by medical history other than tobacco use. The legislation also prohibits payers to deny coverage for individuals, essentially removing the underwriting practice of the traditional commercial individual insurance. Finally, because of the wider availability of healthcare coverage, many previously uninsured Americans will enter the market, which will shift the health risk profile significantly, making traditional actuarial risk assessment practices based on historical data highly ineffective. Because of the new requirements, the traditional risk management approaches in insurance do not carry over to the commercial individual health insurance segment. This has increased the pressure on healthcare payers to manage cost and financial risk through non-traditional means.

To combat the increasing financial risk, payers are putting greater than ever emphasis on engaging individual consumers in health and wellness. For example the payers are:

- Actively engaging individuals in disease management,
- Enhancing their clinician engagement to promote chronic disease management and post-operations support,
- Expanding from healthcare management to wellness management, by offering gym membership, health products and wellness incentives,
- Empowering individuals to make better health and utilization decisions, by providing additional support during product purchasing process to ensure benefits alignment and to increase transparency in coverage and provider network.

In the pre-ACA era, consumers played the role of passive participant in the healthcare system, mainly due to availability of employer-managed healthcare coverage. Most employees paid moderate amounts in out-of-pocket cost, and they typically benefited from nominal co-pays and low deductibles. However, with the advent of consumer-directed healthcare in recent years, consumers found themselves equipped with more decision-making responsibilities. Today, with the implementation of the Affordable Care Act, consumers are being asked to be even more active healthcare participants, and have more at stake, both relative to their personal finances and their overall health. In the resulting consumer-centric healthcare business, in addition to being the end users and receivers of services, consumers will be making more of the decisions around the type of plan and coverage they select, as well as the doctors, hospitals and other providers they patronize. This fundamentally alters all key functional areas of payer operations.

## 23.2.3   Data as the Enabler of Consumer-Centricity

The consumer-centric engagement models and business processes require timely and relevant consumer information and data. Data was the accelerator of consumer-centricity in retail and financial sector, and today with the growth of consumer data in healthcare, it is the lever of change in healthcare industry [7, 19]. In the current market, the sources and types of consumer data relevant to health insurance management are abundant and continue to grow. Beyond the more traditional healthcare data such as claims and electronic medical records, there has been a rise in non-traditional sources, such as retail marketing data, social media data and consumer controlled device data. Table 23.1 highlights the prominent sources of consumer healthcare Big Data and discusses their value in the consumer-centric payer operations.

**Table 23.1** The description of various data relevant to healthcare payers

| | |
|---|---|
| Clinical records | Contain clinical information about the patients from physician encounter notes, prescriptions, medical imaging, laboratory and testing. This information is captured in medical or patient health record |
| | The adoption of electronic records is increasing amongst service providers and in some cases made available to payers [12, 17] |
| Financial and utilization records | Contain healthcare service utilization information for individual health insurance member, associated costs and payment information. This information is typically captured in health insurance member, product and claims data |
| | Claims data includes records related to inpatient services, outpatient services and pharmacy fulfillments. It is submitted by the healthcare providers, and curated and processed by health payers' transactional systems. This data source is traditionally the most matured and available in payer operations |
| Direct consumer engagement records | Contain inbound and outbound member interaction data across channels, including phone calls, direct mail, text messages, emails and web chats. This information is typically captured in unstructured data format, and is rich with information around consumer preferences and concerns. The richness of this data source is growing steadily as payers increase proactive consumer engagement, as well as with the increase in direct communications via digital and mobile channels |
| Government and open data | Publicly available health and wellness statistics for different communities, which typically contain location-specific information gathered by government or non-profit agencies, such as access to care, access to public transportation, environmental data, healthcare benchmarks, disease prevalence, and etc. |
| Third party retail marketing data | Provided by data aggregators like KBM, Axiom and Epsilon, this data contains direct marketing information of individuals, such as retail purchasing history and statistics around socio-economic, education statues. Third party data allows payers to better understand prospects for marketing purposes, and enrich their understanding of members' preferences and attitudes |
| Social media | Contains self-generated data in the social media, including text, graphics and videos. For many active users, this is an extremely rich data source about lifestyle, preferences and behaviors |
| | However, due to privacy issues, it is often difficult to tie the data to individual members or prospects |
| Consumer controlled devices | Contains testing, sensing or self-reported device managed data, generated by consumer controlled digital devices such as blood glucose monitor, activity tracking devices, digital scales; and by consumer reported data from mobile apps and web services (for example iHealth) |

Big Data in consumer healthcare offers tremendous information for payers to understand consumers personally and anticipate their upcoming health and wellness needs. The range of potential applications is broad, spanning all business processes of a payer. For example, healthcare utilization records can be combined with retail marketing data to understand individual's propensity for behavioral change. Consumer communication preferences can be extracted from past engagement records to determine best channel for messaging and engagement. Census, open data and healthcare surveys can indicate general healthcare trends or help benchmark different geographical segments and markets. (In Sect. 23.4, we will discuss several use cases in more details). Payers who successfully manage this diverse data, have capabilities to extract relevant insights and use them effectively in their operations, will have a significant competitive advantage in the new environment.

## 23.3 Consumer-Centricity in Healthcare Insurance

Consumer-centricity in health care payer setting is defined as creating a positive consumer experience at every point of health insurance operations, from sales and marketing, product selection, health insurance utilization, to customer service and care coordination. The emphasis is on providing a personalized experience that is relevant and timely, such that the payer can acquire and retain customers, and engage and empower members to make the best health insurance and care decisions. In the emerging consumer-centric healthcare environment, payers will face a number of challenges and unknowns. For example, because consumers will be making buying decisions, payers must increasingly think like retailers, whether it is in formulating their marketing strategies, performing care management or establishing new billing and payment practices. The emergence of an empowered healthcare consumer calls for payers to develop an entirely new mindset of running the business, focused on winning over consumers and improving outcomes. Some call this paradigm shift the "retailization" of healthcare [3].

The consumer experience starts when an individual is a prospect, a target for the sale of a health insurance product; as the sales cycle matures, the individual is considered a lead, who has expressed an intent to buy and is interested in learning more about the product. As the individual completes the product enrollment process, he/she is an enrollee and transitions into being a member and begins consuming various health insurance services. At the end of the insurance product coverage period, the individual may decide to re-enroll or not. Member who decides to discontinue coverage is considered a dis-enrollee. The stages of prospect, lead, enrollee, member, dis-enrollee constitute the consumer lifecycle. Consumers have different needs and expectations at each stage of the lifecycle, calling for different servicing capabilities.

**Table 23.2** The characteristics of consumer-centric actions and experience throughout the lifecycle of a healthcare customer

| | |
|---|---|
| Prospect | Create the basic profile of the individual to understand key characteristics and tailor relevant marketing messages. Engage through a channel that best resonates with particular individual |
| Lead | Understand individual's personal and family insurance needs, for example, affordability concerns, coverage requirements |
| | Offer product options, for example, the ability to "mix and match" product features |
| Enrollee | Enrich the profile with the information collected at the point of enrollment and (for former members) from historical data. Offer new enrollee orientation, including detailed product and benefits education |
| | Tools and support to enable searching and comparing service providers, and performing financial analysis and planning |
| Member | Enrich the profile with the information collected via service consumption. Provide customer service support best tailored to the individual. Provide access to wellness and care coordination support that is relevant to individual's conditions and lifestyle. Help with life events, including re-alignment to different products, ability to choose new physicians or service facilities |
| Dis-Enrollee | Close out billing in timely manner. Properly archive the member records and ability to retrieve and map past records if/when the individual returns in the future |

Table 23.2 describes the characteristics of a consumer-centric experience throughout the lifecycle.

### 23.3.1 Consumer-Centric Business Processes and Analytics Applications Use Cases

Enabling the consumer-centric experience across the lifecycle requires a new set of analytical capabilities. For example, traditionally, payers relied on direct mail marketing campaigns to target prospects of Individual products in certain geographies. Today, to enhance how they communicate with consumers in the Individual market, payers are expanding their engagement channels to include email, social media, and brick-and-mortar retail stores [2, 4]; this requires new insights on consumers' channel preferences and promotional triggers, the ability to capture responses from these new promotional practices and continuously learn and evolve based on derived insights.

Once an individual makes the purchasing decision and becomes a member of a health plan, the consumer experience continues. While business functions supporting the different stages of the consumer lifecycle vary, payers need to provide consistent and relevant experience throughout the lifecycle, and take advantage of the additional consumer data made available over time. This transformation has significant implication to information management strategy in the payer organization.

It also calls for a range of innovative data and analytics-driven applications in support of the diverse business processes. From improving personalized engagement for care management, to supporting core business functions around flexible risk management and financial planning, there is a broad spectrum of opportunities to create new insights and enhance decision making in a way that has not been done before. Table 23.3 provides examples of analytics use cases at different stages of the consumer lifecycle.

In the following sections, we discuss four analytics use cases in more details. *Prospect Risk Prediction* discusses gaining a predictive view of non-member health risk to improve marketing and product design decisions. *Evolving Consumer Segmentation* highlights the analytics needs and approaches to formulate enterprise wide consumer segments, which are adaptive to the different stages of the consumer lifecycle. *Care Engagement Targeting* focuses on the analytics capabilities to identify "who" the payers should engage with to improve member health. *Behavioral Change Analytics* focuses on analytics supporting insights around "how" to engage the targeted individuals and "what" are the best triggers and enablers to improve wellness.

## 23.3.2   Prospect Risk Prediction

The insights around prospect risks are critical in decisions around market entry and product design and pricing. As discussed in Sect. 23.2, ACA has expanded health insurance access for the previously uninsured individuals and its requirements for health plan benefits are likely to induce different consumption habits compared to previously insured individuals. This will change the risk profiles of the population payers insure, and to mitigate and manage potential financial risk, payers need to improve its ability to understand prospects' risks. Historically, prospect risks are evaluated for different geographies using basic demographic data such as age, gender and tobacco consumption.

However, the predictive ability of models using these basic factors tends to be limited, especially with fundamental shifts in the insured population [9]. To overcome these shortcomings, payers are beginning to explore the use of non-traditional data in modeling consumer risks, such as publicly available location data and retail marketing data. Individual prospect information, such as household size, financial stability, behavioral and life style choices, which can be derived from Census and consumer data, have shown to correlate with healthcare risk [22].

Leveraging these non-traditional datasets poses several predictive modeling challenges. The datasets tend to have hundreds and sometimes thousands of fields that are: (1) sparsely populated (e.g., self-reported health conditions), (2) highly correlated (e.g., estimated income and education level) and (3) have different levels of granularity (e.g., access to care is tied to geography, whereas ethnicity is tied to an individual). As a result, extreme care needs to be taken in selecting analytical methods, in feature engineering and in handling of the missing values.

**Table 23.3** Analytics uses cases at different stages of the consumer lifecycle

| Business functions | Targeted consumer stage(s) | Analytics use case objectives |
|---|---|---|
| Omni channel direct marketing | Prospects | Improve direct marketing effectiveness through more effective prospect targeting and touch point optimization |
| Personalized sales | Leads | Increase sales close rates through insights into "triggers to buy" and communication preferences |
| | | Optimize product-to-individual alignment through insights around individuals' health insurance needs |
| Product design | Lead Enrollee Member | Improve shopping and utilization experience with simple and attractive product offerings |
| | | Empower members to have access to the right care provider at the right price |
| Member engagement and empowerment | Enrollees Members | Improve customer satisfaction and |
| | | loyalty with consistent, timely and relevant communications |
| | | Empower consumers to understand options for health services and insights into provider's quality and cost |
| Customer service | Enrollees Members | Improve self-service offerings to empower consumers and optimize user experience across channels |
| | | Support proactive issue resolution by mining communication data |
| Financial management | All | Predict prospect and member risk and detect early indicators of cost drivers using relevant member information |
| Care coordination | Enrollees Members | Improve patient outcome by sharing relevant and timely patient insights with appropriate healthcare service providers |
| Care and wellness management | Enrollees Members | Improve disease management and promote population wellness through personalized insights on health behavioral change triggers, incentives and intervention effectiveness |

While these non-traditional datasets coupled with new predictive modeling techniques have tremendous potential to help payers understand prospect risk better, the insights derived through analytics need to be leveraged appropriately. The outputs of the predictive models tend to be probabilistic and do not hold the confidence level of medical or clinical data. When lifestyle or socio-economic data are linked to healthcare information, extreme care should be taken to protect patient privacy, and ensure that the insights are not used to disadvantage consumers in any way.

### 23.3.3 Evolving Consumer Segmentation

For a long time, consumer segmentation has been the underpinning to providing consistent and relevant consumer experience to individuals in many industries, including healthcare insurance. In managing prospects and leads, segmentation provides consumer insights for effective marketing. After prospects become members, segmentation is used to understand their healthcare needs and preferences, and to improve customer loyalty and engagement effectiveness. Moreover, understanding how demand drivers and utilization differ from segment to segment allows insurance companies to tailor products and services to meet demand, improve care and retain loyalty. Payers can utilize consumer segment insights to provide value-added services, for example, discounts to health clubs, monthly heart-healthy recipes sent to member email addresses, appointment reminders with GPS directions on mobile phones, mobile reminders for prescription drug schedule updates, applications that track glucose and blood pressure readings, and automatic emails to doctors.

Historically, each business function of a healthcare payer relied on its own consumer segments, thereby creating numerous disjoint consumer segmentations across business units. This often prohibits an enterprise-wide consumer strategy. Different amounts of data about the healthcare consumer are available at different stages of the lifecycle, and the ability to derive insight about the consumer increases from the basic demographic information and third party data, information collected at the enrollment, to detailed health service consumption information once the individual starts utilizing the service. Rather than being a set of disjoint analyses, effective consumer segmentation model needs to reflect this data build-up, while maintaining sufficient stability for cross-business function coordination.

This creates additional requirements on the analytics applications, and calls for the use of robust hierarchical segmentation techniques, capable of handling the increase in member information throughout the lifecycle, and also capable of creating highly targetable segments of various granularity: from a small number of coarse segments used in strategic planning and business assessment, to a large number of actionable micro-segments for use in tactical decision-making.

The segmentation models also need to be capable of handling disparate member data, and creating interpretable insights to support data-driven intelligent member marketing, product design, risk assessment, program design, actuarial pricing, provider and hospital relationship management.

### 23.3.4 Care Engagement Targeting

Engaging members regarding care management has proven benefits in population health management and lowering overall healthcare spent [10, 16]. Payers have access to longitudinal and digitalized records of members' healthcare utilization data across providers, and are financially motivated to engage members to avoid future high cost expenses.

For example, with the goal of minimizing hospital readmission, a Cleveland health plan assigns care counselors to members who have recently been discharged from the hospital to ensure that they understand discharge instructions and identify any potentially unmet needs [8].

Historically, payers identified members for care management efforts by relying on extensive member clams history to conduct retrospective utilization review or predict future high cost claimants [25]. However, with increases in health risk diversity in membership, and with increasing pressure to curb healthcare costs, payers are taking a more proactive role in identifying members for care engagement. The need is intensified with the arrival of previously uninsured or underinsured members, who tend to be less familiar with condition management and might be less knowledgeable about factors and considerations important in choosing the right healthcare providers and treatments.

To take a more proactive and targeted approach in care engagement, payers can incorporate analytics-driven insights focused on early identifications of members who would benefit most from the engagement efforts. For example, payers can greatly improve the effectiveness of the outreach programs by identifying potential high cost individuals shortly after the enrollment, thereby increasing the intervention time window. For example, by analyzing pharmacy data in the first 2 or 3 months of the membership, it is possible to build early risk profiles or apply predictive modeling to identify individuals who are likely to incur high cost in the remainder of the year. Another opportunity to use predictive analytics is in identifying individuals at high risk of progressing in their disease conditions, or identifying members whose chronic condition are likely to deteriorate, thereby enabling more aggressive outreach measures to engage and motivate these members to better manage their conditions. Such highly personalized early insights require analytics capabilities that are capable of deriving longitudinal view of individual members' clinical and behavioral conditions. This also calls for sophisticated data handling and feature-engineering methods, such as data densification and temporal data sequencing [26, 27].

### 23.3.5 Behavioral Modification Analytics

Studies have shown that more than 31 % of US healthcare expenses can be directly attributed to behaviorally-influenced chronic conditions [7].

Healthcare expenses can be avoided with changes in individual behavior, including medication adherence, practicing safety measures, dietary practices, physical exercise, and etc.

While payers have tremendous interest in reducing these avoidable costs and promoting wellness, behavioral modification is fundamentally personal and requires consumer's individual self-regulatory and health enhancing efforts.

To affect behavioral modification effectively, payers cannot simply rely on one-size-fits-all programs or tools, but need to: (a) gain personalized insights around motivations that drive individual behavioral changes, and (b) identify proper incentives that can trigger such changes.

For example, to improve medication adherence in chronic diseases like diabetes, payers need to first understand the non-adherence reasons and potential barriers by mining through population health literature or by conducting observational studies. Some diabetic patients may be non-adherent due to lack of awareness, which can be impacted through consumer monitoring devices, while others may be non-adherent due to financial constraints prohibiting them from getting refills in a timely manner, which can be impacted through discounts programs.

Besides relying on domain expertise and extracting knowledge from the existing literature, personalized insights affecting behavioral change can be derived through mining observational data. For example, by analyzing member response patterns to various interventions, payers can apply predictive modeling techniques to estimate how likely a given member will respond to certain types of interventions. Another opportunity is to combine healthcare utilization and consumer device data to identify the most effective "triggering" moments that influence behavioral change. Furthermore, with sufficient member engagement history, it is possible to utilize stochastic process modeling techniques to determine the most effective "nudge" at any given time to optimize long-term wellness.

Lastly, behavioral modification is also highly social and culturally driven. There are opportunities in mining social media data to understand different consumer segments' perception and motivation of health and wellness.

Moreover, by applying network science, one can identify individuals who can most influence certain community's behavior [23], from determining who in a family network can best improve a child's asthma medication adherence, to identifying the influencer in an employee group to promote physical activities.

## 23.4  The Implications to Information Management Strategy

To enable the consumer-centric transformation, payers need to understand individuals across the consumer lifecycle and the view needs to be coherent and transparent to the various business functions, from marketing, sales, claims management, customer service, to care coordination.

This requires bringing together data across the various business functions, and tapping into data sources both internal and external to the enterprise. Some of these data types are structured, which follow predefined formats like the internal claims data or Census surveys, while other data types are unstructured, such as text, image and video customer service call recordings or social media data.

Figure 23.1 provides the consumer data management landscape for a typical health payer organization, based on the origin of the data (internal vs. external) and format of the data (structured vs. unstructured).

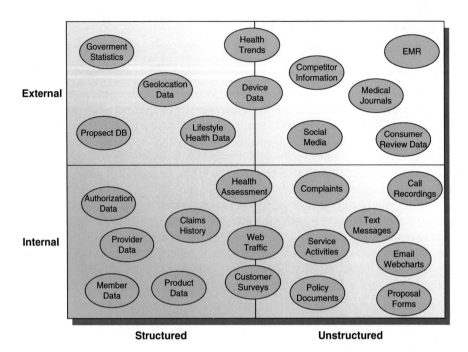

**Fig. 23.1** Data landscape for healthcare payers

### 23.4.1    Consumer-Centric Data Management

Payers had historically relied heavily on internal data for its operations and the corresponding data management method had been group-centric and transactions driven. As illustrated in Fig. 23.1, the internal data is typically derived from administrative function, such as application and policy documents from enrollment, claims history from adjudication and payment processing, and call recordings from customer service.

A common challenge is in turning the internal and structured administrative data from a transaction-centric view to a consumer-centric view.

In a consumer-centric view, data generated throughout the different transactions and contacts are captured and managed around the consumers, and consequently, data about the individuals are made available in a relevant and cohesive manner as different business functions interact with customers or manage consumer-related activities.

Instead of a group-centric approach, the consumer-centric data management strategy needs to transpire across both membership affiliations and business functions. As individuals move between different products, employer groups or between group-based and individual-based plans, they need to be tracked as the same unique consumer and the consumer view is continuously updated and enriched.

This requires data management capability that matches consumer records and reconciles consumer information across disparate sources of data. Many payers have adopted custom or commercially available master data management tools to create and maintain such consumer-centric data view.

With the increasing need to market to prospects and engage with individual members, payers are also expanding their use of external data to gain insights on consumer preferences, health trends and socio-economic characteristics of different geographies and population cohorts. In the US, there has been a significant focus around gathering open data related to healthcare. Data.gov/health provides a collection of Federal, state, local and non-profit collected and derived data related to healthcare. Prominent sources include CDC Health Statistics Report and Census's American Community Survey, which provide population-based information around socio-economic status and healthcare utilization. Other countries have similar initiative (see for example, HSCIC.gov.uk in Great Britain, and data.go.jp in Japan). In addition to open data, payers have also shown successes in leveraging consumer retail databases like Acxiom, KBM and Epislon in their marketing, risk and care management efforts. For example, UPMC utilizes household level retail data, such as education level, marital status, and number of cars, to improve its emergency and urgent care forecasting capabilities [21]. Similarly, an East Coast health insurer identifies patients who are likely to have scheduling and logistical constraints with their regular doctor's appointment, and hence might be at increased risk of hospitalization [14].

In addition to consumer retail data, social media data from social networking sites such as Facebook or Twitter, are another source of timely and personal data about individual consumers, offering insights such as intent to relocate, lifestyle habits and changes, or stress level indicators. Recent advances in information management, text analytics and entity resolution show promising results in linking sparse social media data with customer service records [1].

Despite tremendous potential in leveraging external data to improve consumer experience and personalize service and care, privacy concerns pose limitations in linking external data to individual insured members. Moreover, not all external data can be easily tied to a specific individual or household. For example, open data such as publicly available survey data published by CDC or Census are reported at different geographical summary levels. To effectively derive insight from such data, the data management platform needs to have the flexibility to support integrating external data in an agile manner, depending on different analytical and functional needs and privacy requirements. For example, certain types of analyses will be carried on the consumer location data, while other might operate on the granularity of consumer segments.

Another significant data management challenge includes curating, integrating and analyzing unstructured data from combined internal and external sources. Unstructured data generated from consumer interaction like call center, web chat and email, captures consumers' stated preferences, their perceptions and relationship with the health plans and providers. These insights can be integrated with member record to improve engagement effectiveness like wellness programs and cross selling.

Another major source of unstructured data is clinical or device records like EMR or consumer-driven health mobile apps, which can greatly enrich the transaction-based data like claims records in care coordination and behavioral modification programs.

The nature of unstructured data is highly contextual and the deployment of analytics tends to require heavy involvement of subject matter experts. Recent advances in Natural Language Processing (NLP) technologies provide efficient ways to analyze human languages inherent in data generated throughout consumer and patient interactions. NLP translates between natural and computer languages by identifying text-based concepts, user sentiments, and to find latent meaning and relationships hidden in unstructured data. The information is captured and codified to enhance payers' view of the consumer and can be leveraged to improve predictive modeling efforts.

## 23.4.2  Agile Analytics Platform

In order to transform the growing volume and variety of consumer data into business actions, it is imperative for payers to increase the maturity of analytics technologies focused on mining, analyzing and predicting from consumer insights. Some of the key challenges include:

- The supply chain on consumer data is dynamic and goes through ongoing changes. New data sources of consumer information are constantly made available through new business partners and data providers. Moreover, external data sources differ in quality and can affect the content and schema without notice.
- Different business processes that utilize the same data may require similar but not identical sets of data elements, reports and analytics. However, it is expensive and ineffective to have duplicate data and capabilities.
- Consumer engagement requires timely insight. For example, members expect care management clinician to be aware of their latest medical treatments and wellness program activities. However, many existing analytics platforms rely on batch updates and are not instrumented for near real time performance.
- From the traditional electronic medical records to social media to consumer interaction data, the amount of unstructured data is growing in volume and complexity. The data sources contain tremendous insights around individual consumers' clinical, behavioral and preferential information, but most payers have limited experience in managing and analyzing these types of unstructured data.
- The needs of business user are fluid and constantly evolving. They are highly dependent on changing competitive landscape, business strategy, political environment, consumer trends and emergence of new technologies. To assess the effectiveness of new analytics, prototype of new capabilities needs to be developed and implemented quickly as an enterprise-wide solution to generate

business value. On the other hand, the analytics need to be adaptive to changing business needs.

These challenges call for a new generation of analytics platform, armed with features such as:

- Ability to allow expert users to quickly explore and analyze new data sources. Growing in popularity is the utilization of storage repository like data lake which retains all attributes using light data governance principles. An example of data lake storage is Hadoop-oriented object storage where metadata is captured to facilitate analysis design without pre-specification of data requirements. This allows experts like data scientist and skilled business analysts to work with raw data directly. It enables quick exploration of data value and quality that are use case specific.
- Ability to access the same data and analytics modules for different business needs, enabled by a flexible API services model to allow different users and different business processes to share the same data, reports and analytics.
- Ability to extract insights quickly and effectively, supported by the use of parallelized data processing capabilities to reduce latency (as opposed to the traditional nightly or monthly data warehouse updates), or use of stream processing technologies to aggregate and analyze data in motion.
- Ability to efficiently conduct semantic search and enable content analytics on unstructured data to enrich learning from the more traditional data sources. One way of achieving this is to leverage a data management standard like Unstructured Information Management Architecture (UIMA) to enable interfacing of different text analytics solutions with the enterprise data.
- Ability to accelerate the deployment of complex analytics solutions by leveraging Dev/Ops approach to development and deployment of predictive analytics to facilitate the maturation from prototype to scalable production-grade capabilities. One way of achieving this is via implementing enterprise-wide core analytics foundations, such that data scientists, analysts and developers all utilize the same business-driven data model and common analytics toolsets.

### 23.4.3   Other Implications

More than ever, consumers are seeking the right information delivered in an easy to use decision support tool to assist them in their health care decisions. Consumers' expectations in healthcare are shaped by their consumption experience in other industries, most notably retail, banking, travel and telecommunications, where consumer needs are increasingly influenced by digital channels such as web, mobile and social media. For example, more than 75 % of consumers noted that they are willing to sign up for a mobile app or website to help them adhere to their doctor's treatment plan and track their health goals [13]. To meet such consumer expectations, payers need to compete on multi-channel presence and quality of experience. This includes mobile tools, website content (design), social media participation, consumer surveys and customer support. As a result, in the highly competitive new market, payers need to rethink consumer engagement methods from grounds up, and use growing consumer ownership and accountability to drive sustainable behavioral change, improved outcomes and lower cost of healthcare.

With access to most of the utilization and provider data related to healthcare activities for their insured members, payers are uniquely positioned to act as the information hub and healthcare solution agent. In parallel to maturing their consumer-centric data management and analytics platform, payers are expanding their consumer engagement platforms, ranging from self-service portals, mobile health platforms, social media engagement and gamification, to alternative care delivery platforms.

- **Self-Service Portals:** Omni-channel platform enable consumers to seek information related to their healthcare utilization decisions, from product selection, to healthcare service provider comparison, to wellness choices. Such platforms include information around product features, quality and price of care, delivered via interactive platform that supports diverse queries (e.g. regarding coverage, provider search). Furthermore, the complexity of the ACA and the surge in the number of people seeking insurance is driving the increase in the healthcare plan call center workload, and impacting the quality of service. Many elements of this process can be successfully diverted to the digital channels and self-help mechanisms, which will drive a new wave of digitization of customer care. Examples include: educational aid, online tutorials, online self-service kiosks, insurance calculators, online discussion forums, intelligent virtual shopping assistants, independent consumer surveys, etc.
- **Social Media Engagement and Collaboration Platforms:** Healthcare consumers are seeking information on the Internet and in social media space to make informed decisions on their healthcare choices. An increasing number of individuals are willing to share their healthcare experiences and learn from others. Healthcare payers have increasingly leveraged social media and social collaboration platforms to continuously engage with consumers [20]. They can further enhance consumer experience through collaboration platforms enabling conversation between consumers, providers and prospects. The critical factor shaping the requirements for collaborative platforms in healthcare is HIPAA, which dictates how privacy and personal information is to be managed between various stakeholders in the healthcare industry.
- **Mobile Health Platform:** Utilization of mobile health (mHealth) platform facilitates the exchange of information, diagnosis, treatment, and monitors through phones and mobile devices from millions of individuals, which has enormous potential to lower the cost of health interactions and improve overall quality of care [18].

  - Healthcare, unlike many other industries, is almost entirely delivered by physical interaction between patients and health professionals. Furthermore, many diseases require multiple professionals to be engaged in diagnosis, treatment and follow-up. This need for co-location is manageable for episodic healthcare interactions. However, for chronic diseases, which require constant monitoring, this is not only inconvenient, but also expensive, which often prevents patients for getting ideal care. The promise of mobile health is the ability to achieve co-location through technology solutions, allowing patients and health professionals to interact without the need to be in the same place. mHealth platforms will allow secure connection of multiple devices to data management and storage systems, which can be interrogated remotely by health professionals or expert systems.

- Payer can enable or partner with mhealth platform to enable its member to interact with healthcare service providers, from basic interactions such as voice, video or text-based messages, net-based information resources, or reminders generated by expert systems, all the way to sophisticate ones, such as remote sensors (e.g. heart or glucose monitors), smart pill dispensers, RFID tags which can sense when a pill has been swallowed, or "smart pills" that can monitor vital signs as they pass through the body.
- The ability to have ongoing interactions with multiple service providers via mobile devices is particularly beneficial in managing chronic or high-risk conditions like diabetes, respiratory and cardiac disease.

• **Gamification:** Smartphone users in the US spend an average of 158 min on their phones every day, with gaming taking up to 50 min (32 %) of that time [13]. The ability to apply gaming concepts to real-life tasks, is taking off in many fields, showing potential to improve learning, skill adoption and behavioral change. In healthcare realm, gamification, in form of wellness apps, can be applied to promote healthy lifestyles and improved self-care. Private insurers are beginning to develop mHealth apps, that drive behavioral change, for example, UnitedHealthcare has developed BabyBlocks, a game that incentivizes Medicaid moms to stick to their prenatal checkup appointments, while Aetna has launched CarePass, a platform that aggregates data from different health and wellness applications, within unified dashboard customized to the user.

This anticipated explosion of mHealth and Alternative Care Delivery Platform will result in widespread reliance on distributed file systems (for example, Apache Hadoop) to store vast amounts of personal health data, images, video, GPS data, and chat logs for streamlined indexing and processing. Access to all of this rich, personal data, including sensors, health monitoring readings, and auto-alerts when readings go over thresholds set by physicians, in a real-time shared scenario creates exciting opportunities for traditional healthcare analytics to scale up to meet the big healthcare data challenge.

## 23.5 Conclusion

Health insurance industry in the U.S. has traditionally been group and transaction-focused. With the recent market changes driven by the ACA and the pressures to manage healthcare cost and improve outcomes, many U.S. payers are undergoing the consumer-centric transformation, and making consumer experience and value delivery the number one priority. This transformation requires fundamental shift in how payers manage their businesses, from organizational culture, business processes, to how they use technology as an enabler of more informed and agile operations.

As payers begin to interact with individual consumers throughout the consumer lifecycle, as they take more active role in impacting and changing healthcare behaviors, the need for scalable, timely and agile analytics capabilities to inform and support these dynamic interactions continues to increase. In this chapter, we described how the ever-increasing needs and expectations of healthcare consumers impact different business processes of a healthcare payer, and we highlighted the improvements that can be achieved by applying insights derived with advanced analytics.

While there are some success stories on how payers leverage new data sources or novel analytics methods in this transformation, these successes are not widespread in the industry and tend to impact limited number of business functions within the organization. As payers continue on the journey of consumer-centric transformation, the industry can benefit from in-depth case studies of individual payers' experience and lessons learned from the deployments of enterprise-grade Big Data solutions and predictive analytics platforms.

The primary focus of this work relates to payers' direct engagement with individual consumers. Another potential area for future work is to better understand the role of information technology, advanced analytics and collaborative solutions, as payers engage different players in the healthcare ecosystem to enable consumer-centric business model. The ecosystem players range from traditional service providers (e.g. hospitals, physicians and rehab centers), to social and home services (e.g. social workers and home care), to emerging digital health service providers (e.g. wellness device providers, mobile app developers and data curators).

Payer can greatly benefit from coordinating with these health and wellness providers in motivating and supporting consumer's health journey. There are many open questions, for instance, about how to best gather, synthesize and share information across the magnitude of service providers to improve consumer health and retention, how to improve analytics methods in deriving insights based on data from increasing number of sources, how to leverage the emerging API marketplace to improve payer's consumer-centric operations, and etc.

# References

1. Alexe B. Surfacing time-critical insights from social media, SIGMOD. New York: ACM; 2012.
2. Andrews M. Insurers open stores to peddle health plans. 2012. Retrieved 2 Feb 2015, from http://kaiserhealthnews.org/news/health-insurance-stores-022812-michelle-andrews/.

3. Bank of America, M. Consumer-centric health: treasury impacts on payers and providers. 2014. Retrieved 2 Feb 2015, from http://corp.bankofamerica.com/documents/10157/67594/ ConsumerCentricHealthcare.pdf.
4. Bruell A. Health-insurance providers seek direct-to-consumer connections. 2012. Retrieved 2 Feb 2015, from advertising age: http://adage.com/article/news/health-insurance-providers-seek-direct-consumer-connections/232697/.
5. Deloitte Center for Health Solutions. Health insurance exchanges: a strategic perspective. 2011. Retrieved 2 Feb 2015, from http://www.amcp.org/WorkArea/DownloadAsset. aspx?id=10594.
6. Department of Health and Human Services Office. Health insurance marketplace: summary enrollment report for the initial annual open enrollment period. 2014. Retrieved 2 Feb 2015, from http://aspe.hhs.gov/health/reports/2014/MarketPlaceEnrollment/Apr2014/ib_2014apr_ enrollment.pdf.
7. Dixon-Fyle S, Gandhi S, Pellathy T, Spatharou A. Changing patient behavior: the next frontier in healthcare value. Health Int. 2012;12:65–73.
8. Draper D. Commercial health plans' care management activities and the impact on costs, quality and outcomes. Center for Studying Health System Change. Washington, DC: Congressional Testimony; 2007.
9. Garla S, Hopping A, Monaco R, Rittman S. What do your consumer habits say about your health? Using third-party data to predict individual health risk and costs. SAS global forum. San Francisco: SAS; 2013.
10. Georgetown University. Disease management programs: improving health while reducing costs? Health policy institute. Washington, DC: Georgetown University; 2004.
11. Herman B. Insurers build retail centers to enhance brand image. 2014. Retrieved 2 Feb 2015, from http://www.modernhealthcare.com/article/20141101/MAGAZINE/311019962
12. HIMSS Analytics. Electronic Medical Record Adoption Model (EMRAM). 2014. Retrieved 2 Feb 2015, from http://www.himssanalytics.org/emram/emram.aspx
13. InfoSys Public Services. Healthcare insights – consumer engagement. 2014. Retrieved 5 Feb 2015, from http://www.infosyspublicservices.com/insights/Documents/consumer-engagement. pdf
14. Insurers leveraging Patients' personal data for predictive analytics. 2014. Retrieved 2 Feb 2015, from iHealthBeat: http://www.ihealthbeat.org/articles/2014/6/30/insurers-leveraging-patients-personal-data-for-predictive-analytics.
15. Fox P, Kongstved P. A history of managed health care and health insurance in the United States. In: Peter Kongstvedt, editor. Essentials of managed health care. Burlington, Sixth Edition: Jones & Bartlett Learning; 2013.
16. Mccarthy D, Cohen A, Johnson MB. Gaining ground: care management programs to reduce hospital admissions and readmissions among chronically Ill and vulnerable patients. The Commonwealth Fund Publication. 2013;5:1658.
17. Furukawa M, Patel V. Hospital electronic health information exchange grew substantially in 2008–12. Health Aff. 2013;32(8):1346–54.
18. Parks Associates. Nearly 30% of U.S. broadband households own and use a connected health device. 2014. Retrieved 2 Feb 2015, from ParksAssociate: http://www.parksassociates.com/ events/connected-health/media/chs-2014-pr17
19. Raghupathi W, Raghupathi V. Big data analytics in healthcare: promise and potential. Health Inf Sci Syst. 2014;2(3):2–10.
20. Rao A. Health insurers tune in to twitter for customer service. 2013. Retrieved 2 Feb 2015, from http://kaiserhealthnews.org/news/health-insurers-take-to-twitter-for-customer-service/
21. Singer N. When a health plan knows how you shop. 2014. Retrieved 2 Feb 2015, from NY Times. http://www.nytimes.com/2014/06/29/technology/when-a-health-plan-knows-how-you-shop.html.
22. Stehno C, Johns C. You are what you eat: using consumer data to predict health risk. Contingencies. 2006.

23. Tang L, Liu H. Community detection and mining in social media. Morgan & Claypool Publishers, Synthesis Lectures on Data Mining and Knowledge Discovery; 2010.
24. The Henry J. Kaiser Family Foundation. Health insurance coverage of the total population. 2014. Retrieved 2 Feb 2015, from http://kff.org/other/state-indicator/total-population/.
25. Winkelman R, Mehmud S. A comparative analysis of claims-based tools for health risk assessment. Schaumburg: Society of Actuaries; 2007.
26. Shahar Y, Goren-Bar D. Distributed, intelligent, interactive visualization and exploration of time-oriented clinical data and their abstractions. Artif Intell Med. 2006;38(2):115–35.
27. Zhou J, Wang F, Hu J, Ye J. From micro to macro: data driven phenotyping by densification of longitudinal electronic medical records. 2014. KDD. Association of Computing Machinery.

# Chapter 24
# Interoperability: E Pluribus Unum

David L. Meyers

**Abstract** Healthcare information technology is on a quest for interoperability, driven by the Report of the Commission on Systemic Interoperability: "**Ending the Document Game**", published in 2005. In that document, interoperability was described as "connectivity—constant, instant access to your medical information…" (http://endingthedocumentgame.gov/PDFs/entireReport.pdf) and was viewed as critical to nothing less than transforming health care in the United States. The report exhibits the frustration and, at times, anger over the sorry state of medical information in the US, particularly as it relates to reliance on paper, poor quality of documentation content, the duplication of effort to obtain useful information, lack of availability across platforms and distances and especially the role that this lack of connectedness plays in causing actual harm to patients and huge costs to our economy. The Commission's recommendations reflect the imperative and urgent need for total reconstitution of how we obtain, share and use information in the work of healthcare, especially in patient care, but also in the many other activities which enhance health of individuals, communities and populations. The Commission projected a 10 year timetable to achieve the goals they laid out. We are not there yet, and in fact we still have a long way to go.

This chapter will describe the many terminologies, nomenclatures and classification systems used in healthcare, which ultimately and ideally will be winnowed down, combined, modified, edited and standardized into a single, uniform, encompassing communication tool which permits the exchange of all types of information – clinical, financial, regulatory, demographic, quality- and safety-related, public health and epidemiologic – between and among various digital platforms, institutions, systems, applications, vendors, devices and individuals, **and** makes that information usable without special effort by all who are authorized and need it. In short, **e pluribus unum**.

**Keywords** Interoperability • Ontology • Nomenclature • Terminology • Classification systems

D.L. Meyers, MD, FACEP
Department of Emergency Medicine, Sinai Hospital of Baltimore, Baltimore, MD, USA
e-mail: dm0015@comcast.net

© Springer International Publishing Switzerland 2016                                         421
C.A. Weaver et al. (eds.), *Healthcare Information Management Systems:*
*Cases, Strategies, and Solutions*, Health Informatics,
DOI 10.1007/978-3-319-20765-0_24

## 24.1    Introduction and Overview

Healthcare, like virtually all human activities, is inevitably and immeasurably dependent on communication of useful information. The information exchanged can be clinical, financial, administrative; educational; safety-, quality- and effectiveness-related; of public health significance; and it can be with and among patients and family members, clinicians, researchers, educators, administrators, coders, payers, public health monitors, government regulators and other agencies which review safety, quality and others measures. It can take place using natural and formal languages, structured terminologies, standardized nomenclatures, classification and coding systems, digital 1s and 0s. It is believed that widespread use of electronic health records (EHRs) holds the key to better care and lower costs and, to those ends, substantial investment has been and will continue to be made by government and the private sector in the US to achieve these goals.

To facilitate communication and to serve all the various users of healthcare information in the digital age, numerous methods and approaches have arisen over time to convey and manage information, each with special characteristics pertinent to its users. As Christopher Chute stated over a decade ago, "we are amidst a major revolution in the role and capabilities of health terminologies" [16], and that revolution continues, perhaps with even more ferocity and urgency than when those words were written.

## 24.2    Interoperability, the Holy Grail

In healthcare, one of the fundamental challenges of our age is to create and implement tools for naming, recording, storing and communicating information accurately and effectively to accomplish the goals of our enterprise, namely to foster health and, in its absence, to provide safe, timely, appropriate and effective care to those who need it. Information technology certainly provides the capabilities to handle large amounts of data and to do amazing things with it, and thus the opportunity exists to apply it to the healthcare enterprise to achieve those objectives. Yet we are not where we want to be. Among the reasons are: (1) our information formats are still not as accessible, understandable and mutually comprehensible to all parties as is necessary, that is, the ease-of-use and interoperability problems persist; (2) the absolute costs in money and time related to creating, implementing, using and maintaining them are high and the value proposition is not clearly resolved for the end users – clinicians and others; and (3) we have been overconfident regarding human nature and resistance to change and how long it would take to overcome these challenges.

Although some might criticize the allusion to the Tower of Babel, much work is still needed to bring uniformity and standardization to the various terminologies, nomenclatures, classifications and communication tools used throughout healthcare. The government agency charged with coordinating and overseeing this effort in the

US is the Office of the National Coordinator for Health Information Technology, ONCHIT or ONC for short.

This chapter will introduce the reader to some definitions and tools used to name, describe, classify, transmit and communicate information relevant to healthcare for use throughout the healthcare enterprise. A caveat is in order here: Like so much in our field, our knowledge is constantly changing. Virtually all of these are in evolution, development or decline. Certainly some of the information presented will be out-of-date soon after publication of this text. The reader who wishes or needs to remain knowledgeable will need to work hard to keep up.

## 24.3 Background

Moving from philosophy to theory to practice in health care information technology requires knowledge and understanding of some terms used to define and describe that information. All of the definitions below are subject to various nuances, and different authorities may not all agree on the definitions presented here.

At the most fundamental level, early Greek philosophers used the term "**ontology**", in reference to the nature of existence. In the recent history of artificial intelligence, the word has taken on additional meanings related to naming and cataloging according to their properties, types of things that may exist in a domain or subject matter field, in our case health care [7, 8, 15].

The following definitions and many others as well as a detailed discussion of issues around information technology in health care and patient safety were published by the Institute of Medicine (IOM)/National Academy of Sciences (NAS) in its report "Patient Safety: Achieving a New Standard for Care [6].

"**Classification**": The act of organizing information based on specific characteristics or the result of such an activity. Also, "a taxonomy that arranges or organizes like or related terms for easy retrieval".

"**Code**": A numeric or alphanumeric representation assigned to a term so that it may be more readily processed.

"**Coding**": The process of converting names or terms into codes.

"**Interoperability**" [19, 24, 33]: The extent to which systems and devices used in healthcare can exchange *and* interpret or use shared data. For systems to be interoperable, they must be able to exchange data and subsequently present that data such that it can be understood by a user or across platforms. To accomplish this, the system architectures and standards must make it possible for diverse electronic health record (EHR) systems to work compatibly in a true information network.

"**Nomenclature**": A system of naming or of names, applicable to a particular field or area of interest.

"**Terminology**": A body of words or "terms" used in a particular field of study or application, in this case health care. Examples include findings, diseases, procedures, treatments, drugs, administrative and financial information, any information one may encounter in the provision of health care. Terminologies define, classify, and in some cases code data content.

"**Vocabulary**": is a list of words with their meanings or contexts. This is particularly important because certain words have different meanings depending on the context in which they are used.

## 24.4   The Alphabet Soup of Terminologies, Nomenclature, Coding and Classification Systems with a Few Other Terms of Interest

What follows is a list of terminologies, nomenclatures, classification and coding systems in current use with a brief description of their purposes. The panoply of entities discussed here currently serve many stakeholders and there is certainly overlap among some of these entities. A comprehensive list of resources is published by the American Health Information Management Association [1].

**CDT – Code on Dental Procedures and Nomenclature** [2]: is a coding system created by the American Dental Association (ADA) to report dental services and procedures to dental insurance plans, analogous to the CPT code system, described below, for purposes of billing and reimbursement. It is revised and published annually by the ADA.

**Classification of Death and Injury Resulting from Terrorism** [9]: a set of codes within the framework of ICD and ICD-9 CM (see below), developed following the attacks on the World Trade Center in New York City and the Pentagon in Washington, DC on September 11, 2001, to facilitate recording of deaths from acts of terrorism on death certificates and injuries and illnesses from terrorism reported in healthcare records for statistical purposes and for reimbursement. For these purposes, terrorism is defined as: "… the unlawful use of force or violence against persons or property to intimidate or coerce a government, the civilian population, or any segment thereof, in furtherance of political or social objectives" [38].

**CPT – Current Procedural Terminology** [4]: A medical nomenclature created and maintained by the American Medical Association (AMA) used to report every type of medical procedure and service performed by physicians and other qualified clinicians in all settings (hospital, office, clinic, etc) for reimbursement under public and private health insurance programs. Physicians and other professionals generally bill for their services separately from hospitals and other facilities, and do so based on CPT codes. For example, physician services are covered under Part B of Medicare and are reported for reimbursement using the CPT system. The primary CPT codes are alphanumeric consisting of five digits. It is now in its four Revision (CPT-4). There are several sub-types of codes within the CPT:

- E & M – Evaluation and Management codes: are comprised of seven components, including the three KEY components of patient history, physical examination and medical decision-making. The other four elements under this category are counseling, coordination of care, nature of the presenting problem and time spent in providing the care.
- Numerous modifiers and special codes provide additional information about the services provided.
- Procedure codes – are used to report the wide variety of interventions, operations and other invasive and non-invasive procedures and treatments performed in the provision of care

**DRGs – Diagnosis Related Groups** [13]: is a classification of diseases according to the patient's affected organ system(s), surgical procedures performed, morbidity, and gender. It originally was applied to hospital in-patient services provided to beneficiaries covered under Medicare Part A (the hospital insurance portion of Medicare), and is now used by Medicaid and other payers. The DRG for a patient's care is determined by the "principal diagnosis", i.e., the condition which after evaluation is deemed to have occasioned the hospital admission. These diagnoses are coded using ICD-9 CM terminology; after October 1, 2015, ICD-10 CM/-PCS, assuming it is implemented on that date, will be used (see discussion under "ICD" below). The DRG model was created as part of a "Prospective Payment System (PPS)", mandated by legislation which amended the Social Security Law of 1983 to replace the cost-plus payment methodologies in place since the enactment of Medicare in 1965 and which resulted in burgeoning costs to the program. Under the PPS, a hospital which contracts with Medicare to furnish acute in-patient care to a Medicare beneficiary (patient) is paid a fixed predetermined amount for each such patient. The amount of payment to the hospital is established by the DRG in which the principal discharge diagnosis falls and several other factors which include: a "base rate" determined by Medicare which is the average cost to treat patients with that diagnosis, the hospital's unique "blended" rate which includes the case-mix index (a weighting factor based on that hospital's in-patient average severity of illness across all DRGs) and a number of other factors [18, 32]. Secondary diagnoses, co-existing illnesses, procedures and complications of care also figure into the final payment made for the individual patient's hospitalization. The payment methodology rewards efficient hospitals which can treat a patient for less than the fixed reimbursement. Less efficient hospitals can lose money when the costs of care exceed the Medicare reimbursement for that DRG.

**DSM-5 – Diagnostic and Statistical Manual of Mental Disorders – 5 edition** [5]: After years of preparation, DSM-5 replaced DSM-IV (including the change from Roman numerals to Arabic in the name of the document) in January 2014. The new edition, published by the American Psychiatric Association, is now the official classification of mental disorders and diagnostic tool used by mental and other health professionals in the United States. It contains a listing of diagnostic criteria for every psychiatric disorder and mental health diagnosis recognized in the U.S. healthcare system, and is used in all settings by psychiatrists, other physicians, social workers, nurses and other professionals who provide mental health services. The DSM-5 directs providers to the appropriate codes in the ICD-9 CM (until October 1, 2015) and in ICD-10 CM beginning on October 1, 2015 for determination of diagnosis codes used in billing and reimbursement.

**HCPCS – Healthcare Common Procedure Coding System** [12]: is a two level standardized coding system used by hospitals to bill for services and care. Level I is identical to the CPT coding system developed and maintained by the AMA (see above); it identifies medical services and procedures performed by physicians and other healthcare professionals in hospital outpatient settings. Level II is a standardized coding system for describing and identifying health care equipment and supplies – ambulance services, durable medical equipment, prosthetics and other materials – used in health care encounters outside a physician's office that are not included in HCPCS level I codes. Level 2 codes are alphanumeric with a letter and four digits.

**HCUP – Healthcare Cost and Utilization Project (HCUP, pronounced "H-Cup", not "hiccup")** [23]: is a "family of databases and related software tools and products developed through a Federal-State-Industry partnership and sponsored by the Agency for Healthcare Research and Quality (AHRQ)." The information in HCUP databases is derived from discharge abstracts and contains administrative data as well as encounter-level clinical and nonclinical information including all listed diagnoses and procedures, discharge status, patient demographics, and charges for all patients across all payers – Medicare, Medicaid, private insurance, uninsured, etc. These databases enable research on a broad range of health policy issues, including cost and quality of health services, medical practice patterns, access to health care programs, and outcomes of treatments at the national, state, and local market levels.

**HEDIS – Healthcare Effectiveness Data and Information Set** [31]: is a proprietary tool developed by the National Committee for Quality Assurance used by a large number of health plans, managed care and other healthcare organizations to measure and compare performance on certain aspects of care and service promoted as markers for quality and effectiveness. Meeting certain standards of the NCQA can result in "certification" by the NCQA. The measured parameters, which are updated annually and may be added, changed or removed, are chosen for their application to large numbers of people and/or their relevance to quality and effectiveness of care. The monitored data is obtained from surveys, claims and medical record reviews.

**HIPAA – Health Insurance Portability and Accountability Act of 1996** [14]: In order to protect the privacy and security of individually identifiable healthcare information, this wide-ranging law and the regulations pursuant to it established national standards for the protection and exchange of such information with particular attention to electronic transmission. Enforcement is the responsibility of the federal Office of Civil Rights (OCR). "Covered entities" and "business associates" are defined in the law and required to observe it. Other specified entities are excluded from compliance. The data covered by the law include: claims for payment and encounter information, payment and remittance advice, claim status, eligibility, enrollment and disenrollment, referrals and authorizations, coordination of benefits and premium payment. The following specific code sets for diagnoses and procedures are required to be used in all transactions by a covered entity of business associate: HCPCS, CPT-4, CDT, ICD-9, ICD-10 and NDC. These code sets are described elsewhere in this chapter.

**HL7 – Health Level Seven** [20] is a non-governmental membership organization founded in 1987 for the purpose of fostering a "comprehensive framework and related standards for the exchange, integration, sharing, and retrieval of electronic health information that supports clinical practice and the management, delivery and evaluation of health services". The goal is ease of transmission and communication of clinical and administrative data across disparate healthcare applications and within and across healthcare organizations and international boundaries, in other words to solve the problem of interoperability by promoting specifications to make systems exchange data and present that data such that it can be understood by all users or across platforms. These specifications are developed through collaboration among the members of the organization in various work groups, forums, conferences and educational sessions. Some achievements and projects include:

- The HL7 Consolidated Clinical Data Architecture (C-CDA) [25] is the latest iteration of a base standard for the construction and organization of all kinds of clinical text documents such as discharge summaries, operative and progress notes, narrative reports, etc. It ensures that all text documents maintain the same organization of content to enable sharing between healthcare entities, i.e., interoperability, using vocabularies such as Systematized Nomenclature of Medicine Clinical Terms (SNOMED CT) and Logical Observation Identifiers, Names, and Codes (LOINC) to encode concepts in the documents and also allow for scanned images and other files. It is both machine and human readable.
- HL7 has also taken on responsibility for developing a standardized functional model for EHR systems for use by system builders to help accelerate adoption of EHR systems. The model requires that consistent terminologies be used to provide a standardized language for all EHR systems which will facilitate the mapping of local terminologies to the specified standard terminologies.
- FHIR (pronounced "fire") is a new standards framework created by HL7 for exchanging healthcare information electronically. It combines features of previously developed specifications based on current and emerging web standards and focusing on ease of implementation [21].

**ICD – International Classification of Diseases**: is a system of disease classification, now in use world wide in its 10 revision with the 11 revision under way. The ICD itself is the successor to a long history of efforts to classify causes of death and disease that began, in our current era at least, several centuries ago with early British work by John Graunt who sought to bring order to the process of tracking and recording causes of death in the latter half of the 16th century [16, 45]. While the growing need for a compendium of causes of death and diseases was recognized in the early 1800s, and took on some urgency, it took decades before the international community agreed on establishing such a process. By the late nineteenth century, efforts including a series of international convocations to focus on causes of death led to the International List of Causes of Death, which ultimately evolved to become the ICD, and the approved system was revised and updated every 10 years. The value of a similar classification for morbidity and diseases was also recognized in the mid-nineteenth century, including, in 1860, Florence Nightingale's proposal for adoption of a classification for tracking hospital data. It took several decades more for an international agreement to accomplish this in 1900. Following a period of decennial updates and revision of the system then in place, in 1948, the two classifications were joined into the *International Classification of Diseases, Injuries, and Causes of Death* and accepted by the international community. Decennial updates have continued to the present time when ICD-10 is now the world standard for tracking these conditions.

In 1978, the 9th Revision of ICD (ICD-9) was published followed in 1979 by an adaptation, the Clinical Modification (ICD-9 CM), which included more detail on diseases, especially chronic ones, more frequently encountered in the United States compared to the developing world. In the US, ICD-9 CM is used for the purpose of assigning diagnosis and procedure codes which are in turn used by hospitals, Medicare and other health insurers as the basis for DRGs (see above) and hospital billing and reimbursement.

The 10th revision of ICD (ICD-10), is currently the classification standard in the US for mortality and death certificate data. The version of ICD-10 that is intended to replace ICD-9-CM consists of two subsets of codes, ICD-10-CM to replace the diagnosis code component of ICD-9-CM (volumes 1 and 2) and ICD-10-PCS (Procedure Coding System) to replace procedure codes in ICD-9-CM (volume 3). ICD-10-CM and -PCS have nearly 72,000 codes, while ICD-9-CM has ~17,000 codes.

The original transition from ICD-9 CM to ICD-10-CM/-PCS was to take place October 1, 2013. Objections and concerns about cost and complexity of implementation, raised by various affected parties, especially physicians, critical access hospitals (hospitals certified under a set of Medicare Conditions of Participation (CoP)[1], which are structured differently than the acute care hospital CoP) and others, led the US Congress to pass legislation to delay it for 1 year. As the new deadline of October 1, 2014 loomed, again physicians and other parties raised concerns and objections, leading to another 1 year postponement. The new start date is now scheduled for October 1, 2015 when all entities covered by the Health Insurance Portability and Accountability Act (HIPAA – see above) are scheduled to convert. At the time of this writing, it appears that it will be implemented on that date, although strong opposition continues based on the concerns over anticipated costs, complexity, readiness and the presumed availability of ICD-11 in the near future, possibly as early as 2017.

---

[1] http://www.hrsa.gov/healthit/toolbox/RuralHealthITtoolbox/Introduction/critical.html

**ICF – International Classification of Functioning, Disability and Health** [44]: first published in 1980, this is a World Health Organization classification system for health and functional capability, developed to standardize language and create a framework for describing health and health-related states in terms of body structure and function and relates these elements to "what an individual can do in a standard environment (level of capacity) and what the individual can actually do (level of performance)". These states "are classified from body, individual and societal perspectives by means of two lists: one of body functions and structure, and another of domains of activity and participation. In ICF, the term 'functioning' refers to all body functions, activities and participation, while disability is similarly an umbrella term for impairments, activity limitations and participation restrictions. ICF also lists environmental factors that interact with all these components." An important element of this system is that, rather than a model of health and disability, it views health on a continuum with an individual's level of function as the key determinant of what resources are needed to aid the individual to achieve his or her optimal performance, and a recognition that virtually all of us will at some time function at some level less than our ideal or optimum.

**LOINC – Logical Observation Identifiers, Names and Codes** [29, 30]: is a database for reporting laboratory and other clinical observations in a common language. Originating at the Regenstreif Institute in 1994, its purpose was to create a universal code system for laboratory test names, results and observations in order to facilitate electronic exchange of information and pooling of results. Having been adopted as the federal interoperability standard for lab test orders and drug label section headers, it provides a uniform means of sharing such information between healthcare entities, including facility-based and outsourced laboratories. It is also being used to encode other healthcare information, such as text document titles, mental health instruments, ventilator settings, electrocardiogram parameters, clinical scoring tools, imaging exams and more.

**MU – Meaningful Use** [26]: is a US government program created under the Health Information Technology for Economic and Clinical Health (HITECH) Act, a part of the American Recovery and Reinvestment Act of 2009. Its purpose is to facilitate adoption of electronic health records technology in order to improve quality, safety and efficiency in healthcare and reduce health disparities. The MU program has three components:

1. Use EHR technology to improve care and efficiency;
2. Enhance the electronic exchange of information to improve outcomes;
3. Provide for electronic submission of clinical and quality measures.

Specific objectives are established that eligible professionals (EPs) and hospitals must achieve to qualify for financial incentives and avoid penalties. The program, managed by the Centers for Medicare and Medicaid Services, began in 2011 and is being implemented in three stages to be fully in place in 2016.

**NDC – National Drug Codes**: is a current list of all drugs manufactured, prepared, propagated, compounded, or processed for commercial distribution. Mandated by the Federal Food Drug and Cosmetic Act, drug products are identified and reported using a unique, three-segment number, which serves as a universal product identifier for drugs. It is overseen by the Food and Drug Administration (FDA).

**Newborn Screening Coding and Terminology Guide** [40]: describes electronic health data standards to be used in recording and transmitting newborn screening test results. Included are standard codes and terminologies for such tests as well as the conditions for which they are performed and links to related sites. It is anticipated that "use of these standards can speed the delivery of newborn screening reports, facilitate the care and follow-up of infants with positive test results, enable the use (and comparison) of data from different laboratories, and support the development of strategies for improving the newborn screening process."

## 24.5  Nursing-Related Datasets and Classification Systems

Among these systems, there is a fair amount of overlap or duplication. Some have gained more widespread use than others, but a significant number of nurses do not use any of the standardized tools. It is likely that some will persist and find wider use, others will merge, and still others will ultimately decline and disappear, to be of historic interest only. This listing is not comprehensive, but rather representative of such systems.

**CCC – Clinical Care Classification (formerly HHCC – Home Health Care Classification system)** [39]: was developed by V Saba and colleagues as a standardized framework and a unique coding structure for assessing, documenting, and classifying patient care provided by nurses and other clinical practitioners. CCC has two sets of interrelated terminologies – Nursing Diagnoses and Nursing Interventions. The system consists of 21 Care Components, modeled around the "Nursing Process Standards of Care", namely Diagnosis, Outcome Identification, Planning, Implementation, Evaluation, and Assessment [35].

**ICNP – International Classification for Nursing Practice** [43]: is a system of classification of all the domains of nursing practice. It can be used to compose and represent diagnoses, interventions, and outcomes in a hierarchical manner and includes subsets for selected health priorities, including nursing outcome indicators, pediatric pain management, palliative care and adherence to treatment. Goals are for these data sets and parameters to describe nursing care in a uniform way and to facilitate: (1) communication across languages, settings of care, geography, time and clinical populations; (2) comparison of nursing care; (3) research; (4) identification of trends; (5) policy-making.

**NIC – Nursing Interventions Classification** [36]: developed at the University of Iowa, it is a standardized classification tool consisting of 554 nursing interventions, performed both independently and in collaboration with others. Its uses include "clinical documentation, communication of care across settings, integration of data across systems and settings, effectiveness research, productivity measurement, competency evaluation, reimbursement, and curricular design".

**NOC – Nursing Outcomes Classification** [37]: also developed at the University of Iowa, this tool provides a comprehensive, standardized classification for nearly 500 nursing outcomes. It also has been designed for use in many care settings and patient populations and by non-nursing professionals.

**NMDS – The Nursing Minimum Data Set (NMDS)**: is an early classification system to standardize the collection and recording of nursing care data obtained and/or used by nurses in the delivery of care. It is used in direct patient care settings to provide accurate descriptions of assessments, diagnoses, care and resources used in the provision of nursing services and in public health, policy-making and research, it enables comparison of such data across populations, settings, geographic areas and time.

**OASIS – Outcome and Assessment Information Set (OASIS)** [11]: The Outcome and ASsessment Information Set (OASIS) is a group of data elements that relate to the comprehensive assessment of adult home care patients and the measurement of patient outcomes in the context of outcome-based quality improvement (OBQI) efforts.

**Omaha System** [34]: is a classification system originally developed in the 1970s by the Visiting Nurses Association of Omaha, Nebraska. It consists of three components – a problem classification system based on client assessment, an intervention scheme reflecting care plans and services and a problem rating scale to measure client progress. Its components map to those of the INCP (above).

**RxNorm** [42]: RxNorm is a nomenclature system for generic and branded drugs developed by the US National Library of Medicine (NLM). It provides standardized names including ingredient(s), strength(s), dose(s) and unique identifiers as well as related drug names. These names are linked to other drug vocabularies. The methodology allows different drug and pharmacy systems to communicate reliably and unambiguously. It includes prescription and many over-the-counter drugs and drug packs containing multiple drugs or sequences of drugs available in the US. It does not include radiopharmaceuticals, contrast media, food or dietary supplements or medical devices.

**RBRVS – Resource-Based Relative Value Scale**: is a system of physician payment based on the amount of physician resources expended in providing the services. These amounts were derived from the research of Dr William Hsaio and colleagues at the Harvard School of Public Health published in 1988 [27]. Their study analyzed the many activities physicians do (there are roughly 8000 procedure codes in the CPT-4 code book) and assigned units of relative value to them (Relative Value Units – RVUs) according to three components. First, the physician work RVUs, accounting for ~48 % of the total relative value were based on how much time was required to perform the service, the technical skill, judgment, mental and physical effort required and the stress due to the potential risk to the patient. Second, the practice expense RVUs, accounting for another ~48 %, originally were determined by a formula based on average Medicare charges, a formula since modified to reflect practice costs related to the specific CPT code and site of the service. Third, the professional liability RVU is determined from malpractice premium costs and several other factors; it accounts for ~4 % of the total RVU for each service. The components are combined and multiplied by a conversion factor and adjusted for geography to determine the payment. This system replaced the prior physician payment model.

**SNOMED CT – Systematized Nomenclature of Medicine – Clinical Terms** [28] is a comprehensive, international, multilingual clinical healthcare terminology, originally created by the College of American Pathologists (CAP) and now owned, maintained, and distributed by the International Health Terminology Standards Development Organization (IHTSDO), a not-for-profit association in Denmark of which the National Library of Medicine is a member, allowing free use in the US. With almost a million descriptions for clinical concepts, it provides a common language for indexing, storing, retrieving, and aggregating clinical data across specialties and sites of care, as well as be mapped to ICD-9/10 and other coding systems. SNOMED CT's content is represented by three components:

- **Concepts** representing clinical meanings that are organized into hierarchies
- **Descriptions** which link appropriate human readable terms to concepts.
- **Relationships** which link each concept to other related concepts.

Among its features which have contributed to increasing use are:

- its design and organization allow for use by clinicians, researchers, public health and disease surveillance agencies, auditors and regulators, administrators, management and planning agencies;
- its capacity for expansion as medical knowledge, clinical and other needs evolve;
- machine-readable with ease of entry and retrieval of data and information

**SNODENT** is a similar nomenclature which applies to dental care and services. It is a subset of SNOMED-CT [3].

**UHDDS – Uniform Hospital Discharge Data Set and UACDS – Uniform Ambulatory Care Data Set** [10]: are compendia of standardized data elements and their definitions relating to, respectively, in-patient services provided in acute care hospitals and ambulatory care settings. Originally developed for use by Medicaid and Medicare, they are now used by most payers. For the UHDDS, the elements include patient identifiers and demographic information such as date of birth, age, gender, ethnicity, marital status, address; provider/ hospital or health facility information including unique institution identification number, type of facility, date and type of admission, discharge date, assigned physician(s); and patient specific clinical information such as principal and other diagnoses, services and procedures rendered, disposition of patient; and financial information related to source of payment for services. The UACDS includes similar elements; an exception is the patient's stated reason for the encounter.

**DEEDS – Data Elements for Emergency Department Systems** [22]: now in its three version, is a similar compendium of uniform standardized data for emergency department services developed nearly 20 years ago by the national Center for Injury Prevention and Control.

**UMLS – Unified Medical Language System** [41] is a set of files and software maintained by the National Library of Medicine representing numerous health and biomedical vocabularies and standards made available to facilitate interoperability and the development of computer systems that perform a range of functions across many types of health information.

Although by no means a complete list, many of the nomenclatures, coding and classification systems described here do not meet the two criteria of full interoperability, i.e., they do not exchange information between and among each other nor is the data usable by each entity. Each of these was developed to meet the needs and serve the purposes of a particular set of stakeholders. Some have broadened their utility to accommodate multiple user communities and are fully or close to achieving interoperability. Many simply do not and will not reach that level of performance; they likely will become extinct or used in very limited settings. Others will evolve and mature to finally achieve that heretofore lofty goal. It really is a matter of time and ingenuity, the latter of which is certainly in abundant supply in the healthcare information technology arena, that is you dear readers.

## 24.6 Conclusion

The systems of terminology, nomenclature and, classification described above represent important concepts and tools with which the healthcare IT professional must be familiar, and many of the items are likely to be encountered in some fashion in day-to-day work. Some, of course, play less of a role in daily clinical practice and patient care, but most in some way impact the communication and/or use of important information which drives the healthcare enterprise. While, in some respects, we may be closer to achieving Cimino's desiderata [17], at least for some of the nomenclatures and vocabularies described here, we still face significant challenges to reach those goals. In the future, it is hoped many of these systems can be consolidated into fewer or ideally one universal system and the elements will be completely interoperable. Essential to keep in mind as we go forward is the absolute imperative that healthcare information technology must ultimately make it as easy as possible for patients to get what they need, clinicians to make the right decisions and do the right things for their patients, for the larger community to benefit from lessening the burden of illness and to increase the value for the dollars spent on healthcare. It is incumbent on all of us to remember the end beneficiary of our efforts – the patient, ourselves.

**Acknowledgements** I would like to thank Ellen V Makar, RN at the ONC for her advice, assistance and comments on the manuscript and Marion Ball for inviting me to participate in this important effort.

# References

1. AHIMA. Data standards, data quality, and interoperability. Appendix A: data standards Resource. J AHIMA 78, no. 2: web extra. Feb 2007. http://library.ahima.org/xpedio/groups/public/documents/ahima/bok1_033588.hcsp?dDocName=bok1_033588. Accessed 20 Apr 2015.
2. American Dental Association. CDT: code on dental procedures and nomenclature. 2015. http://www.ada.org/en/publications/cdt/. Accessed 15 Apr 2015.
3. American Dental Association. What is SNODENT? 2015. http://www.ada.org/en/member-center/member-benefits/practice-resources/dental-informatics/snodent. Accessed 20 Apr 2015.
4. American Medical Association. CPT current procedural terminology. 2014. http://www.ama-assn.org/ama/pub/physician-resources/solutions-managing-your-practice/coding-billing-insurance/cpt.page. Accessed 20 Apr 2014.
5. American Psychiatric Association. Diagnostic and statistical manual of mental disorders. 5th ed. Washington, DC: American Psychiatric Association; 2013.
6. Aspden P, et al., editors. Patient safety: achieving a new standard for care; Committee on Data Standards for Patient Safety, Board on Health Care Services, Institute of Medicine of the National Academies. Washington, DC: National Academies Press; 2004.
7. Bodenreider O, Burgun A. Biomedical ontologies. In: Chen H, Fuller SS, Friedman C, Hersh W, editors. Medical informatics: knowledge management and data mining in biomedicine. New York: Springer Science+Business Media; 2005. http://ai.arizona.edu/mis596A/book_chapters/medinfo/Chapter_08.pdf. Accessed 20 Apr 2015.
8. Bodenreider O, Stevens R. Bio-ontologies: current trends and future directions. 2006. http://www.ncbi.nlm.nih.gov/pmc/articles/PMC1847325/pdf/nihms14746.pdf. Accessed 20 Apr 2015.
9. Centers for Disease Control and Prevention. Classification of death and injury resulting from terrorism. 2009. http://www.cdc.gov/nchs/icd/terrorism_code.htm. Accessed 20 Apr 2015.
10. Centers for Disease Control. National Committee on Vital and Health Statistics Preliminary Recommendations for Core Health Data Elements. 1996. http://www.cdc.gov/nchs/data/ncvhs/nchvs94.pdf. Accessed 20 Apr 2015.
11. Centers for Medicare & Medicaid Services. Background. 2012. https://www.cms.gov/Medicare/Quality-Initiatives-Patient-Assessment-Instruments/OASIS/Background.html. Accessed 20 Apr 2015.
12. Centers for Medicare & Medicaid Services. HCPCS—general information. 2014a. https://www.cms.gov/Medicare/Coding/MedHCPCSGenInfo/index.html?redirect=/medhcpcsgen-info/. Accessed 20 Apr 2015.
13. Centers for Medicare & Medicaid Services. Inpatient PPS PC Pricer. 2014b. http://www.cms.gov/Medicare/Medicare-Fee-for-Service-Payment/PCPricer/inpatient.html. Accessed 20 Apr 2014.
14. Centers for Medicare & Medicaid Services. Transaction & code set standards. 2014c. http://www.cms.gov/Regulations-and-Guidance/HIPAA-Administrative-Simplification/TransactionCodeSetsStands/index.html?redirect=/TransactionCodeSetsStands/02_TransactionsandCodeSetsRegulations.asp. Accessed 20 Apr 2015.
15. Chandrasekaran B, Josephson JR, Benjamins VR. What are ontologies and why do we need them. 1999. http://www.csee.umbc.edu/courses/771/papers/chandrasekaranetal99.pdf, Accessed 2 Jan 2014.
16. Chute C. Clinical classification and terminology: some history and current observations. J Am Med Inform Assoc. 2000;7:298–303.
17. Cimino J. Desiderata for controlled medical vocabularies in the twenty-first century. Methods Inf Med. 1998;37(4–5):394–403.
18. Department of Health and Human Services, Centers for Medicare & Medicaid Services, and Medicare Learning Network. Acute care hospital inpatient prospective payment system. Payment System Fact Sheet Series. 2013. http://www.cms.gov/Outreach-and-Education/

Medicare-Learning-Network-MLN/MLNProducts/downloads/AcutePaymtSysfctsht.pdf. Accessed 20 Apr 2015.
19. Fridsma D. Interoperability vs health information exchange: setting the record straight. 9 Jan 2013. http://www.healthit.gov/buzz-blog/meaningful-use/interoperability-health-information-exchange-setting-record-straight/. Accessed 20 Apr 2015.
20. Health Level 7 International. About HL7. 2007–2015a. http://www.hl7.org/about/index.cfm?ref=nav. Accessed 20 Apr 2015.
21. Health Level 7 International 2011. FHIR Specification. www.HL7.org/fhir. Accessed 20 Apr 2015.
22. Health Level 7 International. HL7 version 3 specification: Data Elements for Emergency Department Systems (DEEDS), Release 1—US Realm. 2007–2015b. http://www.hl7.org/implement/standards/product_brief.cfm?product_id=326. Accessed 20 Apr 2015.
23. Healthcare Cost and Utilization Project. Healthcare Cost and Utilization Project (HCUP): what is HCUP? 2015. http://www.hcup-us.ahrq.gov. Accessed 20 Apr 2015.
24. Healthcare Information and Management Systems Society (HIMSS). What is interoperability? 2015. http://www.himss.org/library/interoperability-standards/what-is-interoperability. Accessed 20 Apr 2015.
25. HealthIT.gov. Consolidated CDA overview. 2014. http://www.healthit.gov/policy-researchers-implementers/consolidated-cda-overview. Accessed 20 Apr 2015.
26. HealthIT.gov. Meaningful use definition & objectives. 2015. http://www.healthit.gov/providers-professionals/meaningful-use-definition-objectives. Accessed 20 Apr 2015.
27. Hsiao WC, Braun P, Kelly NL, Becker ER. Results, potential effects, and implementation issues of the resource-based relative value scale. JAMA. 1988;260(16):2429–38. doi:10.1001/jama.1988.03410160105013.
28. IHTSDO. SNOMED CT starter guide. 2014. http://ihtsdo.org/fileadmin/user_upload/doc/download/doc_StarterGuide_Current-en-US_INT_20141202.pdf?ok. Accessed 20 Apr 2015.
29. LOINC. What LOINC is. 1994–2015. https://loinc.org/get-started/02.html. Accessed 20 Apr 2015.
30. McDonald CJ, Huff SM, Suico JG, Hill G, Leavelle D, Aller R, Forrey A, Mercer K, DeMoor G, Hook J, Williams W, Case J, Maloney P, Laboratory LOINC Developers. LOINC, a Universal Standard for Identifying Laboratory Observations: a 5-year update. Clin Chem. 2003;49(4):624–33. http://www.clinchem.org/content/49/4/624.full?ijkey=oUwNonbF33rao&keytype=ref&siteid=clinchem. Accessed 20 Apr 2015.
31. NCQA. HEDIS 2015. 2015. http://www.ncqa.org/HEDISQualityMeasurement/HEDISMeasures/HEDIS2015.aspx. Accessed 20 Apr 2015.
32. Office of Inspector General, Office of Evaluation and Inspections, Region IX. Medicare hospital prospective payment system: how DRG rates are calculated and updated. 2001. https://oig.hhs.gov/oei/reports/oei-09-00-00200.pdf. Accessed 20 Apr 2015.
33. The Office of the National Coordinator for Health Information Technology 2014. Interoperability Basics. http://www.healthit.gov/public-course/interoperability-basics-training/HITRC_lsn1069/wrap_menupage.htm. Accessed 20 Apr 2015.
34. (No authors listed). The Omaha System. 2014. http://www.omahasystem.org/overview.html. Accessed 20 Apr 2015.
35. Saba VK. Clinical care classification system: about. 1994, 2004, 2013-2014. http://www.sabacare.com/About/?PHPSESSID=b9e97459af41b2c80d194d7434aa7800. Accessed 20 Apr 2015.
36. The University of Iowa College of Nursing 2013. CNC—overview: Nursing Interventions Classification (NIC). http://www.nursing.uiowa.edu/cncce/nursing-interventions-classification-overview. Accessed 20 Apr 2015.
37. The University of Iowa College of Nursing 2013. CNC—overview: Nursing Outcomes Classification (NOC). http://www.nursing.uiowa.edu/cncce/nursing-outcomes-classification-overview. Accessed 20 Apr 2015.
38. US Department of Justice, Federal Bureau of Investigation. Terrorism in the United States 1999, Counterterrorism, Threat Assessment and Warning Unit, Counterterrorism Division. 1999. http://www.fbi.gov/stats-services/publications/terror_99.pdf. Accessed 20 Apr 2015.

39. US National Library of Medicine. 2012AA clinical care classification source information. 2012. http://www.nlm.nih.gov/research/umls/sourcereleasedocs/current/CCC/. Accessed 20 Apr 2015.
40. US National Library of Medicine. About the newborn screening coding and terminology guide. 2014. http://newbornscreeningcodes.nlm.nih.gov/nb/sc/about. Accessed 20 Apr 2015.
41. US National Library of Medicine. Fact sheet: unified medical language system®. 2013. http://www.nlm.nih.gov/pubs/factsheets/umls.html. Accessed 20 Apr 2015.
42. US National Library of Medicine. RxNorm overview. 2015. http://www.nlm.nih.gov/research/umls/rxnorm/overview.html. Accessed 20 Apr 2015.
43. World Health Organization. Classifications: International Classification for Nursing Practice (ICNP). 2015. http://www.who.int/classifications/icd/adaptations/icnp/en/
44. World Health Organization. Classifications: International Classification of Functioning, Disability and Health (ICF). 2014. http://www.who.int/classifications/icf/en/. Accessed 20 Apr 2015.
45. World Health Organization 2015. History of the Development of the ICD. http://www.who.int/classifications/icd/en/HistoryOfICD.pdf. Accessed 4 Jan 2014.

# Chapter 25
# Privacy and Data Security: HIPAA and HITECH

**Joan M. Kiel, Frances A. Ciamacco, and Bradley T. Steines**

**Abstract** With the Omnibus Final Health Insurance Portability and Accountability Act (HIPAA) Rule of September 2013, privacy and security of patient health information has been further tightened. Looking back from 2002 when HIPAA was first released, monetary penalties have increased as has the scrutiny surrounding the protection of patient health information. With numerous updates and additions, such as the Health Information Technology for Economic and Clinical Health Act, (HITECH), to the original HIPAA Rule, managers have to be akin to the changes as any day can bring a HIPAA complaint or breach. In this uncertain environment, breach management is a critical part of working with HIPAA. HIPAA and HITECH are laws which are to be operationalized into an organization's standard operating procedures.

**Keywords** HIPAA • Security • Breaches • Risk analysis • Privacy • Patient health information

As focus and emphasis on the privacy and security of patient protected health information (PHI) continues to grow, so do the sanctions associated with a violation of such tenets. The year 2014 saw the largest monetary settlement to date regarding a data breach involving PHI.

J.M. Kiel, PhD, CHPS MPhil, MPA (✉)
HIPAA & HMS Departments, University HIPAA Compliance, Health Management Systems, Duquesne University, Pittsburgh, PA, USA
e-mail: kiel@duq.edu

F.A. Ciamacco, BS, MS, RHIA
Office of Ethics and Compliance, UPMC, Pittsburgh, PA, USA

B.T. Steines, JD
Corporate Services Division, Office of Ethics and Compliance/Office of Patient and Consumer Privacy, UPMC, Pittsburgh, PA, USA

© Springer International Publishing Switzerland 2016
C.A. Weaver et al. (eds.), *Healthcare Information Management Systems: Cases, Strategies, and Solutions*, Health Informatics,
DOI 10.1007/978-3-319-20765-0_25

In the case in point, New York Presbyterian Hospital (NYP) and Columbia University (CU), operating under a joint arrangement, failed to adequately secure the electronic PHI of nearly 7,000 patients, leading to a breach of sensitive patient information. Upon investigation into the matter, the Department of Health and Human Services (HHS) Office for Civil Rights (OCR) determined that neither NYP nor CU had made "data security central to how they manage their information systems." NYP and CU ultimately settled charges stemming from the breach with the OCR in the amount of $4.8 million [1].

Suits and settlements such as the above are becoming more commonplace.

## 25.1   The Emergence of HIPAA, HITECH, and the Omnibus Rule

The Health Insurance Portability and Accountability Act (HIPAA) of 1996 was created to provide health insurance portability for individuals, to protect the privacy and security of patient health information, and to eradicate fraud and abuse. Also known as the Kennedy-Kassebaum Act or the Administrative Simplification Act, HIPAA was enacted on August 21, 1996 (http://www.ihs.gov/hipaa; accessed October 18, 2014). The law applies to all healthcare providers, clearinghouses, and healthcare plans, known collectively as "HIPAA Covered Entities", who conduct 1 or more of 11 transactions electronically, including billing and receiving payment for healthcare services.

The original impetus for HIPAA emanated from both providers and consumers. Providers wanted standardization and simplification of healthcare claims. Multiple healthcare claim forms, both paper and electronic, had previously existed. This inconsistency necessitated that when transmitting claims data, many times the data would thus first be passed through a clearinghouse, formulating the outgoing data from the provider to the receiving payer organization, and vice versa. This "added step" increased both time and cost to the process. HIPAA standardized claim submissions, such that the sender and the receiver would now have the same formage. Consumers demanded privacy and security of their patient health information, including all oral, paper, and electronic notations. HIPAA thus became integral throughout the delivery of quality healthcare, and if not adhered to, raises wide ranging implications.

The standards set forth in the 1996 passage of HIPAA have since been amended and added to via subsequent legislation, all of which has been consolidated under the HIPAA Omnibus Rule (Omnibus Rule), passed in 2013. The intent of the Omnibus Rule was not only to consolidate the ever evolving obligations and technology associated with the delivery of healthcare, but also to promote objectivity and consistency in the analysis of potential breaches patient privacy.

## 25.2  The Timeline of HIPAA

In 1996 HIPAA was passed as federal law with the intents to safeguard the privacy of protected health information, to establish national standards for health care transactions, and to secure the information that are the subject of the transactions. To this end, six rules of HIPAA were released for implementation between 2002 and 2007.

1. Transactions and Code Sets: Has established standard formats and coding of electronic claims and related transactions. Implemented October 16, 2002.
2. Privacy Rule: Has established guidelines for the use and disclosure of patient health information. Implemented April 14, 2003
3. National Employer Identifier Rule: Has established the federal tax identification number as an employer's national identifier. Implemented July 30, 2004.
4. Data Security Rule: Has established technical and administrative protocols for the security and integrity of electronic health data. Implemented April 20, 2005.
5. Enforcement Rule: Has established rules on how the Government enforces HIPAA. Implemented February 16, 2006
6. National Provider Identifier Rule: Has established a national identifier for each provider and the mechanisms for disseminating, storing, and updating the identifier. Implemented May 23, 2007 [2].

In 2009, the Health Information Technology for Economic and Clinical Health Act (HITECH) was passed as a subset of the American Recovery and reinvestment Act (ARRA). Although it focused on the utilization of electronic health records and meaningful use, it also expanded the Privacy and Security Rules of HIPAA. In 2013, HIPAA was further modified and the Final Rule of HIPAA known as the Omnibus Rule was implemented. Some of the highlights include obligations to business associates, increased rights for patients to access and restrict disclosure of their PHI, rules for use and disclosure of PHI, and clarification of the Enforcement Rule [3] (New Privacy and Security Omnibus Rule Released, Robert Tennant and Amy Nordeng, MGMA Connexion, April 2013, page 18 of 18–21).

## 25.3  Security

The HIPAA Security Rule was enacted to prevent patient health information from being accessed by those without a "need to know". It is paramount that the security and integrity of electronic health data must be protected from unauthorized users. Although electronic exchanges and storage of medical information is prevalent, HIPAA security encompasses physical and administrative security in addition to technical security.

The Security Rule challenges that all electronic transmissions maintain a balance between being accessible, but also being secure and confidential. Information technology systems will follow the ANSI (American National Standards Institute) Standards for interfacing with, including storing, accessing, and transmitting data, all systems. In addition, the Security Rule encompasses various technical and operational policies and procedures such as password maintenance and management, incident reporting, periodic reminders to ensure a secure environment, virus protection, and monitoring of log in and user access.

Data intrusion and breaches of privacy and security protocols are not concerns unique to the health care industry. Long gone are the days where customer records exist on a single piece of physical paper locked away neatly in a filing cabinet. Today's world is filled with the ability to immediately access and transmit mass amounts of information of all kinds. Customer information is not only used to facilitate direct transactions, but it is also warehoused and data-mined for downstream use.

As large amounts of information are utilized by the commercial sector such ways, the information is in turn exposed to the risk of intrusion. Further, as the number of individuals whose information an entity utilizes continues to climb, and the detail associated with that information becomes increasingly more detailed, the likelihood that a breach of that information would be a major issue affecting a large population grows exponentially in turn.

An entity's data security measures must be robust enough to combat current threats, while remaining nimble enough to adjust to an ever changing world of risk. Unfortunately, it is tempting to become complacent in times of minimal breach activity, relying on outdated or insufficient security processes. When a technologically savvy criminal element is added to this mix, the setting is ripe for compromise. It was exactly this climate of risk that yielded an epidemic of large-scale data breaches in 2013 and 2014.

Target (2013) – Approximately 110 million people affected
JP Morgan Chase (2014) – Approximately 75 million people affected
Home Depot (2014) – Approximately 56 million people affected
Evernote (2013) – Approximately 50 million people affected
Living Social (2013) – Approximately 50 million people affected
Adobe (2013) – Approximately 40 million people affected [4]

A breach is the acquisition, access, use, or disclosure of protected health information in a manner which compromises the security or privacy of the protected health information (45CFR164.402) [5]. A disclosure to unintended recipients is reportable under HIPAA to the affected individuals and the Department of Health and Human Services. In addition, if the affected number is 500+, the breach must be reported publically and to the media. Breaches must be investigated according to four factors:

(a) The nature, extent, and level of detail of the patient health information involved: In investigating this factor, one would examine if the information was publically available. Was only demographic information sent and does this escalate the risk of identity theft. Are there any embarrassing elements to the patient health information? Lastly, even if a patient name was not used, does the patient health information lead one to have the ability to identify the patient.

(b) Identity of the recipient: Is the recipient a HIPAA covered entity and thus employing privacy and security standards? Would the recipient know what to do with the patient health information in regards to the sender?

(c) Whether the patient health information was actually acquired or viewed: Was the patient health information encrypted? Who saw what and was their further disclosure? How did the covered entity become aware of the situation?

(d) What mitigation steps were taken: If the patient health information was in paper format, was the original copy returned or destroyed; were further copies made? If electronic, was there remote scrubbing of devices and drives. Did law enforcement need to be contacted? [6]

In looking at the four factors, breaches are to be evaluated based on the unique facts and situation. If an allegation or suspicion is substantiated, but a low probability of compromise is legitimately determined, the matter may still be a breach or violation of a standard, but it is not reportable. In contrast, if a risk assessment is not performed, the breach determination reverts to the presumption of the event being reportable.

In 2012, Massachusetts Eye and Ear Infirmary and Eye and Ear Associates (MEEI) settled with the Office for Civil Rights for $1.5 million. It was found that there was theft of an unsecured and unencrypted laptop containing PHI. In addition, MEEI failed to take the necessary steps to comply with the Security Rule [7]. http://www.hhs.gov/ocr/privacy/hipaa/enforcement/examples/meei-agreement.html.

In 2012, the Alaska Department of Health and Human Services (DHHS) settled with the Office for Civil Rights for $1.5 million. It was found that a USB hard drive was stolen out of an employee's vehicle. The portable device was unsecured and unencrypted and thus patient health information could be accessed. In addition, the covered entity did not have HIPAA policies and procedures in place concerning security encryption of devices or appropriate risk analysis for breaches [8]. http://www.hhs.gov/ocr/privacy/hipaa/enforcement/examples/alaska-agreement.html.

In 2014, New York Presbyterian Hospital (NYP) and Columbia University (CU) had a violation while sharing a network and firewall. A physician was able to pull protected health information onto another server without HIPAA compliant technical safeguards. This resulted in the public being able to view patient health information via an internet search engine. Six thousand, eight hundred patients were involved and the resultant fine to the Office for Civil Rights was $4.8 million [9].

HIPAA covered entities must appoint a person to direct their HIPAA security efforts. A major responsibility of the security person is to conduct an information technology security audit. The audit examines how compliant the software and hardware are with the HIPAA mandated ANSI standards and how compliant the organization is in following the standards. The HIPAA Security Rule involves technical, administrative, and physical security and all three are under the auspices of the security person. Technical security involves the information technology security such as passwords. Administrative security involves having the policies and procedures for the HIPAA security Rule. Physical security involves ensuring that patient health information is secure in the physical environment such as having locked cabinets for storage of patient health information. The security person will also determine the employees who have a "need to know" and have role based access to patient health information; they must then undergo training and adhere to HIPAA policies. The Security Rule also mandates about developing a disaster recovery plan and routine back-ups for all electronic information. Facilities must identify a contingency plan to restore any loss of data and to identify safe storage locations such as an off-site mine. Disaster plan testing and recovery are to be performed.

The HIPAA Security Rule is more than information technology, but also how the employees interact and utilize PHI. To this end, a Computer Usage Policy, again based on the "need to know" principle, specifies how the information technology system is to be used in an organization. Computer workstations must be safeguarded such that unauthorized users cannot gain access. In addition the transfer of data must be protected. Employees also agree to certain restrictions such as not accessing information for personal gain, preventing others from using your system, and cooperating with audits and monitoring of technology usage.

Moreso, the Security Rule must become a part of daily operations through policies, procedures, and standard operating practices of all PHI, oral, written, and electronic, including social media. A covered entity's policies and procedures for electronic information systems that hold ePHI are to allow access only to those persons or software programs that have a role based need to know. A covered entity can meet the requirements by doing the following:

1. Require unique user identifications whereby the covered entity assign a unique name and/or number for identifying and tracking user identity.
2. Have emergency access procedures whereby a covered can obtain necessary ePHI during an emergency.
3. Consider using an automatic log-off such that the covered entity can terminate an electronic session after a predetermined time of inactivity.
4. Use encryption and decryption for ePHI [10]. (http://library.ahima.org/xpedio/ groups/public/documents/ahima/bok1_049463.hcsp?dDocName=bok1_ 049463; Accessed October 18, 2014)

Thus far, the security topic has focused on protecting patient health information. But what happens when a facility no longer has to save the health information either as mandated by law or organizational policies and procedures? The answer lies in the destruction and disposal mandates for health information. When disposing of health information, one must ensure that the data is destroyed and cannot be resurrected. Simply removing it from the property or deleting computer files is not adequate. What are needed are strict mandates on the internal and external destruction of health information, and disposal of physical computers and health information. Keep in mind, because healthcare organizations may contract this task to an outside vendor, this vendor must also abide by HIPAA regulations. Here the outside vendor cannot use or disclose the patient health information. In addition, the vendor will use safeguards to ensure that the patient health information is not disclosed during the destruction process, but if a disclosure does occur, the vendor will notify the facility immediately. If the vendor subcontracts to another agent, that agent must be known to this facility and must abide by the HIPAA regulations. Patient health information shall be permanently destroyed such that there is no possibility of reconstruction of the data. Paper records can be destroyed by burning, cross shredding, pulping, and pulverizing. Microfilm and microfiche can be destroyed by recycling and pulverizing. Magnetic data can be destroyed by degaussing [11]. A Certificate of Destruction must then be completed and retained by the organization.

As with the external destruction of health information, all patient health information that is to be internally discarded is to follow a procedure of destruction that will comply with the HIPAA regulation and ensure privacy, security, and confidentiality of all patient health information. Because patient health information is a component of normal business operations, the internal destruction policy mandates that the organization destroy patient health information that no longer has a business function and can rightfully be destroyed under law. Facilities can utilize shredders at the end of each shift or as the information to be destroyed has completed its business function.

The last measure of health information destruction is computer disposal, the actually physical hardware being rendered clear of all health information. Also included here is when a computer is moved and used by another person who does not have the same "need to know" privileges for health information as the former computer terminal user. When information is saved on a computer hard disk, the magnetic characteristics of that disk change in two ways. The first way is for the information that is stored on it (ie. the written file). The second way is for the address or the location of the file being stored on the magnetic disk; thus, the disk holds two identifying elements for each file stored. When a file is "deleted", the only part that is erased on the magnetic disk is the address or location. The information remains even though the disk is used over or formatted, the magnetic characteristics of the disk still hold the information and therefore it is accessible with certain technology tools. The only way to ensure that both the information and address are removed (i.e. change the magnetic characteristics back to their original format) is to overwrite the disk with specific technology tools. Previously DoD 5220.22-M was the standard to follow for data overwrite. But in 2006 and updated in 2012, this standard was replaced with SP800-88 for data erasure compliance for hard drives and other electronic media [12]. After the overwriting is completed, the computer will be dated and initialed as to when and who did the overwrite procedure. The information technology department is to also log the information.

## 25.4  Privacy

The HIPAA Privacy Rule is quite extensive and concerns itself with the use and disclosure of identifiable patient health information and seeks to maintain its confidentiality. The Privacy Rule encompasses protecting the privacy with business associates and users allowing patients to request to amend their medical records, and receiving consent and authorization prior to sharing information. Providers must also publicize their information practices in a "Notice". All personnel who have access to patient health information must be trained on the requirements.

Similar to the Security Rule, the Privacy Rule goes beyond medical records per se as it also includes policies and procedures which impact one's standard operating procedures. Healthcare providers must designate a privacy officer. This person will be responsible for implementing the safeguards to maintain the confidentiality of the information. In addition, they will be the person who performs routine audits and investigates any breaches of privacy and ultimately disciplines those who have committed the breech. The breaches can surface in multiple manners such as through an anonymous complaint line, direct patient or family member complaints, or through the audits. It is the HIPAA Privacy personnel working in concert with the security personnel to protect the covered entity from breaches. Risks must constantly be assessed and measures in place to respond. What is the impact of the risk and what is the probability of occurrence? Although with PHI, all occurrences are problematic, although it is mitigated as all are not a critical risk.

Risks impact the patient, but they do not see it upfront. Other areas of the Privacy Rule have direct impact on patients. For example, patients are able to request to amend their medical records on information that they feel does not represent their health encounter. The key here is that they can make a request which will then be considered, but it does not guarantee that the change will take place. The patient would contact the author of the medical note and request that a change be made and also submit what the wording for the change should be. The provider or a committee will consider the request and make a ruling. With HIPAA as specified in the HIPAA Notice of Privacy Practices is that it is a patient right to be able to request an amendment as the data belongs to the patient. One of the most heralded parts of the HIPAA Privacy Rule is the Right to Request to Inspect, Copy, and Amend Medical Records section. In fact, one of the main purposes of HIPAA from a consumer's perspective is the right to view and possibly amend their record. The physical medical record belongs to the provider, but what is not known by many, is that the information contained within belongs to the individual; therefore under State Privacy Laws, patients have had the right to examine their medical records. HIPAA corroborates that an individual has a right to **request** to inspect, copy, and amend their medical record in most circumstance. Exceptions to this are psychotherapy notes, information to be used in legal proceedings or for forensic matters, information that could cause harm to oneself or another especially when inmates are involved, research information when a patient is in the sample, and if the requestor is judged that they may be further harmed by having seen the information [13].

The facility has the requesting party complete a request form and validate their identification. The request form will ask the patient what needs to be amended, why, and what the new wording should be. The healthcare facility must rule on the matter in a timely manner. If the request is denied, the patient can appeal whereby the facility will have an additional 30 days to further review the case. If the request to amend the record is granted, the healthcare facility will inform the requestor that the amendment was granted, then insert the amended language next to the changed language. The amendment must then be shared with all those who have a "right to know" about the changed language. If the healthcare provider denies the request to amend the record, a written statement in laymen's term of the reason for denial is given to the requestor. The requestor can then counter in writing a statement of disagreement. If it is again denied, the facility must alert the requestor that they can further appeal to the Secretary of Health and Human Services and the facility's complaint line. Also, the facility must make known in the medical record the denied request with any future disclosures of the patient health information.

As introduced above with the request to amend a record, organizations are to issue the Notice of Health Information Practices (Notice). The notice describes how health information about an individual may be used and disclosed and how one can get access to this health information. Many people are already knowledgeable of the fact that health information is shared with insurers and other health care facilities/ providers for treatment decisions and payment. The Notice though covers many other areas related to those that have an interest, for business purposes, in one's health information. Facility departments, such as risk management and quality assurance receive information to analyze the care, treatment, and outcomes of procedures and tests. This health information is used to continually improve the care by analyzing best practices. Information can be extrapolated by physician, procedure, or demographic characteristic. Health care facilities also maintain a directory used by visiting predominantly by clergy. Patients can opt out of being in the directory by stating such prior to signing the notice. Business associates such as pharmacies, medical equipment vendors, and medical laboratories receive patient health information. Business associates must follow HIPAA standards and certify that in writing to the healthcare facility. In the Omnibus Final Rule issued September 23, 2013, business associates needed HIPAA training and must follow the HIPAA policies just as a covered entity does. In teaching hospitals and academic medical centers, health information may be disclosed to researchers if they have appropriate consent forms and the research has been approved by an institutional review board. The researchers will be held to the facility's health information privacy standards and verify that the data being requested is truly needed to accomplish the research objectives. Funeral directors will receive health information in accordance with State laws and for professional purposes only. Consistent with applicable laws, health information may be disclosed to organ procurement organizations or organizations involved in the transplantation of and related services for organs, tissue donation, and transplant [14]. Patient health information being used for marketing has been an area of controversy. Health information can be disclosed to remind patients about treatments and services that may benefit them given their medical condition, but patient data cannot be used for marketing purposes without patient consent. Federal Government agencies, such as the Food and Drug Administration, may be required to disclose health information related to a food recall or outbreak of a food related condition. State Government agencies such as workman's compensation will share health information as it becomes necessary by law and to render a decision on a compensation case. The Federal and State Governments may require health information to be disclosed for public health purposes such as for communicable disease tracking and injury prevention. The Notice specifies, in general, to whom health information can be disclosed to and for what purpose.

An ever increasing challenge for HIPAA is the mobility of data both with portable devices and personnel working from remote locations. It is reported that one-third of healthcare personnel work outside of the healthcare entity at least once per week. In concert with this, 78 % of records breached in security incidents were attributed to stolen or lost mobile devices and 39 % of healthcare security incidents are caused by a stolen and/or lost device [15].

To mitigate issues with mobile devices, organizations can employ several strategies. First, in your information systems strategic plan and disaster plan, know the risks of these devices and plan how they will be used with patient health information. If they are being used to transmit data to external networks, consider that in your information technology risk assessment and HIPAA technical security policies. Develop and manage policies regarding mobile devices. For example, can one use a personal mobile device within the organization. Are there any restrictions on using a mobile device issued by the organization? Ensure that the policies are enforced and make this a routine part of a HIPAA audit [16].

The authors of the Health Insurance Portability and Accountability Act wanted to ensure that providers would not simply put HIPAA in place and then forget about it. Rather, the authors wanted HIPAA to be operationalized into a provider's daily operations. To do such, they required that an organization institute operational audits, a reporting mechanism, and discipline procedures. Operational audits are an evaluation mechanism to measure compliance with the stated policies and regulations of HIPAA. The Compliance Officer and staff will conduct monthly (or more frequent) audits on various measures such as computer logins, medical record documentation, coding and billing, adherence to confidentiality policies, adherence to security policies, HIPAA training for employees, and a review of personnel access to patient health information. These, among others, will be conducted to assess system weaknesses such that corrective action can be taken to ensure that HIPAA is being adhered to. Audits can be announced or unannounced, but predominantly they will become a part of the facility's operations such that employees will see them as a part of routine business. If the audits detect problems, then an action plan must be specified on how to reeducate the affected employee(s) and/or department(s). Second, the employee(s) and/or department(s) must be re-audited. Even if on the next audit, there is not a problem, one must continue to routinely re-audit them such that a problem does not reoccur. All of this must be documented on the audit forms. If the facility fails to reeducate and re-audit, or fails to document it, they can be held liable for not correcting a situation that they were aware of [17].

Another way to detect non-adherence to HIPAA is via a reporting mechanism system. Here, employees and other constituents can confidentially report violations or suspected violations of HIPAA without retaliation. The facility must publicly advertise its reporting mechanism system in all of its locations. The reporting mechanism system can include a hotline telephone number, paper reporting system, or electronic reporting system. The most important criteria is that the reporting system must be conducive for all levels of employees to use. The employee and/or constituent can only report violations or credible, suspected violations of criminal conduct in relation to HIPAA; thus, this is not a general complaint line. Employees must also know that HIPAA is a Federal mandate and false reporting can lead to a criminal penalty. The reporting system must maintain the confidentiality of the reporting individual and no retribution can be taken against the reporting individual. If the reporting individual tells of any retribution, the facility must document it and have a follow-up investigation immediately. When an employee or constituent files a complaint, the reporting mechanism call log is to be completed immediately. The complaint has a statute of limitations of 180 days. An initial investigation must begin immediately on the complaint with the action and response being documented. After the investigation is complete, follow-up must ensure that credible violations are not repeated. In addition, the facility must cooperate with any outside investigation including sharing records in a timely manner and allowing access to pertinent records [18]. As shown in Table 25.1, complaints and follow-up have increased exponentially since HIPAA began, but it is this due diligence that is required to protect patient health information.

When operationalizing HIPAA, a covered entity is to develop and implement a disciplinary system for HIPAA violations. With this, all breaches must be fully investigated and if warranted disciplinary measures taken, including termination from and non-rehire to the organization. Disciplinary measures are taken on those who violate the HIPAA mandate and those who are responsible to monitor, detect, and report an offenses, but fail to do so; therefore covering acts of commission and omission.

All breaches and sanctions in violation of HIPAA must be clearly documented and substantiated. During the investigation, as warranted by the compliance person, the employee(s) under investigation can be moved to another position whereby access to patient health information is not warranted. If the investigation reveals a

**Table 25.1** Enforcement results by year

| Year | No violation | | Resolved after intake and review | | Corrective action obtained | | Total resolutions |
|------|--------------|---|----------------------------------|---|----------------------------|---|-------------------|
| Partial year 2003 | 79 | 5 % | 1,177 | 78 % | 260 | 17 % | 1,516 |
| 2004 | 360 | 7 % | 3,406 | 71 % | 1,033 | 22 % | 4,799 |
| 2005 | 642 | 11 % | 3,888 | 68 % | 1,162 | 21 % | 5,692 |
| 2006 | 897 | 14 % | 4,128 | 62 % | 1,574 | 24 % | 6,599 |
| 2007 | 727 | 10 % | 5,017 | 69 % | 1,494 | 21 % | 7,238 |
| 2008 | 1,180 | 13 % | 5,940 | 63 % | 2,221 | 24 % | 9,341 |
| 2009 | 1,211 | 15 % | 4,749 | 59 % | 2,146 | 26 % | 8,106 |
| 2010 | 1,529 | 17 % | 4,951 | 54 % | 2,709 | 29 % | 9,189 |
| 2011 | 1,302 | 16 % | 4,466 | 53 % | 2595 | 31 % | 8,363 |
| 2012 | 979 | 10 % | 5,068 | 54 % | 3,361 | 36 % | 9,408 |
| 2013 | 993 | 7 % | 9,837 | 69 % | 3,470 | 24 % | 14,300 |

Source: Department of Health and Human Services. Office for Civil Rights. Enforcement Results by Year. http://www.hhs.gov/ocr/privacy/hipaa/enforcement/data/historicalnumbers.html

violation of civil or criminal, federal or state law, the violation must be reported to Government authorities immediately. If the investigation reveals an overpayment to a facility, the overpayment must be returned immediately. Organizations must then discipline the individual according to their chain of discipline. For example, individuals who use health information for malice, personal gain, and or intimidation can be terminated. Breaches which involve accessing patient health information not related to one's job responsibilities can be suspended without pay for 3 weeks, be put on a 90 working day probationary period, and undergo HIPAA training. A second offense can result in immediate termination. Organizations will need to determine if their present discipline procedures are stringent enough for the violation of health information privacy.

HIPAA violations need not occur if the organization develops a "culture" to adhere to HIPAA by all employees. This can occur through orientation sessions, email reminders, staff meetings, payroll reminders, and diligence among all employees.

## 25.5 Summary

The keys for compliance to the Health Insurance Portability and Accountability Act is to operationalize it into the organization's daily functions and to be very current on changes. In fact, know of proposed changes and enter into the public comment foray. HIPAA must be integrated to not only protect information, but also to deliver quality health care when data are needed. With so much in healthcare depending on accurate data and information, the protection of those data and information are paramount.

## References

1. Department of Health and Human Services. News release. http://www.hhs.gov/news/press/2014pres/05/20140507b.html. Accessed 7 May 2014.
2. Department of Health and Human Services. HIPAA security series. Volume 2, paper 1, March 2007. http://www.hhs.gov/ocr/privacy/hipaa/administrative/securityrule/security101.pdf.
3. Robert Tennant and Amy Nordeng. New privacy and security omnibus rule released. MGMA connexion, Apr 2013, page 18 of 18–21.
4. The Wall Street Journal. Home depot's 56 million card breach bigger than target's.http://www.wsj.com/articles/home-depot-breach-bigger-than-targets-1411073571. Accessed 18 Sept 2014.
5. Department of Health and Human Services. HIPAA final rule, 45CFR164.402. 25 Jan 2013.
6. Downing K. Navigating a compliant breach management process. J AHIMA. 2014;85(6): 56–8.
7. US Department of Health and Human Services. Massachusetts provider settles HIPAA case for $1.5 million. http://www.hhs.gov/ocr/privacy/hipaa/enforcement/examples/meei-agreement.html. Accessed 20 Apr 2015.

8. US Department of Health and Human Services. Alaska DHSS settles HIPAA security case for $1,700,000. http://www.hhs.gov/ocr/privacy/hipaa/enforcement/examples/alaska-agreement.html. Accessed 20 Apr 2015.
9. US Department of Health and Human Services. Data breach results in $4.8 million HIPAA settlements. 2014, May 7. http://www.hhs.gov/news/press/2014pres/05/20140507b.html. Accessed 21 Apr 2015.
10. AHIMA. Mobile device security (updated). J AHIMA. 2012;83(4):50–5. http://library.ahima.org/xpedio/groups/public/documents/ahima/bok1_049463.hcsp?dDocName=bok1_049463. Accessed 20 Apr 2015.
11. Office for Civil Rights. The HIPAA privacy and security rules. Frequently asked questions about the disposal of protected health information. http://www.hhs.gov/ocr/privacy/hipaa/enforcement/examples/disposalfaqs.pdf
12. Department of Defense Media Sanitization Guidelines 5220.22 M. http://www.destructdata.com/dod-standard/
13. Department of Health and Human Services. Standards for privacy of individually identifiable Health Information. 45CFR164.508.
14. Office for Civil Rights. Understanding the HIPAA notice. http://www.hhs.gov/ocr/privacy/hipaa/understanding/consumers/understanding-hipaa-notice.pdf
15. Sherman C, Shey H, with Balaouras S, Duong, J. Brief: stolen and lost devices are putting personal healthcare information at risk. Forrester Res. 2014:3.
16. Department of Health and Human Services. Managing mobile devices in your health care organization. http://www.healthit.gov/sites/default/files/fact-sheet-managing-mobile-devices-in-your-health-care-organization.pdf
17. HIPAA Privacy, Security, and breach notification audit program. http://www.hhs.gov/ocr/privacy/hipaa/enforcement/audit/
18. Department of Health and Human Services, Office of the Secretary. Standards for privacy of individually identifiable health information. 45 CFR 160.306(b)(3).

# Part IV
# Looking Towards the Year 2025

## Introduction

In this fourth and final section, we look at research and development work in healthcare information technology and how it is actively being translated from visions to the realistic embodiments of the Institute for Healthcare Improvement's Triple Aim of improving the care of individual patients, of improving the health of populations, and of reducing the cost of healthcare.

Healthcare IT work is now expanding vertically upward to studying and impacting on population health (using big data techniques) and downwards to continuous remote monitoring of individual patients (using mobile sensor technology in critical and primary care). Another dimension into which work is progressing is the management of complexity, from the incorporation of new types of data (patient generated health data, genetic/genomic information, environmental exposures and other types of data yet to be defined) to automated processing and novel visualization technologies and decision support tools. At the core of all of these is focus on the needs of users, providers and patients, to present new views, controls, and problem-solving tools, for health and disease, as healthcare moves into an era of participatory medicine.

- Informatics and healthcare pioneer, Lawrence Weed (and son) present the case for the need to transform the way we prepare future medical practitioners, couple knowledge to assessment and treatment, and use technology to provide care based in evidence and appropriate to the individual patient. The Weeds' message in Chapter 26 is a clarion call for fundamental change that is consistent with Dr Weed's entire career and body of work.
- Silva and Ball (IBM) describe a Complex Adaptive System (CAS) architecture that addresses current limitations in health IT in Chapter 27.
- In Chapter 28, David McCallie (Cerner Corp) presents the new and emerging technologies for clinical decision support with case study examples that offer hope for more effective and helpful support to clinicians across the complex needs of knowledge and decision support in clinical settings; while Chapter 29, Jim Fackler by James Fackler (Johns Hopkins) explores novel uses of API technologies and new applications that sit on top of EHR systems to organize and present data to support real-time decision support at the individual patient level in ways that improve medical cognition and patient safety
- Chapter 29 by Daby Sow (Exploratory Clinical Analytics and Systems, IBM), Chapter 30 by Hu and colleagues (Healthcare Analytics, IBM) and Chapter 32 by Devarokonda and Mehta (Watson Health, IBM and Cleveland Clinic, respectively) respectively look at uses of new technologies that are actively being explored and tested within the IBM laboratories: wearable sensors for patient-generated health data, data-driven analytics and cognitive computing to create an active patient-centered learning healthcare system
- In Chapter 33, Robert Greenes (Arizona State University and Mayo Clinic) closes Part IV as well as the book with his critical overview of our field and relating these key areas as they are addressed by the authors and chapters throughout this book.

# Chapter 26
# Building a Reliable and Affordable System of Medical Care

**Lawrence L. Weed and Lincoln Weed**

**Abstract** In this critical review of our approach to medical education, medical practice and decision-making in medicine, the authors draw upon the disciplined thinking of Francis Bacon (mid 1600s), Battista Morgagni (late 1700s), and others to advocate for recognition of the limitations of the human mind as applied in the way medical learning is imparted and the way physicians practice. The authors outline how medical students acquire scientific knowledge, but not scientific behaviors. A scientific approach to diagnosis begins with using information tools to identify all diagnostic possibilities for the presenting problem and the initial findings needed to determine which possibilities are worth investigating in the patient. If the initial findings do not reveal a clear diagnostic solution, then information tools must be employed as part of a system of care to enforce highly organized follow-up processes, that is, careful problem definition, planning, execution, feedback, and corrective action over time, all documented under strict standards of care for managing the complexities involved.

**Keywords** Intellectual behaviors of modern science • Transforming medical education • Fallacies in medical decision-making • Medical error/diagnostic failures • Clinical decision-making technology • Knowledge development system • Individualized healthcare delivery • Patient's problem oriented medical record

L.L. Weed, MD (✉)
Department of Medicine, University of Vermont, Underhill, VT, USA
e-mail: ll.weed@comcast.net

L. Weed, MD, JD
Axiom Resource Management Inc., Oakton, VA, USA
e-mail: ldweed424@gmail.com

© Springer International Publishing Switzerland 2016
C.A. Weaver et al. (eds.), *Healthcare Information Management Systems:
Cases, Strategies, and Solutions*, Health Informatics,
DOI 10.1007/978-3-319-20765-0_26

## 26.1    Introduction

It was 300 years ago that Battista Morgagni gave to the world a systematic treatise in two volumes containing the records of some 640 dissections along with the symptoms during the course of the illness, with precision of statement and exhaustiveness of detail [5]. Morgagni was the first to understand and to demonstrate the absolute necessity of basing diagnosis, prognosis and treatment on an exact and comprehensive knowledge of anatomical conditions. His treatise began the era of steady and cumulative progress in pathology and practical medicine (as stated in the 1911 Encyclopedia Britannica at the time of the 1910 Flexner report which produced the modern medical school). From Morgagni's time on, disease began to be viewed as "the cry of the suffering organs". Many of the false notions of the nature of disease, for example the humor theory of surpluses of fluids (e.g., blood and bile) that had held sway since the times of Hippocrates and Galen were discredited.

The practical application by practicing physicians of Morgagni's insights would require that each practicing physician could and would elicit and then recognize in each patient the combination of symptoms and physical findings, the cry of a specific suffering organ, the diagnosis. The public has been led to believe that a degree from a medical school and a license from a state to practice medicine enable the mind of a physician to do what Morgagni's insights required. But the present reality is that the unaided mind of a licensed physician is not capable of remembering, keeping up-to-date and processing all the combinations of symptoms and physical findings of all the diseases described by Morgagni and his successors. Yet, physicians are willing to act as if they have those capabilities because they have a license to practice medicine. That license was given because they sat through courses and passed exams in medical school. They were never given the right tools to recall and process the appropriate knowledge from the literature and data from the patient at the time of actual practice. Unsurprisingly, mistakes in medicine are now the third most common cause of death [1]. Francis Bacon told us 100 years before Morgagni that when we extol the powers of the human mind, we do not search for its real helps [2]. And deaths—for example from an undiagnosed ruptured appendix or a fatal case of Addison's disease—that could have been avoided had the diagnosis been made will continue to occur if the practice of medicine is left to the unaided minds of autonomous physicians. As Francis Bacon said: "Our only remaining hope and salvation is to begin the whole labor of the mind again; not leaving it to itself, but directing it perpetually from the very first, attaining our end as it were by mechanical aid" [2].

## 26.2    Medical Education

The "real helps" for the mind advocated by Bacon are not provided in the present system of medical care, but they are known, written about and ignored [8, 9]. The question we should explore here is how is it that the medical schools and a medical education system initiated by the Flexner report [3] over a century ago produce so many physicians who are willing to make medical decisions that are in error so often. The answer is that the Flexner report led to medical schools based on the premise that requiring students to sit through courses in the basic sciences such as biochemistry, physiology, pharmacology etc., followed by 2 years of seeing patients on wards and in clinics, they would enable students to do what Morgagni's insights required. But the reality is that the student does not see connections between what he is learning in the basic science courses and the care of patients and would not remember them even if he did 2 or 3 years later when seeing a patient in a busy clinic. Nor would the PhD teaching him biochemistry be any help because he does not see the connections either and never has been required to operate under the time constraints of medical practice. What Flexner missed was that medical students need to learn a core of behavior, the intellectual behaviors essential to modern science. First identified by Francis Bacon four centuries ago, these behaviors include the habitual use of external tools and techniques and standards to produce and manipulate complex information. Yet, in medical education, credentialing and practice these scientific behaviors are conspicuously absent. This gap between the behaviors of scientific and medical practitioners becomes all too obvious when one compares the training and examination of basic science PhD candidates with that of medical students [6].

What we are witnessing now is a spectacle of "fragments of intention" that leads to passing exams, getting licenses to practice medicine and finally to the multiple deaths from errors. But the damage to the student and the patients he will see in the future is deeper and longer lasting than we realize. Not only does the faulty system fail to give the tools and the competence that good care requires, but it does give authority to the physician so trained to go on making mistakes and eventually for some to acquire leadership positions that defend the system that produced them.

A critical point in the journey of a medical student through medical school is the day he is asked to actually work-up a patient with a problem. For example if the problem is a complaint of abdominal pain, does the student know the 70 plus causes of abdominal pain and the combination of findings on history and physical examination for each cause as he starts to work up the patient. Since no one could know all that, does the student hesitate and say to the resident in charge, "I feel anxious and insecure because I do not know all I should know to serve this patient properly," and then refuse to go on? Does the resident say "be a big boy and do the best you can. We all have to go through these clerkships to develop clinical judgment and become a physician."? How many of us in our training have answered: "It is not a question of my being willing to keep going and becoming a physician that tried to learn clinical judgment from experience. It is a question of whether I want to stay in a faulty system that puts patients at risk while I advance my career and lose my scientific integrity."

How many colleges focus just on MCAT scores and getting their pre-med students into medical school, and ignore having them understand what is going on in medical schools before they ever get into the position of the student just described. Pre-med students should be reading Francis Bacon and preparing themselves to recognize phrases like "clinical judgment" as one of Bacon's "Idols of the Mind" that lead us into fallacies. They should be reading the philosopher Whitehead who wrote in 1911: "It is a profoundly erroneous truism that we should cultivate the habit of thinking about what we are doing. The precise opposite is the case. Civilization advances by extending the number of important operations which we can perform without thinking about them" [10]. They should be studying the realities described in our recent article [7] on diagnostic error:

> *Diagnostic failure results from misplaced dependence on the clinical judgments of expert physicians. The remedy for diagnostic failure involves defining standards of care for managing clinical information (medical knowledge and patient data), and implementing those standards with information tools designed for that purpose. These standards and tools are external to the minds of physicians, thus bypassing two inherent constraints on human cognition: limited capacities for information retrieval and processing, and innate heuristics and biases. Medical education and credentialing socialize physicians into misplaced acceptance of these constraints. Medical students acquire scientific knowledge, but not scientific behaviors. A scientific approach to diagnosis begins with using information tools to identify all diagnostic possibilities for the presenting problem and the initial findings needed to determine which possibilities are worth investigating in the patient. If the initial findings do not reveal a clear diagnostic solution, then information tools must be employed as part of a system of care to enforce highly organized follow-up processes, that is, careful problem definition, planning, execution, feedback, and corrective action over time, all documented under strict standards of care for managing the complexities involved.*

## 26.3   The Role for Information Technology

The thoughtful pre-medical student who reads the above may conclude that he does not want to be a traditional physician that goes through the present system of medical education and care. He would rather learn to function within a system of care, much as a pilot learns to function safely within the transportation system. A system of care would provide information tools adequate to meet high standards of care and training programs adequate to make individuals competent in the use of those tools in the part of the system where they choose to function.

Before presenting a diagram of what a transformed system of medical education and care should look like, let us review the need for, and difficulties in achieving, such a transformation. Consider a distinction between two different types of health information: patient data and medical knowledge. Patient data resides in medical record repositories, while medical knowledge is transmitted from external text repositories (medical libraries and journals) to the minds of physicians. Their minds serve as intermediate knowledge repositories for use in patient care. Then, in patient care, physician minds perform an information processing function: matching knowledge with patient data.

These repository and processing functions far exceed the capacities of the human mind. Moreover, even in situations where the mind's information processing capacities are sufficient, reliance on the mind introduces disorder and undermines transparency, coordination, productivity, feedback, and improvement. The outcome is to cripple the entire health care system. Misguided reliance on the human mind causes a fatal voltage drop in transmission of medical knowledge from its original repositories in libraries and journals to its intended beneficiaries in patient care.

The apparent solution to this voltage drop is information technology. Technology's superior capacity to perform repository and processing functions has led everyone to hope that IT will somehow generate huge gains in quality and efficiency. All that is needed, on this view, is to define "meaningful use" of IT, as a condition for subsidizing its purchase.

Yet, the current hopes for health IT are doomed to disappointment. Misguided reliance on the human mind is deeply embedded in the formative social institutions of medical practice—graduate medical education, credentialing systems, reimbursement, entitlements, the doctor-patient relationship. A wrenching transformation in those institutions would be the outcome of demanding truly "meaningful use" of health IT. That is far from happening. On the contrary, the culture of medicine is in a state of denial about the breadth and depth of the transformation that must come about—a transformation that ends the era of autonomous physicians and the medical schools that the Flexner report led to and begins the era of a system of medical care where knowledge is in tools and where people are trained to use those tools and trained to perform the actions chosen in light of what the tools reveal.

Other fields of expertise have found that external tools do not destroy what is best in those fields. Beryl Markham discussed this phenomenon in her reminiscences about flying. On the attitude of an older pilot who resisted instrument-controlled flying, she wrote:

> After this era of great pilots has gone, as the era of great sea captains has gone—each nudged aside by the march of inventive genius, by steel cogs and copper discs and hand thin wires on white faces that are dumb, but speak—it will be found, I think, that all the science of flying has been captured on the breadth of an instrument board, but not the religion of it. [4]

## 26.4   The Transformative Changes Needed

Figure 26.1 shows what the transformed system would look like. In understanding this diagram, one should keep in mind the following assertions:

1. The medical care system should be like the travel system, in which from childhood the traveler learns how to use the system to reach goals and destinations. Knowledge is built into the tools used to function within the system. It is not built into the traveler's head or into the head of someone who is paid to guide the traveler through the system.
2. All users of the medical care system should understand what we have called "Scientific principles that tell us why people must manage their own health care." (See Appendix B of *Medicine in Denial* [8]).

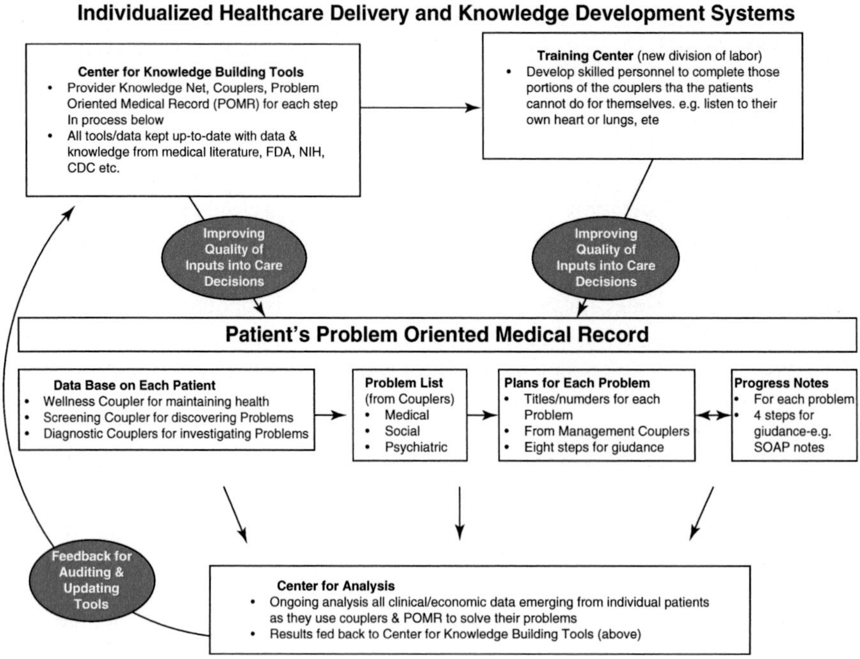

## Individualized Healthcare Delivery and Knowledge Development Systems

**Fig. 26.1** What a transformed system of medical education and care should look like. **Explanation of terms: Knowledge Net**: an organized collection of the entities (objects) of medical knowledge and the relationships among them, with commentary on the relationships. **Couplers:** a specific implementation of a generic concept, referred to as knowledge coupling tools. A Coupler is oriented around a problem, and is concerned with the diagnosis or the management of that problem. It is built from knowledge components drawn from the Knowledge Net. Most importantly, the relationships captured there become "voting" relationships in a Coupler, between possible findings, and possible diagnoses (as evidence or risk factors) or options for management (as "pros" or cautions)

3. Practitioners are trained to do for the patient tasks and procedures that are chosen based on system guidance but that the patient cannot do for himself.

For a detailed operational description of actual use of the Knowledge Coupler and POMR tools referenced in Figure 26.1, see Chapter 13 , authored by Dr. Kenneth Bartholomew, in *Knowledge coupling: new premises and new tools for medical care and education* [9]. The volume *Medicine in Denial* [8] provides a detailed analysis of the need and basis for the system of care depicted in Figure 26.1.

To be safe and effective and productive, software and knowledge bases of this kind must be designed to implement rigorous standards of care for selection and analysis of patient data in light of medical knowledge. These standards are based on a combinatorial approach (as distinguished from judgmental, algorithmic, and probabilistic approaches) to generating hypotheses and evidence. Together, the combinatorial standard for knowledge coupling and the POMR standard for medical records constitute generic standards of care for managing clinical information. These are standards that apply universally to medical problems and practice settings of all kinds.

The notion of such universality may seem simplistic and naïve in the context of health care, with its extraordinary diversity and complexity. But the science of complex adaptive systems shows that simplicity and universality are essential goals for a complex activity such as health care. And part V of *Medicine in Denial* shows how these goals have been attained in two complex domains where health care operates—science and commerce. Health care lags centuries behind these two domains in its lack of simple, universal standards of care for managing information. The universal standards for managing healthcare information must be specific, operational and yet generic. And corresponding information tools must be usable jointly by all caregivers, by patients/consumers and by third parties (clinical researchers, regulators, payers). Standards and tools of that kind provide a necessary foundation for health care reform in general and, in particular, a foundation for reform concepts such as "patient-centered" and "consumer-driven" care, "medical home," "pay-for-performance," "comparative effectiveness research," and "meaningful use" of health IT.

What needs to be built on that reform foundation is a unified system of patient-driven care, medical education, and clinical research, a system that harvests continuous feedback on provider performance, patient behaviors and medical knowledge. Medical education would mean instilling a core of behavior, not transmitting a core of knowledge, producing trustworthy practitioners, not fallible repositories of knowledge. Feedback for practitioners would be based on defined inputs and audit of performance under defined rules. Feedback for patients would be based on intelligible medical records revealing the exact connections between their own behaviors, their social environments and their medical problems. Feedback on medical knowledge would be continually harvested from medical records, coupled with scientific research and translated into precisely relevant, usable, new knowledge, accessed instantly through continually updated knowledge coupling tools. "Evidence-based medicine" would be transformed from standardized into highly individualized guidance for decisions. The surrounding support systems for patient care—regulators such as the Federal Drug Administration, public health agencies such as the Center for Disease Control, drug and device vendors, educational and credentialing institutions, third party payers—all could function in a coordinated way, with better information than ever before. A patient-driven marketplace could evolve where advanced medical technologies would be selected not for raising provider incomes bur rather for their power to improve patient outcomes and lower everyone's costs. Above all, patients could navigate a transparent and trustworthy system of care, empowered to manage their own health and their own care.

**Acknowledgements**   The authors wish to acknowledge Chris Weed's assistance in the planning and preparation of this paper and to thank him for all his support in his editorial reviews of the manuscript.

# References

1. Allen M. How many die from medical mistakes in U.S. hospitals? 2013. ProPublica, 19 Sep. Accessed 20 Jan 2014: http://www.propublica.org/article/how-many-die-from-medical-mistakes-in-us-hospitals.
2. Bacon F. Novum organum, 1620; ed. by Joseph Devey, M.A. (New York: P.F. Collier, 1902). Available at: http://oll.libertyfund.org/titles/1432. Accessed 19 July 2015.
3. Flexner A. Medical education in the United States and Canada. Pittsburg: Carnegie Foundation for Advancement of Teaching; 1910.
4. Markham B (1942) West with the Night. Berkeley: North Point Press
5. Morgagni, GB. De Sedibus et Causis Morborum per Anatomen Indagatis (The seats and causes of diseases investigated by anatomy. Published in Italy. 1761. Available at: https://archive.org/details/seatscausesofdis02morg. Accessed 19 July 2015.
6. Weed LL. Medical records, medical education, and patient care. Cleveland: Case Western Reserve University Press; 1969, pp. 4–5.
7. Weed LL, Weed L. Diagnosing diagnostic failure. Diagnosis. 2014;1(1):13–7. doi:10.1515/dx-2013-0020.
8. Weed LL, Weed L. Medicine in denial. 2011. Charleston: CreateSpace. Table of contents, overview and introduction available at: http://www.thepermanentejournal.org/files/MedicineInDenial.pdf. Available for purchase at: Amazon.com or www.createspace.com/3508751.
9. Weed LL, Abbey LM, Bartholomew KA, et al. Knowledge coupling: new premises and new tools for medical care and education, Computers in Health Care series. New York: Springer; 1991. Chapter 13, pp. 235–277.
10. Whitehead AN. An introduction to mathematics; 1911. Project Gutenberg at: http://www.gutenberg.org/files/41568/41568-pdf.pdf. Available in paperback edition 2009 from Bibliobazaar.

# Chapter 27
# Engineering the Next Generation of Health Systems

John S. Silva and Marion J. Ball

*"Insanity, doing the same thing and expecting different results"*
*Albert Einstein*

**Abstract** This chapter focuses on three changes that will dramatically affect the rapidly evolving health ecosystem. It highlights today's high value/high usability computing paradigm, the explosion of information within the Web and the challenges for EHR systems as they try to face the data tsunami. The chapter proposes that a Complex Adaptive System (CAS) framework will be essential for an inclusive health ecosystem that meets the needs of clients, consumers and health workers. The authors suggest that a person-owned wellness-health record (POWR) will be required in the new ecosystem. It postulates that a Smart point of need system for all users should replace the current point of care systems that are limited to healthcare workers. The chapter concludes with a description of a community-based health ecosystem that adopts the behaviors of a CAS, incorporates continuous quality improvement and exploits new technologies to support decision-making for all individuals within the community.

**Keywords** Complex adaptive system • Health ecosystem • Person owned health/wellness record • Smart point of need support • Continuous quality improvement • Community-based health

J.S. Silva, MD FACMI (✉)
Chief Architect, Silva Consulting Services, 2055 Conan Doyle Way,
Eldersburg, MD 21784, USA
e-mail: Jc-silva-md@att.net

M.J. Ball, Ed.D
Healthcare and Life Sciences Institute, IBM Research, Johns Hopkins University,
5706 Coley Court, Baltimore, MD 21210, USA
e-mail: marionball@us.ibm.com

© Springer International Publishing Switzerland 2016    461
C.A. Weaver et al. (eds.), *Healthcare Information Management Systems:*
*Cases, Strategies, and Solutions*, Health Informatics,
DOI 10.1007/978-3-319-20765-0_27

## 27.1    Introduction

This fourth edition of *HIMS* details many of the components of electronic health record (EHR) systems as they exist today, how an EHR and its components might evolve in the near future, and aspects of implementing and sustaining these systems at the local, regional and national levels. This chapter focuses on three changes that will dramatically alter current healthcare systems:

- The explosive move towards a "trillion sensor world… in which you'll be able to know anything you want, anytime, anywhere and query that data for answers and insights" [9]
- The move towards a more holistic, person-owned wellness-health record (POWR) that support the needs of all health workers, clients and consumers and away from today's sick care record systems [the EHRs of today] that support only the needs of healthcare workers, managers and payers
- The move towards vibrant health and wellness in the community and home and away from traditional healthcare in hospitals and other healthcare settings; i.e. towards the national "Triple Aim" of Better Care, Healthy People/Communities and Affordable Care but from individuals and their community [10].

## 27.2    The Future Is Here

The Internet and World Wide Web (Web) are disruptive technologies that have transformed the way we learn, work, play and even think. These technologies have evolved and expanded very rapidly from the 'read-only' Web 1.0 of the 1990s to the 'connected' Web 2.0 of the early 2000s. Crowdsourcing, social power [20] and user-generated content developed spontaneously and proliferated rapidly within the Web. It is estimated the Web handled 4 Zettabytes of data ($4 \times 10^{21}$) in 2013 and is doubling every 2 years. By comparison, the healthcare ecosystem generated an estimated 150 Exabytes ($1.5 \times 10^{20}$) in 2011 [29]. Individual patient home monitoring/rapid diagnostic test data and the Internet of Things (IoT) for health and wellness sensor data [5] will increase the total health data even more dramatically. Beecham Research has provided an early view of the potential transformations that will occur in all industrial sectors [6], Fig. 27.1.

These twenty-first century data sources already exceed the capacity of most systems to gather and analyze it, further exacerbating the ability of EHRs to provide relevant and usable information to health workers and consumers/clients. The next-generation Web 3.0, the Semantic Web, is just beginning to understand, link, and convert the Web's data tsunami into information so that we and technologies can rapidly co-evolve towards not-yet-imagined businesses, practices, and knowledge.

The Internet is a prime example of a complex adaptive system that has transformed nearly every sector of the global economy and introduced "social power" to industry and politics. Complex Adaptive Systems are characterized by a high degree

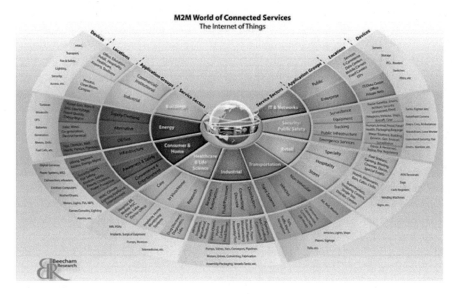

**Fig. 27.1**   M2M world of connected services (Reproduced with permission of Beecham Research Ltd)

of adaptive capacity, giving them the ability to succeed and flourish in the face of change. They are adaptive, communicative, cooperative, specialized, spatially and temporally organized, and reproduce, often with new parts that are more resilient and effective than earlier ones (Wikipedia, complex adaptive system, accessed 1/12/2015). One clear manifestation of the Web's adaptive behavior is the rapid emergence of cloud computing. These vast grids of always-on computing resources are fundamentally changing how companies purchase IT components and services. In many cases, fairly robust versions of software products are free, like Google Analytics, web conferencing systems, or the phone service Skype. As a result, today's users expect their "point of need" devices to access whatever information they need, wherever and whenever they need it, and conduct **useful** transactions **with no learning curve**; i.e., on Internet Time. For example, it is expected that a person can access their online banking services from their Smartphone or tablet, deposit checks, pay their bills and manage their finances in a completely transparent way, all without taking a single training class or having to change their behavior. This high user value for minimal user cost (high value/high usability) computing paradigm has enabled Smartphone and tablet computing to become the dominant model for user interactions with the Web. In fact, users expect these sorts of experience from their interactions with any IT. The health ecosystem must learn to play by these rules.

Twenty-first century manufacturing approaches have shrunk medical devices and their costs, making them significantly more affordable and pervasive. These devices, which require a fraction of the maintenance, supplies and technical support of their counterparts even a decade ago, are commonly available in doctor's offices.

In the home, a rapidly expanding set of inexpensive sensors of all kinds are monitoring diseases, medications, vital signs, saliva, urine and numerous other signals. Intel, Qualcomm, Freescale and many others have implemented unique solutions to collect and transmit home acquired sensor/diagnostic information to monitoring systems and/or physicians' mobile devices and office systems [31]. In addition to the mostly passive sensor data collection efforts described above, there are a few attempts to combine rapid diagnostic devices and linked Smartphone apps. One company has combined mobile technology, clinical and behavioral science and validated clinical outcomes to bring "mobile integrated therapy" to clients with Type 2 diabetes. They achieved very significant average decrease in A1c of 2 % [35]. These combined approaches start addressing the need for immediacy of actionable health and wellness to their clients. It certainly holds the promise to be an extraordinary game-changer for chronic disease management. In summary, these technologies are ushering in a new age that moves from receiving care in a doctor's office to the customer/client doing care themselves, at home or their workplace [22]. The critical question is: how can the health ecosystem adopt the behaviors of a CAS so as to exploit these new technologies and evolve toward 'health and wellness in the community' approaches that are more resilient and effective than earlier ones that were 'focused on sick care'? A recent National Research Council (NRC) report of a symposium honoring the 200th anniversary of Charles Darwin addressed this issue in the large: "Understanding and managing such complex systems requires ongoing adaptive cooperation and collaboration among disciplines and across jurisdictions, both public and private, as knowledge continues to evolve [26].

## 27.3   The Path Forward

At the turn of the twenty-first century, the IOM (Institute of Medicine) concluded that healthcare professionals needed to interact effectively with their EHRs to perform their daily tasks. At that time it was assumed that EHRs could effectively and efficiently support the needs of its users [13]. It was assumed that these systems of systems would result in significantly improved outcomes for patients and decreased healthcare costs. While there have been some isolated successes, these goals have not been realized in the large. A recent IOM report summarized it thusly:

> More than a decade since the Institute of Medicine's (IOM's) *To Err Is Human*: *Building a Safer Health System* was published, the U.S. healthcare system continues to fall far short of its potential. Although *To Err Is Human* and other IOM reports, including the *Crossing the Quality Chasm* series, have helped spark numerous efforts to improve practices, persistent health care underperformance and high costs highlight the considerable challenge of bringing isolated successes to scale. The nation has yet to see the broad improvements in safety, accessibility, quality, or efficiency that the American people need and deserve. [16]

A continuous learning systems approach was proposed to address the lack of success [16]. A follow-on IOM workshop on Integrating Research and Practice [17] has elaborated on requirements of a continuous learning system.

In a continuously learning health system, data from sources such as electronic health record systems used to manage patient care, claims data necessary for billing purposes, and increasingly patient-generated sources of data such as patient portals, surveys, and online communities are used to inform questions of operations, to guide care, to further scientific understanding, and to power innovation. This approach differs from traditional approaches to clinical research, which are often removed from the clinical experience both in terms of the questions asked and the environment in which they are carried out, require large amounts of additional data collection, can take several years to complete, can be very expensive, and are often criticized for producing evidence that is not easily generalizable to broader populations or easily implementable in real-world settings.

By realizing the potential of knowledge generation that is more closely integrated with the practice of care, it should be possible not only to produce more usable evidence to inform decisions, but also to increase the efficiency and decrease the costs of doing clinical research. Delivering on this promise will depend on certain technical capabilities, but, more importantly, **ensuring the sustainability of this approach will require the delivery of value to stakeholders who are engaged in these processes**. [17]

The important elements from the above IOM report drive home: (1) the need to provide relevant information at the points where health decisions are made; (2) the need to make "evidence" relevant to the specific contexts of client/health consumer and health worker; and (3) the need to significantly decrease the latency and costs of generating useful knowledge. The Roundtable on Value & Science-Driven Health Care clearly recognized the intimate relationship between providing value to the users and the sustainability of the infrastructure (bolded text above). These features are very similar to the characteristics of a CAS and the high value/high usability systems described above.

The failure to improve outcomes for patients and decreased healthcare costs may be related to the fact that the interactions between healthcare professionals and their EHRs may not be effective or efficient as previously believed. The authors have reported that the lack of adequate provisioning of healthcare professionals was a principal reason for the very slow adoption of EHRs [4]. The HIMSS EHR Usability Task Force reported that "Electronic medical record adoption rates have been slower than expected in the United States... A key reason is lack of efficiency and usability of EMRs currently available" [11]." A National Academy of Science report was more direct – current EHRs (in 2009) do not support clinical users, are not designed for usability and may even set back the vision of twenty-first century health care [34]. The lack of a usable point of care system for clinicians makes their work harder [4] and may actually introduce errors [3, 8, 36] (Authors note: Chaps. 8 and 9 in this book address these issues in detail.)

Realizing a system that provides utility and usability to clinicians, consumers and administrators is still an unfulfilled vision. Recognizing the importance of the "Cognitive Window" (*vide infra*), the Office of the National Coordinator, HHS, has funded projects that were focused on cognitive support issues. A recent report from one of these projects, SHARPC, detailed a number of features to make a better EHR [37]. However, efforts are focused primarily on users of EHRs and not the broad set of clients, health consumers or health workers outside of traditional health care settings. The authors suggest that failure to address the information needs of all health ecosystem users will not realize Triple Aim vision. We use the term point of need (PON) rather than point of care to emphasize this critical requirement.

In addition to the problems with usability, the lack of data interoperability amongst the myriad of data systems, both within and across health systems, continues to be one of the most vexing problems that negatively impacts usefulness [18, 28]. For clinicians, this lack translates into a less than complete picture of their patients who received health services in multiple settings. For clients and health consumers (aka patients), this necessitates collecting and maintaining copies of records, usually paper, from each health provider. This situation will continue to worsen as health services move more from hospital and clinic settings to community and home settings. Recent efforts by the Office of the National Coordinator (ONC) within the Department of Health and Human Services have focused on improving the interoperability of electronic health record systems and health information exchanges. ONC has released its 10 year vision for an interoperable health system [27]. In addition, the HL7 standards organization has released its Fast Healthcare Interoperability Resources (FHIR) specification to accelerate exchanging healthcare information electronically [12]. Taken together, funding from ONC and support for rapid standards evolution by HL7 will be a key factor in realizing data interoperability. It remains to be seen if and how these national efforts, focused on the current healthcare systems and associated EHRs, will be able to evolve towards the high value/high usability systems that today's users expect.

After all, high value/high usability systems do make it easier for us to accomplish our tasks. Thus, the authors believe that the major objective of health IT should be to subtract work not to add work or make our work harder. Clinicians, clients, consumers and health workers in general want systems that support and enhance their work – in short, that ease it, not complicate it" [4]. The next section describes the conceptual architecture for a Smart PON system that is designed to specifically address value and usability for all clients, consumers and health workers.

## 27.4   Vision and Value of Smart Point of Need Support System

Imagine a "clients, consumers and health workers support system" that: (1) knows and uses the PON user's context to increase the user's "cognitive window"; (2) supports the coordination and scheduling tasks – based on locally relevant outcomes and measures; (3) is customized based on what information is entered, what the user needs to see, what s/he does and closely replicates the way s/he thinks; (4) moves from device to device – installing automatically on whatever PON device is being used; (5) insulates the user from the quirks of systems, EHRs or person-owned wellness health record systems (POWR) to which the Smart PON sends or receives data; and (6) connects securely to whatever source of information is required by the user [32].

The client, consumer and health worker communities have the same need for relevant information, anywhere, anytime and on any device (Fig. 27.2). The Smart PON must support intelligent provision of data and information from a very diverse set of data sources, including:

- Traditional healthcare sources
- Home, personal and community medical or health sensors
- Rapid diagnostic devices
- Social media conduits, and
- The myriad of wearable/fixed devices via the IoT.

> From these sources, it must enable the efficient fusion and analysis of continuously improved clinical, health and wellness practices (*vide infra* for feedback loops) and other relevant information to support a client, consumer or health worker's activities. The Smart PON expands its users' 'cognitive window' where the users will have more time to evaluate the relevant facts and analyses. Under explicit user controls, it purposefully exploits the power of social interactions, crowdsourcing, and collaboration to augment its users' decision-making by reaching out to others in the health ecosystem. The Smart PON produces required documentation and records of acquired data, analyses and decisions as a by-product of its use. It then distributes these user-owned artifacts to POWRs, EHRs and Payors, Public Health, and other entities and individuals, as appropriate. The anticipated result is better decisions across the entire spectrum from persons, healthcare and wellness workers, managers and policy-makers. It becomes an active CAS platform for engagement of individuals into the wellness, health and healthcare ecosystem as it evolves.

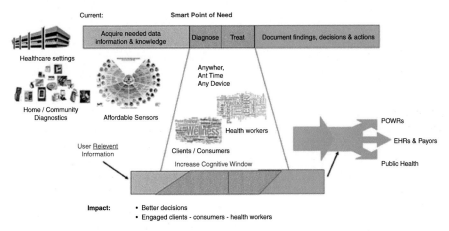

Used with permission of Consulting Services, LLC

**Fig. 27.2** Changing how clients, consumers and health workers work (Used with permission of Silva Consulting Services, LLC)

The Smart PON system described above has other key attributes, namely:

- It anticipates its user's needs – has data/information waiting for users
- It has a minimal learning curve as it continuously adapts to its user
- It hides all the complexity of underlying POWR and EHR systems with simplicity ('magical' IT), and
- It is built to bring immediate value to its user

A conceptual architecture for Smart PON support is shown below in Fig. 27.3 [30]. The three components operate within a services oriented architecture and exchange data within the Smart PON and to external information sources (such as local POWRs and EHRs, health information exchanges (HIE) and knowledge sources) using standardized messages.

The Context/Task Manager (C/TM) is the "heart" of the architecture. It monitors user's activity to determine context, uses models of user's tasks and current/ expected context to anticipate activities, tasks and necessary data exchanges with the User Interface Manager (UIM) and the Information Broker (IB) components, and maps user activities and tasks to the most appropriate decision-support and analytic application for a true extensible software-as-a-service framework. The IB component is the data/information cache for its users as well as the connection point to external systems. The set of services required by the IB are available in many commercial HIE or SOA offerings from vendors. Exchanges between the IB and external systems should be mediated by HL7's FHIR [12]. Both the C/TM and IB are modeled from CAS design patterns and attributes. The C/TM and IB have analytic engines that monitor the efficacy and efficiency of user and system tasks versus

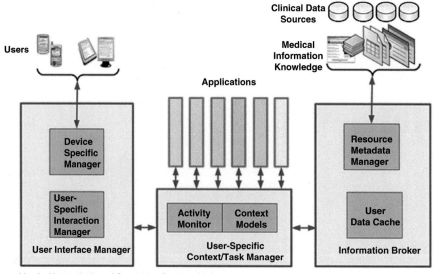

Used with permission of Consulting Services LLC

**Fig. 27.3** Conceptual architecture of the smart PON environment (Used with permission of Silva Consulting Services, LLC)

outcomes to continuously enhance best practices and system performance by giving feedback directly to its users. The UIM component presents relevant data, information and health, wellness and clinical knowledge to users and gathers data from them. It has presentation strategies to achieve communication goals that depend upon current context, criticality of message and device being used, and adapts to the unique style of the user. It provides a consistent set of metaphors regardless of the user's location.

The Smart PON system is designed to:

- Automatically present relevant data and information via pre-filled "Health/ Wellness/Care Widgets"
- Offer "Executable" care/health/wellness plans for its users
- Unobtrusively collect data from users
- Generate relevant POWR and/or EHR documentation as well as charge or billing information as a by-product
- Continuously adapts to the user's and their communities' best practices

The value proposition to users is that they have support system designed for them that implements a systems engineering approach, using CAS design patterns, for the collection, distribution and maintenance of best practices, health/wellness/clinical data and system performance. This context-aware Smart PON uses user-specific and continuously-adapting practice patterns that have the potential to dramatically enhance the quality and efficiency of all health, wellness and healthcare service delivery. The UIM component directly addresses issues of usability via its feedback systems to continuously evolve an efficient and effective interface. The Smart PON is specifically designed to meet requirements of high value/high utility. This approach addresses the very thorny and expensive issue of how to make practice guidelines/best practices relevant to local context and, at the same time, solves the "how can we maintain, sustain and evolve the practices that we have implemented" question [17]. The built-in business intelligence and analytic tools provide users and managers the "What's Been Done" versus "What Should be Done" based on context and outcomes. This near real-time feedback loop simultaneously provides analyses for informed decisions about:

- What is best for me – at the individual (client, consumer or health worker)
- What is best for our community, our state and our nation (population-level)
- Best practices that are adaptive to the unique context of the individual and their location

It is one path towards "realizing the potential of knowledge generation that is more closely integrated with the practice of care" [17].

## 27.5 A Bottom Up Model for the Health Ecosystem

Our health care system is a very large $2.9+ trillion enterprise with many diverse "business units". Each of these business units are firmly entrenched within the system and has a vested interest in ensuring that its portion of revenue increases or, at worst, does not change. There is significant pressure to keep the status quo and continue to focus on treating disease in patients.

Other industrialized countries have found that delivering a majority of health services through primary care physician practices, and focusing on health by keeping people healthy, work quite well [33]. These systems do not require over 17 % of their GDP as the U. S. healthcare system does. Since wholesale changes to our healthcare system are unlikely, is it possible to use the above principles, dramatic changes in technologies, and social power [20] to lead us to a "health and wellness Spring"? The authors believe we can. We need to use design principles of complex adaptive systems (*vide supra*) to enable an adaptive evolution from today's disparate healthcare systems towards a next-generation health ecosystem that embodies the Triple Aim of Better Care, Healthy People/Communities and Affordable Care [10]. These activities needs to begin at the grass roots, in communities that will partner with its citizens and health and public health workers. The partnership needs to nurture high levels of community and personal well-being via individual citizen participation, social power and transparent, continuous evaluation of the effectiveness, usefulness and efficiency of their entire community's ecosystem.

This evolution is already underway. The Patient-Centered Medical Home (PCMH) model, as defined by the "Joint Principles of the Patient-Centered Medical Home" [1], is a physician-directed practice that provides accessible, continuous, comprehensive and coordinated care that is delivered in the context of family and community [7]. Like systems in many other industrialized countries, the PCMH is based in primary care physician practices and focuses on keeping its participants healthy. The PCMH model has already developed substantial traction in both the private and public sectors, including support from a number of Fortune 100 companies and other organizations to promote and foster its implementation via Patient-Centered Primary Care Collaborative (www.pcpcc.org). The National Committee for Quality Assurance (NCQA) depicts the rapid growth of recognized PCMHs from 2008 when the first PCHM were established to January, 2015, when there were 8,828 – over 10 % of primary care practices in the US [24]. It recently summarized what a PCHM must do to meet receive NCQA recognition:

> ...offering access afterhours and online so patients get care where and when they need it. PCMHs get to know patients in long-term partnerships, rather than hurried, sporadic visits. They make treatment decisions together with patients based on individual preferences. They help patients become better engaged in their own healthy behaviors and healthcare. Everyone in the practice – from clinicians to front desk staff – works as a team to coordinate care from other providers and community resources. [24].

Both organizations have recently summarized the success of the PCMH model and noted reductions in costs and in appropriate utilization, improved population health with more frequent use of preventative services, better access to and continuity of primary care, and improved patient and physician satisfaction [24].

In addition to PCMHs, Accountable Care Organizations (ACO) have emerged as key elements of the evolution of the healthcare landscape. The Affordable Care Act of 2010 introduced a series of incentives to pay for value rather than volume and reward organizations for realizing savings while improving quality. Under the Act,

ACOs will be responsible for both the quality and cost across the entire spectrum of healthcare services for a defined population. The ACOs are often comprised of many primary care provider, PCMHs, hospitals, specialists and associated services; accountability and risk are shared among all its participants [23]. The Brookings Institute analyzed the results of the initial 2 years of the Pioneer ACO Model. The participating ACOs saved $96 million in the second year, shared savings of $68 million, and improved mean quality scores by 19 % [21].

It is important to note that for both PCMH and ACO's measuring and reporting quality is an essential component, as the Act mandated that HHS and stakeholders formulate a National Quality Strategy for quality improvement [2].

PCMHs and an ACO's primary care providers promote shared decision-making among its staff and the client. In this context, it is envisioned that the client will transition from a passive "patient" that is told what to do to an engaged client that is active in his/her care. There is a strong anticipation that a client's PCMH will be the connection point for all interactions between the client, their health workers and the 'medical neighborhood' [25]. Berenson described the implications of these relationships thusly: "It [a full-featured medical home] requires developing processes and systems (including IT) to support high levels of access for and communications with patients, coordination of patients' care within and outside the practice, capturing and using data for care of patients and populations and evaluation of performance, and support for evidence-based decision-making [7]."

The above discussions represent the traditional view of the healthcare system from those who provide, manage or pay for care; i.e., at the point of care where healthcare workers interact with their "patients". Certainly, many PCMHs and ACOs are moving towards patient engagement as an essential component of their practices. However, clients and health consumers use many other sources of information, including home, personal and community medical or health sensors, rapid diagnostic devices, social media conduits, and the myriad of wearable/fixed devices via the IoT (*vide supra*), hence the authors recommendation that individuals have and maintain their own holistic, person-owned wellness-health record (POWR) that is separate from, but interoperates with EHRs and other health data stores. From an individual's perspective, s/he needs relevant information anytime, anywhere **s/he** makes a decision about their wellness, their health, their prevention, or their social and personal activities; i.e., their point of need. The client's and health consumer's point of need is not limited to visits to a clinic or interactions with a health worker. Rather, their point of need is always with them and always on – wherever they are, whatever they are doing – to support their decisions and behaviors. They are active on Facebook, Twitter, Amazon and other Internet channels where they are able to conduct **useful** transactions **with no learning curve**. Interactions with their health worker or healthcare services are exceptions to their daily life; they seldom use a personal health record (PHR) system, if one is available. PCMHs and ACOs need to rethink the most effective way to provide their clients with access to clinical information and to support understanding the choices for therapeutic and preventative plans. After all, for PCMHs and ACO's to be successful, the client or health consumer must 'live' their specific therapeutic, preventative and/or wellness plans, taking the pills, modifying behaviors and lifestyle, and monitoring their outcomes.

The person-centric nature of these new business practices, POWRs that need be supported, the information exchanges that will be required, and the capabilities to support them are not well understood in the current healthcare system. Most of these capabilities do not exist in current EHR systems. Unfortunately, absent appropriate and useful IT support for these critical components, it is unlikely that PCMH or ACO efforts will achieve the anticipated benefits.

The last section in this chapter describes a possible pilot of a community-based, mesoscale version of a health ecosystem that adopts the behaviors of a CAS and exploits new technologies to support decision-making for all individuals within a community.

## 27.6   County/Community-Based Pilot Project

Our exemplar County Public Health Department (CPHD) is planning a new initiative they call "County 3.0" that will nurture high levels of community and personal well-being via individual citizen participation and social power. The County Public Health Officer and team decided to focus their efforts on the county's Federally Qualified Health Centers (FQHC). These FQHCs, community clinics and safety net clinics serve citizens of communities within the county who are near or below the poverty line, who have few resources and who have significant barriers to accessing healthcare services. Many must use public transportation to get to the clinic and other necessary health services, such as laboratories or pharmacies. Many are non-English speaking and are often unable to understand instructions in English. And, many have negative perceptions about their healthcare services. A key goal of the project is to improve the performance of the county's FQHCs by maximizing the time a patient is within the clinic – which the team has called the "Golden Hours". The FQHC staff plan to reengineer their workflows to build trust and optimize information about their clients conditions and associated treatments, in a culturally sensitive and effective manner.

A second key goal for the project is to ensure, within the "Golden Hours," that:

- Health workers have sufficient, relevant historical and diagnostic data they need for diagnosis and treatment planning
- Clients participate in decisions and receive all appropriate disease, treatment and medication information and training and any questions are answered
- Clients are interviewed prior to departure from the clinic to ensure that they participated and were successfully informed; and, if there are any identified problems, these are resolved prior to the client leaving the clinic
- Provide each client with their own POWR

Measuring progress and assessing how well the patient response system and reengineered clinic workflows have improved patient outcomes and clinic performance is fundamental to the approach. Results would be fed back frequently to all involved parties for their evaluation; successful ones would be accelerated and the FQHCs would adopt best clinical and management practices while avoiding IT solutions or practices that do not work.

The FQHC team, in collaboration with CPHD's obesity and diabetes awareness programs, has decided to start its efforts on reengineering its workflow for diabetic patients. It plans to provide FQHC staff with a Smart PON system to interface with their existing EHR and to incorporate practice guidelines and the results of rapid diagnostic tests. They intend to use the Smart PON to produce the set of clinical and patient measures they have selected as a by-product of using it for managing visits and interactions with their clients. They will incorporate rapid diagnostic testing, electronic capture of vital signs and a client response system (see Chap. 20 for more details on patient reporting) into the clinic workflow as shown in Fig. 27.4 below.

The team anticipates that the Smart PON system and the IT infrastructure will enable the FQHC to collect appropriate clinical, administrative, and client outcome information as a by-product of providing and orchestrating health services. At a later date, the IT infrastructure and Smart PON will ingest client-selected data from their POWR that has stored data from their home, other sources and self-entered information. As a result, best practices, local clinical guidelines and clinical decisions would be linked directly to patient outcomes. These data, the HIE infrastruc-

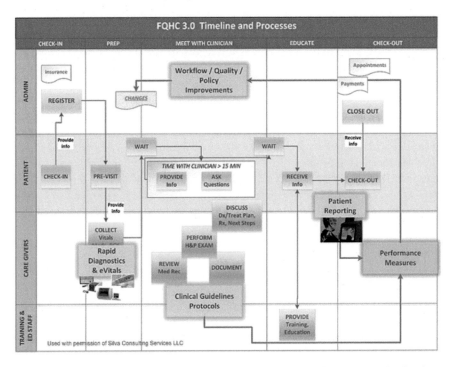

**Fig. 27.4** FQHC 3.0 workflow and feedback (Used with permission of Silva Consulting Services, LLC)

ture and associated clinical and business intelligence tools come together as a disruptive technology platform that could revolutionize evaluation processes and research. FQHC and CPHD staff, management and clients will know – what are the best practices, what practices are not effective or not safe and what practices are more expensive without added value, all of which are continuously updated.

This approach seems to be just what the IOM has outlined in its report on comparative effectiveness research (CER):

> "CER is the generation and synthesis of evidence that compares the benefits and harms of alternative methods to prevent, diagnose, treat, and monitor a clinical condition or to improve the delivery of care. The purpose of CER is to assist consumers, clinicians, purchasers, and policy makers to make informed decisions that will improve health care at both the individual and population levels" and that "consumers, patients and caregivers as well as their health care providers must be involved in all aspects of CER to ensure its relevance to everyday health care delivery." [15]

The fully integrated evaluation framework is fundamental to the design of 'the community-based, mesoscale version of a health ecosystem that adopts the behaviors of a CAS and exploits new technologies to support decision-making for all individuals within a community.' That is, the county/community 3.0 system is designed to provide immediate feedback of performance, metrics, KPIs and other analyses, directly and transparently to local participants, clinicians and consumers and to record decisions about what changes need to be made. This information continuously informs decisions by all participants so they can adjust their local practices and behaviors to continuously improve their performance. Absent readily available CER data at the nexus of decision-making, the CER enterprise will not achieve its stated goal of "better decision making by patients and providers" [15].

Lastly, this approach for the county/community 3.0 is designed to address the maintainability and sustainability of guidelines. Guidelines are implemented within the Smart POC system, then continuously adapted, evolved and communicated to the local practice setting by feeding back the county/community outcomes, costs and utilization data and new biomedical knowledge onto the guideline itself. It should be a fascinating story for the science of CER to observe and analyze the time-oriented adaption and evolution of guidelines both within and across communities and special populations. After all, as Sir William Osler stated: "It is much more important to know what sort of patient has a disease than what sort of disease a patient has."

# References

1. AAFP, American Academy of Pediatrics, American College of Physicians, and American Osteopathic Association. Joint principles of the patient-centered medical home. Mar 2007. http://www.medicalhomeinfo.org/Joint%20Statement.pdf.
2. AHQR. Accessed January 24, 2015 at http://www.ahrq.gov/workingforquality/agencyplans/ahrq-specific-plan-nqs2014.pdf

3. Ash JS, Berg M, Coiera E. Some unintended consequences of information technology in health care: the nature of patient care information system-related errors. J Am Med Inform Assoc. 2004;11(2):104–12.
4. Ball MJ, Silva JS, Bierstock S. Failure to provide clinicians useful IT systems: opportunities to leapfrog current technologies. Methods Inf Med. 2008;47:4–7.
5. Booker, E. Can IoT slash healthcare costs? 22 Oct 2014. http://www.informationweek.com/healthcare/mobile-and-wireless/can-iot-slash-healthcare-costs/d/d-id/1316841.
6. Beecham Research Ltd. M2M sector map; 2011. http://www.beechamresearch.com/download.aspx?id=18. Accessed 29 Jan 2015.
7. Berenson RA, et al. A house is not a home: keeping patients at the center of practice redesign. Health Aff. 2008;27:1219–30.
8. Campbell EM, Sitting DF, Ash JS, et al. Types of unintended consequences relation to computerized provider order entry. JAMIA. 2006;13(5):547–56.
9. Diamandis P. Singularity hub; 2014. http://singularityhub.com/2014/12/23/know-anything-you-want-anytime-anywhere/.
10. Health and Human Services. National quality strategy; 2014. http://www.ahrq.gov/workingforquality/about.htm#aims. Accessed 8 Jan 2015.
11. HIMSS. Defining and testing EMR usability: principles and proposed methods of EMR usability evaluation and rating. Jun 2009. Available at: http://www.himss.org/content/files/HIMSS_DefiningandTestingEMRUsability.pdf. Accessed 10 Jul 2009.
12. HL7. FHIR, DSTU 1. http://www.hl7.org/implement/standards/fhir/overview.html. Accessed 30 Sep 2014.
13. IOM. Crossing the quality chasm: a new health system for the 21st century. Washington, DC: National Academy Press; 2001.
14. IOM. Knowing what works in healthcare: a roadmap for the nation. Washington, D.C.: National Academy Press; 2008.
15. IOM. Initial national priorities for comparative effectiveness research report brief. Washington, DC: National Academy Press; 2009.
16. IOM. Best care at lower cost: the path to continuously learning health care in America. Washington, DC: The National Academies Press; 2013.
17. IOM. Integrating research and practice: health system leaders working toward high-value care: workshop summary. Washington, DC: The National Academies Press; 2014.
18. JASON. A Robust health data infrastructure; 2013. http://healthit.ahrq.gov/sites/default/files/docs/publication/a-robust-health-data-infrastructure.pdf – 397k. Accessed 17 Apr 2014.
19. Jonsson A. How open source initiative can influence the internet of things; 2014. http://evothings.com/how-open-source-initiatives-can-influence-the-internet-of-things/. Accessed 29 Jan 2015.
20. Kirkpatrick D. Social power and the coming corporate revolution. Forbes, 26 Sep 2011, p. 74–81.
21. Kocot L, White R, Katikaneni P, et al. Blog: a more complete picture of pioneer ACO results. 13 Oct 2014 10:08am. http://www.brookings.edu/blogs/up-front/posts/2014/10/09-pioneer-aco-results-mcclellan. Accessed 30 Jan 2015.
22. Lefrak M. Diagnosing Disease from Home. InnovationHub December 12, 2014, accessed January 12, 2015 at http://blogs.wgbh.org/innovation-hub/2014/12/12/diagnosing-disease-home/>
23. McClellan M, McKethan A, Lewis J, et al. A national strategy to put accountable care into practice. Health Aff. 2010;29:982–90.
24. NCQA. Growth of medical homes. Accessed Jnauary 30, 2015 at http://www.ncqa.org/.
25. Nielsen M, Gibson L, Buelt L, et al. The Patient-Centered Medical Home's Impact on Cost and Quality, Review of Evidence, 2013–2014. Accessed January 13, 2015 at https://www.pcpcc.org/resource/patient-centered-medical-homes-impact-cost-and-quality.
26. NRC. Twenty-first century ecosystems: managing the living world two centuries after Darwin. Washington, DC: The National Academies Press; 2011.

27. ONC/HHS. Connecting health and care for the nation: a 10 year vision to achieve an interoperable health IT infrastructure. n.d. http://www.healthit.gov/sites/default/files/ONC10yearInteroperabilityConceptPaper.pdf.
28. PCAST. Realizing the full potential of health information technology to improve healthcare for all Americans; 2010. http://www.whitehouse.gov/sites/default/files/microsites/ostp/pcast-health-it-report.pdf.
29. Raghupathi W, Raghupathi V. Big data analytics in healthcare: promise and potential. Health Information Science and Systems. 2014;2:3.
30. Silva J, Ball M. Next generation health professional workstations, Yearbook of Med Inform 1994: Advanced Communications in Health Care. Stuttgart: Schattauer; 1994. p. 78–84.
31. Silva JS, Ball MJ. Prognosis for year 2013. Int J Med Inform. 2002;66:45–9.
32. Silva JS, Seybold N, Ball MJ. Creating usable health IT for physicians – the smart point of care system. Healthcare informatics, July 2010. p. 40–3.
33. Starfield B, Shi L, Macinko J. Contribution of primary care to health systems and health. Milbank Q. 2005;83(3):457–502.
34. Stead W, Linn H. Computational technology for effective health care: immediate steps and strategic directions. Washington, DC: National Academies Press; 2009.
35. WellDoc. Accessed January 12, 2015 at http://www.welldoc.com/Clinical-Trials.aspx.
36. Weiner JP, Kfuri T, Chan K, Fowle JB. "e-Iatrogenesis": the most critical unintended consequence of CPOE and other HIT. JAMIA. 2007;14(3):387–8.
37. Zhang J, Walji M, editors. Better EHR. Usability, workflow and cognitive support in electronic health records. 2014. ISBN: 978-0-692-26296-2.

# Chapter 28
# Emerging Clinical Decision Support Technology for the Twenty First Century

David P. McCallie Jr.

**Abstract** Chapter 1 reviewed key aspects of the history of Clinical Decision Support (CDS), describing the significant progress achieved as well as calling out some of the limitations that have diminished the expected benefits of CDS despite increasingly widespread use of EHR technology. This chapter will describe emerging approaches and new technologies that show promise for addressing some of the current limitations of the field, and which hold hope for more widespread realization of the benefits of CDS.

**Keywords** Cloud-based CDS • Machine learning • Infobutton manager service • Predictive analytics • Service-oriented CDS • SMART Apps • Knowledge models • Automatic chart summarization • FHIR Resources

## 28.1  Emergence of New CDS Knowledge Models: Machine Learning

A characteristic of many of the CDS systems described in Chapter 1, such as systems based on Arden-like Medical Logic Modules (MLM) or on declarative, rule-based implementations, used human-readable logic statements or rules to encapsulate the clinical knowledge. This made it relatively easy for the knowledge engineer to understand and explain the logic of the CDS. If the system was not working as expected, a human expert could readily debug it. With the advent of "big data" analytics, and the explosion of new tools for machine learning, informaticists have begun to change the assumption that human readability of the knowledge base was required. In its place, informaticists have begun to use a variety of techniques that capture the decision support logic as a mathematical formulation (e.g., a matrix

D.P. McCallie Jr., MD
Medical Informatics, Cerner Corp., Kansas City, MO, USA
e-mail: dmccallie@cerner.com

© Springer International Publishing Switzerland 2016    477
C.A. Weaver et al. (eds.), *Healthcare Information Management Systems:
Cases, Strategies, and Solutions*, Health Informatics,
DOI 10.1007/978-3-319-20765-0_28

of coefficients, etc.) that may well be opaque to human comprehension. This is potentially a profound shift in CDS knowledge modeling, since the knowledge source becomes more of a "black box" whose inner workings are not readily inspected. New approaches to validation of the accuracy of the knowledge model will be required. Some of these new approaches are outlined below.

Many of these new "black box" models for CDS are based on the application of statistical mathematical techniques frequently described as "machine learning" [41]. A common type of machine learning is called *supervised learning* [11], which can be summarized as follows: first, a set of curated training data is collected by experts. Typically hundreds or even thousands of example training cases should be used to get a good learning result. The training data contains cases where the learnable decision is known to be "true" as well as cases where the learnable decision is known to be "false." An appropriate machine-learning algorithm is selected to process the training data, which then uses a well-defined mathematical process (e.g., regression, support vector machines, rule-induction, etc.) to induce a set of parameters that optimally distinguish the "true" cases from the "false" cases. Typically, before the training starts, the raw clinical data is processed to generate "features" that capture the essence of the case at hand. Those features are often pre-processed using techniques to reduce the dimensionality (complexity) of the input data. After pre-processing, the learning algorithm is applied to the training data. At that point, the system is said to have "learned" how to reach the desired decision. In some learning algorithms, such as C4.5 rule-induction, the training process may create human readable classifiers [25, 42] but in many of the more commonly used algorithms, the induced parameters are simply coefficients describing an abstract mathematical function, and are thus are not readable by human review.

Regardless of which type of machine learning is performed, the trained system is then validated against test data containing previously unseen cases in which the correct answers are also known. If the predictions of the learned parameters are accurate enough, the trained system can then be put into service to predict the outcomes of unknown cases. A recent study [14] provides a good example – they developed a system that predicts lactate levels and mortality from sepsis using four different mathematical learning models (naïve Bayes, support vector machines, Gaussian mixture models, and hidden Markov models) instead of the traditional "if-then-else" hand-coded algorithm approach. Their machine-learned model was able to achieve good predictive power while relying on fewer data elements than traditional approaches. As adoption of electronic health records spreads, and more digitized clinical data becomes available for analysis, machine-based learning will likely play a growing role in the development of sophisticated CDS systems.

## 28.2   Predictive Analytics

An important use of machine-learned knowledge in CDS is the growing field of *predicative analytics* [4]. In this approach, a machine learning process is used to train an algorithm that can predict a particular outcome, often via generation of a score where the higher the score, the more likely the outcome. The inputs used to train the algorithm may come from EHR data, claims data, or other sources. A threshold is calculated that maximizes the accuracy of the prediction, such that the algorithm can be used to identity patients that are "positive" for the predicted outcome. Regression models are commonly used to develop the score, but more complex machine learning models can also be used. A common use of predictive analytics is to assess *readmission risks*. The Centers for Medicare and Medicaid Services (CMS) will penalize hospitals for preventable readmissions, so hospitals have developed predictive models to identify the patients at high risk of readmission. Patients at high risk may receive extra interventions with a goal of reducing the number of preventable readmissions. Readmission scores can be calculated for "all causes" (any disease) or can be targeted to specific diseases or procedures. For example, a recent collaborative project between Cerner and Advocate Hospital (Chicago) was able to combine claims data and EHR data to predict readmissions with clinically useful accuracy (C-statistic of 0.78) [6]. Recent work [5] has demonstrated that inclusion of data that capture the social and behavioral determinants of health (such as home living situation) can significantly increase the accuracy of these predictive tools. The growing understanding of the impact of social and behavioral factors on health outcomes has led to calls for EHRs to routinely capture this data [1]. In general, the more data available, the better the predictive models will perform.

## 28.3   Other Non Arden Knowledge Models

Numerous other types of non Arden decision-support tools have been developed using technologies other than the ones detailed in this chapter. For example, *Bayesian Nets* have been applied to diagnosis of community acquired pneumonia [3], and *Decision Trees* have been applied to numerous CDS and diagnostic problems [32]. Despite the power of these many tools for decision support, many commercial EHR vendors have chosen to rely heavily on Arden-like "if-the-else" models as their core CDS service, primarily because Arden-like systems are relatively easy to implement and are easy to understand. However, as will be described below, new methods of delivering more complex CDS services should lead to increased use of these powerful "post Arden" methods.

## 28.4   Visual Methods for Diagnostic Decision Support

Approaches to diagnostic decision support were described in Chap. 1. Those approaches focused on textual display of diagnostic assistance. A relatively new approach to diagnosis assistance are the *visual differential diagnosis* tools, typified by the commercial product VisualDx® [36, 38]. These visual diagnostic assistants contain a large database of images that are linked to diagnostic criteria. For example, VisualDx® contains more than 100,000 peer-reviewed images. A clinician can use these tools to rapidly narrow a potential diagnosis and then verify by comparing the patient to the online images. An obvious target for these tools is dermatology, but they are also relevant to radiology and other image-intense specialties.

Diagnostic decision support is likely to become necessary in the domains of medicine where the knowledge base is so large or so rapidly evolving that it is impossible for a clinician to keep it in memory. For example, in genomic medicine, where new diagnostic tests emerge on a rapid basis, and interpretation of whole-genome or whole-exome sequences require access to massive databases that correlate genetic variants to clinical syndromes, clinicians will have little choice but to depend on genomic CDS tools [35]. Standards and CDS frameworks are just beginning to be proposed for this new field of genomics and personalized medicine [39].

## 28.5   Advanced Literature and Knowledge Retrieval

Providing expedited access from within the clinical workflow to relevant clinical literature is an important type of CDS. This is certainly not a new capability. One of the first tools to support bedside access to the clinical literature was the ground-breaking PaperChase system [21] developed at the Beth Israel Hospital in Boston. The obvious value of ready access to medical literature led the National Library of Medicine to invest in free literature search tools like PubMed [27] – tools now considered invaluable by clinicians and patients alike. Important commercial products such as *UpToDate®* or *ClinicalKey®,* which combine the literature indexing of PubMed with curated summaries of key clinical information and full text access to key journals have emerged as indispensable providers of CDS, and are now being widely integrated directly into EHR products, due in part to incentives created by the United States'(US) Meaningful Use program.

Providers raise many questions during a patient's workup [8]. Unless tools are present that make it easy to find answers to those questions, as many as 70 % of the questions will remain unanswered [12]. Early approaches to bedside literature retrieval relied on custom EHR interfaces. Providing access to the many available external resources led to complex menus, slowing providers down. In response to this problem, the *Infobutton* model, developed at Columbia [7] provided a uniform, context-aware approach to invoking the available resources. A standardized Infobutton icon is placed near key clinical facts in the patient's record, such as lists of the patient's problems, medications, and procedures. When the user clicks on the icon, an Infobutton manager service automatically collects the local context of the icon (e.g., the diagnosis code, medication, or lab) as well as demographic data about the patient (age and gender). The Infobutton manager service then automatically links the user to the most relevant available medical literature, and presents the information back to the clinician via a pop-up web browser. More sophisticated Infobutton implementations are capable of using the clinical context to automatically select the best decision support resource from among similar resources. Some Infobutton services can prompt the clinician with additional questions that help select the most relevant information (such as whether to jump directly to standard ranges for a lab test, or to contraindications for a medication, etc.) Many of the more popular information retrieval services (such as UpToDate® and ClinicalKey®) also support searching from within the tool itself, such that if the Infobutton target was not what the clinician needed, "smart search" can facilitate quick navigation to the sought-after knowledge. Literature access tools play a major role in clinical decision support. By reducing barriers to accessing expert information, and by improving retrieval accuracy, these tools allow the clinician to leverage their own clinical judgment with access to high-value information at the click of a button. The Infobutton model has become an HL7 standard that is now a required component of certified EHR technology under the US EHR Meaningful Use program [16].

## 28.6   Automatic Summarization and Semantic Chart Search as Aids for CDS

The tools described above help address the problem of accessing relevant reference information from the vast array of medical literature. However, as EHR systems have become replacements for the complete paper record, finding the right *patient* data from the growing amount of data available in a typical EHR can be as challenging as searching the reference literature. Numerous researchers have tried to address this problem of "too much data" by creating systems for *automatic summarization* of key aspects of the patient's record, in order to ensure that the provider can quickly review the most important content in the patient's record [13, 37]. Typically these systems allow the clinician to select a key concept (such as a problem) at which point the systems generate a dynamic summary of the most important data in the patients record related to the selected problem.

An alternate approach to automatic summarization is to create semantically enabled "chart search" tools which can find and prioritize relevant information from anywhere in the record. By using the same clinical ontologies that power literature searches, these tools can locate important data in the patient's record, even if the provider doesn't know exactly where the data was captured in the record, or the precise term used to describe the finding. Cerner's Chart Search is one such example. This tool uses natural language parsing (NLP) tools to extract important clinical concepts from the entire record, even if the concepts are buried inside free-text documents, deep in the record. These extracted concepts are then cross-linked with clinical ontologies derived from SNOMED CT® and other sources to create a comprehensive index of the record. The search can be triggered by a provider's query or by clicking on an item in the problem list, medication profile, or any other clinical term in the patient's record. Using the clinical connections represented in the ontologies, the tool can also find all of the occurrences of the concept as well as key related concepts, such as mentions of the drugs that treat a particular problem, as

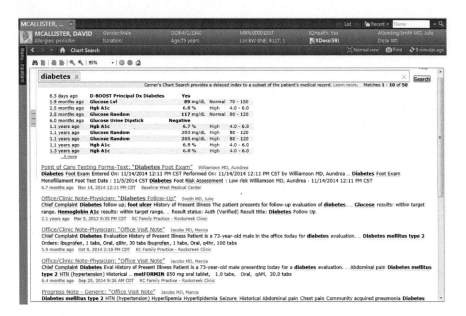

**Fig. 28.1** Cerner Chart Search product showing semantic content fetched on query for "diabetes" (Reproduced with permission of Cerner Corp)

well as documentation of key related physical findings, common symptoms, etc. Figure 28.1 shows an example of a semantic chart search for "diabetes" where documents that mention relevant labs, medications, and quality measures are quickly located. Providing easy access to this relevant chart information is an important new form of clinical decision support for the entire care team.

## 28.7 New Delivery Models: Clinical Decision Support as a Service

Given the difficulty of defining standards for encoding CDS knowledge (as was outlined in the Chap. 1), it is natural to consider an obvious alternative. Since it should be easier to create standards for key components of a patient's record than to standardize complex CDS knowledge models, the easier solution would be to standardize the patient's data and send it to a remote CDS service. This approach, called *service-oriented CDS*, addresses the problem of requiring that all EHRs be able to embed complicated CDS knowledge. In service-oriented CDS, the patient's data is abstracted out of the EHR and sent to a CDS system that is running as a remote service, possibly outside of the EHR entirely.

Halamka described an early experience of using a remote CDS service at the Beth Israel Hospital in Boston [15]. He describes sending an arbitrary XML data structure containing patient information to a remote service that then responds with the requested advice. In similar approach, members of the Clinical Decision Support Consortium [9, 31] demonstrated a shared CDS service based on sending patient data using a Clinical Document Architecture (CDA) document [17] – a standards-based XML-encoded patient summary document. Participating EHR systems generated a patient-specific CDA and sent it to an external CDS service. The remote system unpacked the XML-encoded clinical data, used an existing rules engine to generate a recommendation, and then delivered the result back to the originating system. The team demonstrated that a single shared implementation of a rules engine could easily support multiple clients and different EHR vendors, by leveraging existing CDA standards.

Using CDA documents to send data to the cloud is a logical approach, since all EHRs qualified under Meaningful Use are required to produce a standard Consolidated CDA (CCDA) [18]. However, the CCDA can be a large and unwieldy document, which may not contain the data that the remote CDS service needs [40]. Initial standards work on defining the data structures that could be sent to a CDS service focused on the development of HSSP, the Healthcare Services Specification Project [23], jointly developed by HL7 and the Object Management Group® (OMG.) HSSP, more commonly known has HL7 DSS, uses the vMR to specify the necessary clinical data structures that are matched to a corresponding set of Service Oriented Architecture (SOA) services provided by the CDS system [26]. An authorized EHR can populate the vMR data structures, send the data to the DSS instance, and await the reply. The DSS service invokes internal decision logic, using whatever techniques are desired. A number of pilot implementations of the HL7 DSS standard exist, most notably the Open CDS project [22].

However, given the relative lack of uptake of the DSS standard, the Office of the National Coordinator for Health IT (ONC) created the Health eDecisions (HeD) project in 2013 to improve the standardization of the data messages for remote CDS services [30]. The HeD team has proposed simplifying the HL7 SOA-style DSS standards to better support remote service implementations that don't require a tightly coupled service bus (SOA) architecture. They also proposed using simplified vMR data structures instead of sending the full CCDA. A number of Health eDecisions pilots have been deployed, such as an "immunization calculation engine" [20] which used a cloud-based service to return immunization advice to clinicians inside their EHR. The emergence of HL7's new FHIR standard (Fast Healthcare Interoperability Resource) [19] is likely to cause the HeD recommendations to be revised in the future. The important new role of FHIR in CDS will be described in more detail below.

## 28.8 New Delivery Models: Cloud-Based CDS: A More Scalable Approach

"Cloud computing," defined loosely as the use of a network of remote computer servers made available over the Internet, has come to be broadly accepted and adopted in healthcare [34]. Cloud computing approaches can be used to deliver a complete EHR, but they can also be used to deliver specific services such as remote

CDS. Cloud-based CDS has a number of advantages over traditional deployments that embed the CDS system inside each EHR, and over SOA-style services that require use of a local enterprise service bus. One obvious benefit is that a single, cloud-based service can be shared across many implementations, allowing vendors to spread the costs of the service over many more users. Centralization of the service also enables vendors to keep the CDS knowledge up to date without having to manage large numbers of distributed knowledge bases, spread out over many local EHRs. Implementation of a sharable cloud-based system is also considerably easier than implementing local rules across many different sites. Cloud-based CDS can be implemented and maintained by a central authority of experts, relieving local EHRs from the maintenance and upkeep of the increasingly complex knowledge models required by more advanced CDS that goes beyond simple Arden-like systems.

Another important advantage of cloud-based CDS is that it is often easier and faster for vendors to deploy the service to their client base. Cerner's recent experience with a cloud-based sepsis alerting system provides a relevant example. The Cerner sepsis system is known as the "St John's Sepsis Agent" in honor of St John Medical Center (Tulsa OK) where it was initially developed [2]. Prior to the advent of the cloud-based model, only a small number (fewer than 10) of Cerner's clients had implemented the fairly complex logic that underlies the alert. In an attempt to increase the number of clients who could benefit from sepsis alerts, Cerner implemented a cloud-based sepsis detection engine. The sepsis engine is deployed in Cerner's secure data center. A small "data crawler" service is installed at each participating client site. The data crawler monitors the local system for arrival of sepsis-relevant patient data and sends it to the cloud-based sepsis system. The data is processed in a multi-tenant service in the cloud, organized so that a single engine can simultaneously monitor many hospitals. If the sepsis alert fires, a message is sent back to that hospital's EHR. At that point, the hospital uses the local rules engine to route the alert to the appropriate users.

Cerner's approach is an example of a *hybrid local/cloud CDS model* that combines the use of a local rules engine to do data capture and alert routing along with a cloud-based engine to manage the actual logic of sepsis detection. Figure 28.2 shows the overall logic of the cloud based sepsis system. By shifting to a cloud-based approach, more than 400 hospital sites have been able to deploy the alerting system, with a fraction of the effort than a local approach would have required.

This cloud-based sepsis model has also benefited from fine-tuning and improvements based on continuous evaluation of sensitivity and specificity of the alerts, based on data from all of the deployment sites. More than a dozen iterative improvements of the sepsis decision logic have been shared with the participating clients since the system go-live. These upgrades can occur without any required actions by the client. It should be noted that a cloud-based model does not eliminate the potential for local control and local tuning. Cerner's sepsis clients use a web-based console to optimize the alert thresholds for each hospital's particular patient mix, and to decide how they prefer to route the alerts. Some clients route the alert to a dedicated rapid response team, whereas other clients choose to send the alert to the primary nurse associated with the patient. Relatively few have elected to send the

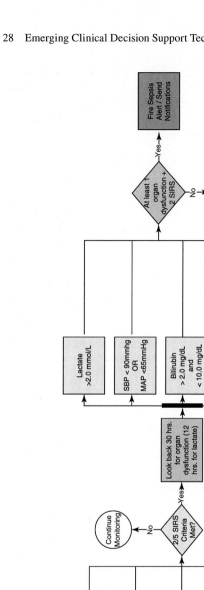
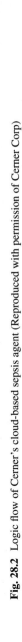

**Fig. 28.2** Logic flow of Cerner's cloud-based sepsis agent (Reproduced with permission of Cerner Corp)

alert directly to the physician, thus minimizing physician "alert fatigue" and improving the likelihood of a timely response to the alert. The advent of CDS as a service, delivered using cloud-computing approaches represents a powerful step forward in high-scale delivery of sophisticated CDS, while at the same time minimizing burdens on busy hospitals to implement and maintain increasingly complex local systems.

## 28.9   New Delivery Models: "SMART Apps" for CDS

"App stores" have revolutionized smart phones and many other consumer computing platforms, but not until recently have apps stores emerged as an option for healthcare computing platforms. [29] suggested that "substitutable apps" could play a role in expanding the capabilities of commercial EHR products, following the paradigm of app stores in other computing domains. In this model, EHRs would become "platforms" that supported standards-based, "plug-in" apps that allow for customization of the EHR beyond the vendor's native offering. Two emerging standards that are likely to have a significant effect on CDS are making this concept a reality. The first standard is FHIR – Fast Healthcare Interoperable Resource, being developed by HL7 [19]. FHIR uses core internet standards (HTTPS – hypertext transfer protocol) to define an API (application programming interface) standard that can be used to move information encoded using simple data structures (called "resources" in FHIR) from place to place. FHIR resources represent a major simplification compared to the HL7 V3 RIM. Early experience with FHIR suggests that it is quite feasible for an EHR vendor to expose a FHIR-based API that provides comprehensive read and write data access to the clinical data contained in the EHR [33]. The breadth of data access provided by FHIR opens many possibilities for new kinds of CDS. For example, using FHIR, a remote CDS service could fetch necessary lab data, vital signs, and other information necessary to make a more accurate CDS recommendation than if the EHR merely sent a predefined, fixed set of clinical data to the service. If the EHR exposes the FHIR API, then the decision support service can ask for whatever it needs, as it evaluates the decision logic. The profound implications of this shift should not be underestimated. The ability for a remote CDS service to easily request whatever data it needs, without requiring custom programming, should rapidly expand the scope of CDS services that remain EHR vendor-neutral and thus available to more providers.

The SMART Platform [28], on the other hand, specifies a standard way to embed a web-based *application* directly into any EHR capable of exposing a web browser interface. An embedded SMART application can use standard HTML to create any desired user visual experience, while running integrated into the clinician's workflow, and while preserving patient context. SMART apps can also be deployed to smart phones and tablet devices, as long as web pages are supported. The combination of SMART and FHIR together creates the technology necessary to create "SMART on FHIR" app stores. SMART apps are relevant to CDS in a number of

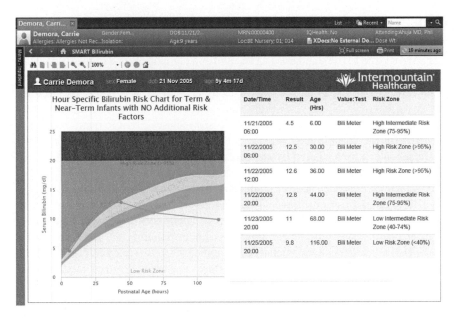

**Fig. 28.3** Neonatal bilirubin decision support using a SMART on FHIR app (Reproduced with permission of Intermountain Healthcare)

ways. First, many of the complexities that have made standardization of complex CDS rules so difficult (e.g., Arden, vMR, HL7 DSS, Health eDecisions, etc. as described earlier) are mitigated by use of a simple plug-in app that brings an external CDS conversation right into the clinical workflow. FHIR provides the necessary data access, and the SMART app delivers the visual presentation and user conversation, allowing for arbitrarily complex remote CDS interventions to be embedded into any compliant EHR.

One use of SMART apps is for *CDS visualizations*. A number of studies have suggested that condition-specific data visualizations may facilitate complex decision making, by organizing the data using an appropriate visual metaphor to expose key relationships that might get lost in tabular displays of data [10, 24]. Complex visualizations are often specific to a narrow range of clinical conditions, which would make it costly for each EHR vendor to create the required libraries of condition-specific visualizations. However, the SMART on FHIR app approach enables third-party developers to create custom visualizations that can then be "plugged in" to SMART on FHIR compliant EHRs. For example, a SMART app developed at Intermountain Healthcare (Fig. 28.3) shows a graphical representation that helps clinicians manage neonatal hyperbilirubinemia by graphically representing the change in bilirubin as a function of time under phototherapy lights. At a glance, the clinician can determine when sufficient phototherapy has been delivered. This customized visualization app could be used by any EHR that supports the SMART and FHIR standards.

## 28.10    SMART on FHIR to Deliver Remote CDS

The SMART and FHIR standards can be used as a component of a powerful remote CDS service that could supplement a vendor's built-in CDS tools. The orchestration could flow as follows: First, the EHR uses its internal tools to detect the need to invoke the external CDS service (likely running as a cloud-based service). Secondly, once contacted by the EHR, the remote CDS service uses FHIR to query back into the EHR for the specific data necessary to answer the contextual question. This conversation can be mediated by standard FHIR services, thus relieving the EHR vendor from the need to create custom code for each remote CDS service. Thirdly, if the remote CDS service needs to "talk" to the clinician to get more data, it can ask the EHR to invoke a specific SMART app. And fourthly, once all the data is present, the remote CDS can make a recommendation, which it sends back to the EHR using FHIR standards. This process can be done without requiring the EHR vendor to have knowledge of the internal details of the remote CDS service, while also freeing the CDS vendor from requiring custom interfaces to each EHR. Implementation of remote CDS services that follow this model should be easier and more robust compared to previous approaches that required the EHR vendor to understand and embed complex CDS logic. In other words, move the data to the service, not the knowledge to the EHR. Note that the EHR vendor must still exercise careful design in deciding when and how to invoke the remote service, to avoid excessive pop-up alerts and "alert fatigue."

## 28.11    Summary

In Chap. 1, we reviewed the history of clinical decision support, with a focus on the most widely deployed paradigm, Arden-like scripting rules. We reviewed the efforts to standardize CDS, with the focus mostly on standardizing the knowledge models and knowledge encoding. We reviewed the strengths and weaknesses of current approaches, noting that "alert fatigue" remains a key barrier, despite efforts to improve the accuracy of rules, and the workflow of rule delivery. We noted the inherent limitations of the simple rules used in Arden-like models, and the difficultly in trying to embed complex CDS knowledge bases in each of the many EHR platforms.

In this chapter, we called out some emerging technologies that should help address these current limitations. In particular we note the increased alert accuracy that should be available to systems that explore post-Arden knowledge models, such as those based on machine learning and data-driven analytic technologies. We highlighted the shift in focus from locally embedded systems to remote, cloud-based CDS, with the attendant increase in scale and scope of what can be deployed. We also highlighted the shift away from trying to standardize CDS knowledge encoding, to instead standardizing the data that needs to be exchanged with service-oriented, remote decision services. We highlighted the promise of FHIR, as a major simplification over the previous generation of standards based on the cumbersome

**Table 28.1** Summary of evolution of clinical decision support

| CDS Category | Current CDS | Future CDS |
|---|---|---|
| Location of CDS rules: | Embedded in local EHR | Services running in cloud |
| CDS Standards: | Focus on encoding the knowledge model and rules | Focus on encoding the clinical data to send to the remote service |
| Workflow for CDS alerts: | Interruptive, reactive, not personalized | Ambient, anticipatory, personalized to user preferences |
| CDS Knowledge encoding: | Human curated rules and scripts | Mix of human curated and machine learning |
| Focus of CDS: | Safety, reminders, treatment | Adds differential dx, diagnostic workup, chronic management |
| CDS Intervention: | Alerts | Pluggable apps, visualizations, literature search, chart search |
| Disease focus of CDS interventions: | Single conditions, one at a time | Multiple diseases, via machine learned multi-condition patterns |
| Recipient of the interventions: | Deliver to the current user (MD) usually with only one try | Route to best clinician, with escalation to ensure deliver |
| Clinical data standards | Complex: RIM and vMR | Simple: FHIR resources |

HL7 RIM. We concluded with an introduction to embeddable CDS "apps" that follow new standards such as SMART on FHIR. In closing, in Table 28.1 we contrast the Arden-like models in current EHRs to the future possibilities using twenty first century web and cloud technologies. In this table, we summarize many of the changes that are occurring with an eye to the future that holds promise for more accurate, widespread, and powerful clinical decision support.

# References

1. Adler NE, Stead WW. Patients in context — EHR capture of social and behavioral determinants of health. N Engl J Med. 2015;372:698–701. doi:10.1056/NEJMp1413945.
2. Amland RC, Hahn-Cover KE. Clinical decision support for early recognition of sepsis. Am J Med Qual. 2014. doi:10.1177/1062860614557636.
3. Aronsky D, Haug PJ. Diagnosing community-acquired pneumonia with a Bayesian network. Proc AMIA Symp. 1998;632–6.
4. Bates DW, Saria S, Ohno-Machado L, et al. Big data in health care: using analytics to identify and manage high-risk and high-cost patients. Health Aff (Millwood). 2014;33:1123–31. doi:10.1377/hlthaff.2014.0041.
5. Calvillo-King L, Arnold D, Eubank KJ, et al. Impact of social factors on risk of readmission or mortality in pneumonia and heart failure: systematic review. J Gen Intern Med. 2013;28:269–82. doi:10.1007/s11606-012-2235-x.
6. Choudhry SA, Li J, Davis D, et al. A public-private partnership develops and externally validates a 30-day hospital readmission risk prediction model. Online J Publ Health Inf. 2013;5:219. doi:10.5210/ojphi.v5i2.4726.
7. Cimino JJ, Elhanan G, Zeng Q. Supporting infobuttons with terminological knowledge. Proc AMIA Annu Fall Symp. 1997;528–32.

8. Covell DG, Uman GC, Manning PR. Information needs in office practice: are they being met? Ann Intern Med. 1985;103:596–9.

9. Dixon BE, Simonaitis L, Goldberg HS, et al. A pilot study of distributed knowledge management and clinical decision support in the cloud. Artif Intell Med. 2013;59:45–53. doi:10.1016/j.artmed.2013.03.004.

10. Dolan JG, Veazie PJ, Russ AJ. Development and initial evaluation of a treatment decision dashboard. BMC Med Inform Decis Mak. 2013;13:51. doi:10.1186/1472-6947-13-51.

11. Duda RO, Hart PE, Stork DG, Wiley-Interscience. Pattern classification. 2nd ed. New York: Wiley-Interscience; 2000.

12. Ely JW, Osheroff JA, Chambliss ML, et al. Answering physicians' clinical questions: obstacles and potential solutions. J Am Med Inform Assoc. 2005;12:217–24. doi:10.1197/jamia.M1608.

13. Feblowitz JC, Wright A, Singh H, et al. Summarization of clinical information: a conceptual model. J Biomed Inform. 2011;44:688–99. doi:10.1016/j.jbi.2011.03.008.

14. Gultepe E, Green JP, Nguyen H, et al. From vital signs to clinical outcomes for patients with sepsis: a machine learning basis for a clinical decision support system. J Am Med Inform Assoc. 2013;21:315–25. doi:10.1136/amiajnl-2013-001815.

15. Halamka J. Life as a healthcare CIO: decision support service providers. 2010. http://geekdoctor.blogspot.com/2010/06/decision-support-service-providers.html. Accessed 13 Jan 2015.

16. HL7. HL7 context aware knowledge retrieval application ("Infobutton"), knowledge request, release 2. 2014. http://www.hl7.org/implement/standards/product_brief.cfm?product_id=208. Accessed 28 Mar 2015.

17. HL7. Clinical document architecture release 2; 2006. http://www.hl7.org/implement/standards/product_brief.cfm?product_id=7. Accessed 1 Jun 2015.

18. HL7. HL7 standards product brief - HL7 implementation guide for CDA® release 2: IHE health story consolidation, release 1.1 - US Realm; 2012. http://www.hl7.org/implement/standards/product_brief.cfm?product_id=258. Accessed 28 Mar 2015.

19. HL7. FHIR; 2014. http://www.hl7.org/implement/standards/fhir/. Accessed 18 Dec 2014.

20. HLNConsulting. HLN: Immunization Calculation Engine (ICE); 2015. https://www.hln.com/ice/. Accessed 13 Jan 2015.

21. Horowitz GL, Bleich HL. PaperChase: a computer program to search the medical literature. N Engl J Med. 1981;305:924–30. doi:10.1056/NEJM198110153051605.

22. Kawamoto K. OpenCDS Home; 2015. http://www.opencds.org/. Accessed 13 Jan 2015.

23. Kawamoto K, Honey A, Rubin K. The HL7-OMG healthcare services specification project: motivation, methodology, and deliverables for enabling a semantically interoperable service-oriented architecture for healthcare. J Am Med Inform Assoc. 2009;16:874–81. doi:10.1197/jamia.M3123.

24. Klimov D, Shahar Y. A framework for intelligent visualization of multiple time-oriented medical records. AMIA Annu Symp Proc. 2005;405–9.

25. Lamy J-B, Ellini A, Ebrahiminia V, et al. Use of the C4.5 machine learning algorithm to test a clinical guideline-based decision support system. Stud Health Technol Inform. 2008;136:223–8.

26. Loya SR, Kawamoto K, Chatwin C, Huser V. Service oriented architecture for clinical decision support: a systematic review and future directions. J Med Syst. 2014;38:140. doi:10.1007/s10916-014-0140-z.

27. Lu Z. PubMed and beyond: a survey of web tools for searching biomedical literature. Database Oxford University Press 2011:baq036. doi: 10.1093/database/baq036.

28. Mandl KD, Mandel JC, Murphy SN, et al. The SMART platform: early experience enabling substitutable applications for electronic health records. J Am Med Inform Assoc. 2012;19:597–603.

29. Mandl KD, Kohane IS. No small change for the health information economy. The New England Journal of Medicine. 2009;360(13):1278–81. doi:10.1056/NEJMp0900411.

30. ONC S and I. Health eDecisions Homepage; 2013. http://wiki.siframework.org/Health+eDecisions+Homepage. Accessed 17 Mar 2015.

31. Paterno MD, Maviglia SM, Ramelson HZ, et al. Creating shareable decision support services: an interdisciplinary challenge. AMIA Annu Symp Proc. 2010;2010:602–6.

32. Podgorelec V, Kokol P, Stiglic B, Rozman I. Decision trees: an overview and their use in medicine. J Med Syst. 2002;26:445–63.
33. Raths D. Trend: standards development. Catching FHIR. A new HL7 draft standard may boost web services development in healthcare. Healthc Inform. 2014;31(13):16.
34. Schweitzer EJ. Reconciliation of the cloud computing model with US federal electronic health record regulations. J Am Med Inform Assoc. 2012;19:161–5.
35. Segal MM, Abdellateef M, El-Hattab AW, et al. Clinical pertinence metric enables hypothesis-independent genome-phenome analysis for neurologic diagnosis. J Child Neurol. 2014. doi:10.1177/0883073814545884.
36. Tleyjeh IM, Nada H, Baddour LM. VisualDx: decision-support software for the diagnosis and management of dermatologic disorders. Clin Infect Dis. 2007;43:1177–84. doi:10.1086/508283.
37. Van Vleck TT, Stein DM, Stetson PD, Johnson SB. Assessing data relevance for automated generation of a clinical summary. AMIA Annu Symp Proc. 2007;761–5.
38. Vardell E, Bou-Crick C. VisualDx: a visual diagnostic decision support tool. Med Ref Serv Q. 2012;31:414–24. doi:10.1080/02763869.2012.724287.
39. Welch BM, Loya SR, Eilbeck K, Kawamoto K. A proposed clinical decision support architecture capable of supporting whole genome sequence information. J Pers Med. 2014;4:176–99. doi:10.3390/jpm4020176.
40. Zhou L, Hongsermeier T, Boxwala A, et al. Structured representation for core elements of common clinical decision support interventions to facilitate knowledge sharing. Stud Health Technol Inform. 2013;192:195–9.
41. Dua S, Archarya U, Dua P. Machine learning in healthcare informatics. Intelligent Systems Reference Library. 2014;56:40017. doi: 10.1007/978-3-642-40017-9.
42. Zorman M, Stiglic MM, Kokol P, Malcić I. The limitations of decision trees and automatic learning in real world medical decision making. J Med Syst. 1997;21:403–15.

# Chapter 29
# Beyond Current HIMS: Future Visions and a Roadmap

James Fackler

## 29.1   Introduction

This chapter explores a future vision for technologically supported healthcare beyond where current health information management systems (HIMS) have taken us. This vision is informed from over three decades of experience as a Pediatric Intensivist working in academic medical centers; as well as being a Medical Informatician engaged for the past 20 years in system design for a major EHR vendor and multiple consulting roles for smaller niche and start-up health information technology (HIT) companies. Based on these experiences and supported by the HIT literature [1] and health policy bodies [2], I believe:

1. The current health care system is not safe,
2. The billions of dollars spent designing, testing, and implementing HIMSs have been spent instantiating the same workflows that created the unsafe current health care system.
3. It is not just unlikely, but rather *impossible*, that current HIMSs can improve the value of care delivered.
4. The primary way HIMS can improve the value of care delivered [3] is by improving the clinical decisions leading to an improvement in patient outcomes.

The cliché that insanity is repeatedly doing the same processes but expecting different results is quite relevant here. Thus, this chapter describes a significant deviation from the United States healthcare industry's current HIMS strategy built as it is upon a few monolithic electronic health record (EHR) vendors with the

J. Fackler, MD
Pediatric Anesthesiology and Critical Care Medicine,
The Johns Hopkins University School of Medicine, Baltimore, MD, USA
e-mail: fackler@jhmi.edu

© Springer International Publishing Switzerland 2016                    493
C.A. Weaver et al. (eds.), *Healthcare Information Management Systems:
Cases, Strategies, and Solutions*, Health Informatics,
DOI 10.1007/978-3-319-20765-0_29

inherent limitations associated with monolithic size. Instead, what is envisioned here is an altogether different technology support road that has been started by others and importantly, presents solutions built on twenty-first century technologies. Three more predicates will guide this new journey:

1. Current HIMSs can play a valuable role in the data collection process.
2. The data collected by these HIMSs must be augmented with data not now routinely captured in HIMSs.
3. The data collected by these HIMSs must then be made accessible to vendor-agnostic patient-centric applications.

## 29.2 The Imperative for Clinical Decision Support Begun by Others…

Two meta-analyses reviews on clinical decision support (CDS) systems, published independently in 2005, concluded that for a CDS to be effective, the system must be automated [4] and must interrupt workflow [5]. Pushing these two points to their logical extensions, for technology to support our clinical decisions, there must be a tight coupling of the clinician and the computer. There must be more than good human computer interfaces; there must be human-computer symbiosis. In 1960 (yes, 55 years ago), JCR Licklider, a psychologist and pioneer in computer science coined the concept of "man-computer symbioses" [6], noting that while none existed in 1960:

> The hope is that, in not too many years, human brains and computing machines will be coupled together very tightly, and that the resulting partnership will think as no human brain has ever thought and process data in a way not approached by the information-handling machines we know today. [6]

Licklider's vision of the tight coupling of man and computers is closer to being realized, but not yet a reality. We may be on the threshold of Licklider's vision, if the opinions of Kurzweil [6] and others predicting the "singularity" state – the time when there will be no distinction between human and machine – are correct. It would be a fair bet that clinicians in their early 1940s have a good chance of making clinical decisions in a setting of true human-computer symbiosis.

## 29.3 Decision Support …

Looking at what's involved in decision support must begin with a discussion of what decisions clinicians make, how those decisions are made, and how the decisions are best supported. Broad, often excellent, theoretical guidance is published on clinical decisions [7], but again little guidance is available in the literature cataloging the decisions clinicians actually make. A 2010 study of ten faculty pediatric cardiologists found that each physician made close to 160 decisions per day, and of these, 80 % were made without any basis in published data [9]. The authors further reported that fewer than 3 % of decisions were based on a study relevant to the specific decision [8]. Even less guidance in the form of evidence-based data is available to entrepreneurs and developers of clinical decision support systems in terms of pointing to which decisions *should* be supported.

The best place to start deciding where to start should follow from the work of Daniel Kahneman whose book "Thinking, Fast and Slow" should be required reading for any developer of future clinical decision support applications [9]. Kahneman suggests a dichotomy between System One (fast) thinking and System Two (slow) thinking. System One operates automatically and quickly with little or no effort and no sense of voluntary control. In contrast, System Two allocates attention to the effortful mental activities that demand it, including complex computations or in a clinical context, puzzling through a complicated patient.

At the bedside, a System One decision is often what is euphemistically called "the art of medicine" but is better recognized as intuition. Gary Klein has long studied intuition in experts [10] lauding the expert's pattern recognition capabilities. Again, pattern recognition is a core cognitive task and senior physicians perform better than do junior physicians [11, 12]. However, given that the vast majority of clinical decisions are based on precious little data and the most senior clinicians do not often make these decisions, it begs the question whether CDS can support the System One, intuition-based pattern recognition decisions. The answer is – yes; but few such solutions, even as prototypes exist [13]. The reader is referred to a recent review on the subject of supervised classifiers that may have applicability to medical diagnosis [14].

The operations of System Two are often associated with the subjective experiences of choice and concentration. The highly diverse operations of System Two have one feature in common: they require attention and are disrupted when attention is drawn away. In the medical context, System Two decisions are those that demand thought, often because a well-established pattern is not recognized and even partial patterns are not obvious or are conflicting. Data may be missing, wrong, and/or are conflicting. Rarely, is there time in a busy clinical environment to engage System Two thinking. While there are strengths and weaknesses associated with System One and System Two thinking, both used at the right times, are crucial for optimal patient care [15]. IT support of the clinical decisions will differ depending on which System is being supported.

At the most fundamental level, CDS should help protect clinicians, and the patients they serve, from cognitive biases. The formal study of cognitive biases was launched in 1974 by Amos Tversky and Daniel Kahneman [16]. Although there are a number of excellent references in the medical literature describing cognitive biases [17–20], a better place for CDS developers to start deciding which apps to build is with a crosswalk of an anti-bias checklist proposed for business decisions [21] into medical decisions. Twelve bias checks are proposed (e.g. check for groupthink, check for saliency bias, check for availability bias – which is also called, below, WYSIATI). Whether deciding to build a new manufacturing facility or whether to initiate an invasive surgery for cancer, the decision should seek dissenting opinions (to avoid groupthink), be certain the recommendation is based on more than the memory of a recent success (to avoid saliency bias) and be certain there isn't a better option not yet considered (to avoid availability bias). CDS developers will do well focusing on as many of the twelve categories of bias as outlined by Kahneman, and his colleagues as is possible.

## 29.4    Getting the Data in …

Although it sounds too mundane an issue for a discussion of future HIMS systems, accuracy of the clinical documentation by nurses, physicians and other team members is an under appreciated problem. The cliché of garbage in – garbage out (GIGO) continues to be a major contributor to unsafe systems and renders clinical decision support ineffective, or worse, dangerous. If we are to improve outcomes, we cannot do so if the primary data that clinicians use for their decisions are wrong. Yes, the electronic data are legible, they can be graphed and used in calculations, but unfortunately, all too often the data are erroneous due to omissions, incorrect readings, or disparities between human and medical device readings. Finding evidence for problems with nursing documentation is not hard. One notable study reported on a quality improvement effort in an Italian emergency department and found that triage vital signs were missing in acutely ill trauma victims 10 % of the time even *after* their quality improvement intervention [22]. Mentioning this is not to suggest these adults received poor care – but it does mean as decision support solutions are created with triage vital signs (to, for example, focus the attention of clinicians in a busy environment) that trauma victims might be inappropriately classified by the decision support solution and then these patients might be harmed. Another small survey of trauma resuscitation documentation with a HIMS showed that serial vital signs were not documented a quarter of the time and fully half of the time the Glasgow coma scale and the fluid input-output data were missing [23]. Imagine trying to create a decision support solution for trauma resuscitation without input-output data! However, at this time, HIMSs flow sheets will always be necessary for clinicians to input relevant data that cannot be captured automatically. Level of consciousness, Glasgow coma scale, and capillary refill are extremely important parameters that machines cannot, yet, accurately acquire. The workflow for clinicians (e.g. with voice-based data input) must be augmented and routine use of data error checking routines should be incorporated. HIMSs should prohibit entry of biologically impossible data (e.g. a weight of 874 kg when 87.4 is correct) as well as "implausible" data (e.g. a weight of 87.4 lbs when the patient's most recent weight was 87.4 kg). These implausible data elements should be based not on population norms for healthy people, but based on that specific, individual patient's norms and that person's trends as one would expect to find in a patient-centric system.

Another category of error occurs when other sources of data that are available are just wasted. For example, clinicians periodically do record heart rate – at shorter time intervals when physiological instability demands. Often, EMRs interface with the physiological monitors and some therapeutic devices to automate data entry into the HIMS system. Doing so requires use of Medical Device Data Systems (MDDS) and these "middle-ware" solutions have well-established regulatory [24] requirements and are commercial availability from a number of vendors. MDDS interface with existing bedside medical devices and offer the clinician a time-stamped value for them to verify and then store in the HIMSs data tables. Because, for example, the electrocardiogram (ECG) is routinely available as a 240 Hz waveform signal, even verifying and recording the data every 5 min (as is done routinely in by anesthesiologists) means that almost one million data points are lost per patient per hour for just this one signal. That there is value in this single example of wasted data is evidenced by heart rate variability (HRV) analysis and its proposed ability to predict disparate conditions like extubation readiness [25] and subarachnoid hemorrhage [26]. HRV analysis has been shown in a randomized controlled trial to allow early detection of sepsis in low-birth-weight newborns and that with early detection newborn lives are saved [27].

It is important to dig a bit deeper into the challenges of manual data entry biases and the waste of high-fidelity data. A detailed look into the MIMIC II (Multiparameter Intelligent Monitoring in Intensive Care) database work by Hug and Clifford (2007) is in order [28, 29]. Best described on the PhysioNet website (http://www.physionet.org/), the MIMIC-II research database has three defining major characteristics: it is publicly and freely available; it encompasses a diverse and very large population of [mostly adult] ICU patients; and it contains high temporal resolution data including lab results, electronic documentation, and bedside monitor trends and waveforms. Developers should also note that because it is built on open source, it allows volunteers to continuously build, refine and share data management and analysis apps. Hug and Clifford (2007) first wanted to determine if the electrocardiogram, systemic arterial blood pressure, and systemic oxygen plethysmography waveform data recorded outside the HIMS (from automated downloads from the physiological monitors) differed from the nursing documented data in the EHR [28]. After developing a filtering algorithm to reject some artifacts, Hug and Clifford found that the monitoring and vital sign data automatically captured as compared to nurse-captured recordings differed not just statistically, but also differed by clinically significant ranges. For example, they found that the least error for each of the four measurements studied occurred on Wednesdays, the highest error rate occurred on Fridays, and errors were most prevalent on the weekend. Diurnal differences were seen as well. And significantly, they detected a significant variation in errors (mean and variance) between data entered by clinicians who logged in anonymously (not now allowed in most mainstream EMRs) compared to those clinicians who were logged in appropriately [28].

In their follow-up paper, Hug and colleagues (2011) analyzed MIMIC II records with both nursing documented data and the automatically captured waveform data not available with the EHR in their 2007 study [29]. For each patient they determined baseline states and then used either the EHR data or the waveform data in an algorithm to predict hypotension. Again in short, the automated data filtered out major artifacts and better predicted episodes of hypotension. Thus, it is not just interesting that there is variability in the quality of EHR data rather the data quality has potential patient outcome effects. Assuming others confirm these investigator's findings, there are crucial ramifications for restructuring documentation workflows in all areas using continuous vital sign monitors. The takeaway from this research, suggests that clinicians should be viewed as "annotators" of these continuous waveforms rather than arbiter of "truth".

## 29.5    Federal Drug Administration and Medical Devices Regulation

The above discussion on reliable vital sign capture and recording has comingled two critically distinct regulatory issues. The issue of how to obtain device data (e.g. physiological monitor data and/or therapeutic device data) via an automatic interface for clinician validation and storage within an EHR is regulated as Medical Device Data Systems (MDDS). However, the issue of how to obtain and use the "raw" data from monitors and devices in clinical decision support solutions is not as cleanly described.

In 2011, the Federal Drug Administration (FDA) finalized a rule describing MDDSs stating:

> Medical Device Data Systems (MDDS) are hardware or software products that transfer, store, convert formats, and display medical device data. An MDDS does not modify the data or modify the display of the data, and it does not by itself control the functions or parameters of any other medical device. MDDS are not intended to be used for active patient monitoring. [24]

This MDDS rule does not cover the routine use of filtering algorithms and hypotension prediction as illustrated above in the MIMIC II work of Hug and Clifford. The FDA has issued the Food and Drug Administration Safety and Innovation (FDASIA) Health IT Report and delayed a definitive position on the regulation of clinical decision support systems [30]. The report clearly implied a hands-off approach as long as any recommendations passed from a CDS go to a "learned intermediary", meaning any clinician who assumes responsibility for any actions taken [31]. The regulation of an artifact-filtering algorithm used by Hug et al. [29] and any closed-loop CDS solutions will likely be regulated as are current medical devices [31].

Finally, were all these issues not enough as problems in need of solutions in future HIMSs, actually getting the data acquired remains a challenge. A diatribe asking why consumer electronics are increasing often "plug-and-play" whereas medical devices wallow in a proprietary morass has been done many times by every clinician. As of this writing, there are two well-organized and funded efforts to bring true plug-and-play to medical devices. Most long standing is the Medical Device Plug-and-Play effort spearheaded by Julian Goldman [32, 33]. Work is in part focused on an integrated data environment [33] and dissemination of practical language for health care organizations to use during request for proposals and contracting that would demand vendors support plug-and-play. West Health is also expending substantial effort in the domain of interoperability (see: http://www.westhealth.org/initiative/our-research).

So far, the discussion of getting the data in has focused solely on the data collected by clinicians (largely nurses) using standard clinical parameters often facilitated with standard medical equipment. However, there is also a massive untapped trove of data streaming from consumer products. Connected pedometers, scales, pulse oximeters, sphygmomanometers are mainstream consumer devices and are becoming far more common. Location tracking coupled with environmental data and consumer-grade air quality monitors will add previously unavailable data (and might, for example, be useful in an asthma CDS solution). Consumer focused genetic data is also available and although not without problems [34], has broader acceptance than might be guessed [35]. The "Quantified Self" movement has a devoted but still rather small community (see an excellent discussion in the context of a broader vision of the future [36]). Consumers are putting substantial effort into data acquisition, visualization, and analysis. There is some data suggesting the use of consumer device data can improve outcomes [37]. Skepticism should remain high as these early successful reports emerge; the Hawthorne effect can be powerful [38]. However, it seems likely that as sensors improve and become more smoothly incorporated into normal consumer workflow (e.g. by being built into clothing or, maybe, watches) that data quality and availability will improve. Consumer electronics companies, fitness clothing companies and a wide array of startup companies are pushing efforts in this area. HIMSs companies are noticeably absent in this arena, again, making the integration of consumer-generated data with HIMSs data ripe for creation of patient-centric applications that are HIMS vendor agnostic.

Somewhat more established is the use of patient entered data; and "more established" still means efforts less than 10 years old. Consumers have been sharing health stories for millennia if only at the level of chicken soup, garlic necklaces etc. But in early 2006, the social website, *PatientsLikeMe,* opened to the public (http://www.patientslikeme.com/). There are hundreds of other such consumer-focused sites but *PatientsLikeMe* has shown some extraordinary successes. From their website, they have about 300,000 members who are recording health data for more than 2,300 conditions and have accumulated 25 million data points [39]. Most extraordinary, if "patientslikeme" is used as a PubMed search term, 46 articles are retrieved. This link between research and social media dynamic is illustrated by this example of lithium and Amyotrophic Lateral Sclerosis patients (ALS). An early (2007) article focused on the story behind an early success understanding on the use of lithium for suppression of symptoms of ALS [40]. In brief, a randomized trial of 44 patients with ALS followed a cohort of 16 who were treated with lithium [41]. No disease progression was reported in this small sized, ALS patient study population when it was published in February 2008. Before then, however, the data had been presented in a conference format and was picked up by the *PatientsLikeMe* social-media community. Working with the investigators from the report, around the time the article was publically released, 116 patients with ALS were already reporting their symptoms within *PatientsLikeMe* while taking doses of lithium much like those reported at the conference. Thereafter, a complete analysis of the *PatientsLikeMe* data was done based on a dataset finalized in February 2010, when 149 patients were eligible for analysis having taken lithium for a part of a year and 78 patients who took lithium for a full year. In short, the analysis showed lithium had no effect on the progression of ALS (albeit with a low side effect profile) [42]. In an extraordinary waste of resources, a larger randomized controlled trial enrolled patients between 2009 and 2011 and showed the same result as the completely patient entered data from the *PatientsLikeMe* analysis. This randomized clinical trial was published in 2013 [43]. An accompanying editorial [44] simply dismissing the patient entered data analysis should itself be dismissed [45]. To bring this discussion back to point from which it was launched, HIMSs of the future must better acquire accurate data that effectively tells the patient story. But HIMSs must also morph to accommodate this massive consumer-patient data treasure.

## 29.6   The Future Roadmap Builds on Twenty-First Century Technologies for Vendor-Agnostic Patient-Centric Applications…

If there is a single message readers should take from this chapter it is this: the future of health care information technology is in the dissemination of applications (or "apps") in a fashion completely analogous to the Android and iOS platform devices. These apps may be as "simple" as gathering data from worn sensors or as "complicated" as combining diagnostic, laboratory, and device data into specific clinical recommendations – even to the point of passing closed-loop instructions to therapeutic devices. Building these apps will require the same entrepreneurial passion and follow through that has gone, and continues to go, into the Angry-Birds-like enterprises. Health care apps, however, must be built with the experience of seasoned clinicians who have the odd combination of out-of-the-box thinking who can entertain the "impossible", coupled with a 20-something developer partner but with the clinicians' wisdom to keep the programmer out of clinical trouble.

This concept of the dissemination of apps in a fashion completely analogous to the Android and iOS platform devices for healthcare was first proposed by Ken Mandl and Zak Kohane in an 2009 opinion piece in the New England Journal of Medicine [46]. In that article, Mandl and Kohane wrote:

> As we seek to design a [HIM] system that will constantly evolve and encourage innovation, we can glean lessons from large-scale information-technology successes in other fields. An essential first lesson is that ideally, system components should be not only interoperable but also substitutable. The Apple iPhone, for example, uses a software platform with a published interface that allows software developers outside Apple to create applications.

Pushing further in a 2012 opinion piece, aptly titled, "Escaping the EHR Trap – The Future of Health IT" [47], Mandl and Kohane urge Health IT vendors to adopt modern technologies wherever possible, and argue that "…" Incentive Programs should not be held hostage to EHRs that reduce…efficiency and strangle innovation. New companies will offer bundled, best-of-breed, interoperable, substitutable technologies…that can be optimized for use in health care improvement. Properly nurtured, these products will rapidly reach the market,

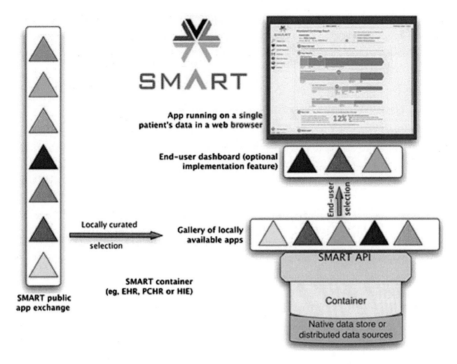

**Fig. 29.1** The SMART Platform. Central to the success of the SMART platform is the SMART API that delivers to developers a consistent way to acquire data (from the Container) upon which CDS apps can be built. See text for further details (Reproduced from Mandl et al. [48], with permission of Oxford University Press and the authors)

effectively addressing the goals of 'meaningful use', signaling the post-EHR era, and returning to the innovative spirit of EHR pioneers.

What has emerged from Mandl and Kohane's concepts is the SMART Platform [48] illustrated in Fig. 29.1. A SMART platform enabled HIMS (because, yes, this does describe a post-EHR Health Information Management System) is built on a data container. Writing in 2012, Mandl and colleagues [45] reflected that the SMART data models were still very much a work in progress and limited in scope. The authors further explained that the goal of their data modeling work is not to provide a detailed model for every possible aspect of a patient's medical history; but rather, to provide highly consistent views for the most common data elements. Because the SMART data models are freely available, this foundational work is accessible to other innovators as well. The SMART model is evolving and now incorporates the Fast Healthcare Interoperability Resources within the Health Level Seven standards organization (or HL7 FHIR pronounced "fire" [49]). As shown in Fig. 29.1, the application program interface (API) also now leverages FHIR. Most remarkable is, within this platform, the wise clinician and 20-something developer dyad can create apps and place them in a public exchange. Local organizations (e.g. hospitals, group practices, payers) can vet applications and then individuals (clinicians and/or consumers) can further decide which apps to use. Today, SMART enabled applications are being used clinically and in environments beyond those of the original developers [50, 51].

## 29.7   Using Humans to the Best of Their Ability …

So now that more and better data is into a vendor-neutral patient-centric platform so the wise clinician/20-something developer dyad can build and disseminate apps, what should they build? According to Licklider, the answer lies in what he called the "man-computer symbiosis" and, therefore, demands an understating of what humans do best. Humans are masters of pattern recognition. In a cognitive task analysis focused on critical care physicians, Fackler and colleagues (2009) identified five broad categories of cognitive activities: pattern recognition; uncertainty management; strategic vs. tactical thinking; team coordination and maintenance of common ground; and, creation and transfer of meaning through stories [35]. Pattern recognition is, however, the prime task after which all other cognitive tasks follow. Additionally, the authors found that while many members of a critical care team used the term 'pattern', most physicians could neither define what they meant by 'patterns' nor give specific examples of a 'pattern'. Regardless that clinicians could not be explicit about just what a pattern is, the cognitive task analysis, however, found that pattern recognition did happen in two forms. One pattern was of a complete 'template'. Asthma is one such complete template based on a minimal history, appearance and breath sounds. A typical template of severe asthma includes the constellation of cues of a patient who is in an upright position, sweaty, speaking in one word answers, exhibiting labored breathing and attentive to his or her own breathing. However, such 'classic' complete templates are uncommon.

The second but distinct cognitive task is the real-time merging of pattern fragments (also called 'packets') into unique (patient specific) templates. Observed more frequently than identifying a complete template, these packets are recognized as cues that are postulated to be related. It is only through a flexible and dynamic integration of these packets that a complete (or a more complete, but still, partial) template can be created. These templates are context specific. The cue of systolic blood pressure of 80/40 mmHg is quite different in a patient with respiratory failure than in a patient with renal failure, chronic hypertension and altered mental status. Two other cognitive themes from our research [11] are also related and will tie into the decision support discussion below. Critical care clinicians may be uncertain, for example, about missing or possibly erroneous laboratory values. They may be uncertain if a patient's symptoms do, or do not fit a complete pattern or even partial template. What is often lost in all these discussions, however, is that regardless of this uncertainty, decisions are made, actions are taken, and outcomes may then be equally as uncertain.

Finally, inter-clinician communication is built on pattern recognition but in our study the cognitive theme was identified as creation and use of stories. The term 'story' was used explicitly during rounds as senior clinicians often ask, "What's the patient's story?" Reference was also made to the patient's 'picture'. Despite differences in terminology, the observational and interview data suggest a common cognitive activity that is closely related to patterns. In both settings, health care teams develop a framework of causal connections and a central theme that tied the various packets of patient data (medical history, test results, etc.) together in a meaningful way.

## 29.8   Using Machines to the Best of Their Ability …

So in the man-computer symbiosis, if man is a pattern recognition master, what in a man-computer symbiotic relationship should be the role of computer? In brief, the computer should be a bias-fighter. Pulling again from Kahneman's book [9], the bias best initially tackled by computers is the "What You See Is All There Is" (or WYSIATI, also called as mentioned above, "the availability bias" [21]). This particular bias is easily understood as its definition is nicely described in its name. It's equally relevant in what Donald Rumsfeld so famously called "unknown unknowns" or, "you can't know what you've not seen and you don't even know what you're missing". Croskerry (2013) provides an excellent critique of cognitive bias in clinical decision making [52]; and Hough (2013) extends this topic to examine irrationality in decision making throughout our healthcare systems [53]. Again, the reader is referred to the checklist of Kahneman and his colleagues [21].

## 29.9   Advances in Computer Science and Artificial Intelligent Machines …

As of this writing (and within my WYSIATI bias) the best potential vendor-agnostic patient-centric decision support solution is exemplified by Watson from IBM. Watson became famous in 2011 when the system crushed the two reigning human champions in *Jeopardy!*. Watson uses a combination of mathematical and computer science techniques applied to massive amounts of unstructured facts. Watson parsed clues of puns and slang and most importantly ranked the confidence of potential answers. Watson meets Licklider's man-computer symbiosis as it is described on the IBM website (see http://www.ibm.com/smarterplanet/us/en/ibmwatson/) as being "a cognitive system that enables a new partnership between people and computers that enhances and scales human expertise." When Watson approaches a question, "Watson relies on hypothesis generation and evaluation to rapidly parse relevant evidence and evaluate responses from disparate data." Again, because Watson is handling natural language and most its available data is unstructured text (think textbooks and the medical literature), vast tracks of what to any human is an unknown then become available. Further (and again quoting from the IBM website above), "Through repeated use, Watson literally gets smarter by tracking feedback from its users and learning from both successes and failures. Watson 'gets smarter'

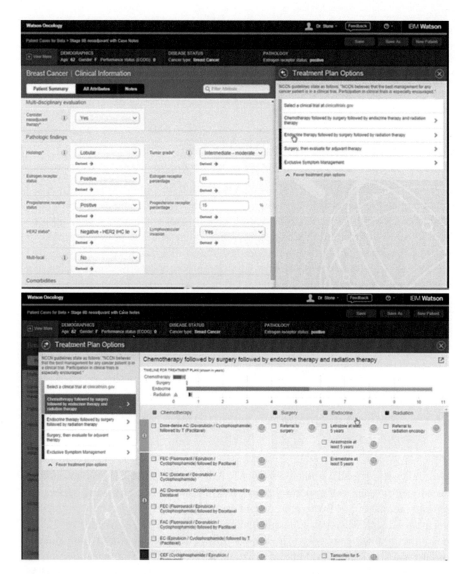

**Fig. 29.2** Two screen shots from Watson Oncology. Watson summarizes the EMR data and then suggests the best treatment option based on a diagnosis made solely by the clinicians. Watson is then able to display the available supporting literature including local expert knowledge and patient preferences (Reproduced with permission of IBM)

in three ways: by being taught by its users, by learning from prior interactions, and by being presented with new information."

The two frames in Fig. 29.2 shows a hypothetical encounter between an expert clinician and Watson for Oncology symbiotic dyad as treatment options are optimized after a diagnosis has been established. Watson for Oncology offers case information, test options, and treatment options. This example shows both the power of Watson, but also the crucial role of the expert clinician. To be purposely redundant, this must be a symbiotic interaction.

Watson presents the clinical facts as it knows them. These data may come from patient entered data, specific EMR data fields (e.g. age and smoking history) and/or from natural language processed clinical notes. As discussed elsewhere in this chapter these data may be right, wrong, and/or incomplete. The expert clinician must always be cognizant the primary data may be wrong making to avoid the bias of premature closure. Said differently the expert clinician must repeatedly question the primary diagnosis.

In the second frame Watson for Oncology suggests potential treatment plans (along with the hyperlinks to the data and literature supporting the recommendations). Patient preferences can be incorporated into the treatment plan decisions. Yet again, in the symbiotic relationship between the clinician and the computer, it is the human that that will help the patient balance the options.

However, it is important to again emphasize all the work shown in the above example is done to optimize treatment and is not at all focused on the much harder problem of making the correct diagnosis. Diagnostic decision support has long been a focus of clinical informatics [54] but after 40 years of work diagnostic decision support systems remain poorly penetrated [55]. While integration of available data is certainly a problem, even more problematic is the inability of current systems to integrate into the workflow [56]. Said differently, the current diagnostic support systems do not operate in a symbiotic relationship.

Further, although focus on therapy for cancer is laudable and will undoubtedly contribute to adherence to both application of best therapies as well as to patient personalization, there are far more complex problems the approach Watson embodies has the potential to revolutionize. Actually assisting the expert clinician make the diagnosis would yield far more benefit. In only the domain of pediatric critical care, children arrive with a wide array of critical illness that are beyond the full understanding of even the most seasoned clinician [57]. Tests and procedures are done based on precious little data [58]. Diagnostic errors are significant [59].

One need only morph the frames in Fig. 29.2 to imaging the workflow associated with a CDS solution assisting clinicians with diagnostic precision. (And the use of the word "only" in this last sentence is not to trivialize the computer science and engineering necessary.) This CDS solution would first pull data from the EMR and present the available data. Before moving from a case overview workflow to recommendations for testing workflow, many interactions of questions might be necessary. It is the clinician's role to elicit symptoms and work with the CDS to create as complete a pattern as is possible. As new data becomes available, CDS might assigns new confidences to each potential diagnosis. The CDS solution might "ask" for specific data elements if the solution learns its diagnostic model confidences would be enhanced with additional specific data elements. As more data becomes available, (e.g. family history and a patient's past medical history) even if no new diagnoses become relevant the confidences the CDS assigns to each diagnosis might fluctuate. With the addition of medication data, side effects and drug-drug interactions can be added to the problem list. To an experienced clinician even a to rather obvious diagnosis, the CDS has the potential to add diet and life style counseling and/or medication changes to minimize side effects. To be purposefully redundant, in the man-computer symbiosis, will let the clinician be the human touch, the translator of the computer generated confidences, and the overall pattern recognition guru and let the computer make unknown unknowns, known. Again quite cognizant of WYSIATI, there is only one reference to Watson within PubMed [60] and is primarily a descriptive manuscript of work within oncology.

The title of this chapter includes the phrase "a Roadmap". It is not hyperbole to suggest that opportunities are endless for the wise-clinician/developer dyad to improve patient outcomes. The path should use the SMART platform to build apps that incorporate Watson-like cognitive de-biasing characteristics, and as mentioned in the opening of the chapter, place them within the clinician's workflow [5]. Not at all parenthetically, as apps are built and evaluated, the outcome analyses must include *patient-centric* measures.

## 29.10   Data visualization: A Special Instance of Man-Computer Symbiosis

Finally, with good data in both a SMART platform and Watson-consumable forms, data visualization techniques hold a special place in the man-computer symbiosis and decision support efforts of any future HIMS. Again, because humans are pattern recognition masters, presentation of data in a picture is often an effective way

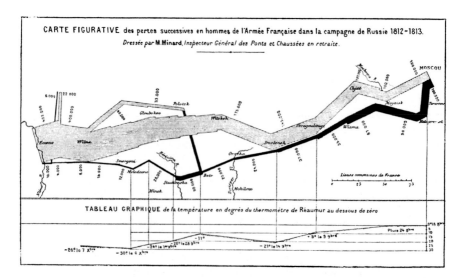

**Fig. 29.3** Napoleon's 1812 Russian Campaign showing devastation of French army as drawn by Charles Minard. Note there are six dimensions of data presented: direction of travel, the global position, time, the soldiers alive and temperature; the latter being responsible for many soldiers' deaths. Reprinted from Wikimedia Common: https://commons.wikimedia.org

for data to be presented to facilitate full or partial template recognition by the clinicians, and also to allow the clinician to see new patterns. Much has been written on data visualization both in the lay press [61] as well as the medical literature. This brief review will highlight only two examples.

Many authors believe the 150-year-old visualization shown in Fig. 29.3 to be the best graphic of all time [62]. The map, drawn by Charles Joseph Minard, shows the losses suffered by Napoleon's army during the Russian campaign of 1812. The size of the top, light-colored band shows the location between the Polish-Russian border and Moscow and the thickness of the band represents the number of soldiers. It is obvious from the diminishing gold bandwidth that the French sustained substantial losses on their march to Moscow. The retreat from Moscow is shown in the black on the bottom, distance is fixed on the "x-axis", and temperature is added to the graphic in the French troops' retreat from Moscow. The narrow black line on the bottom right corner captures the devastation of Napoleon's army at a glance.

Books, too numerous to reference, have been written about data visualization and about medical data visualization (see [63, 64]). The points to make here, in a discussion of the future of HIMSs and a roadmap to the future, are that: (1) there are no current "main-stream" data displays that should be emulated and (2) data visualizations must push not just to present data, but should push into interactive visualizations that allow visual explorations into both patient-centric and population-level data sets with the intent to discover new patient-centric and population-level insights [65]. This latter point will not be explored further here except to point out yet again that the wise-clinician/developer/designer (now) triad must have access to unfettered vendor-agnostic patient-centric data.

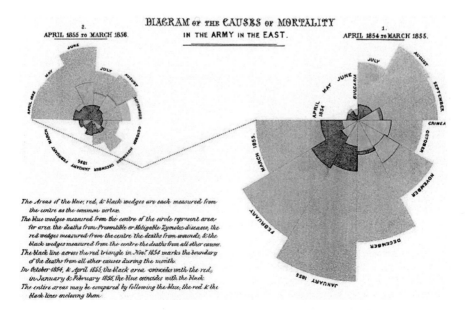

**Fig. 29.4** Causes of death among the English during the Crimean war as drawn by Florence Nightingale. Reprinted from Wikimedia Common: https://commons.wikimedia.org

## 29.11   Conclusion

I will close this roadmap discussion by highlighting one very and two other rather old visualizations that I believe should serve as "headlights" as the road to the future

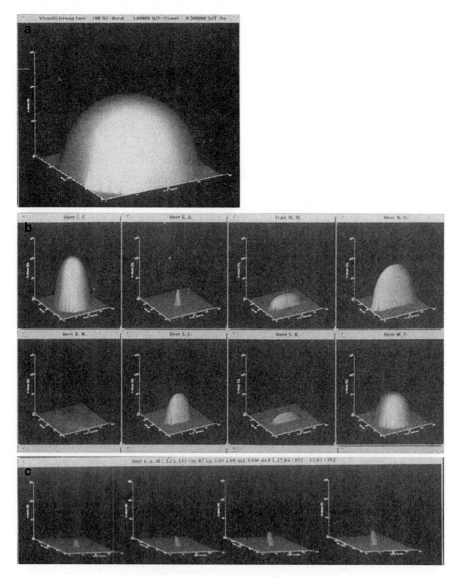

**Fig. 29.5**  An example of a novel visualization that promotes rapid understanding of complex data (in this case renal function) (Reproduced from Wenkebach et al. [66], with permission of the American Medical Informatics Association, Inc. Frame **a** is normal. Frame **b** shows 8 abnormal patterns. Frame **c** shows a time series of one abnormal pattern. Frame **d** labels the 3 axes)

**Fig. 29.5**  (continued)

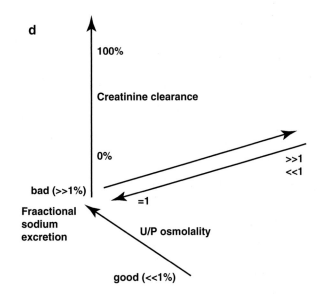

is travelled. Figure 29.4 is now famously about 170 years old from the pen of Florence Nightingale and it still, instantly, tells a story. The distance from the center represents mortality from all causes (in this case during 1 year of the Crimean War). Because the text does not reproduce well here, certainly the reader should ask what is represented by the red, black and blue? The blue wedges represent "Preventable or Mitigable Zymotic Diseases". The black wedges represent "all other causes". Only the relatively small wedges actually represent death from "wounds". Future visualizations should tell so much so "simply". Enhance the graphic with 2015 available interactions. Allow drill downs into sub-populations such as those dying of cholera, or from a different war, the flu. Drill into the causes of wound mortality to identify patterns so soldier protection can be improved.

In addition, there are two relatively old papers from the medical literature that are worth special mention. First, please look at Fig. 29.5 and assume that the hemisphere drawn in Fig. 29.5a represents normal function. Without knowing anything about the axes, you can then look at the eight patients in Fig. 29.5b and know that none of them are "normal" and that each vary from normal in a different pattern. Finally, in Fig. 29.5c a fourth dimension (time) is added by the sequence of plots for a single patient. Yes, in 2015 this might be animated and additional dimensions may be added with color/shading. But from 1992 when this was published [66], the reader knows that from Fig. 29.5c that function is changing (and either improving or not depending on the direction of time between the pictures). That this was drawn to show renal function is irrelevant (Fig. 29.5d) because the wise-clinician/developer/designer triad, with unfettered vendor-agnostic patient-centric data can create any number of these novel visualizations.

The second paper that the wise-clinician/developer/designer triad with unfettered vendor-agnostic patient-centric data should know about is from Powsner and

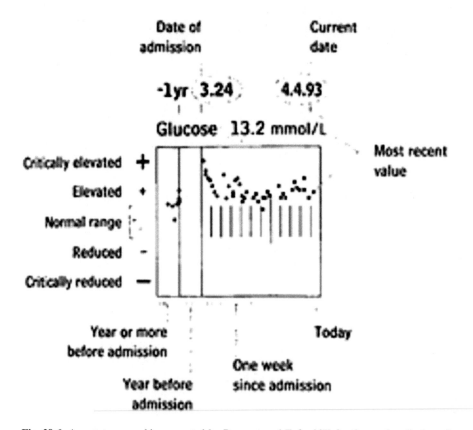

**Fig. 29.6** A prototype graphic suggested by Powsner and Tufte [67] for the routine display of medical data. To fully appreciate the power of this representation cover the text explanations and realize how much information is transmitted with very few pixels (Reproduced from Powsner and Tufte [67], with permission of Elsevier)

Tufte (1994) also from about 20 years ago [67]. Powsner and Tufte describe design characteristics that can be oversimplified as that can be and in brief, "transmit as much information with as few pixels as is possible." See Fig. 29.6 as a prototypical representation of serum glucose over time. Note that time on the x-axis is not linear. Much like the example in Fig. 29.5 where pattern recognition in easily supported, here the user quickly knows this particular result that was critically high on hospital admission had not been tested in the previous year, but also that it was normal more than once a year or more before admission. An app designer would do well to heed the design principles these authors espouse. So too, the wise-clinician should encourage the designer to use new visualization techniques.

In conclusion I would like to reproduce the concluding paragraph of the Powsner-Tufte paper and add to it a challenge. Twenty-one years ago, Powsner and Tufte concluded their paper with,

Medical computer systems will soon be able to print a fresh summary for each patient every day. Our proposal for a graphical summary should encourage doctors and nurses to reshape, perhaps re-invent, the medical record *before computer programmers cast institutional convenience into silicon.* Legal and organizational demands for detailed information will not disappear, but these demands need not compromise clinical needs for accessible patient information.

The emphasis is added in the above quote to highlight that Powsner and Tufte saw coming not just the instantiation of 100 year-old, paper-based, data entry and analysis workflows cast into silicon, but also that the codifying these ancient paper-based workflows would compromise accessibility of patient information. Thus the challenge is now even greater, because the roadmap to the future of HIMSs must be disruptive in the every sense of the word [68, 69] The challenge for entrepreneurs plus the wise-clinician/developer dyad or wise-clinician/developer/designer triad is now not merely to undo what the main-stream HIMSs have codified in silicon but to use the data HIMSs record, augment the data as is possible and build apps (including novel visualizations) on the vendor-agnostic patient-centric data. A self-perpetuating cycle must be created as more apps are built and users (again, clinicians and consumers) will clamor for more. As more apps are used they will become more refined. As this cycle spins, there can be optimism that the ultimate goal – improved patient care – will be realized.

# References

1. Middleton B, Bloomrosen M, Dente MA, et al. Enhancing patient safety and quality of care by improving the usability of electronic health record systems: recommendations from AMIA. JAMIA. 2013;20(e1):e2–8.
2. Institute of Medicine. Health IT and patient safety: building safer systems for better care. Washington, DC: The National Academies Press; 2012. p. 1–235.
3. Gordon JE, Leiman JM, Deland EL, Pardes H. Delivering value: provider efforts to improve the quality and reduce the cost of health care. Annu Rev Med. 2014;65(1):447–58.
4. Garg AX, Adhikari NKJ, McDonald H, et al. Effects of computerized clinical decision support systems on practitioner performance and patient outcomes: a systematic review. JAMA. 2005;293(10):1223–38.
5. Kawamoto K, Houlihan CA, Balas EA, Lobach DF. Improving clinical practice using clinical decision support systems: a systematic review of trials to identify features critical to success. BMJ. 2005;330(7494):765.
6. Kurzweil R. Human 2.0. New Sci. 2005;187(2518):32–7.
7. Fox J, Glasspool D, Patkar V, et al. Delivering clinical decision support services: there is nothing as practical as a good theory. J Biomed Inform. 2010;43(5):831–43.
8. Darst JR, Newburger JW, Resch S, Rathod RH, Lock JE. Deciding without data. Congenit Heart Dis. 2010;5(4):339–42.
9. Kahneman D. Thinking, fast and slow. New York: Macmillan; 2011.
10. Klein G. Sources of power: how people make decisions. Cambridge: MIT Press; 1999.
11. Fackler JC, Watts C, Grome A, Miller T, Crandall B, Pronovost P. Critical care physician cognitive task analysis: an exploratory study. Crit Care. 2009;13(2):R33.

12. Custer JW, White E, Fackler JC, et al. A qualitative study of expert and team cognition on complex patients in the pediatric intensive care unit. Pediatr Crit Care Med. 2012;13(3): 278–84.

13. Shirts BH, Bennett ST, Jackson BR. Using patients like My patient for clinical decision support: institution-specific probability of celiac disease diagnosis using simplified near-neighbor classification. J Gen Intern Med. 2013;28(12):1565–72.

14. Amancio DR, Comin CH, Casanova D, et al. A systematic comparison of supervised classifiers. PLoS ONE. 2014;9(4):e94137. Shen H-B, ed.

15. Kahneman D, Klein G. Conditions for intuitive expertise. Am Psychol. 2009;64(6): 515–51526.

16. Tversky A, Kahneman D. Judgment under uncertainty: heuristics and biases. Science. 1974;185(4157):1124–31.

17. Dawson NV, Arkes HR. Systematic errors in medical decision making: judgment limitations. J Gen Intern Med. 1987;2(3):183–7.

18. Aberegg SK. Omission bias and decision making in pulmonary and critical care medicine. Chest. 2005;128(3):1497–505.

19. Berner ES, Graber ML. Overconfidence as a cause of diagnostic error in medicine. Am J Med. 2008;121(5 Suppl):S2–23.

20. Croskerry P, Singhal G, Mamede S. Cognitive debiasing 1: origins of bias and theory of debiasing. BMJ Qual Saf. 2013;22 Suppl 2:ii58–64.

21. Kahneman D, Lovallo D, Sibony O. Before you make that big decision. Harv Bus Rev. 2011;89(6):50–60. 137.

22. di Martino P, Leoli F, Cinotti F, et al. Improving vital sign documentation at triage: an emergency department quality improvement project. J Patient Saf. 2011;7(1):26–9.

23. Bilyeu P, Eastes L. Use of the electronic medical record for trauma resuscitations. J Trauma Nurs. 2013;20(3):166–8.

24. Medical Device Data Systems, Medical Image Storage Devices, and Medical Image Communications Devices. 2015. Available at: http://www.fda.gov/MedicalDevices/ProductsandMedicalProcedures/GeneralHospitalDevicesandSupplies/MedicalDeviceDataSystems/default.htm. Accessed 22 Mar 2015.

25. Seely AJ, Bravi A, Herry C, et al. Do heart and respiratory rate variability improve prediction of extubation outcomes in critically ill patients? Crit Care. 2014;18(2):R65.

26. Park S, Kaffashi F, Loparo KA, Jacono FJ. The use of heart rate variability for the early detection of treatable complications after aneurysmal subarachnoid hemorrhage. J Clin Monit Comput. 2013;27(4):385–93.

27. Moorman JR, Waldemar AC, Kattwinkel J, et al. Mortality reduction by heart rate characteristic monitoring in very low birth weight neonates: a randomized trial. J Pediatr. 2011;159(6):900-6.e1.

28. Hug CW, Clifford GD. An analysis of the errors in recorded heart rate and blood pressure in the ICU using a complex set of signal quality metrics. Comput Cardiol. 2007;34:641–4.

29. Hug CW, Clifford GD, Reisner AT. Clinician blood pressure documentation of stable intensive care patients: an intelligent archiving agent has a higher association with future hypotension. Crit Care Med. 2011;39(5):1006–14.

30. FDASIA Health IT Report. 2014:1–34. http://www.fda.gov/downloads/AboutFDA/CentersOffices/OfficeofMedicalProductsandTobacco/CDRH/CDRHReports/UCM391521.pdf. Accessed 23 Mar 2015.

31. Karnik K. FDA regulation of clinical decision support software. J Law Biosci. 2014;1(2): 202–8.

32. Goldman JM. Solving the interoperability challenge: safe and reliable information exchange requires more from product designers. IEEE Pulse. 2014;5(6):37–9.

33. Arney D, Goldman JM, Bhargav-Spantzel A, et al. Simulation of medical device network performance and requirements for an integrated clinical environment. Biomed Instrum Technol. 2012;46(4):308–15.

34. Yim S-H, Chung Y-J. Reflections on the US FDA's warning on direct-to-consumer genetic testing. Genom Inform. 2014;12(4):151–5.

35. Carere DA, Couper MP, Crawford SD, et al. Design, methods, and participant characteristics of the Impact of Personal Genomics (PGen) Study, a prospective cohort study of direct-to-consumer personal genomic testing customers. Genome Med. 2014;6(12):96.
36. Swan M. Health 2050: the realization of personalized medicine through crowdsourcing, the quantified self, and the participatory biocitizen. JPM. 2012;2(4):93–118.
37. Caulfield B, Kaljo I, Donnelly S. Use of a consumer market activity monitoring and feedback device improves exercise capacity and activity levels in COPD. Conf Proc IEEE Eng Med Biol Soc. 2014;2014:1765–8.
38. McCambridge J, Witton J, Elbourne DR. Systematic review of the Hawthorne effect: new concepts are needed to study research participation effects. J Clin Epidemiol. 2014;67(3):267–77.
39. Available at: https://www.patientslikeme.com. Accessed 30 Mar 2015.
40. Frost JH, Massagli MP, Wicks P, Heywood J. How the social Web supports patient experimentation with a new therapy: the demand for patient-controlled and patient-centered informatics. AMIA Annu Symp Proc. 2007;6:217–21.
41. Fornai F, Longone P, Cafaro L, et al. Lithium delays progression of amyotrophic lateral sclerosis. Proc Natl Acad Sci U S A. 2008;105(6):2052–7.
42. Wicks P, Vaughan TE, Massagli MP, Heywood J. Accelerated clinical discovery using self-reported patient data collected online and a patient-matching algorithm. Nat Biotechnol. 2011;29(5):411–4.
43. UKMND-LiCALS Study Group. Lithium in patients with amyotrophic lateral sclerosis (LiCALS). Lancet Neurol. 2013;12(4):339–45.
44. Chiò A, Mora G. The final chapter of the ALS lithium saga. Lancet Neurol. 2013; 12(4):324–5.
45. Wicks P, Vaughan T, Heywood J. Subjects no more: what happens when trial participants realize they hold the power? BMJ. 2014;348(jan28 9):g368.
46. Mandl KD, Kohane IS. No small change for the health information economy. N Engl J Med. 2009;360(13):1278–81.
47. Mandl KD, Kohane IS. Escaping the EHR trap – the future of health IT. N Engl J Med. 2012;366(24):2240–2.
48. Mandl KD, Mandel JC, Murphy SN, et al. The SMART Platform: early experience enabling substitutable applications for electronic health records. J Am Med Inform Assoc. 2012; 19(4):597–603.
49. Introducing HL7 FHIR®. hlorg. 2014:1–2. http://hl7.org/implement/standards/fhir/fhir-summary.pdf. Accessed 29 Mar 2015.
50. Bosl W, Mandel J, Jonikas M, Ramoni RB, Kohane IS, Mandl KD. Scalable decision support at the point of care: a substitutable electronic health record App for monitoring medication adherence. Interact J Med Res. 2013;2(2):e13.
51. Klann JG, McCoy AB, Wright A, Wattanasin N, Sittig DF, Murphy SN. Health care transformation through collaboration on open-source informatics projects: integrating a medical applications platform, research data repository, and patient summarization. Interact J Med Res. 2013;2(1):e11–8.
52. Croskerry P. From mindless to mindful practice – cognitive bias and clinical decision making. N Engl J Med. 2013;368(26):2445–8.
53. Hough D. Irrationality in health care: what behavioral economics reveals about what we do and why. Stanford: Stanford Economics and Finance, Stanford University Press; 2013.
54. Barnett GO, Cimino JJ, Hupp JA, Hoffer EP. DXplain. An evolving diagnostic decision-support system. JAMA. 1987;258(1):67–74.
55. Bond WF, Schwartz LM, Weaver KR, Levick D, Giuliano M, Graber ML. Differential diagnosis generators: an evaluation of currently available computer programs. J Gen Intern Med. 2011;27(2):213–9.
56. Henderson EJ, Rubin GP. The utility of an online diagnostic decision support system (Isabel) in general practice: a process evaluation. JRSM Short Rep. 2013;4(5):31.
57. Fackler JC, Wetzel RC. Critical care for rare diseases. Pediatr Crit Care Med. 2001;3(1): 89–90.

58. Fackler J, Lehmann HP, Wetzel RC. Critical care for rare diseases (and procedures). Pediatr Crit Care Med. 2015;16(3):297–9.
59. Cifra CL, Jones KL, Ascenzi JA, Bhalala US, Bembea MM, Newman-Toker DE, Fackler JC, Miller MR. Diagnostic errors in a PICU. Pediatr Crit Care Med. 2015;16(5):468–76.
60. Doyle-Lindrud S. Watson will see you now: a supercomputer to help clinicians make informed treatment decisions. CJON. 2015;19(1):31–2.
61. Carey B. Learning to see data. NY Times. 2015;164(56,820):SR1.
62. Worth a thousand words. The economist. 2007. Available at: http://www.economist.com/node/10278643.
63. Wurman RS. Understanding healthcare. Newport: Top; 2004.
64. Holzinger A. Biomedical informatics. New York: Springer International Publishing; 2014. doi:10.1007/978-3-319-04528-3.
65. Rind A. Interactive information visualization to explore and query electronic health records. FNT Human Comput Interact. 2013;5(3):207–98.
66. Wenkebach U, Pollwein B, Finsterer U. Visualization of large datasets in intensive care. *Proc Annu Symp Comput Appl Med Care.* 1992:18–22.
67. Powsner SM, Tufte ER. Graphical summary of patient status. Lancet. 1994;344(8919): 386–9.
68. Christensen CM, Bohmer R, Kenagy J. Will disruptive innovations cure health care? Harv Bus Rev. 2000;78(5):102–12. 199.
69. Hwang J, Christensen CM. Disruptive innovation in health care delivery: a framework for business-model innovation. Health Aff (Millwood). 2007;27(5):1329–35.

# Chapter 30
# Big Data Analytical Technologies and Decision Support in Critical Care

Daby M. Sow

**Abstract** Intensive care units use sophisticated patient monitoring systems that produce massive amounts of physiological streaming data. Critical care physicians manage several hundred of time-critical health-related variables a day in the course of their work, using data from multiple disjoint systems, running in silos. Patient monitoring devices produce hundreds of alarms per day for each patient, with approximately 90 % being insignificant. These have introduced a significant data and decision overload problem. We present state- of-the-art big data analytical approaches that address these problems. We describe how the combination of "at rest" data mining analytics and streaming analytics is transforming critical care by enabling applications that improve clinicians' situation awareness at the bedside. We describe novel system architectures together with real-world deployments of big data analytical technologies in critical care environments that are helping physicians to be more proactive in delivering timely care.

**Keywords** Physiologic sensors • Critical care • Intensive care • Electronic medical records • Real-time physiologic data • Big data analytics • Situation awareness • Clinical decision support • Data overload • Data mining • Online healthcare analytics

## 30.1 Introduction

Advances in sensor technologies have transformed many industries, including healthcare. Today, medical institutions are extensively using various forms of sensing technologies at different levels of clinical care, particularly in critical care, arguably the branch of medicine that is the most dependent on sensors. Modern intensive care units (ICUs) use sophisticated patient monitoring systems able to produce

D.M. Sow, PhD
Exploratory Clinical Analytics and Systems, IBM T. J. Watson Research Center,
Yorktown, NY, USA
e-mail: sowdaby@us.ibm.com

© Springer International Publishing Switzerland 2016                                        515
C.A. Weaver et al. (eds.), *Healthcare Information Management Systems:*
*Cases, Strategies, and Solutions*, Health Informatics,
DOI 10.1007/978-3-319-20765-0_30

massive amounts of physiological streaming data that continuously report on the state of patients.

Merging incoming streams of real-time data with accumulated Electronic Medical Record (EMR) data has resulted in the creation of large, dynamic data sets that providers must cognitively process and manage in an ongoing and timely manner. On a daily basis, critical care physicians deal with over 200 temporal variables [16] produced by medical equipment assessing the ongoing health of their patients. In many cases, these data points are redundant and noisy, produced by disjoint IT systems running in silos systems.

It is estimated that intensive care units (ICUs) and operating rooms (ORs) contain 50 to over 100 different pieces of electronic equipment which do not communicate [26]. These systems produce hundreds of alarms per day per patient, with an estimated 90 % being false or clinically insignificant [8]. While these monitoring systems aim at improving patient care and staff productivity by delivering better insights on patients, they introduce a significant data overload problem, alarm fatigue and thereby new patient safety risks. The recognition of data overload as a systemic problem [23] has caused the Joint Commission to make reduction of harm associated with clinical alarm systems a National Patient Safety Goal (NPSG.06.01.01) for hospitals, mandating organizational prioritization of identification and management of important alarms, with a second phase (2016) of implementation of specific policies, procedures and staff education [17]. Using analogies from calm computing (technologies that reduce information overload [38]), critical care IT systems need to enable and support users by running calmly and silently in the background and not at the center of user workflows (where the patient should be).

Critical care is currently in a state similar to one in which aviation was a few decades ago, in which pilots operated in cockpits filled with round gauges providing disjoint pieces of information that they integrated unaided [7]. Airline safety has dramatically improved with the introduction of Situation Awareness (SA) concepts [10] into the design of modern cockpits where data is now carefully integrated and presented to pilots in a comprehensive fashion, with little ambiguity and redundancy.

Similarly, SA is finding its way into patient safety in ICUs and other clinical environments to modify current workflows that are highly distractive and interruptive. Big data analytics techniques are being developed to deliver the right insights to the right people and at the right time. State-of-the-art analytical approaches and systems are bringing SA to the critical care bedside, and proper combinations of "at rest" data mining analytics and streaming analytics are transforming critical care. In what follows, we derive requirements for such systems from well-known SA concepts, before presenting system architectures and real-world research deployments that demonstrate the power of big data analytics in critical care environments.

## 30.2    Bringing Situation Awareness to the Bedside

An intuitive definition of Situation Awareness (SA) is "the perception of the elements in the environment within a volume of time and space, the comprehension of their meaning and the projection of their status in the near future" [10]. From a clinician perspective, **perception** is the awareness at all times of the current state of the patients for which they are providing care [19]. While various patient monitors provide physiological observations such as electrocardiograms, respiration rates, etc., these variables require inference to estimate the clinical state of a patient. For instance, a discrete score (0–4) obtained from consideration of respiration rate, heart rate, body temperature and white blood cell count may be used to evaluate a patient for the likelihood of sepsis as inferred by the Systemic Inflammatory Response Syndrome (SIRS) score [35].

**Comprehension** is the ability to understand the significance of perceived elements. Using the SIRS score example described above, clinicians should be able to understand the implications of perceived or collected data, e.g., an elevated SIRS score being an indicator for sepsis. In another example, perception or detection of a reduction in heart rate variability may be indicative of a general loss of health for a patient, possibly due to nosocomial (i.e. hospital acquired) infections [11]. In another context, a perceived reduction of heart rate variability may be due to other complications such as delayed cerebral ischemia [33]. The context of perceived observations is essential to comprehension in SA.

With good comprehension of the state of patients, clinicians can make short term **predictions**. Using a GPS analogy from Dr. Timothy Buchman (Emory University) [29], once clinicians comprehend the health of a patient in a complex multi-dimensional physiological map, they can estimate/predict the possible trajectories of a patient's health and course. Without specifically suggesting actions, SA intend to help physicians make well informed decisions through short term predictions, just as a GPS system helps a driver understand the consequences of her actions and helps her decide when and where to turn to reach a specific destination.

These three fundamental stages of SA impose the following functional requirements on any infrastructure bringing SA to the bedside:

- *Sensing*: the ability to generate data from the real-world phenomena or observations through instrumentation. While it is common practice to restrict sensing operations to device sensing, we use the term here in a broader sense that includes the generation of data/observations from devices and humans (e.g., nursing reports captured in an EMR). Sensing is a core requirement for SA perception.
- *Acquiring*: the ability to extract and integrate data from sensors. This function is challenging in critical care where a large number of heterogeneous sensors are used in silos, often temporally desynchronized [22] and producing readings in various (and often proprietary) formats. Acquiring complements sensing for SA perception.
- *Analyzing*: the ability to transform data into actionable information leading to knowledge gain. This requires the ability to make sense of the data perceived. Analyzing supports the SA comprehension and prediction steps.
- *Presenting*: the ability to close the gap between computers and humans. Presentation comes with requirements for visualization and seamless integration with existing workflows. In critical care settings, clinicians should not be burdened with unnecessary cognitive tasks (such as calculations or graphing) to get the analytical benefits, neither should they be burdened with manipulation of complex IT systems. Nurses and physicians should focus on their patients with systems

operating silently in the background to facilitate tasks without distractions. Designing such systems requires adoption of concepts from Cognitive Informatics (CI) [28]. CI is a branch at the intersection of multiple disciplines such as human factors and human-computer interaction. It provides a framework for modeling human performance, focusing specifically on human interaction with technology to design presentation layers that are well integrated with workflows.

Figure 30.1 shows a functional diagram for a system that brings SA to the bedside. It consists of two process loops: the decision support process loop and the knowledge discovery process loop.

The decision support process loop *exploits* all data available at the bedside together with existing analytical knowledge to support and deliver SA. Data is sensed, acquired and analyzed at the bedside before being presented to physicians in a timely fashion to help them take the right actions. All analytical operations are driven by models either obtained from existing knowledge (e.g., existing well understood acuity scoring models such as SOFA, the Sequential Organ Failure Assessment score or MEWS, the Modified Early Warning Score [2, 30]) or obtained in a data driven way via the knowledge discovery process loop.

The knowledge discovery process loop in a data driven way requires the *exploration* of data after sensing and acquisition steps. After acquisition, the process goes through the Analyze and Discover stages where data sets are mined to discover interesting relationships and produce new predictive models. Machine Learning and Data Mining techniques provided by software packages such as R [31], Matlab [25], Weka [21], SPSS [15] can be used to perform these analytical steps. After testing of these newly discovered models, analysts may decide to promote them in the decision support process loop for the exploitation of this new knowledge at the bedside.

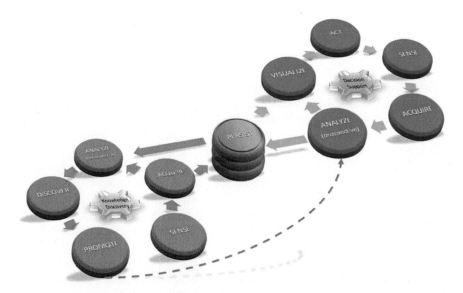

**Fig. 30.1** Bridging translational research with decision support

## 30.3 The Online Healthcare Analytics Infrastructure for Critical Care

Figure 30.2 shows a high level architecture for an infrastructure called the Online Healthcare Analytics (OHA) [34], developed at IBM Research to address the SA functional requirements described in the previous section. The main design philosophy behind OHA is to provide an open platform for analytics that bring SA to the bedside. "By "open", we mean that OHA needs to cope with an open set of sensing, acquisition, analytics and presentation technologies while providing the infrastructural underpinning required to handle high volumes of data in real-time with low latencies and high integrity". OHA supports both the decision support and the knowledge discovery process loops.

### 30.3.1 Decision Support in OHA

As shown in Fig. 30.2 the decision support process starts with sensing functions. In OHA, sensing data sources belong to an open set consisting of monitoring devices and Electronic Medical Records. Monitoring devices measure physiological signals (e.g., electrocardiograms, electroencephalograms, respiration signals, pulse oximetry, blood pressures) and produce alerts when the physiological state of the patient appears

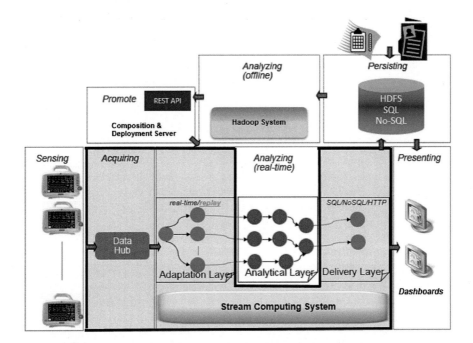

**Fig. 30.2** High level system architecture of the online healthcare analytics infrastructure

to be out of range. State of the art patient monitors allow physicians to program abnormal thresholds and alerts for physiological parameters (For example, a monitor can be set to produce an audible alarm if the oxygen saturation level of the blood drops below 85 %). The values of these thresholds are typically obtained from general guidelines or from data mining processes. Such simple alerting schemes produce large numbers of false alarms. Regardless, the OHA platform is able to ingest both these derived alerts, the raw physiological event and waveform data. The set of data elements sensed via EMR systems is also open ended. It typically consists of laboratory results (e.g., blood tests) nurse and physician notes and assessments. The aggregate data elements sensed in OHA may either be structured or unstructured.

With this open approach to sensing comes acquisition challenges. Data coming from an open set of sources may be represented differently and accessed using different and potentially proprietary protocols. Analyzing these data points requires complex integration steps where external data are accessed and mapped into a common data model. In OHA, these challenges are resolved with third party solutions. There are several vendors in the market that specialize on data acquisition and integration in critical care.[1] With the lack of wide scale adoption of standards to represent and transmit patient monitoring data in real-time, most commercially available solutions have developed their own schemes with some providing support to the HL7 standard. Consequently, OHA extends its openness philosophy to allow the infrastructure to be tailored to data acquisition systems found in the real world in medical institutions but at the cost of software engineering required to build adapters to these acquisition systems. OHA provides an adaptation API for this matter.[2] This loose integration has allowed tailoring of OHA for several real-world critical care environments in leading critical care research institutions such as the Emory Center for Critical Care, the Columbia Medical Center Neurological ICU and the UCLA Ronald Reagan Center for Critical Care. More recently, OHA components are being adopted by the Michigan Center for Integrative Research in Critical Care at the University of Michigan to drive their ambitious critical care research agenda and develop analytics for SA in critical care.

From an analysis stand point, OHA is also open. It is a programmable framework facilitating the authoring and deployment of real-time analytics. OHA is built on top of the IBM InfoSphere Streams product [14], a distributed stream computing middleware for the real-time high-performance analysis of structured and unstructured data [9]. This stream computing platform in OHA is the back bone for the decision support process loop. Big data analysts use this stream computing platform to design sophisticated analytics that can extract nuggets of information from real-time patient data flows. The design and implementation of these analytics re-uses statistical and computing building blocks from product toolkits for time series, machine learning and data mining [9].

---

[1] Notable examples of data acquisition systems for ICU monitoring devices are Excel Medical Electronics (with their BedMasterEX and BedCom products), CapsuleTech, Airstrip (with their Airstrip ONE product), iSirona and IBM (with its Healthcare Integration Bus product).

[2] Excel Medical Electronics offers today a research platform based on OHA that interfaces its BedMasterEX and BedCom data acquisition products with IBM InfoSphere Streams, the stream computing runtime of OHA. Airstrip announced recently its plan to integrate its Airstrip ONE product with InfoSphere Streams.

OHA was prototyped in 2008 and deployed for the first time at the Hospital for Sick Children in 2009 to allow analysts to compose and deploy an open set of analytics, assembled graphically to address their analytical goals [27]. While other research groups have been developing custom real-time analytic solutions for the monitoring of specific critical care conditions [37], the OHA platform differs significantly from these systems with its programmability and agility. With OHA, as analysts discover new real-time analytics that they would like to deploy, they are able to promote these discovered analytics to the bedside. To enable this, OHA makes full use of the InfoSphere Streams programming model designed to be extensible. This programming model provides application programming interfaces (APIs) where external system and legacy software can be integrated. This extensibility of the OHA programming model facilitates the inclusion of analytics written in several common languages ranging from high level languages such R and Matlab to lower level languages like Python, Java, C++ and C.

## 30.3.2   Discovery in OHA

The knowledge discovery loop in OHA is supported with "at rest" analytical platforms ranging from standalone application software like Weka and SPSS to Big Data infrastructures like Hadoop. Analytic models developed using these platforms can be promoted for prospective use by leveraging the extensibility of the InfoSphere Streams programming model. Toolkits have been designed to take models produced by the knowledge discovery process and seamlessly incorporate them in the decision support process loop. The ability to incorporate analytics to use data from similar groups of patients has also been designed to help physicians make more informed clinical decisions. Similarity models are developed on a Hadoop installation while the scoring of models takes place prospectively inside InfoSphere Streams as part of the decision support loop [18]. Details on such similarity analysis have been described [36] where the authors describe a system allowing physicians to query proactively for similar patients and use their records to make predictions on the health evolution of a patient in question. An in-silico study using physiological sensor data streams from over 1,500 ICU patients obtained from the Physionet MIMIC II database [24] shows how this approach may be used to forecast the trajectory of blood pressure trends and help predict acute hypotensive episodes in ICUs.

## 30.4   Real World OHA Solutions

The OHA platform has been use for the development and research deployment of several real-world critical care applications in medical research institutions such as the Hospital for Sick Children in Toronto, the Columbia Medical Center Neuro ICU in New York, the Emory Center for Critical Care in Atlanta and the UCLA Ronald Reagan Institute. We present a sample of these real-world applications with high level descriptions of the analytical capabilities supported by OHA.

### 30.4.1  Modeling Patient Health with Heart Rate Variability

While users of OHA are focusing on different use cases, a common theme in most of these applications is that they intend to provide SA by modeling patient states and tracking state changes. It is important for clinicians to have awareness on the current state of their patients at all time, and many would argue that it is even more informative for them to be notified when the states of these patients are changing for better or worse [6].

Many applications incorporate analytical techniques deriving features from physiological time series to model and predict the inflammatory response of the body, as it is highly correlated with early signs of complications in general. The inflammatory response is a reaction from the body to different harmful stimuli such as pathogens, various irritants or even damaged cells. Hence, accurate modeling of its changes enables a wide range of early detection applications in intensive care. In particular, devastating complications such as sepsis are known to produce an inflammatory response well before the appearance of overt clinical findings [1].

The inflammatory response is known to be influenced by the autonomic nervous system: the sympathetic and parasympathetic nervous systems. These systems regulate involuntary and measurable phenomena such as heart rate, respiration, salivation, and transpiration. Inflammation results in poor regulation of these systems, and is often correlated with the Systemic Inflammatory Response Syndrome (SIRS). Poor regulation manifests itself as a loss of variability associated with physiological sensor streams. Consequently, researchers have hypothesized and verified experimentally that modeling the inflammatory response can be performed by computing measures of signal variability of the heart rate and the respiratory rate of patients [4]. The frequencies where these variations occur require instantaneous and precise measures of heart rate values that are derived from electrocardiograms (ECGs). Reductions in heart rate variability (HRV) have been linked to the early onset of disorders of the central and peripheral nervous system that induce a pro-inflammatory response. Currently, most efforts to model the inflammatory response are focused primarily on the one dimensional HRV analysis, due to a large body of work on ECG waveform processing. Variability metrics use techniques such as spectral analysis [39], sample entropy [32] and fractal analysis [5]. These ECG routines are composed with operators computing various forms of variability to model the inflammatory response.

The OHA infrastructure enables users to derive convenient measures of heart rate variability from ECG processing in real time. Many users of OHA are reusing the same ECG processing tools to extract precisely the QRS complex portions of the waveform by using well established signal processing algorithms [12].

### 30.4.2  OHA and the Artemis Project at the Hospital for Sick Children, Toronto

At the University of Virginia, Lake [20] pioneered and demonstrated how sample entropy on heart rate measurements can predict the onset of sepsis in neonates. This work recently led to a large scale clinical trial that is a prime example of SA in critical care. This trial demonstrates how the appropriate bedside display of an HRV derived score indicating the likelihood of a neonate becoming sick, increased SA and reduced mortality by more than 20 %. While this specific work does not use the OHA platform, a similar study using OHA has been performed at the Hospital of Sick Children in Toronto Canada (SickKids) under the supervision of the University of Ontario Institute of Technology (UOIT) [27]. This study leverages the OHA infrastructure to extend the analysis and monitoring beyond ECGs and incorporate in real-time other vital signs such as respiration rate, arterial blood pressure, oximetry and other observations from the hospital EMR. In this study, OHA was used for both decision support and discovery. Proprietary discovery analytics developed at UOIT were implemented and used for knowledge discovery. The OHA system went live at the SickKids NICU in 2009. Sample clinical results of the work have been published [27], showing how detected state changes preceded the appearance of sepsis clinical findings several hours if not days ahead of the event. Since then, UOIT has been expanding this study in other research hospitals inside and outside of Canada.

### 30.4.3 OHA at the Ronald Reagan UCLA Medical Center

The application of OHA at the University of California Los Angeles (UCLA) has focused on the real-time analysis of continuous high-volume and high-frequency brain signals that are commonly collected by bedside monitors in neuro-critical care. While such signals often carry early signs of neurological deterioration, detecting these signs in real-time has been challenging as conventional data processing methods have been designed principally for retrospective analysis and not for handling large volumes of waveform data produced by bedside monitors. In a joint pilot study between UCLA and IBM, an OHA application has been developed to detect in real-time unstable intracranial pressure (ICP) dynamics. This application continuously receives ECG and ICP waveform signals and analyzes the ICP pulse morphology looking for deviations from a steady-state, according to novel algorithms developed at UCLA (using MATLAB). The IBM team incorporated these algorithms inside InfoSphere Streams operators and externalized the results to a Web interface. With this interface, physicians are able to receive real time patient status updates in a web browser and gain direct insight and interpretation of real-time ICP waveforms, viewable through their hospital network. The prototype system has been successfully tested prospectively on hospitalized patients [3].

### 30.4.4 OHA at the Columbia University Medical Center

At Columbia University, under a partnership with IBM Research, the OHA platform has been used to address several problems. This extended team developed predictive models for the early detection of the onset of complications in neurological intensive care units. The targeted population for this work consists of patients with subarachnoid hemorrhages (SAH). Complications of interest included: nosocomial infections (e.g., sepsis, urinary tract infections, pneumonias), vasospasms, delayed cerebral ischemia and infarctions. The InfoSphere Streams engine encapsulated in OHA was used to extract features from the collected data, including HRV metrics computed on ECGs before merging them with additional relevant features such transcranial Doppler frequency features of blood flow. The predictive model discovery used the Weka data mining library. Ahis study [33] demonstrated the ability to predict complications 24 h ahead from this ocean of physiological data with good sensitivity and specificity, with the area under the receiver operating characteristic curve (the AUC of the ROC) for this classification problem at 83 %.

This research team also addressed the auto-regulation of the inter-cranial pressure (ICP) for SAH patients by developing novel real-time analytics able to compute and display regression lines between ICP and Mean Arterial Pressure (MAP) after detecting patient states using time series analysis techniques. This end-to-end solution increases SA significantly by allowing clinicians to access key physiologic parameters in real-time. Without the application, it takes up to 30 min per bed to obtain similar regression plots on retrospective data with the help of an experienced resident.

### 30.4.5 Exploring Alarm Data with OHA at the Columbia University Medical Center

IBM Research and Columbia have also been developing OHA related technology to address the ICU alarm fatigue problem. As mentioned earlier, studies have shown that 85–99 % of medical device alarm signals are false and/or clinically insignificant, resulting in desensitization and alarm fatigue in critical care staff. The discovery loop in OHA has been applied to this problem to analyze the temporal relations between time series of alarm events with the intent to identify clusters of events that relate to the same physiological phenomena. OHA has been equipped with novel time series analytical techniques for measuring and visualizing such temporal relationships across time series. Early results obtained on over a million alarms from 572 neurological ICU patient admissions have shown that the system can detect "obvious" patterns (e.g., strong association of bradycardia and heart rate low alarms), but also patterns attributed to artifact events and also to important physiological conditions. Definite quantitative results evaluating the ability of these approaches to tackle the alarm fatigue problem are underway.

## 30.5 Conclusion

Big data analytic approaches and techniques are bringing much needed SA to the bedside by addressing the data and decision overload facing practicing clinicians in critical care. An open state-of-the-art infrastructure has been presented together with an overview of existing research pilots applying this infrastructure in the real-world. While this technology is quite mature from an analytical stand point, several challenges need to be addressed to allow its widespread deployment in critical care.

- The first challenge is a lack of data standards and protocols for the representation and access of clinical data and analytics. Without such standards, the deployment of infrastructures like OHA requires significant customization at the different sites.
- A second challenge is the integration of advanced analytical capabilities within existing workflows with little disruptions to clinicians. While a good amount of insight can be extracted through data analysis, delivering these insights in the right way remains a challenge that must be overcome. More research is needed to ensure that results of complex real-time analytics can be consumed and digested seamlessly within cognitive and clinical workflow.
- A third challenge is the remaining gap between the data-driven approaches described herein and knowledge-driven approaches able to provide additional reasoning capabilities for better situation awareness. There is a large body of medical literature in unstructured text that could produce a vast amount of knowledge that has not been integrated yet with the operational knowledge extracted by OHA-like platforms in real-time. Research in cognitive computing is needed to bridge this gap.

Addressing these challenges to bring SA to the bedside in critical care is a significant task requiring the involvement of several key players, ranging from device manufacturers, small and large IT companies, clinicians, academics, data scientists, regulators and hospital administrators. Under the supervision of Excel Medical Electronics and IBM, a growing discussion forum called "Streaming Analytics" has been created in 2012 to bring together these key players. The goal of this group is to develop transformative technology for proactive critical care. The group holds workshops twice a year [13]. While the impact of these meetings has been constrained to research deployments at this point, it is also helping with the emergence of new startup companies developing and offering services that helping bring situation awareness closer to the bedside.[3]

# References

1. Ahmad S, Tejuja A, Newman K, Zarychanski R, Seely A. Clinical review: a review and analysis of heart rate variability and. Crit Care. 2009;13:232.
2. Arts DG, de Keizer NF, Vroom MB, de Jonge E. Reliability and accuracy of Sequential Organ Failure Assessment (SOFA) scoring. Crit Care Med. 2005;33(9):1988–93. Retrieved from Medscape: http://www.medscape.com/viewarticle/512520_1.

---

[3] Example companies participating in the Streaming Analytics workshops are CleMetric (http://www.clemetric.com/), Synchronicity In Motion (http://synchronicityinmotion.com/) and UNSCRAMBL (http://unscrambl.com/).

3. Bai Y, Sow D, Vespa P, Hu X. Real-time processing of continuous physiological signals in a neurocritical care unit on a stream data analytics platform. In: Beng-Ti Ang C, (ed) Intercranial Pressure and Brain Monitoring XV, 1st Edition, Acta Neurochirurgica Suppl. Springer International Publishing, 2016;122(1), DOI 10.1007/978-3-319-22533-3.

4. Bradley B, Green GC, Batkin I, Seely AJ. Feasibility of continuous multiorgan variability analysis in the intensive care unit. J Crit Care. 2012;27(2):218.e9–20.

5. Bryce R, Sprague B. Revisiting detrended fluctuation analysis. Sci Rep. 2012;2:315. doi:10.1038/srep00315.

6. Buchman T. Novel representation of physiologic states during critical illness and recovery. Crit Care. 2010;14:127.

7. Buchman T. How one hospital is making intensive care smarter with analytics. 2013. Retrieved from A Smarter Planet Blog: http://asmarterplanet.com/blog/2013/11/smarter-care-analytics.html

8. Cvach M. Monitor alarm fatigue: an integrative review. Biomed Intrum Methodol. 2012;46(4): 268–77.

9. Ebbers M, Abdel-Gayed A, Budhi VB, Dolot F, Kamat V, Picone R, Trevelin J. Addressing data volume, velocity, and variety with IBM InfoSphere Streams V3.0. 2013. Retrieved from IBM Redbooks: http://www.redbooks.ibm.com/abstracts/sg248108.html?Open

10. Endsley MR. Toward a theory of situation awareness in dynamic systems. Hum Factors. 1995;37(1):32–64.

11. Gopal Reddy S. Big data saves small babies by detecting nosocomial infections earlier than clinicians. 2014. Retrieved from nuviun connecting great minds: http://nuviun.com/content/news/big-data-saves-small-babies-by-detecting-nosocomial-infections-earlier-than-clinicians

12. Hamilton PS, Tompkins WJ. Quantitative investigation of QRS detection rules using the MIT/BIH arrhythmia database. IEEE Trans Biomed Eng. 1996;33(12):1157–65.

13. Hunter D. Excel medical electronics – #BigData for healthcare. 2013. Retrieved from IBM Innovation Center – Chicago: https://www.ibm.com/developerworks/community/blogs/Chicagoiic/entry/excel_medical_electronics_bigdata_for_healthcare?lang=en

14. IBM. Capture and analyze data in motion. (no date a). Retrieved from InfoSphere Streams: http://www-03.ibm.com/software/products/en/infosphere-streams

15. IBM. SPSS software: predictive analytics software and solutions. (no date b). Retrieved from http://www-01.ibm.com/software/analytics/spss/

16. Imhof M. Dimension reduction for physiological variables using graphical modeling. AMIA annual symposium. AMIA; 2003. p. 313–17.

17. The Joint Commission. The Joint Commission Announces 2014 National Patient Safety Goal. 2013. Retrieved from Joint Commission Perspectives, ®, Volume 33, Issue 7: http://www.jointcommission.org/assets/1/18/jcp0713_announce_new_nspg.pdf

18. Kirchner P, Böhm M, Reinwald B, Sow D, Schmidt M, Turaga D, Biem A. Large scale discriminative metric learning. In: IPDPS workshops. Phoenix: IEEE; 2014. p. 1656–63.

19. Koch SH, Weir C, Haar M, Staggers N, Agutter J, Görges M, Westenskow D. Intensive care unit nurses' information needs and recommendations for integrated displays to improve nurses' situation awareness. J Am Med Inform Assoc. 2012;19(4):583–90.

20. Lake DE, Richman JS, Griffin P, Moorman R. Sample entropy analysis of neonatal heart rate variability. Am J Physiol. 2002;283(3):R789–97.

21. Machine Learning Group at the University of Waikato. Weka 3: data mining software in Java. (no date). Retrieved from http://www.cs.waikato.ac.nz/ml/weka/

22. M.H. The economist: Babbage science and technology. 2012. Retrieved from Medical devices: a ticking time-bomb: http://www.economist.com/blogs/babbage/2012/05/medical-devices

23. Manor-Shulman O, Beyene J, Frndova H, Parshuram CS. Quantifying the volume of documented clinical information in critical illness. J Crit Care. 2008;23(2):245–50.

24. Massachusetts Institute of Technology. MIMIC II. (n.d.). Retrieved from mimic.physionet.org: https://mimic.physionet.org/

25. Mathworks. MATLAB: the language of technical computing. 1994–2014. Retrieved from http://www.mathworks.com/products/matlab/

26. Matthews SC, Pronovost PJ. The need for systems integration. J Am Med Assoc. 2011;305(9):934–5.
27. McGregor C, James A, Eklund M, Sow D, Ebling M, Blount M. Real-time multidimensional temporal analysis of complex high volume physiological data streams in the neonatal intensive care unit. Stud Health Technol Inform. 2013;192:362–6.
28. Patel VL, Kaufman DR, Cohen T, editors. Cognitive informatics in health and biomedicine. Case studies on critical care, complexity and errors. London: Springer; 2014.
29. Patrizio A. Helping doctors stitch together real-time data to help intensive care patients. 2013. Retrieved from citeworld.com: http://www.citeworld.com/article/2115650/big-data-analytics/helping-doctors-stitch-together-real-time-data-to-help-intensive-care-patients.html?null
30. Pohlman,TH. Trauma scoring systems. 2014. Retrieved from Medscape: http://emedicine.medscape.com/article/434076-overview
31. The R Foundation. The R project for statistical computing. (no date). Retrieved from http://www.r-project.org/
32. Richman JS, Moorman R. Physiological time-series analysis using approximate entropy and sample entropy. Am J Physiol Heart Circ Physiol. 2000;278(6):H2039–49.
33. Schmidt JM, Sow DM, Crimmins M, Albers D, Agarwal S, Claassen J, Mayer SA. Heart rate variability for preclinical detection of secondary complications after subarachnoid hemorrhage. Neurocrit Care. 2014;20(3):382–9.
34. Sow D, Turaga DS, Schmidt M. Mining of sensor data in healthcare: a survey. In: Aggarwal C, editor. Managing and mining sensor data. New York: Springer; 2013. p. 459–504.
35. Stony Brook Medicine. Severe sepsis/septic shock recognition and treatment protocols. 2013. Retrieved from http://www.survivingsepsis.org/SiteCollectionDocuments/Protocols-Sepsis-Treatment-Stony-Brook.pdf
36. Sun J, Sow D, Hu J, Ebadollahi S. A system for mining temporal physiological data streams for advanced prognostic decision support. In: International conference on data mining (ICDM). Sydney: IEEE; 2010. p. 1061–6.
37. Terry K. ICU platform first to integrate, analyze monitoring data. 2013. Retrieved from informationweek.com: http://www.informationweek.com/healthcare/clinical-information-systems/icu-platform-first-to-integrate-analyze-monitoring-data/d/d-id/1109600?
38. Weiser M, Brown JS. Designing calm technology. Powergrid J. 1996;1(1):75–85.
39. Winchell RJ, Hoyt DB. Spectral analysis of heart rate variability in the sepsis syndrome. J Surg Res. 1996;63(1):11–6.

# Chapter 31
# Data Driven Analytics for Personalized Healthcare

**Jianying Hu, Adam Perer, and Fei Wang**

**Abstract** The concept of Learning Health Systems (LHS) is gaining momentum as more and more electronic healthcare data becomes increasingly accessible. The core idea is to enable learning from the collective experience of a care delivery network as recorded in the observational data, to iteratively improve care quality as care is being provided in a real world setting. In line with this vision, much recent research effort has been devoted to exploring machine learning, data mining and data visualization methodologies that can be used to derive real world evidence from diverse sources of healthcare data to provide personalized decision support for care delivery and care management. In this chapter, we will give an overview of a wide range of analytics and visualization components we have developed, examples of clinical insights reached from these components, and some new directions we are taking.

**Keywords** Data driven healthcare analytics • Learning health system • Practice based evidence • Real world evidence • Clinical decision support • Machine learning • Data mining • Data visualization

## 31.1 Introduction

In recent years we have witnessed a dramatic increase of electronic health data, including extensive Electronic Medical Records (EMR) recording patient conditions, diagnostic tests, labs, imaging exams, genomics, proteomics, treatments, outcomes, claims, financial records, clinical guidelines and best practices etc.

J. Hu, PhD (✉) • A. Perer, PhD
Healthcare Analytics Research Group, IBM T.J. Watson Research Center,
Yorktown Heights, NY, USA
e-mail: jyhu@us.ibm.com; adam.perer@us.ibm.com

F. Wang, PhD
Computer Science and Engineering, University of Connecticut, Storrs, CT, USA

© Springer International Publishing Switzerland 2016                            529
C.A. Weaver et al. (eds.), *Healthcare Information Management Systems:*
*Cases, Strategies, and Solutions*, Health Informatics,
DOI 10.1007/978-3-319-20765-0_31

Healthcare professionals are now increasingly asking the question: what can we do with this wealth of data? How can we perform meaningful analytics on such data to derive insights to improve quality of care and reduce cost?

Healthcare Analytics needs to cover the whole spectrum including both Knowledge Driven Analytics and Data Driven Analytics. Knowledge driven approaches operate on knowledge repositories that include scientific literature, published clinical trial results, medical journals, textbooks, as well as clinical practice guidelines. Traditionally the gold standard of evidence in healthcare has been produced through the randomized controlled trial process. Results of such trials get published and then healthcare professionals consult those publications to bring to the point of care nuggets of evidence that apply to the scenario at hand. This process of knowledge diffusion can take as long as 17 years [2, 10].

Innovations such as Watson Discovery Advisor [32] can dramatically reduce that time frame to close the knowledge diffusion gap. In tools such as WDA, the deep NLP and Q&A capabilities such those developed in the original Watson Jeopardy machine are leveraged to teach the computer to learn medical domain knowledge from unstructured data captured in the knowledge repository, and then make intelligent inference from such knowledge to bring the most relevant pieces of information to the finger tips of the practitioners.

Complementary to this knowledge dissemination processing, data driven healthcare analytics is about making the computer learn from observational data collected in the process of delivering care. This is important because published guidelines typically target a single disease and the average patient, so by themselves don't provide sufficient insight into how to best manage a real world patient with multiple comorbidities and complex conditions. By tapping into the vast real world observational data collected at the individual patient level, we can leverage the collective experience of a healthcare delivery system, to extract insights that can be used to fill in that personalization gap, and in that process continuously enhance and refine our knowledge on best practices. Such insights are referred to as Practice Based Evidence, or Real World Evidence, and are at the center of the vision of "Learning Health Systems" advocated by the Institute of Medicine [11].

The focus of this chapter is on data driven healthcare analytics. In line with the vision of LHS, the healthcare analytics research group at IBM has been working on applying advanced machine learning, data mining and data visualization techniques in the context of real world healthcare data and use cases to build up a data driven healthcare analytics framework. An earlier version of this analytics framework, called Intelligent Care Delivery Analytics (ICDA), was reported in AMIA 2012 [6]. We have continued to expand this framework by adding more machine learning and visualization components since then, and expect to continue to do so in the future.

Figure 31.1 gives an overview of the current snapshot of ICDA. At the center of this framework is Patient Similarity Analytics. The objective of this component is to develop methodologies that can be used to identify patients who are similar to a patient of interest in a clinically meaningful way, so that insights derived from longitudinal records of the similar patients can be used to help determine personalized

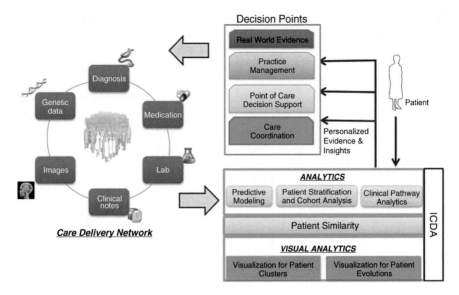

**Fig. 31.1** Intelligent Care Delivery Analytics (ICDA) – the data driven healthcare analytics platform at IBM research

prognosis and treatment plans for this specific patient. Building on and around this central component, we have developed a suite of analytics and visualization components to address challenges and use cases encountered in different aspects of the care process, and deliver insights in an interactive, consumable manner.

Throughout the rest of the chapter, we will describe some of the key elements, and provide concrete examples of novel algorithms that have been developed in this framework. Due to the limited space, we focus on describing the functionalities and high-level approaches of these analytics and visualization components. In-depth technical details and discussions can be found in the numerous publications cited throughout the chapter.

## 31.2   Patient Similarity Analytics

Existing EMR systems typically store data in a manner that makes it difficult for clinicians to extract what is necessary to make clinical decisions at the point-of-care. Most of EMR systems are primarily used to record clinical events for book-keeping and claim purposes as opposed to be used as a decision support tool for better diagnosis and treatment. Constructing a patient network with nodes representing patients and edges connecting clinically similar patients could be very helpful to such a clinical decision support system, as the physician can look at the treatments and disease condition evolutions of the similar patients to come up with a better care plan for the current patient.

Besides decision support systems, there are also other areas in medical informatics where such patient network could be very helpful. For example, Comparative Effectiveness Research [1], which is the direct comparison of existing health care interventions to determine which work best for which patients and which pose the greatest benefits and harms [w1]. In this case, if we can first stratify the patients into different cohorts according to their clinical similarity, then CER can be performed on the patients within the same cohorts [13]. Under a similar setting, patient risk stratification aims to stratify the patients according to their disease condition risks. This is a crucial step for effective management of patients because for patients with different risks, we may have different treatment plans. Furthermore, if we can construct an undirected patient network using such patient similarity, we can expect to discover clinically meaningful insights such as disease evolution patterns and care or treatment patterns.

## 31.2.1   Patient Similarity Metric Learning

While traditional patient cohort generation tools such as i2b2 [16] address some aspects of patient similarity, they are limited in that cohorts have to be identified through database queries using a few pre-selected attributes. To fully realize the power of patient similarity analytics, a big data approach is needed where all known attributes about patients are taken into consideration, in order to account for all potential confounding factors. This poses two challenges. First, since the number of attributes can be very large (e.g., in the order of tens of thousands), how to define distance, or similarity metric, in this high dimensional space is a challenging mathematical problem. Second, the notion of patient similarity is context dependent. For example, the factors that are important for identifying similar patients in the context of determining best treatment for hyperlipidemia may be completely different from the ones for evaluating different chemotherapies for a cancer patient. To address these challenges, machine learning approaches called metric learning are needed to derive from data the most appropriate similarity metric, i.e., most important attributes along with the weighting factors for a specific clinical context.

Patient EMRs contain a large amount of features coming from heterogeneous sources, such as demographic information, diagnosis, medication, lab tests and so on and so forth. To facilitate the process of similarity learning, researchers have proposed constructing a profile for each patient, which is a feature vector with the dimensionality equal to the number of different features. Before constructing such a vector, a time period of interest is defined, within which the features are aggregated to obtain the entries in the patient profile (e.g., the average value of a specific lab test, or the count of a specific diagnosis code). In this way, after profiling, each patient is represented as a feature vector [27, 28].

Local Supervised Metric Learning (LSML) is a supervised metric learning approach that has been proved to be useful in patient similarity evaluation [3, 23, 24].

This algorithm was initially proposed in [30] for face recognition. The basic idea of LSML is to maximize the local separability of the data vectors from different classes.

We applied the LSML in the context of monitoring patients in the Intensive Care Unit (ICU) [3]. ICUs are data rich environments where patients are continuously being monitored for several aspects of their health. Alerts that can indicate the likely onset of an imminent adverse condition based on the behavior of patients' temporal data provide important support mechanism for physicians in this environment. Accompanying those alerts with insight regarding the likely behavior of patient KPIs can further qualify and clarify them. In this setting, our goal is to retrieve patients who display similar evolution patterns in their ICU data to the patient being monitored and use the future trend of the cohort of similar patients to predict if the patient being monitored is going to experience a medical event within a specific time horizon. The insight provided to the clinician through the projections of the patient's physiological data into the future could further clarify and qualify the generated alerts. The proposed approach and system were tested using the MIMIC II database, which consists of physiological waveforms, and accompanying clinical data obtained for ICU patients.

## 31.2.2   Inference Over Multiple Similarity Networks for Personalized Medicine

Using patient similarity analytics methods such as the described above, one can construct patient similarity networks where each node represents a patient and the edge between a pair of patients represent the degree of similarity between the two patients represented by their key clinical indicators. In a recent work, we augmented this patient similarity network with a drug similarity network, and developed a machine learning approach to make inferences over this heterogeneous network to derive Real World Evidence for personalized drug response prediction [36]. To compose the drug similarity network, we used chemical structure extracted from PubChem, and drug target protein information extracted from DrugBank [34]. Links between patients and drugs were then constructed to represent the prior associations between patients and drugs, which were measured by the Tonimoto Coefficient between ICD9 diagnosis codes of patients and ICD9-format drug indications from MEDI database [33]. Finally, a machine learning technique called label propagation [31] was applied to infer, for any given drug, the likely effectiveness of this drug on any of the patients who have not yet received this drug. Intuitively, this allows us to infer the likely response of a patient to a particular drug based on observations of how similar patients have responded to similar drugs in the past. Experimental evaluation results on a real-world EMR dataset of 110,157 hyperlipidemia patients demonstrate the effectiveness of the proposed method and suggest that the combination of appropriate patient similarity and drug similarity analytics can help identify which drug is likely to be effective for a given patient.

### 31.2.3  CareFlow: Data-Driven Visual Exploration of Similar Patients

Patient similarity analytics can be combined with advanced visualization techniques to provide physicians with the most relevant information in a consumable manner. One example of such a tool is CareFlow, for the exploration of care pathways from similar patients. When a patient is diagnosed with a disease, their doctor will often devise a care pathway, a sequence of medical treatments to help manage their disease or condition. When doctors devise care pathways, they often must rely on their education, experience, and intuition [25]. The goal of CareFlow [17] is to leverage the rich longitudinal data found in Electronic Medical Records (EMRs) to empower clinicians with a new data-driven resource for the design of personalized care plans. Using the relevant clinical data of a specific patient, CareFlow mines the EMRs to find clinically similar patients using our patient similarity analytics. CareFlow then visualizes all of the different care pathways that these similar patients have undergone, while providing context on which care pathways were successful and which were not. The resulting visualization supports the identification of the most desirable and most problematic care plans.

### 31.2.4  Mining Care Pathways from Data

In order to model the care pathways for the similar patient population, CareFlow mines the EMRs for relevant patient events. For each similar patient, CareFlow will extract records of performed treatments and their associated dates by querying the EMR database for relevant medical events. The result of this query is a complex dataset describing the details of various treatments given to the entire similar patient population.

Of course, each similar patient underwent treatments at different points in time. In order to unify them, CareFlow aligns all treatments by the time at which each patient was first diagnosed with the disease of interest. CareFlow defines the care pathway as the sequence of treatments after diagnosis. In addition to deriving care pathways, outcomes are also derived from the EMRs for each of these similar patients. By associating each care pathway with an outcome, it is possible to infer which care pathways lead to statistically better outcomes. CareFlow makes this outcome information visually prominent to inform medical decisions.

### 31.2.5  Visualizing Care Pathways

While a doctor may be able to make sense of a care plan for a single patient (e.g. [20]), doing so for a similar patient population is much more challenging. Care pathways may have a large number of different types of treatments, and the sequence

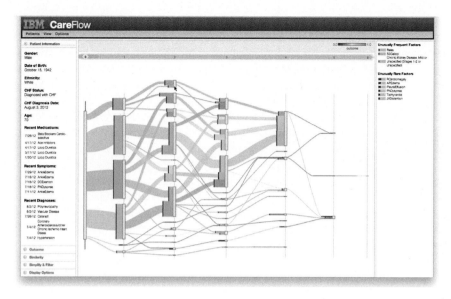

**Fig. 31.2** CareFlow's visual interface. The *left panel* displays a summary of the patient's relevant medical history. The *center panel* displays a visualization of the care plans of the 300 most similar patients. The *right panel* displays the factors associated with a selected subset of patients

of these treatments often varies as well. CareFlow provides a visualization of the temporal sequence of treatments. As shown in Fig. 31.2, treatments are represented as nodes and positioned along the horizontal axis, which represents the sequence of treatments over time. The diagnosis of a disease occurs on the far left of the visualization, and treatments in the care plan extend to the right. The height of each node is proportional to the number of patients that took a given treatment. Link edges are also present to connect nodes from their previous and future nodes in the care pathway. The visual elements are colored according to the average outcome of all patients represented by the node or edge. Elements that are colored green represented parts of the care plan where patients remained healthy, whereas elements that are colored red indicate care plans of patients who ended up in poor health.

## 31.2.6   Use Case: Congestive Heart Failure

This use case involves a doctor who has recently diagnosed a patient with congestive heart failure and wishes to use CareFlow to examine the historical outcomes of possible care pathways. CareFlow connects to a longitudinal EMR database of over 50,000 patients with heart conditions spanning over 8 years.

On the left-hand side of Fig. 31.2, a summary of the patient's relevant medical history is shown, including recent medications, symptoms, and diagnoses. In the center panel of Fig. 31.2, a visualization of the care plans of the 300 most similar patients is shown. The left-most node represents these similar patients at their point of diagnosis with heart failure. As the visualization extends to the right, the various treatment sequences of similar patients are shown. The care pathways are colored according to a continuous color scale,; pathways that are colored red implies most patients within that node ended up being hospitalized, whereas green pathways means most patients managed to stay out the hospital.

In addition to gaining an overview of all care pathways, a doctor can also focus on the most successful treatment plan. By selecting the appropriate button, the care plan that leads to the best outcomes for patients is highlighted.

CareFlow provides doctors with the ability to get more information about the patients who undertook a particular care plan. By selecting a Treatment node, doctors can view a precise count of the number of patients the node represents, as well as the average outcome for these patients. In addition, the right panel of the interface displays summary information about a set of patients by displaying factors common to this cohort, as well as factors rare in this group.

## 31.3   Predictive Modeling

Healthcare analytics research increasingly involves the construction of predictive models for disease targets across varying patient cohorts using observational data such as EMR. A common workflow for predictive models is a five-step process: (1) cohort construction, (2) feature engineering, (3) cross-validation, (4) feature selection, and (5) classification/model selection. We have developed novel machine learning and visualization methods to help address the challenges faced in each of these steps.

### 31.3.1   Feature Engineering

Feature Engineering, which is about inferring phenotypic patterns from population-scale clinical data, is a core computational task in the development of personalized medicine. One important source of data on which to conduct this type of research are patient EMRs. However, the patient longitudinal EMRs are typically sparse and noisy, which creates significant challenges if we use them directly to represent patient phenotypes. We developed a data driven phenotyping framework called Pacifier (PAtient reCord densIFIER) [37], where we interpret the longitudinal EMR data of each patient as a sparse matrix with a feature dimension and a time dimension, and derive more robust patient phenotypes by exploring the latent structure of those matrices. Specifically, we assume that each derived phenotype is composed of a subset of the medical features contained in original patient EMR, whose value evolves smoothly over time. We propose two formulations to achieve such goal. One is Individual Basis Approach (IBA), which assumes the phenotypes are different for every patient. The other is Shared Basis Approach (SBA), which assumes the patient population shares a common set of phenotypes. We developed an efficient optimization algorithm that is capable of resolving both problems efficiently. Pacifier was validated on two real world EMR cohorts for the tasks of early prediction of Congestive Heart Failure (CHF) and End Stage Renal Disease (ESRD). Our results showed that the predictive performance in both tasks can be improved significantly by the proposed algorithms (average AUC score improved from 0.689 to 0.816 on CHF, and from 0.756 to 0.838 on ESRD respectively).

### 31.3.2  Large Scale Feature Selection Algorithms

Another key challenge in developing risk prediction models from observational healthcare data is how to effectively identify, form the larger number (typically thousands to tens of thousands) of features the salient risk factors, i.e., the subset of features that are most predictive. Knowledge driven and data driven strategies reflect two ends of the spectrum of risk factor identification or feature selection. More specifically, a knowledge driven approach is based on evidence of varying quality, guidelines, and experts' opinions, while a data driven approach is solely based on the observational data. We developed a hybrid strategy that starts with prior knowledge, then extends to a more comprehensive model by selectively including an additional set of features that both optimize prediction and complement knowledge based features. In particular, we extended a sparse feature selection method called Scalable Orthogonal Regression (SOR) [12] to expand a set of knowledge driven risk factors with additional risk factors from data [22]. The method was designed specifically to select less redundant features without sacrificing the quality, for which redundancy is measured by an orthogonality measure added as a penalty term in the objective function. The approach was validated using a large dataset containing 4,644 heart failure cases and 45,981 controls. The proposed method was shown to identify complementary risk factors that are not in the existing known factors and can better predict the onset of HF. In other words, the combined risk factors between knowledge and data significantly outperform knowledge-based risk factors alone. Furthermore, those additional risk factors were confirmed to be clinically meaningful by a cardiologist [22].

### 31.3.3  Scalable Model Exploration

To develop an appropriate predictive model for healthcare applications, it is often necessary to compare and refine a larger number of models derived from a diversity of cohorts, patient-specific features, feature selection algorithms, and classifiers/ regression methods. An efficient and scalable computing platform is required to facilitate such large scale models exploration. To support this goal, we developed a

PARAllel predictive MOdeling (PARAMO) platform [15] which (1) constructs a dependency graph of tasks from specifications of predictive modeling pipelines, (2) schedules the tasks in a topological ordering of the graph, and (3) executes those tasks in parallel. We implemented this platform using Map-Reduce to enable independent tasks to run in parallel in a cluster computing environment. Different task scheduling preferences are also supported.

We assessed the performance of PARAMO on various workloads using three datasets derived from the EMR systems in place at Geisinger Health System and Vanderbilt University Medical Center and an anonymous longitudinal claims database. We demonstrate significant gains in computational efficiency against a standard approach. In particular, PARAMO can build 800 different models on a 300,000 patient data set in 3 hours in parallel compared to 9 days if running sequentially.

This work demonstrates that an efficient parallel predictive modeling platform can be developed for EMR data. Such a platform can facilitate large-scale modeling endeavors and speed-up the research workflow and reuse of health information.

### 31.3.4  Visual Analytics for Predictive Modeling

When data is high-dimensional, feature selection algorithms are often used to remove non-informative features from models. Here the analyst is confronted with the decision of which feature selection algorithm to utilize, and even if the analyst decides to try out multiple types, the algorithmic output is often not amenable to user interpretation. This limits the ability for users to utilize their domain expertise during the modeling process. To improve on this limitation, INFUSE (INteractive FeatUre SElection) [9], was designed to help analysts understand how predictive features are being ranked across feature selection algorithms, cross-validation folds, and classifiers.

### 31.3.5  Use Case: Diabetes Prediction

In order to demonstrate the promise of visualizing predictive models, we describe an example scenario with clinical researchers interested in using predictive modeling on a longitudinal database of electronic medical records. Their database features over 300,000 patients from a major healthcare provider in the United States. The team is interested in building a predictive model to predict if a patient is at risk of developing diabetes, a chronic disease of high blood sugar levels that causes serious health complications.

From this database, the team constructs a cohort (Step 1) of patients. Fifty percent of these patients are considered incident cases with a diagnosis of diabetes. Each case was paired with a control patient based on age, gender, and primary care physician resulting in control patients without diabetes. From the medical records of these patients, they extract four meaningful types of features (Step 2): diagnoses, lab tests, medications, and procedures. Next, in order to reduce the bias of the predictive models, the team uses ten cross-validation folds (i.e. random samples) (Step 3) to divide the population randomly into ten groups. After cohorts, features, and folds are defined, the clinical researchers are ready to use feature selection. The team has four feature selection algorithms implemented and available to them (Step 4): these include Information Gain, Fisher Score, Odds Ratio and Relative Risk. Finally, the team evaluates each selected feature set as a model using four classifiers (Step 5): Logistic Regression, Decision Trees, Naive Bayes, and K-Nearest Neighbors.

Typically, this team executes a pipeline of multiple feature selection algorithms and chooses the model that ends up with the best scores from the classifier. However, while this approach allows the team to find the model with the highest accuracy score, they do not have direct access to view the features that make up the model. This is the goal of INFUSE: to make those features automatically selected more visible.

## 31.3.6   Visualizing Features

As described, the features are ranked by multiple feature selection algorithms and across multiple cross-validation folds. INFUSE's visual design embeds all of this information in a circular glyph that shows all the rankings obtained from each algorithm/fold pair. As shown in Fig. 31.2 INFUSE (a), the glyph is divided into equally-sized circular segments; where each segment represents one of the ranking algorithms. For instance, in Fig. 31.2 INFUSE (b), the feature was ranked by four feature selection algorithms, so the circular glyph is divided into four sections. These sections are then divided further into a fold slice for each cross-validation fold. For instance, in Fig. 31.2 INFUSE (c), each feature selection algorithm was executed on ten cross-validation folds, therefore there are tenfold slices. Within each fold slice, there is an inward-growing bar (that is, starting from the perimeter and growing towards the center) that represents the rank of the feature in a particular fold. For example, in Fig. 31.2 INFUSE (c), the feature is higher ranked in Fold 3 than in Fold 4 as the bar in Fold 3 stretches closer towards the center than in Fold 4. Features that are unranked, because their scores are too low to meet the minimum threshold requirement of the algorithm, are represented as empty slices with no bars.

The feature glyphs are displayed inside a zoomable visualization that allows users to find the features of interest. For instance they can group all features by type (e.g. medication, diagnosis, lab type, as seen in Fig. 31.3 INFUSE) or display the features on a scatterplot (e.g. average of features vs how many times a feature was picked by an algorithm, as seen in Fig. 31.4 INFUSE).

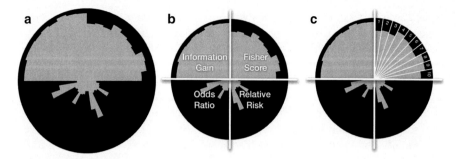

**Fig. 31.3** (**a**) An illustration of how features are visually represented as circular glyphs. (**b**) Multiple models for each feature are represented as *model sections*. In this example, the feature is divided into four sections, as it was ranked by four feature selection algorithms (Information Gain, Fisher-Score, Relative Risk, and Odds Ratio.). (**c**) Each section is further divided into *fold slices* representing each of the cross-validation folds. Each fold slices features an inward-filling bar that represents the rank of this feature in that fold. A longer bar implies the feature has a better rank. If no bar appears, the feature was unranked in the fold, and thus did not meet the importance threshold

### 31.3.7   Finding Clinically Relevant Features

The following is an example of the types of insights that can be reached with INFUSE. When examining the scatterplot view (the top of Fig. 31.4 INFUSE), all of the medications that were ranked by all feature selection algorithms and folds and found that they were antihyperglycemic medications, which are common treatments to lower the blood sugar of diabetes patients, and made clinical sense to be ranked high.

However, looking towards the center of the scatterplot, where the features are only ranked by half of the algorithms and folds, it is noticeable that a cluster of medications that had half-circle patterns like those described above. This region is highlighted in the red box of Fig. 31.4 INFUSE. By mouse-hovering these features to read their names, it shows that those ranked high by the upper-half of the circle (Information Gain and Fisher Score) were as clinically relevant and similar as those ranked by the bottom-half algorithms (Relative Risk and Odds Ratio). This provided feedback that in predictive modeling it is not safe to assume that one single feature selection algorithm is able to detect all possible interesting features and also

→

**Fig. 31.4** CAVA supports an iterative search process as described in the use case. This sequence shows several snapshots from the scenario where a clinician expands and refines an initial high-risk cohort using a mix of visual filters and patient similarity analytics. The end result is a targeted cohort of candidate patients for a new treatment regimen. (**a**) The sequence begins with a cohort overview showing age, gender, and diagnosis distributions. (**b**) Interactive visual filters are used to focus the analysis to narrower cohort. (**c**) Because the filtered group is too small, patient similarity analytics are requested to expand the cohort by retrieving additional clinically similar patients. The newly retrieved patients are visually integrated into the display for further analysis

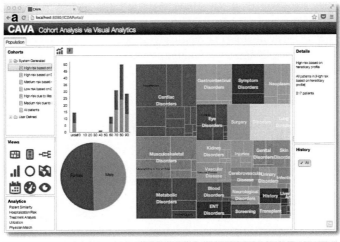

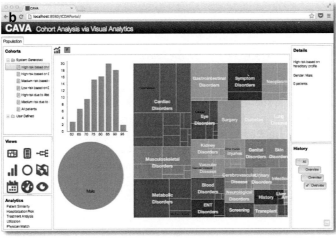

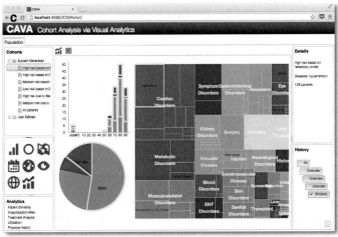

that having a system like INFUSE allows them to build a much richer picture of what kind of feature sets may lead to effective modeling. Without such a tool they would be restricted at evaluating one single algorithm at a time or, at best, restricting the comparison to a small number of features. Without such knowledge, the efficacy of the predictive models could be reduced.

## 31.4 Patient Stratification and Cohort Analysis

Patient stratification and cohort analysis are important techniques used in healthcare to study risk factors within population groups. The cohort study is a foundational tool that helps experts uncover correlations between specific risk metrics and the underlying attributes of individuals within the study population. Cohort studies are often performed prospectively using techniques that are statistically mature and powerful. However, the analytical process is often slow and expensive when collecting data prospectively. Retrospective analyses, which use previously collected data, are a possible alternative. Unfortunately, the use of retrospective studies has been relatively limited due to the historical difficulty in collecting and analyzing very large datasets. However, as more and more data become electronic, very large repositories suitable for retrospective cohort analysis are becoming increasingly common. These data warehouses can contain comprehensive historical observations of millions of people over time spans of many years. The increasing availability of such data helps overcome the fundamental limitations of the retrospective approach. In theory, domain experts can use these data to perform interactive, exploratory cohort studies without the overheads associated with prospective techniques. In practice, however, interactive cohort studies exploring large-scale retrospective data collections produce their own set of challenges. Data management, analysis, and summarization all become more difficult and typically lead to the use of more advanced technologies. Instead of relying on a spreadsheet and some basic statistics, users must also use technologies such as machine learning, data mining, and visualization tools to help make sense of the large scale of data they wish to examine.

### 31.4.1 Actionable Risk Stratification

A key step in providing personalized care is to segment the patient cohort into more homogeneous groups in terms of risk factors, so that a customized treatment plan can be constructed for each group. We term this process *Actionable Risk Stratification* because it goes beyond the traditional approaches of stratifying patients based on a single risk score. While that approach can effectively identify the group of high-risk patients to focus resources on, it does not provided insights into what are the most important risk factors to manage for these patients. Specifically, patients with the same (high) risk score may have incurred that high risk for different reasons (e.g., different comorbidities) and thus need to be managed differently.

A major challenge for actionable risk stratification is the heterogeneity of patients' clinical conditions. For example, CHF patients may have different comorbidities, such as diabetes, kidney diseases, or lung diseases. In different comorbidity groups, the medical features that contribute to the risk, or risk factors, are different. One way to perform patient stratification while taking into consideration of the most important factors is to construct a patient similarity network using techniques discussed earlier in this chapter, and then perform graph based clustering over this similarity network. However such an approach has the limitation that there is often inherent ambiguity in part of the network, due to the complexity of patients' conditions. As a result a purely data-driven approach would often lead to results that are unstable (i.e., different segmentation could emerge with slight perturbation of the attributes) and difficult to interpret.

One way to address the inherent ambiguity in data is to bring in prior knowledge from domain experts and literature. Such knowledge can be used to guide the data driven segmentation process such that the results conform with crucial clinical insights that have already been validated through extensive clinical studies, and are thus more interpretable and actionable. To this end we have developed an approach called RISGAL (RISk Group anALysis), which is a novel semi-supervised learning framework for data- and knowledge-driven patient risk group exploration [29]. The input of RISGAL is a graph with nodes as patients and edges as patient similarities, as well as a set of knowledge-driven risk factors or groups provided by domain experts or extracted from literature. The output is a set of patient risk groups that align with those provided risk factors. The approach was applied to a real-world electronic medical record database to stratify a set of patients with respect to their risk of CHF onset and was show to be able to identify both data- and knowledge-driven risk groups with rich clinical insights.

## 31.4.2   Healthcare Utilization Analysis and Hot Spotting

Another area where patient stratification has important applications is in healthcare utilization analysis. Utilization analysis based on observational healthcare data collected through normal course of care delivery and carried out in a systematic manner can be leveraged to improve care delivery in many ways. For example, through "hot spotting", we wish to identify patients, in a timely manner, who are heavy users of the system and their patterns of use, so that targeted intense intervention and follow up programs can be put in place to address their needs and change the existing, potentially ineffective, utilization pattern [4]. In anomaly detection, the goal is to identify utilization patterns that are unusual given patients' clinical characteristics, including both underutilization and overutilization. The former may indicate a gap in medical service that if left unaddressed could result in further deterioration of patient's condition leading to situations requiring more costly and less effective interventions. The latter incurs unnecessary cost and waste of precious healthcare resources that could have been directed towards cases in real need.

We have developed a novel framework for utilization analysis designed to address these needs. The first component of the framework is Utilization Profiling and Hot Spotting. Here we use a vector space model to represent patient utilization profiles, and apply advanced clustering techniques to identify dominant utilization groups within a given population. The second component of the framework is Contextual Anomaly Detection for Utilization. Here we developed a novel method for *contextual anomaly detection* designed to detect utilization anomalies while taken into consideration the patients' clinical characteristics. In this method we first build models trained from observational data to compute the expected utilization levels for each patient given his/her clinical and demographic characteristics. We then examine the difference between the expected and actual levels based on well-established statistical testing methods to identify anomalies. This utilization analysis framework was tested and evaluated using outpatient data for a population of 7,667 diabetes patients collected over a 1 year period, and was shown to be effective in identifying clinically meaningful instances for both hot spotting and anomaly detection [8].

## 31.4.3 Interactive, Visual Cohort Analysis

CAVA—a platform for Cohort Analysis via Visual Analytics—was designed to help clinical researchers work faster and more independently when performing retrospective cohort studies Zhang et al. [35]. Motivated by the needs of real-world analysts working in the healthcare domain, CAVA follows a novel system design centered around three primary types of artifacts: (1) cohorts, (2) views, and (3) analytics. Cohorts are CAVA's fundamental data construct and represent a set of people and their associated properties. Views are visualization components that graphically display a cohort and allow users to directly manipulate or refine the underlying cohort. Analytics are computational elements that create, expand, and/or alter the contents of a cohort. In this way, CAVA treats both Views and Analytics as functional components that operate on an input cohort and produce an output cohort. Building on this design principle, CAVA allows users to chain together complex sequences of steps that intermix both manual and machine-driven cohort manipulations.

## 31.4.4 Use Case: Iterative Cohort Analysis

The CAVA platform enables a wide range of cohort analysis workflows. As an example, suppose a clinician who has recently become aware of a new preventive technique that has been shown to help delay or prevent certain types of patients from developing heart disease. In particular, the treatment has been studied most in male hypertensive patients between 60 and 80 years of age. Due to limited resources and potential side effects, the clinician wants to focus this new treatment regimen on only those patients who are both (a) at high risk of developing the disease and (b) best fit the selection criteria for which the treatment is most effective. The clinician uses CAVA to find a cohort of candidates for the treatment following a usage pattern that we call iterative search.

To start, the physician selects a high-risk group from the cohort panel that has been generated by a risk stratification analytic. The user then drags and drops the cohort onto the demographic overview visualization icon. This results in the visualization shown in Fig. 31.4a, which displays linked views of age, gender, and diagnosis distributions. The user interactively selects various elements in the visualizations to explore how these three demographic criteria are correlated.

Next, the clinician interacts with the visualization to select and filter the age group in which the treatment has been studied: 60–80 years of age. By selecting the age range in the histogram and clicking the filter button, the user modifies the cohort to exclude those outside the specified range. The clinician then selects the men in the cohort and applies an additional filter. The result is shown in Fig. 31.4b. As a result of the filters, the initial cohort has been reduced to a group roughly one-third in size. However, the clinician presumes that there are likely additional patients—missing from the current cohort—who are clinically similar to the visualized patients and could benefit from the treatment even if they do not strictly meet the inclusion criteria. Therefore, the clinician decides to search for similar patients by dragging the current cohort from the active view to the Patient Similarity entry in the analytic panel. In response, CAVA binds the visualized cohort to the analytic and presents the user with a dialog box to gather the needed input parameters. In particular, the clinician indicates that she wants to retrieve enough similar patients to double the size of the cohort. After clicking OK, CAVA runs the analytic and updates the visualization with the newly expanded cohort.

The visualization now shows the additional similar patients, but the clinician is still not finished. Because the treatment was designed for patients with hypertension, she selects the hypertension subgroup in the visualization (as shown in Fig. 31.4c) and applies one last filter. The clinician has now used a combination of ad hoc filters and analytics to identify an initial set of candidate patients to target with the newly available treatment. Moreover, they have accomplished this without the help of a technology team to write SQL queries, run analytics, or produce reports.

## 31.5 Care Pathway Analytics

Extracting insights from temporal event sequences, such as mining frequent patterns, is an important challenge in healthcare. However, despite the availability of temporal data and the common desire to extract knowledge, mining patterns from temporal event sequences is still a fundamental challenge in data mining [14].

Frequent Sequence Mining (FSM) techniques have emerged in the data mining community to find sets of frequently occurring subsequences. However, these algorithms often have constraints that limit its applicability to real-world data.

First, they may not take into account the multiple levels of detail present in healthcare data. For example, ICD-9 diagnostic codes (which encode symptoms, causes, and signs of diseases using ICD-9 standards) are organized according to a meaningful hierarchy. In EMRs, temporal events are often recorded at a specific level-of-detail to record maximum information about an event's type. FSM techniques applied to data with a large dictionary of event types will often suffer from computational complexity. Perhaps even more of a fundamental problem is that patterns extracted from a specific level- of-detail may impair an interpretable overview of patterns for users.

A second issue is that FSM techniques ignore the temporal context associated with data, and instead focus on the pure sequentially of events. However, for medical scenarios, if a certain amount of time elapsed between events, the events should not be considered as part of the same sequence, even if events are technically sequential in the event log.

A third issue is concurrency. Many FSM algorithms suffer from pattern explosion when there are many concurrent events. This is particularly troubling for medical data, as many systems may record data in low-resolution precision, such as a day, and many events may occur on the same day.

A fourth issue is outcome. Many FSM algorithms are agnostic to the types of patterns mined. However, in healthcare data, analysts may not just need a list of patterns but instead how each of the patterns correlate to an outcome measure.

A recent system, Frequence [19], address these issues by featuring a novel frequent sequence mining algorithm to handle multiple levels-of-detail, temporal context, concurrency, and outcome analysis. Frequence also features a visual interface designed to support insights, and support exploration of patterns of the level-of-detail relevant to users.

### 31.5.1   Visual Representation of Frequent Patterns

In order to make the description of the system understandable, the characteristics of our visualization are illustrated in Fig. 31.5. In this example, the patterns are sequences of clinical events, and each patient has an outcome measure.

Events in the frequent sequences are represented as nodes, and event nodes that belong to the same sequence are connected by edges. The nodes and edges are positioned using a modified Sankey diagram layout [9].

Thus, in Frequence, subsequences are represented as individual edges. For instance, the simple pattern **Diagnosis → Medication**, is visualized as a **Diagnosis** node connected to a **Medication** node, as shown at the bottom of Fig. 31.5. Patterns that share similar subsequences, such as **Lab → Diagnosis → Medication** and **Lab → Diagnosis → Lab**, involve two edges from **Lab** to **Diagnosis** representing each

| Sequence | Outcome |
|---|---|
| Vital → Diagnosis → Medication | positive |
| Lab → Diagnosis → Medication | positive |
| Lab → Diagnosis → Lab | negative |
| Diagnosis → Medication | neutral |

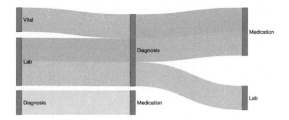

**Fig. 31.5** An example of Frequence's visual encoding for a set of frequent patterns. Patterns are represented by a sequence of nodes (events) connected by edges (event subsequences). Patterns are colored according to their correlation with users' outcomes

subsequence. Thus, prominent subsequences also become visually prominent due to the thickness of the combined multiple edges.

Of course, not all event subsequences are equal as some correlate to a positive outcome, whereas others correlate to a negative outcome, as determined by Frequence's outcome analytics. The visualization uses color to encode each pattern's association with an associated outcome. For this scenario, the patterns that occur more often with healthy patients are more blue. The patterns that occur more often with unhealthy patients are more red. The neutral patterns that appear common to both healthy and unhealthy patients are gray.

## 31.5.2   Use Case: Lung Disease and Sepsis

As an illustrative example, we briefly present a use case involving a team of clinical researchers interested in determining if there are particular patterns that lead to patients with lung disease developing sepsis, a potentially deadly medical condition. Additional details about this use case are presented in [19].

The institution used a set of 2,336 patients diagnosed with lung disease, each with longitudinal events of ICD-9 diagnostic codes. Of the patients with lung disease, 483 developed sepsis within 6 months of their diagnosis of lung disease, whereas 1,853 managed to not contract the condition.

At the top of Fig. 31.6, the coarsest patterns for all of the lung disease patients are shown. The clinician was particularly interested in cardiovascular complications, and noticed that the pattern **CardiacDisorders → SymptomDisorders** was common yet neutral (that is, this pattern was common to patients who did and did not end up contracting sepsis). After selecting this pattern in Frequence and filtering by cohort to see the matching patients, the finer level of detail (Level 1) allowed the clinician to see more detailed cardiac conditions, such as cardiac dysrhythmia and heart failure. Other complications, such as acute renal failure (which medical literature suggests is linked to developing sepsis), also appear. However, the clinician is interested in the patterns that led to patients not developing sepsis, and filtered to the positive patterns in the middle of Fig. 31.6. Surprised to see the pattern **HeartFailure**

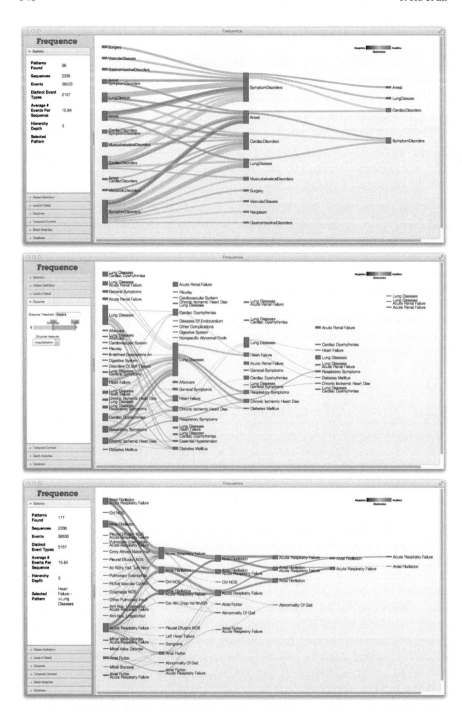

**Fig. 31.6** The *top figure* shows an overview of the coarsest patterns in Frequence using the Lung Disease and Sepsis dataset. The *middle figure* shows the positive patterns at a finer level-of-detail for the cohort who matched the CardiacDisorders → SymptomDisorders sequence. The *bottom figure* shows the patterns at the finest level of detail, after selecting HeartFailure → LungDiseases

→ **LungDiseases**, the clinician filtered to the cohort that matched this pattern and pivoted to Level 2, as shown in the bottom of Fig. 31.6. The clinician immediately noticed that patterns that featured both Atrial Fibrillation and Acute Respiratory Failure are red, which is sensible, as medical literature suggests both are risk factors for sepsis. However, the clinician found it interesting that patterns beginning with Acute Respiratory Failure alone were not predictive of sepsis, but rather what happened next in the sequence was more predictive. From the Acute Respiratory Failure node in the first column of the visualization, the patterns diverge into red and blue, making it clear that what happens immediately after such Acute Respiratory Failure will likely determine if the patient will get sepsis or not.

## 31.6  Disease Modeling

Chronic diseases usually follow a long and slow progression. For example, Chronic Obstructive Pulmonary Disease (COPD) may take around 10 years to evolve from stage I (mild) to stage IV (very severe) [5]. It may also take 10 years for Congestive Heart Failure (CHF) progressing from stage I (mild) to stage IV (severe). Detection of such chronic diseases at its early stage is of key importance for effective treatment or intervention.

Disease Progression Modeling (DPM), which aims at modeling the entire progression procedure of a disease with computational technologies, is one important technique that can help realize disease early detection. Key challenges in developing DPM methodologies include: (1) Multiple Covariates. The progression of disease usually involves the evolution of many different types of covariates. In general it is not know which one or which group of variables are important. (2) Progression Heterogeneity. The patient disease conditions can progress differently for different individuals, and the patient records are not necessarily aligned. (3) Incomplete Records. The patient records are not complete, meaning that in most of the cases we are not able to get the patient records from the beginning stage of the disease to its end stage. (4) Irregular Visits. The patient only has medical records when he/she pays visit to medical facilities. Most of the times patients visits are at irregular time stamps due to various reasons. (5) Discrete Observation. Although the disease progression is a continuous time procedure, the patient records are only observed on certain discrete time stamps or intervals. (6) Limited Supervision. For most of the diseases we only have very limited knowledge on which observed events should belong to which disease stage.

As an initial step towards addressing these challenges, we developed an machine learning approach to infer probabilistic disease progression models from the longitudinal clinical findings of a cohort of patients who have developed, or are at risk developing such disease [26]. First of all, we use a Markov Jump Process to model the transition of disease stages/states, which implies (1) the progression is continuous-time; (2) the transition probability to the future state only relies the current state and the time span.

Second, we use the onset pattern of comorbidities to drive the transitions of the Markov Jump Process. Generally speaking, a comorbidity is a disease or syndrome that co-occurs with the target disease. For example, hypertension is a common comorbidity of diabetes and osteoporosis is a common comorbidity of COPD. Since the onset of a new comorbidity often signifies the exacerbation of the target disease, we use the onset pattern of multiple comorbidities to collectively capture the state transitions of the target disease. Finally, in order to infer the presence of the comorbidities from the observed clinical findings, we use a bipartite noisy- or Bayesian network [7, 20]. Simply speaking, given a set of comorbidities and a set of clinical findings, we assume an observed clinical finding was "activated" by the presence of any of the comorbidities with a certain activation probability. Such structure is especially well suited to our setting due to its flexibility in modeling sparse and noisy observations.

We validated our model on a data warehouse from a real-world longitudinal EMR database of 3,705 confirmed COPD patients over the course of 4 years. For each patient encounter ICD- 9 codes were recorded to indicate what medical conditions that patient had at that time point. Other information, such as drug prescription, lab test results, was also recorded. The results demonstrated that the proposed method can detect the episodes corresponding to different disease stage of every patient [26].

### 31.6.1   Visualizing Disease Progression

In order to better understand the progression of diseases, researchers can use tools like MatrixFlow. MatrixFlow is designed to help aid medical decision makers and researchers by making the subtle trends of disease progression more obvious. The goal is that by unearthing the hidden patterns in patient health records, emerging health risks may become more discoverable and earlier diagnoses of diseases can occur so clinicians and patients can proactively develop preventative strategies to reduce negative future outcomes.

The analytics work by extracting clinical event sequences from patient EMR data and then constructing a temporal network of co-occurring events to model the relationships between events as a disease progresses over time. The patterns in the evolution of the disease are then revealed in our interactive visualization as a temporal flow of matrices, MatrixFlow. MatrixFlow provides several interactive features for analysis: (1) one can sort the events based on the similarity in order to accentuate underlying cluster patterns among those events; (2) one can compare co-occurrence events over time and across cohorts through additional line graph visualization.

### 31.6.2   Clinical Event Networks

This work aims at discovering meaningful patterns from clinical event sequences of patients. Clinical event sequences are simply a series of time-stamped events from a patient's medical record, such as disease diagnoses, patient symptoms, lab results, and medication orders. However, what if researchers are interested in determining the co-occurrence of event—that is, when events simultaneously occur. Co-occurrence can be modeled by creating a network of clinical events, where events are nodes, and co-occurring events are connected by an edge.

Instead of using a traditional node-link diagram, MatrixFlow [18] relies on its namesake visualization: the adjacency matrix. In matrix visualizations, the columns and rows represent the nodes of the network, whereas each cell in a matrix represents the edge between the two nodes.

## 31.6.3   Use Case: Heart Failure

One motivating example is the clinical complexity and heterogeneity of heart failure (HF). HF has posed challenges to developing standardized criteria for its diagnosis. The Framingham HF criteria, originally published in 1971, were based on clinical data acquired in the 1950s and 1960s. In that study, two or more major criteria or one major and two or more minor criteria are used as the diagnosis criteria for HF. The challenges for making the correct HF diagnosis earlier are (1) how to correlate the sparse signals of a single patient across time and encounters, and (2) how to leverage historical data of other similar patients to identify the emerging pattern earlier.

We illustrate the capabilities of MatrixFlow with a dataset of over 50,625 patients. A total of 4,644 incident HF cases were identified between 2003 and 2010. Up to ten control patients were selected for each case. Controls were clinic-matched, sex-matched, and age-matched to the corresponding case but did not meet operational criteria for HF on or before the corresponding case's diagnosis date. Note that two different cases can share common controls, in this design. For this study, we extracted the clinical notes portion of the EMRs for 4,644 case patients and for 45,981 control patients. Additionally, we have 1,200 confirmed HRrEF (reduced ejection fraction) and 1,615 confirmed HFpEF (preserved ejection fraction) cases, and the rest are HF cases without a confirmed subtype.

Figure 31.7a shows the evolution of co-occurrence matrices of positive Framingham symptoms in the HFrEF patients, where patients are aligned by their diagnosis date. Each matrix displays co-occurrence events in a 3-month window. The rightmost matrix corresponds to the window right before diagnosis and the leftmost one the window 15–18 months before the diagnosis. From left to right as time evolves, it is possible to observe the percentage of patients having co-occurring Framingham symptoms is increasing, which confirms with the degrading clinical status of those patients. Notably, as patients gets closer to HF diagnosis, multiple Framingham symptoms starts to appear more frequently. A similar temporal pattern is observed in HFpEF patients Fig. 31.7b, which seems to suggest that despite the pathophysiological differences, both HF types seem to develop the same co-occurrence patterns on Framingham symptoms. On the other hand, control groups

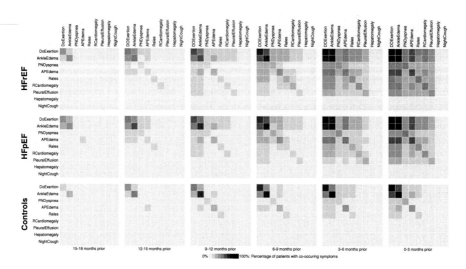

**Fig. 31.7** The temporal evolution of the Framingham symptoms in MatrixFlow. (**a**) The *top row* of matrices represents the patterns the HFrEF patient cohort. (**b**) The *middle row* represents the HFpEF patient cohort. (**c**) The *bottom row* represents the Controls cohort

Fig. 31.7c have much less obvious patterns, except a slight increase of prevalence on common symptoms like DOExertion and AnkleEdema, presumably due to the normal aging process.

## 31.7 Conclusions

Healthcare has undergone a tremendous growth in the use of EMR systems to capture patient disease and treatment histories. This and other rich observational data being captured in the healthcare system provide the foundational source material for realizing the vision of Learning Health Systems. However, to truly realize this vision, advanced data driven analytics and visualization methodologies and systems need to be developed in order to convert the source material into meaningful insights. In this chapter we described some initial progresses we have made in applying advanced analytics to derive insights to support smarter, more personalized care, and the journey continues. We are continuing to develop cutting edge innovations that will take us to the next level. One direction we are exploring is the integration of health and social programs. Specifically, we are working on developing comprehensive risk assessment models to better predictive risk in a cross domain environment, linking together physical health with mental health, behavioral factors, and overall quality of life, in order to drive successful integrated care. Another direction we are focusing on is the better understanding of the drivers of risk through disease modeling. Here we have efforts underway to better model phenotype representation from complex data, and to develop machine learning approaches to derive disease progression models. Finally, we are working on developing a *Visual*

*Analytics Workbench*, where advanced analytics can be tightly integrated with interactive visualizations tools to support dynamic, comprehensive and efficient data-driven hypothesis generating and testing. Our vision here is to provide a powerful tool that can be leveraged by researchers everywhere to speed up the development of data-driven analytics that can lead to better deliver of care at lower cost.

# References

1. Alexander GC, Stafford RS. Does comparative effectiveness have a comparative edge? JAMA. 2009;301:2488–90.
2. Berwick DM. Disseminating innovations in healthcare. JAMA. 2003;289:1969–75.
3. Ebadollahi S, Sun J, Gotz D, Hu J, Sow D, Neti C. Predicting patient's trajectory of physiological data using temporal trends in similar patients: a system for near-term prognostics. AMIA Annu Symp Proc. 2010;2010:192–6.
4. Gawande A. The hot spotters. New Yorker, Jan 2011.
5. Global Initiative for Chronic Obstructive Lung Disease. Global strategy for the diagnosis, management, and prevention of COPD. 2014. http://www.goldcopd.org/guidelines-global-strategy-for-diagnosis-management.html. Accessed 21 Apr 2015.
6. Gotz D, Starvropoulos H, Sun J, Wang F. ICDA: a platform for intelligent care delivery analytics. Am Med Inform Assoc Annu Symp AMIA. 2012;2012:264–73.
7. Halpern Y, Sontag D. Unsupervised learning of noisy-or bayesian networks. In: Proceedings of the twenty-ninth conference on uncertainty in artificial intelligence (UAI2013). Bellevue, WA, USA. 2013. p. 272–81. arXiv:1309.6834 [cs.LG].
8. Hu J, Wang F, Sun J, Sorrentino R, Ebadollahi S. A healthcare utilization analysis framework for hot spotting and contextual anomaly detection. Am Med Inform Assoc Annu Symp (AMIA 2012). 2012;2012:360–9.
9. Krause J, Perer A, Bertini E. INFUSE: interactive feature selection for predictive modelling of high dimensional data. Paris: IEEE Visual Analytics Science and Technology (VAST 2014); 2014.
10. Lenfant C. Clinical research to clinical practice – lost in translation. N Engl J Med. 2003;349: 868–74.
11. LHS. Institute of Medicine Report: best care at lower cost: the path to continuously learning health care in America, released on 6 Sept 2012. 2013. http://www.iom.edu/Reports/2012/Best-Care-at-Lower-Cost-The-Path-to-Continuously-Learning-Health-Care-in-America.aspx.
12. Luo D, Wang F, Sun J, Markatou M, Hu J, Ebadollahi S. SOR: scalable orthogonal regression for non redundant feature selection and its healthcare applications. SIAM Data Mining. 2012. http://www.research.ibm.com/healthcare/papers/sorSDM2012.pdf.
13. Markatou M, Kuruppumullage Don P, Hu J, Wang F, Sun J, Sorrentino R, Ebadollahi S. Case-based reasoning in comparative effectiveness research. IBM J Dev Res. 2012;56(5):468–79.
14. Mitsa T, editor. Temporal data mining. 1st ed. Boca Raton: Chapman & Hall/CRC; 2010.
15. Ng K, Ghoting A, Steinhubl SR, Stewart WF, Malin B, Sun J. PARAMO: a PARAllel predictive MOdeling platform for healthcare analytic research using electronic health records. J Biomed Inform. 2014;48:160–70.
16. Partners Healthcare. i2b2. 2014. https://www.i2b2.org/.
17. Perer A, Gotz D. Data driven exploration of care plans for patients. Paris: ACM CHI; 2013.
18. Perer A, Sun J. MatrixFlow: temporal network visual analytics to track symptom evolution during disease progression. Am Med Inform Assoc Annu Symp (AMIA 2012). 2012;2012: 716–25.
19. Perer A, Wang F. Frequence: interactive mining and visualization of temporal frequent event sequences. In: IUI '14 proceedings of the 19th international conference on intelligent user interfaces. New York: ACM; 2014. doi:10.1145/2557500.2557508.

20. Plaisant C, Mushlin R, Snyder A, Li J, Heller D, Shneiderman B. Lifelines: using visualization to enhance navigation and analysis of patient records. In American Medical Informatics Association Annual Symposium (AMIA), AMIA 1998 (1998), 7680.
21. Shwe MA, Middleton B, Heckerman D, Henrion M, Horvitz E, Lehmann H, Cooper G. Probabilistic diagnosis using a reformulation of the internist-1/qmr knowledge base. Methods Inf Med. 1991;30:241–55.
22. Sun J, Hu J, Luo D, Markatou M, Wang F, Edabollahi S, Steinhubl SE, Daar Z, Stewart WF. Combining knowledge and data driven insights for identifying risk factors using electronic health records. AMIA. 2012;2012:901–10.
23. Sun J, Sow DM, Hu J, Ebadollahi S. A system for mining temporal physiological data streams for advanced prognostic decision support. In: IEEE international conference on data mining. 2010. p. 1061–66. http://www.research.ibm.com/healthcare/papers/05694085.pdf.
24. Sun J, Sow DM, Hu J, Ebadollahi S. Localized supervised metric learning on temporal physiological data. In: International conference on pattern recognition. 2010. p. 4149–52. http://www.research.ibm.com/healthcare/papers/05597728.pdf.
25. Tracy CS, Dantas G, Upshur R. Evidence- based medicine in primary care: qualitative study of family physicians. BMC Fam Pract. 2003;4(1):6.
26. Wang X, Sontag D, Wang F. Unsupervised learning of disease progression models. In: Proceedings of the 20th ACM SIGKDD international conference on knowledge discovery and data mining. New York: ACM; 2014. p. 85–94.
27. Wang F, Sun J, Hu J, Ebadollahi S. iMet: interactive metric learning in healthcare applications. In: SIAM Data Mining Conference. 2011. pp. 944–55. http://www.research.ibm.com/healthcare/papers/304.pdf.
28. Wang F, Sun J, Ebadollahi S. Integrating distance metrics learned from multiple experts and its application in inter-patient similarity assessment. In: SIAM Data Mining Conference. 2011. p. 59–70. http://www.research.ibm.com/healthcare/papers/113.pdf.
29. Wang X, Wang F, Wang J, Qian B, Hu J. Exploring patient risk groups with incomplete knowledge. 2013 IEEE 13th international conference on data mining (ICDM). New York: IEEE; 2013. p. 1223–28.
30. Wang F, Zhang C. Feature extraction by maximizing the average neighborhood margin. In: Computer Vision and Pattern Recognition, New York: IEEE; 2007. p. 1–8.
31. Wang F, Zhang C. Label propagation through linear neighborhoods. In: Proceedings of the 23rd international conference on machine learning, Pittsburgh, 2006, p. 985–92. http://www.autonlab.org/icml_documents/camera-ready/124_Label_Propagation_th.pdf.
32. WDA. What is Watson? 2014. http://www.ibm.com/smarterplanet/us/en/ibmwatson/discovery-advisor.html.
33. Wei WQ, Cronin RM, Xu H, Lasko TA, Bastarache L, Denny JC. Development and evaluation of an ensemble resource linking medications to their indications. J Am Med Inform Assoc. 2013;20(5):954–61.
34. Wishart DS, Knox C, Guo AC, Shrivastava S, Hassanali M, Stothard P, Chang Z, Woolsey J. DrugBank: a comprehensive resource for in silico drug discovery and exploration. Nucleic Acids Res. 2006;34(Database issue):D668–72.
35. Zhang Z, Gotz D, Perer A. Iterative cohort analysis and exploration. Journal of Information Visualization, March 19, 2014. doi: 10.1177/1473871614526077. http://ivi.sagepub.com/content/early/2014/03/19/1473871614526077.abstract
36. Zhang P, Wang F, Hu J, Sorrentino R. Towards personalized medicine: leveraging patient similarity and drug similarity analytics. Am Med Inform Assoc (AMIA) Jt Summit Transl Sci Transl Bioinforma (TBI). 2014;2014:132–6.
37. Zhou J, Wang F, Hu J, Ye J. From micro to macro: data driven phenotyping by densification of longitudinal electronic medical records Proceedings of the 20th ACM SIGKDD international conference on knowledge discovery and data mining. New York: ACM; 2014. p. 135–44.

# Chapter 32
# Cognitive Computing for Electronic Medical Records

Murthy V. Devarakonda and Neil Mehta

**Abstract** The explosive growth of data has led to a situation where the human brain is overloaded with more information than it can process. It is particularly dire in healthcare where critical information may be buried in the mountains of data in the Electronic Medical Record systems (EMR systems) and healthcare workers struggle to make sense of this information to provide the best care for their patients. Cognitive computing, exemplified by Watson, offers the promise of transforming EMR systems from mere data storage to intelligent systems that help physicians in providing improved patient care. When seeing a patient, a physician needs to quickly grasp the summary of the patient's medical history from the EMR to prepare for the visit and to put the patient's complaints in context. During the visit, there may be a need to supplement, confirm, and investigate the information that the patient provides with information from the EMR. These information needs can be fulfilled by a cognitive system using advanced analytics on the patient record data. Some of the ways this can happen are a problem-oriented summary of a patient record, precisely answering natural language questions about the patient record content, automatically identifying urgent abnormalities, and by providing precise causes for such abnormalities. In this cognitive computing view, an EMR is an active entity that leverages the vast knowledge of the medical sciences, drug information, and medical ontologies in the context of the patient medical records to meet the information needs of the healthcare provider.

M.V. Devarakonda, PhD (IBM) (✉)
Research Staff Member and Manager, IBM T.J. Watson Research Center,
Yorktown Heights, NY, USA
e-mail: mdev@us.ibm.com

N. Mehta, MBBS, MS
Education Institute and Medicine Institute, Cleveland Clinic,
Cleveland Clinic Lerner College of Medicine of Case Western Reserve University,
Cleveland, OH, USA

© Springer International Publishing Switzerland 2016
C.A. Weaver et al. (eds.), *Healthcare Information Management Systems:
Cases, Strategies, and Solutions*, Health Informatics,
DOI 10.1007/978-3-319-20765-0_32

## 32.1 Introduction

The potential for health information technology to support clinical care and transform the health care delivery system has long been recognized [13]. The HITEC Health Act of 2009 and Meaningful Use incentives starting from 2013 have encouraged integration of health information technology in the clinical setting. While some benefits due to the technology have been observed with the introduction of Electronic Medical Record systems (EMR systems),[1] physicians continue to struggle with potential workflow disruptions and the resulting decrease in productivity in using EMR systems [2]. A recent American Medical Association study has identified reducing cognitive load as one of the priorities for improving usability of electronic health records [1]. This presents a clear need and an opportunity to use advanced analytics, such as those demonstrated by IBM Watson, to improve physician's efficiency and effectiveness in using EMRs.

Expert systems have been developed for medical applications in the past. However, very few have been adapted for practical use, and even fewer have been designed to improve the use of EMR. For example, MYCIN [3] is one of the first research attempts in 1970s to apply artificial intelligence to identify bacterial infections and recommend antibiotics. While it was a successful experiment, it was never used in practice. Isabel [14] is a modern symptom checker system which identifies likely diagnoses from symptoms described in natural language. It does not provide other features of a cognitive computing system mentioned earlier like a semantic search or a problem-orientated medical summary. Recent research work on IBM Watson [8] adapted the system to the medical domain and showed that it can answer medical questions, such as the American College of Physicians' Doctor's Dilemma questions and United States Medical Licensing Examination Step 1 questions, with a high degree of accuracy.

So, why can't the existing expert systems address the cognitive load on physicians in patient encounters? The missing piece of the puzzle is the integration with the EMR data. In all the medical diagnostic expert systems, a user is expected to extract relevant data from an EMR and present it to the system as an input, and there lies a major challenge. This takes precious additional time and effort and it is not easy to determine exactly what information to include. Patients don't have just one medical problem. Providing input relevant to one potential disease may lead to a solution for that one disease but not a holistic solution for patient care. A system that hopes to reduce a physician's cognitive load must be applied to where the key information exists, i.e. the patient's EMR.

In this chapter, we present an approach to applying cognitive computing to EMRs using IBM Watson. We demonstrate the value and feasibility of the approach with an application of IBM Watson called Watson EMRA (Electronic Medical

---

[1] Computer stored and managed patient data is referred to by multiple names, such as, EHR and EMR, often with little or no difference between the terms. To avoid possible confusion, we consistently use the term EMR to refer to a patient medical record and EMRs as its plural. Furthermore, we use the term *EMR system(s)* to refer to the software and hardware system that stores and provides access to the contents of EMRs.

Record Analysis). We begin by providing a background on the concepts of cognitive computing; and then summarize a physician's cognitive needs in an outpatient setting based on interviews with physicians at two major hospital systems. We next discuss a model of patient record summarization based on an automated problem list generation and the use of semantic search within an EMR. The discussion includes a user perspective of the impact of these capabilities alleviating cognitive load. We explore the full potential of cognitive computing for enhancing the use of EMRs and conclude the chapter with a brief summary.

## 32.2  Cognitive Computing

According to IBM, cognitive computing marks a new era of computing where computers interact with users in a natural way, learn continuously, and expand human cognition [15]. Cognitive computing systems are built from techniques developed over past several decades in many areas of computer science research including, natural language processing, information retrieval, knowledge representation, machine learning, and advanced data analytics. It is a confluence that is enabled by continuous development in computing hardware, software engineering, and many decades of research in algorithms for natural language processing and machine learning. The resulting cognitive computing systems can analyze, predict, reason, and interact with humans in ways that are natural to us. These cognitive computing systems do not aim to eliminate humans in the decision process but instead attempt to augment human intelligence and cognition.

IBM Watson [7], by winning the Jeopardy championship [24], has become *an opening to an era of cognitive computing* according to Kelly and Hamm [15]. Since the Jeopardy event, research has continued at IBM to adapt Watson to the medical domain [8] and to solve realistic problems in patient care. This effort created a powerful foundation, using which new applications can be built to address the cognitive needs of physicians in patient care. Before discussing these applications, let us first explore the cognitive needs of a physician in the next section.

## 32.3  Physicians' Cognitive Needs

Physicians for the most part follow a typical *workflow* in a patient contact. The concept of workflow was first introduced by Frederick Taylor and Henry Gantt, in late nineteenth century, to bring scientific principles to management of manufacturing [23]. This work gave raise to time and motion studies which became a systematic methodology to optimize manufacturing processes and service delivery. While specific details of a clinical workflow distinctly varies from specialty to specialty and from one individual physician to another even in the same specialty, there are certain high level steps that are consistently repeated in a typical patient contact.

A closer examination of these workflow steps help us identify a physician's cognitive needs and how solutions to these cognitive needs impact the overall outcome of physician efficiency and patient care. Since patient care takes place in many settings, in order to arrive at a practical solution let us examine a physician's workflow in one common setting, i.e. in outpatient care. Shartzer divides clinical tasks performed by a physician [19] into four distinct steps:

1. Visit Preparation
2. Patient History and Examination
3. Assessment and Plan
4. Visit Wrap-up

These four steps form a general workflow for an outpatient clinical setting. These tasks along with the transitory steps are the key to understanding physicians' information needs. An ongoing study [17], developed from interviews with physicians of two major hospital systems from a broad range of specialties, further breaks down the information needs at each step.

The first step, the visit preparation, involves a review of patient profile, problems list, event notifications, and routine activities. Here a physician is seeking information such as: "What was done at the last visit? What data has accumulated since the last visit? What is overdue or needs to be addressed today?" It is necessary for a physician to be able to find important information without being overwhelmed with irrelevant information. At this stage an *abstracted* summary would be useful as it would avoid physician having to read through several previous notes, lab results, procedures, and medication orders to formulate the abstraction in their own minds.

In the second (history and physical) step, a physician's information needs can be broadly described as filling gaps in the patient's history (*supplementation*), verification of something either reported by the patient, stated in the medical record, or suspected by the physician (*confirmation*), and exploring how or why a diagnosis or treatment evolved (*investigation*)..

In the "Assessment and plan" step, as the physician is evaluating test results, coming up with a diagnosis, contemplating further tests, and developing a treatment plan, she may rely on various sources of knowledge. Of course, one of the key sources is their own medical knowledge, but they may also want to look up information that could be relevant, such as current guidelines, newly developed treatment options, and ongoing clinical trials. The information available to the physician in this situation should be highly focused on the specific issue at hand and contextually related to the specific patient, and not a general document or web page with broad (and possibly irrelevant) information. Lack of precision and relevance in the available information at this stage leads to distraction, irritation, and inefficiency instead of intelligent assistance.

At the end of the visit, physicians want to make sure that everything that is needed to be addressed has been addressed. This includes not only the reason for the visit or the chief complaint which is typically addressed with a treatment or management plan in the earlier step, but also any routine activities or outstanding health maintenance items. In addition, physicians strive to provide a clear decision and communication to the patient on what the next steps are. It is also the time to document or at least prepare for documentation of the patient visit at a later time. In this stage of the workflow, the cognitive needs are highly focused around what steps the patient needs to take (such as medications and preparation for diagnostics if any) and could significantly impact the outcome from proposed plans and documentation thereof.

While this workflow describes only one patient contact scenario, i.e. an outpatient visit, it is a concrete example of a physician's information needs, and therefore, a prime target for cognitive computing solutions. One such solution, an automatically generated problem-oriented patient record summary [6] is described in the next section. It is intended to help physicians in the patient visit workflow by providing a quick summary of a patient record and the ability to browse for specific information.

## 32.4    Problem-Oriented Patient Record Summary

As Weed [21] pointed out several decades ago, a medical record should be organized by a patient's medical problems for it to be useful in their diagnosis, treatment, and management. He called it a problem-oriented medical record. Given the centrality of the medical problems, it would be natural and effective to model patient record summary around them. But, the problem list is rarely well maintained and so physicians find it usually unreliable. A reliable problem list is needed as a part of patient record summary, and we will discuss an automatic extraction of a problem list using natural language processing and machine learning later in the chapter.

Previous approaches to clinical summarization involved applying a succession of aggregation, organization, reduction/transformation, interpretation, and synthesis to a specific patient data. Linear abstraction works well for a lab result or a single patient problem, but a summary of an entire EMR needs to go beyond this. For example, it also needs to inter-relate such individual data as we discuss below. So, the natural way to achieve coverage while maintaining brevity is to start with aggregates of key patient data types such as problems, medications, labs, encounter notes, and procedures, and then provide additional semantics over them.

EMRA summarization therefore consists of multiple clinical aggregates, including the problem list, medications, clinical encounters, and lab results. Elements of each of these may be aggregated to some level by themselves. For example, results of a lab may be organized, transformed and interpreted such that the summary shows the latest value and an indication as to whether it is now, or has ever been, out of the normal range.

As mentioned above, there are also important relationships between the data aggregates and need to be surfaced. For example, a problem is treated by one or more medications. Neither the problem data aggregate nor the medications data aggregate reliably contains such clinical associations. These relationships may not be explicitly documented in a visit note either, even though they are the result of a

**Fig. 32.1** The Watson patient record summary model showing the generated problems list and other clinical data aggregates along with clinical relationships among them

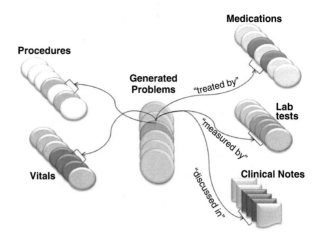

physician's judgment and actions. So, identifying such relationships between the problem list and other clinical aggregate are a part of the summarization.

Do elements of a clinical aggregate have an association? For example, two of a patient's medications may be closely related by the fact that they both treat the same problem. There are also other aspects such as the pharmacologic mechanisms of action of a medication and pharmacologic effects on human physiology, and so intra-relationships among medications are complex, and similarly two problems on the problem list may be related in multiple ways. In general, however, some elements of a list may have a closer relationship with each other than with the others. Physicians make these associations instinctively and based on their training. An intelligent summary of a patient record should present data aggregates in a clinically meaningful manner. EMRA summarization produces a nearness score based on multiple intrinsic relations among elements of an aggregate which identifies how closely an element is related to the other elements of the aggregate. For example, this analysis allows us to present the medications list in a clinically meaningful manner.

Encounter notes are a unique data aggregate in an EMR. They are the notes written by physicians, nurses, and other clinicians on every contact with the patient. Some of them may simply capture notes of a telephone call with the patient, and the others may involve detailed notes of a physician in a comprehensive visit. From the information content view point, not only is the data within a clinical note valuable, but the existence of the note and the data describing it (known as *meta-data*) are also equally valuable. The existence of notes in a time period indicates the amount of care provided. The meta-data may include the specialty and the note's author and the type of the note (i.e. whether it is a Progress Note or a Discharge Summary) further expanding on what of type of care received and who provided it. Therefore, our summarization organizes the clinical notes by specialty and by timeline, identifies the note type, and relates them to the problem list. Watson EMR analytics (specifically, the automated problem list generation algorithm) produces the association between each of the problems listed and one or more clinical notes. Figure 32.1 shows an abstract model of our summarization comprehensively

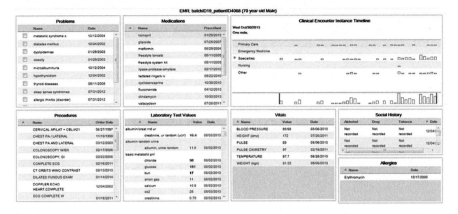

**Fig. 32.2** A dashboard-style visualization of the Watson patient record summary, showing clinical data in tables and patient contacts as a timeline

representing the analysis and the organization of clinical data discussed so far. A Web-based Graphical User Interface view, implementing the summarization model, is shown in Fig. 32.2 for an actual patient record.

## 32.5  Using Patient Record Summary for Patient Care

This patient record summary can meet important cognitive needs identified earlier in the chapter. Let us consider an Internal Medicine physician seeing a patient with diabetes.. The physician may not have seen the patient before or it may have been several months since the last visit. The physician needs to learn or recall the patient's medical history somewhat quickly prior to the visit. The Watson EMRA patient record summarization helps the physician in visit preparation by presenting an accurate and reliable problem list, along with the active medications, labs, vitals, and recent visits to physicians and hospitals. In preparing for this patient visit, physician notices that the patient has Diabetes Mellitus Type II along with comorbidities Dyslipidemias, Obesity, and Microalbuminuria from the summary view (Fig. 32.2). Noticing related comorbidities is made easier because Watson EMRA shows them close to Diabetes in the problem list.

Next, the physician observes clinical associations of the Diabetes with other clinical data of the patient by clicking the checkbox next to Diabetes in the problem list. As shown in Fig. 32.3, upon selecting the problem, related patient's medications – Metformin and Glipizide, in this case – are highlighted and shown at the top of the list. Figure 32.4 shows an isolated view of the problem – medications association. In addition, related labs and clinical encounters are highlighted. The highlighted lab results show the most recent value and indicate if the value is within the normal range

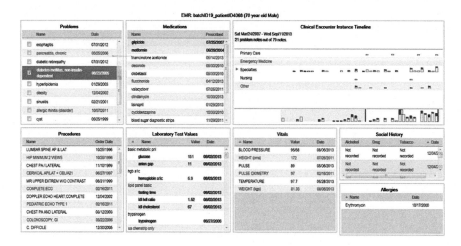

**Fig. 32.3** When a medical problem is selected, the dashboard highlights related patient data including medications, labs, patient contacts, and procedures

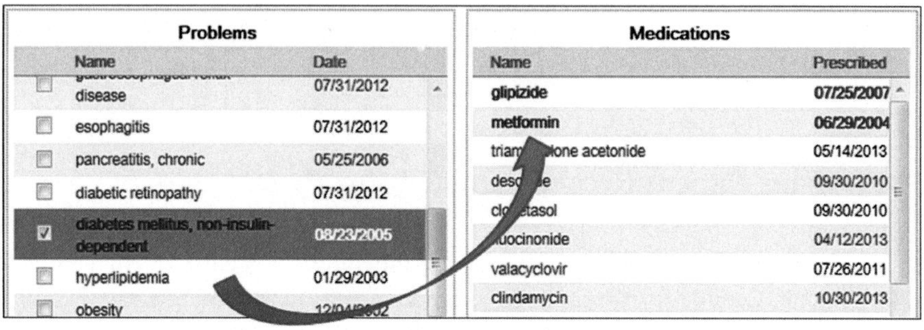

**Fig. 32.4** The problem and medication relationships are isolated here for clarity, and note that the related medications are highlighted and moved to the top of the list

as per the ranges defined in the lab test panel. Viewing this summary provides a rapid understanding of the patient's treatments and labs for the problem and relevant notes from previous encounters. We should note that the problem to clinical data associations are not in the EMR but are generated by Watson EMRA using novel analytics based on natural language processing techniques adapted for the medical domain.

In the history and physical step, the physician needing help with supplementation, confirmation, and investigation can find the necessary clinical data details either directly in the summary view or by detailed data by at most two clicks. For instance, let's say the physician would like to investigate historic glycemic control as indicated by Hemoglobin A1c over time, he/she can click on Hemoglobin A1c in the labs table, which opens a new window showing the historical values of the lab (see Fig. 32.5).

Now the physician wants to confirm what was planned by the primary care physician or Internal Medicine specialist in the most recent visit related to Diabetes, the

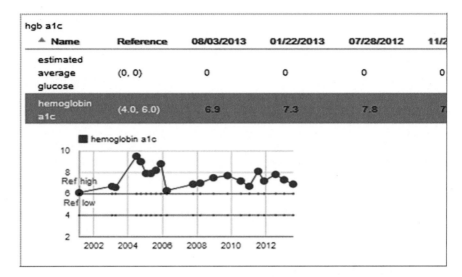

**Fig. 32.5** From the summary dashboard, one click enables access to detailed lab test results, for example, here Hemoglobin A1C data is shown as a plot over time along with reference high and low values, and as a table

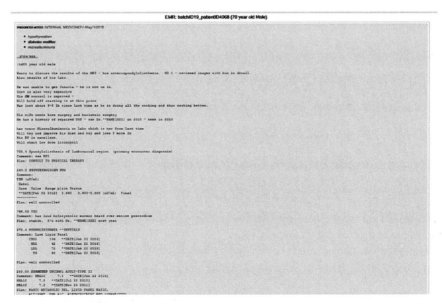

**Fig. 32.6** Access to physician notes is also available with one click from the summary dashboard, and the selected note is shown with relevant problems highlighted

physician goes to the clinical encounters table, finds the encounter categorized under primary care and highlight as related to Diabetes, and clicks the marker which opens a window showing the clinical note (See Fig. 32.6). The note provides the information needed the physician is looking for. The same note can also be accessed by clicking on the problem (Diabetes) from the problem list. A list of relevant clinical notes appears, each with a brief synopsis, and the physician can preview the synopsis and then click to fully open the needed clinical note. In each clinical note, Watson EMRA highlights references to the problem and so reading the note for details on Diabetes history, observations, assessment and plan is made easier. This association between a problem and clinical notes is also enabled by the Watson EMRA analytics.

In the assessment and plan stage, the physician needs highly focused information as they decide on a course of action. Let's say, the physician in this case is thinking of introducing an additional medication to improve A1c and blood sugar levels. He/she might want to see if the patient was on the medication before. The medications table allows switching to discontinued medications so that the physician can see if the medication was given and discontinued before. If the physician wants to know why it was discontinued he/she can use another function Watson EMRA called Semantic Find, which will be described later in the chapter. In addition, the physician wants to ensure the patient is prescribed medication for hypothyroidism (which he notices as comorbidity from the problem list) and that TSH levels are at desirable levels, which he/she do by clicking the box next to hypothyroidism in the problem list.

In the final visit wrap up, the summary view provides the physician with the necessary context to write the new encounter note. This context includes the problem list, active medications, and current labs. If necessary, he/she can review previous notes selected by the specialty and timeline. Later in the chapter we will discuss a semantic search functionality of Watson EMRA, which will also be useful in these visit workflow steps. In the next section, we will take a deeper look at how Watson EMRA generates the problem list [5] and how physicians can use this understanding in making the best use of the generated problem list.

## 32.6   Automatic Problem List Generation

Most EMR systems allow physicians and clinicians to enter and maintain the problem list manually. However, this problem list is not usually well maintained and as a result physicians almost always ignore it [4, 11, 12, 18]. There are many reasons for this state of affairs which include lack of proper support from the EMR systems, lack of clarity of what goes on the list and what comes off of the list, multiple authors populating the list, and many intended uses of the list, at least some of which are contradictory. Perhaps the fundamental reason, which is often missed in the discussions of the EMR systems, is that the problem list maintenance is a knowledge and time intensive task requiring significant investment of an experts' time. If for the sake of argument we set aside the difficulty of the problem list creation and maintenance, it is indisputable that the potential value of an accurate problem list is considerable.

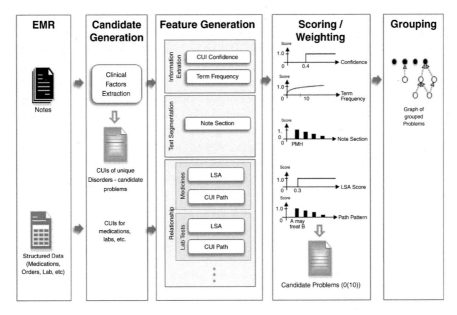

**Fig. 32.7** The Watson problem list generation uses natural language processing to extract features from the patient record that are used with a machine learning model to generate the problem list

The EMRA problem list generation starts with an automated step of identifying a large pool of medical disorders mentioned in the encounter notes of a patient's EMR. It then goes through additional steps of algorithmically gathering evidence for each potential problem, and then in the final two steps the candidate list is reduced to a final and presumably an accurate problem list and closely related problems are merged (See Fig. 32.7). The EMRA method uses NLP and machine learning. These steps are described in some detail below.

Watson EMRA recognizes the words and phrases denoting medical disorders in the encounter notes and assigns one or more Concept Unique Identifiers (CUIs) from the UMLS Metathesaurus [20]. This internal representation of words and phrases allows reasoning about them as medical concepts, such as recognizing medical synonyms, i.e. recognizing that HTN, high blood pressure, and hypertension all represent the same disease. In fact, Watson EMRA recognizes all medical terms in the clinical text, not just disorders, and categorizes them into UMLS semantic groups, e.g. as Disorders, Chemicals and Drugs, and Procedures. Each of these groups is further subcategorized, for example, Disorders are sub-grouped as Diseases or Syndromes, Signs or Symptoms, Findings, and others. Mapping terms (i.e. words or phrases) to CUIs is, in itself an interesting research task because the mapping between terms and CUIs is many-to-many, and the correct CUI may depend on the context. So, in addition to using the standard natural language processing methods and UMLS lookup, Watson takes advantages of additional context and sentence structure to obtain better mapping, and uses a numerical score to indicate the confidence that a CUI represents a given term. This confidence score is one of many features used in the problem list generation as discussed below.

In the first step of the method Watson EMRA identifies a term in an encounter note as a candidate problem if the term is categorized in the above CUI mapping process as a diseases or a syndrome, or one of a select set of findings. For a typical EMR, this results in identifying a few hundred candidate problems. When compared to the final list, the list of candidate problems has high recall (>90 %) but poor precision (<10 %). We note that recall represents the percentage of correct problems reported and precision represents the percentage of reported problems that are correct. So, this initial step attempts to capture all the correct problems but it may also include many problems that are not correct. The subsequent steps attempt to improve precision of the problem list without a substantial loss of recall.

In the next step, the method produces a set of feature values which will be used in a machine learning model in the next step. Longitudinal EMRs are a rich source of information and extracting and aggregating the information into the features is crucial to success. We used many types of features – lexical, medical, frequency, structural, and temporal features – each which we will describe below.

### 32.6.1   Lexical Features

We used the standard TF-IDF (term frequency – inverse document frequency) formulation, where the term frequency is number of occurrences of a term (candidate problem) normalized using the maximum frequency of any term in the document and the inverse document frequency is the inverse of the fraction of documents with the term in the corpus. Depending on the goal, a document can be a note or an EMR. When generating the problem list for a patient, an EMR is a document and the entire collection of EMRs is our corpus. When deciding which encounter note is relevant to a selected problem, the encounter note becomes the document and an EMR becomes the corpus. For the problem list generation, IDF is calculated using the entire de-identified EMR collection.

Unlike a normal text document, an EMR is a longitudinal record and therefore, more recent notes are likely to better represent the patient's medical problems. Also, each note in the EMR has implicit sections and so a term (e.g. hypertension) appearing in different sections (e.g. family history vs. assessment and plan) may have significantly different meanings. Because of this, in addition to calculating TF at the EMR level, TF is also calculated for each note section and for a few different time periods.

### 32.6.2   Medical Features

Terms in the EMR semi-structured data are also mapped to UMLS CUIs so that we can use the UMLS relations. Medications turn out to be one of the most important features, whereas lab tests and procedure orders were less useful. One reason is that the medication names are relatively standardized, even while mixing the generic and brand names, and a UMLS CUI can be reliably found. Conversely, labs and procedures are often specified in institution specific abbreviations instead of CPT codes and LOINC codes, and are therefore harder to accurately map to UMLS concepts. Another reason is that while medications are prescribed to treat problems, some lab tests are very general and the others are very specific. For example, Hemoglobin A1c is used only to check for blood sugar control while a Basic Metabolic Panel could be ordered for glucose, calcium, potassium, renal function, and others. The relation between a problem and a medication is derived from a weighted confidence score obtained from distributional semantics and UMLS relationships.

### 32.6.3  Problem Frequency Features

Certain problems occur commonly among a patient population, and thus the frequency of a problem can be thought of as the prior probability that the patient is likely to have it. Two sources of frequency are used in our method. The first is the SNOMED CORE usage, which represents the frequency in a broad population. The second is calculated using all diagnosed problems (as ICD-9 codes) in our collection of EMRs, which represents the frequency in a particular institution.

### 32.6.4  Structural Features

The concept "diabetes mellitus" appearing in the assessment and plan (informal) section in a patient's progress note is a much stronger indicator that the patient has the disorder than the same concept detected in the family history section in a nursing note. Since notes are in plain text and note metadata is optional, the structures have to be learned. Watson EMRA detects informal sections in a note using regular expressions and heuristics, and the informal section in which a term appears is used as a feature.

### 32.6.5  Temporal Features

The span of an EMR varies from a single day to several decades. Most temporal features in our experiments are normalized to prevent bias towards longer EMRs, but the absolute value is also used to define certain features, e.g. note *recency*, where the recency is defined as the number of days from the most recent patient contact.

Temporal data elements are used in three ways. First, they are used as features directly. Temporal features considered include the first/last mention of a problem, and the duration of a problem. Second, the temporal data is used to align semi-structured data and unstructured data, e.g. a medication prescribed before a problem is mentioned in a note is not considered as evidence to the problem. Third, temporal data is used to divide notes into bins on the timeline so that frequency can be counted by intervals, e.g. term frequency in recent notes vs. term frequency in earlier notes.

### 32.6.6  Machine Learning Model

Once all feature values are generated, they are converted to numerical values and normalized to a standard 0–1 scale. Subsequently a machine learning algorithm, the Alternating Decision Tree [9] generates a confidence score for each potential problem, and problems with a confidence score above a threshold are accepted as the entries on the patient's problem list. Both the machine learning model and the confidence threshold are *learned* using a gold standard we developed with the help of medical experts.

### 32.6.7  Gold Standard

To evaluate the accuracy of the Watson problem list generation method, we tasked medical experts to create a gold standard using initially 199 EMRs (which later grew to 400 EMRs) acquired from the Cleveland Clinic under an IRB protocol for the study. The medical experts, mainly medical students in the fourth year of their medical degree program, studied the EMR, including the encounter notes, medications ordered, labs, procedures, and allergies, created a problem list. Each EMR was reviewed by at least two medical students and they separately created two problem lists. Next a physician has reviewed the lists and adjudicated any differences between the two lists.

The final gold standard still needs further refinement to be useful in training and testing our method. The problem lists created by the medical experts are usually in English terms that require mapping to UMLS concept unique ids or CUIs. We decided to use SNOMED CT CORE (US National Library of Medicine 2014) as the vocabulary for the problem list as this vocabulary has been developed for the express purpose of being used for the problem list. Therefore, we needed to map the gold standard developed by the medical experts to the SNOMED CT CORE, and usually this mapping required further review because of the many-to-many mapping between textual problem terms and the SNOMED CT subset. We set aside a test set of 20 % of random EMRs from the gold standard and used them to assess the accuracy of the Watson method.

### 32.6.8  Candidate Problems

Figure 32.8 shows a distribution of the number of candidate problems generated per EMR (across all EMRs in our test and train set). We see a nearly normal distribution, with an average of 135 candidate problems and a standard deviation of 33. The

**Fig. 32.8** The candidate problems per patient record in the data have a near normal distribution with a median of about 140 candidate problems per patient

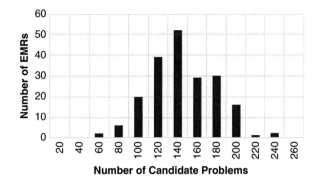

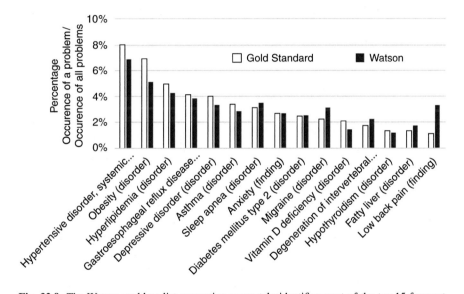

**Fig. 32.9** The Watson problem list generation accurately identifies most of the top 15 frequent problems occurring in the gold standard as seen in the bar chart below

machine learning model reduces these candidate problems to an average of 9 predicted final problems, a reduction by over 93 %.

## 32.6.9 Most Frequent Problems

Figure 32.9 shows the 15 most frequently occurring problems and their frequency in the gold standard. Juxtaposed against them, Fig. 32.9 also shows how closely Watson EMRA's prediction tracks the gold standard for these most frequent problems. Watson EMRA is mostly accurate in predicting frequently occurring problems. However, our model does not do well with lower back pain. A problem like

**Table 32.1** An accuracy analysis of the Watson problem list generation method indicates promising results with a recall (sensitivity) of 80 % when optimized for high recall

| Model prediction objective | Recall (%) | Precision (%) | F1 score | F2 score |
|---|---|---|---|---|
| Tuned for maximum F1 score | 70 | 67 | 0.69 | 0.69 |
| Tuned for maximum F2 score | 80 | 53 | 0.64 | 0.73 |

**Fig. 32.10** The top two levels of the alternating decision trees machine learning model used in the Watson problem list generation

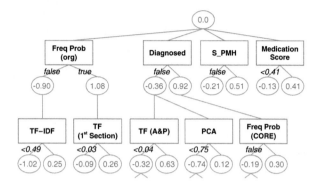

this is usually a challenge for our model. Physicians often prescribe medications for this especially when it is acute or severe, but subsequently if it is chronic a patient may be taking over the counter medications that may not be listed in the medications list or controlling this with back exercises. In including the problem in the gold standard medical experts used somewhat non-specific reasons, such as the severity and there not being another problem that explains the finding. Overall, EMRA accuracy on the most frequent problems is very good.

## 32.6.10   Overall Accuracy

At this time, the Watson EMRA achieves a recall of 70 % and the precision of 67 % on this gold standard as shown in Table 32.1. What it implies is that on average roughly 70 % of actual problems are captured in the list generated and 67 % of the problem list entries are correct. It is possible to tune the method so that it provides a higher recall and slightly lower precision while keeping the overall "accuracy" same, which ensures more of the actual problems at the risk of introducing more noise in the problem list generated.

## 32.6.11   Features with the Strongest Contribution

Which machine learning features have the strongest positive contribution for correct predictions in the Watson EMRA method? Figure 32.10 shows the top two levels of the Alternating Decision Tree machine learning model used in the

Watson EMRA method. From the Figure we see that the problem frequency (i.e. how common a problem is), whether it is in the diagnosis codes of the EMR, whether the problem is in the previous medical history of a note (S_PMH), and whether the patient is being treated with a medication for the problem are the features with strongest influence on the model. This observation shows that our model well captures the basis a physician might use in reviewing an EMR to identify the patient's problem list.

## 32.7    How to Use and Interpret the Generated Problem List?

There will always be a margin of error in a computed result, but with the help of evidence created for a problem selection in the problem list generation process, it is possible to examine the evidence and use human judgment before accepting the results for patient care. A part of the evidence for a problem is the set of clinical notes that mention the problem or its clinical synonym. An examination of the notes would reveal if the problem was identified by a physician or if it was a false positive. In the latter case it, the physician would instruct the system to ignore it and the system would learn from the feedback.

Another part of the evidence is the feature values of the machine learning model for problems. An examination of the weighted feature values typically reveals which features were responsible for a candidate problem to become a problem list item. A closer examination of the dominant feature reveals whether the score was justified or not. If the score seems inappropriately high, a physician can once again provide feedback to the system which will help correct the selection. In spite of the need to verify the results, the generated problem list offers a practical and efficient way to maintain and use the problem list in clinical practice.

## 32.8    Semantic Search for Clinical Information

Summarization described above may not address all the information needs of the physician. Studies [10] indicate that while browsing is a predominant mode of information seeking, search is often employed when browsing fails to produce the desired result. So, when a physician is looking for specific information that is not provided in the summarization, a search function is needed to fulfill the information need. For example, if a diabetic patient's previous labs indicate microalbuminuria, a physician treating the patient may now want to know if the patient was an ACE inhibitor. If not, why not? In general, this is a level of detail that is not usually available in the summary. But a search of the patient record can provide this information. Manually scanning through the record is not only tedious but also error prone.

Watson EMRA provides a search function that takes a set of words as input and finds matches for the search terms on many *semantic* dimensions. We call this Semantic *Find* to emphasize its similarity to finding matches in a document based on clinical similarities, not just textual matches. For example, Semantic Find identifies exact ("literal") matches of the search terms just as any standard document search, but even more importantly it also finds clinical synonyms. Searching for "hypertension" would match clinically equivalent terms such as "BP Elevated", "high blood pressure", and even a report of blood pressure measure of 147/95 in the EMR.

Semantic Find also finds other useful types of matches such as more general and more specific matches. If one enters "back pain", it will of course returns instances of semantic matches to "backache" but it also returns instances of "lower back pain" as a more specific match and instances of "pain" as a more general match. These matches help in seeing a broader scope of matches related to the search terms, and may be helpful in determining a new treatment or modifying an existing one.

In medicine, absence of certain findings is almost as important and may be even more important than the presence of the findings. Take for instance, the finding of Deep Vein Thrombosis (DVT) in a patient after a recent surgery. Determining its absence is important for treatment as well as for gathering quality metrics. Semantic Find therefore searches for negated instances (such as "no DVT") when searching for a term (i.e. DVT) and identifies them as negated results in the output.

To provide rapid response, Semantic Find builds an internal index of all medical concepts recognized in an EMR. The index construction is made possible by the Watson analytics that recognize all words and phrases which represent medical concepts in an EMR. When a search is initiated on an EMR, the search terms are also mapped to one or more medical concepts using the Watson analytics and the concepts are "looked up" in the EMR's medical concepts index. Different ways of looking up or comparing the search concepts yields a different facet of the search results. For instance, synonymy comparison of the search concepts with the concepts index yields semantic matches. The hyponym relationship yields more general matches and the hypernym relationship yields more specific matches. This matching takes place in the context of UMLS – i.e. depends on the relationships UMLS defines for a pair of concepts. See Fig. 32.11 for the results of Semantic Find for the search term "back pain" in an EMR, and notice how different tabs provide matches along different dimensions.

Multiple hyponym/hypernym relationships may be defined in UMLS which results in multiple matches along this dimension. Furthermore it is possible to mix synonymy with hyponym/hypernym relationships and find even more indirect but still relevant matches. These complex matches can quickly become expensive and slow the response time, and so we employ heuristics to limit the search. Semantic Find also provides matches for the terms in the semi-structured data in an EMR such as in the Ordered Medications list. The "treats" relationship from UMLS is used when the search term is a disease or a symptom.

## 32.9    Using Semantic Find to Meet Cognitive Needs

The overall value of the semantic find can be seen in its ability to complement the patient record summary in meeting a physician's information needs in the workflow of a patient contact. While the patient summary provides a quick way to understand

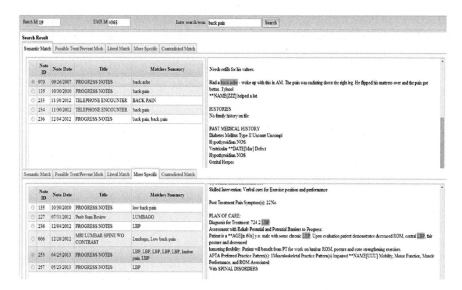

**Fig. 32.11** The Watson patient record Semantic Find matches search terms to the contents of a patient record on several dimensions, including medical semantic match, more specific and less specific matches, and contradicted matches

the patient's overall clinical status, Semantic Find helps to probe the record for specific information that may not be available in the summary. This can be particularly important in supplementation, confirmation, and investigation during the history and examination phase.

Semantic Find is also useful in finding specific information during Assessment and Plan. For example, if the physician is looking for an answer to the question – Why did the patient stop taking medication *Sitagliptin?* (After the physician finds that the patient discontinued the medication from the patient summary.) The physician enters the medication name as a search query, and when the results are presented, he/she looks for the most recent (by date) result in the literal or semantic matches returned by the search.

Similarly, to find an answer to the question: Did the patient complain about sleeplessness before December 2013? The physician enters the symptom (in this case *sleeplessness*) and looks at the literal, semantic, more specific, and more general matches up to the specific month and year. The semantic find Graphical User Interface helps this process by displaying results for each type of match in a different tab and by listing results in reverse chronological order.

## 32.10   Looking into the Future

From these current capabilities we can build new and more sophisticated capabilities in the system to expand the assistance a cognitive system can provide to a physician. These advanced capabilities reduce the amount of work a physician needs to do in using an EMR for patient care, and the cognitive system takes on an increasing responsibility to provide highly specific and targeted cognitive help.

## 32.11 Natural Language Question Answering on an EMR

Semantic Find is a powerful capability in finding clinically semantic matches in an EMR for given search term or terms. When the search terms succinctly capture the information needs, it delivers the needed results. However, when the information need can only be specified as a natural language question with all its inherent nuances, an advanced Question Answering capability is needed including the system capability to understand the question correctly and then find the relevant answer(s) precisely. Watson has demonstrated this ability even in the medical domain when the target of the question is the medical knowledge as represented by the text corpus provided to Watson. However, answering questions in a similar way when the target of the question is a single EMR is a distinctly different challenge at a technical level, and is an active area of research at IBM.

## 32.12 Advanced Patient Summary

The patient record summary presents the problem list for a patient and relates it to other clinical data aggregates, but a physician may need more detailed information about a specific problem in the list. For example, if the problem is the hypertensive disease, the physician may want to know what the duration of the disease was, and if there was any end organ damage such as its manifestations on kidneys or heart. The physician may want to know the timeline of blood pressure readings and if any medications were added, removed, or changed overtime. For some other types of problems like headache, it is important to understand if the problem is recurrent, chronic, or acute. Is there a plan in place, is there a definite diagnosis, or is there a need to monitor and follow up on the problem? From a cognitive computing perspective, these are advanced information extraction and abstraction challenges. Some of the data such as the medication time line is available from the semi-structured data but the majority of the information needs to be identified in the unstructured text, abstracted as necessary, and reasoned about. Watson EMRA is an excellent foundation to build these additional capabilities.

## 32.13 Guidance on Treatment Options

Weed proposed Knowledge Couplers as a way to improve physician's decision process during patient care. The idea behind the Knowledge Couplers is that they automatically apply rules representing the medical knowledge to patient care workflow steps. At the history and physical step of the visit, this knowledge guides a physician on what data to collect. The collected data plus additional medical knowledge helps physician decide on a set of diagnostic tests needed. Subsequently, the history and physical data and the assessment from the diagnostic tests as well as additional medical knowledge helps the physicians decide on treatment plans. This powerful conceptual model can be realized using Watson core capabilities of reasoning with medical knowledge [16] and Watson EMRA capabilities of analyzing an EMR. When realized using the Watson technology, this capability can help a physician by prompting "have you considered this?" as they are exploring the next steps in diagnosing and treating a patient condition. It can bring a wealth of latest treatment guidelines, medical knowledge, and specific patient data such as comorbidities, symptoms, and current medications to bear upon the consideration of next steps.

## 32.14   Guideline Extraction from Documents

In determining the treatment options, how will the medical knowledge become available in a form that can be used in automated reasoning? Some efforts are directed towards a manual process of human experts creating these knowledge rules. While at first it seems a reasonable and expedient way to do so, one realizes very quickly that it is highly human resource intensive, brittle, and difficult to update and correct. After N rules exist in the system, adding a new rule requires understanding and assessing its impact on various combinations of existing N rules. The number of combinations to consider grows very quickly even for small numbers of N, eventually leading to combinatorial explosion that is way beyond human cognition. Therefore, our approach to generating machine usable knowledge from guidelines document is to use natural language processing for extracting the knowledge. There is early work demonstrating the feasibility of this approach [22].

## 32.15   Summary

In this chapter, we discussed how the principles of cognitive computing are realized in Watson EMRA, a patient record summarization and semantic search capability built on the foundations of Watson. The functionality of the Watson EMRA is driven by the information needs of physicians in patient care. Watson EMRA takes a longitudinal patient record and creates a summary of the record, centered about an automatically generated problem list. The problem list is generated using natural language processing and machine learning. The summary also includes semantic relations between the problems and other clinical data aggregates such as medications ordered. For the times when the patient summary is not adequate for finding specific details, Watson EMRA also provides a semantic search which finds matching semantic medical concepts in the semi-structured and unstructured EMR contents, along several dimensions, including more general, more specific, and negated instances. The future work in this area includes advanced summary of problem status, natural language question answering on an EMR, and cognitive assistance to a physician in terms of next steps in diagnostic testing and treatment. The technology described here is a proof point of cognitive computing for Electronic Medical Records, and an indication of future promise.

**Acknowledgements** We thank the physicians and IT staff at Cleveland Clinic who guided definition of the requirements for the functionality discussed here and provided de-identified EMRs under an IRB protocol for the studies. Watson EMRA is a next higher level function built on the medical-domain adapted *Jeopardy!* Watson. All three, the Jeopardy! Watson, Medical Watson, and Watson EMRA, are the results of an extraordinary team of research, engineering, and support staff at IBM. We gratefully acknowledge their work and contributions which are discussed here.

# References

1. American Medical Association. Improving care: priorities to improve electronic health record usability. 2014. [Online]. https://download.ama-assn.org/resources/doc/ps2/x-pub/ehr-priorities.pdf. Accessed 9 Oct 2014.
2. Bowens FM, Frye PA, Jones WA, 2010. Health Information Technology: Integration of Clinical Workflow into Meaningful Use of Electronic Health Records, Perspectives in Health Information Management / AHIMA, American Health Information Management Association, 7(Fall), 1d.
3. Buchanan GB, Shortliffe HE. Rule based expert systems: the MYCIN experiments of the Stanford Heuristic Programming Project. Boston: Addison-Wesley Longman Publishing Co; 1984.
4. Campbell JR. Strategies for Problem List Implementation in a Complex Clinical Enterprise. Lake Buena Vista, FL, American Medical Informatics Association (AMIA). 1998.
5. Devarakonda M, Tsou C-H. Automated problem list generation from electronic medical records in IBM Watson. Austin: AAAI (Innovatibe Applications of AI Track); 2015.
6. Devarakonda M, Zhang D, Ching-Huei T, Bornea M. Problem-oriented patient record summary: an early report on a Watson application. Natal: IEEE Healthcom; 2014.
7. Ferrucci D, et al. Building Watson: an overview of the DeepQA project. AI Mag. 2010;31(3): 59–79.
8. Ferrucci D, et al. Watson: beyond jeopardy!. Artificial Intelligence. 2013;199(200):93–105.
9. Freund Y, Mason L. The Alternating Decision Tree Algorithm. San Francisco, Proc. of the 16th Int'l Conf on Machine Learning. 1999.
10. Gibbs WJ. Examining users on news provider web sites: a review of methodology. J Usability Stud. 2008;3(3):129–48.
11. Holmes C. The Problem List beyond Meaningful Use, Part I. Journal of American Health Information Management Association, 2011a;81(2), 30–3.
12. Holmes C. The Problem List beyond Meaningful Use, Part 2. Journal of American Health Information Management Association, 2011b; 81(3), 32–5.
13. Institute of Medicine. Crossing the quality chasm: a New Health System for the 21st century. Washington, DC: The National Academics Press; 2001.
14. Isabel Healthcare. Isabel symptom checker. 2014. [Online]. http://symptomchecker.isabel-healthcare.com/. Accessed 22 Dec 2014.
15. Kelly JE, Hamm S. Smart machines: IBM's Watson and the era of cognitive computing. 2013. s.l.:Columbia Business School Publishing, New York, NY.
16. Lally A, et al. WatsonPaths: scenario-based question answering and inference over unstructured information. Yorktown Heights: IBM Research; 2014 (Report No. RC25489).

17. Liang J, Devarakonda M, Mehta N. Cognitive needs of physicians: a study based on interviews at two major hospitals s.l. 2015. IBM Research Report (Manuscript in Preparation).
18. Meystre SM, Haug PJ. Randomized controlled trial of an automated problem. International Journal of Medical Informatics, 2008;77,602–12.
19. Shartzer LJ. Health IT and workflow in small physicians' practices. Quest Answer Brief. 2005. http://www.nihcm.org/pdf/AHRQ-QandA.pdf [Accessed: 7/21/15]
20. US National Library of Medicine, 2009. UMLS Reference Manual. [Online] Available at: http://www.ncbi.nlm.nih.gov/books/NBK9675/ [Accessed 15 04 2014]
21. Weed LL. Medical records that guide and teach. New Engl J Med, 1968;278(11):593–600.
22. Wenzina R, Kaiser K. Using TimeML to support the modeling of computerized clinical guidelines. In: Lovis C, et al., editors. e-Health – for continuity of care. s.l.:2014 European Federation for Medical Informatics and IOS Press. Washington, DC.
23. Wikipedia – Workflow. Workflow. 2014. [Online]. http://en.wikipedia.org/wiki/Workflow. Accessed 24 Dec 2014.
24. Wikipedia. Jeopardy!. 2014. [Online]. http://en.wikipedia.org/wiki/Jeopardy!. Accessed 14 Dec 2014.

# Chapter 33
# Health Information Systems 2025

Robert A. Greenes

**Abstract** The next generation of health IT is poised to both evolve from the present and be quite different. We are in the early stages of an inevitable and much to be desired transition from a siloized, fragmented *health care* "non-system" to a more articulated, comprehensive *health* system. Information technology is both an enabler of the goals of this new system and a *forcing function* creating the technology imperative that is itself a driver. In this chapter we pull together many of the aspects of health and health care and the IT system to support them that have been discussed throughout this book. Our discussion will focus on eleven disruptive factors that together are creating a sort of "perfect storm" that will make the health system of 10 years from now quite different from, although derived from and combining significant parts of, our current system. The disruptive forces variously have scientific, technology, policy, regulation/standards, or social/cultural origins, but all have significant IT architecture and function implications. The mantra going forward can be summed up by three words: integration, interoperability, and innovation. As we continue to move ahead in the disparate developments and innovations of this field, there will be increasing emphasis on aligning our efforts, making them interoperable, and creating a more integrated ecosystem aimed at optimizing health.

**Keywords** Clinical information systems • Health system • Health care system • Health IT • Health care IT • Health care transformation

## 33.1 Introduction: A Period of Significant Transformation

As of early 2015, we are at a remarkable point in time in terms of the process of health IT adoption and use. The adoption of electronic health record (EHR) systems has evolved over a period of 50–60 years, with many of the commercial systems

R.A. Greenes, MD, PhD
Department of Biomedical Informatics, Arizona State University and Mayo Clinic,
Scottsdale, AZ, USA
e-mail: greenes@asu.edu

© Springer International Publishing Switzerland 2016      579
C.A. Weaver et al. (eds.), *Healthcare Information Management Systems:
Cases, Strategies, and Solutions*, Health Informatics,
DOI 10.1007/978-3-319-20765-0_33

existing today having an actual 20–30 year history, and before that having roots in academic medical center home-grown implementations on which they were based that go back to the 1960s and 1970s. Yet we are poised for significant change.

The EHR systems available today are largely vertically integrated. By this, I refer mainly to the fact that they are built on a proprietary database with internal business processes and orchestration of functionality to support applications that are also part of the system. A considerable amount of customization is possible in terms of configuration of templates, screen views and layouts, order sets, decision support logic, and other capabilities, usually with dedicated editing tools within the proprietary environment. A number of the vendors have acquired, through mergers and acquisitions, or built subsystems and developed various strategies such as APIs (application program interfaces) for integrating these subsystems. But from an external perspective, EHR systems are "walled gardens".

In the past decade, government incentive programs have greatly increased the adoption and use of such systems in the US and other nations. In the U.S. as of February 2015, well over 90 % of primary health care providers (and smaller but growing numbers of specialty providers) and at least 60 % of hospitals/medical centers are now using EHRs [20]. But partly as a result of such top-down programs and incentives (with their associated time constraints), the adoption has mainly been of these large vertically integrated legacy EHR systems.

A dilemma that has arisen is that the urgency to deal with a number of pressing health and healthcare challenges has begun to force a need for a transformation of our health system and to convert it to a truly integrated "learning health system" [27]. These forces are building at the very time that the legacy health IT infrastructure is also becoming entrenched as a result of the accelerated push for broad adoption.

What are the issues? EHR systems have several shortcomings in today's transforming health environment. Their vertical integration impedes customization in ways that are needed by health care organizations and practices that go beyond the configuration capabilities provided. These needs also include horizontal integration with other systems and data sources. This is particularly important as health care organizations and practices increasingly must interface actively with other care providers and with their patients directly to coordinate and provide continuity of care and provide connected care services to patients in their own environments. Payne (Chapter 4), Kim et al (Chapter 5), Koppel (Chapter 6), and Edmunds et al (Chapter 7).

Data sharing needs frequently cut across health care organization/practice boundaries and vendor proprietary systems and they rarely (if ever) embrace the incorporation of patient-generated and sensor-generated data that are increasingly becoming important. Legacy systems also do not provide ready means for incorporation of analytics that foster optimal management of particular health care problems or categories of patients, or tracking of performance of providers, practices or organizations. Such analytic feedback and reporting are of growing importance in quality measurement, as a basis for health care services payment, and as part of a learning health system. Chapter 16 by Minetti et al.; Chapter 17 by Gibbons and Shaikh; and Chapter 21 by Hsueh, Chang and Ramakrishnan.

Data sharing must also be timely, be central, and must contribute to high-quality care. Health Information Exchange (HIE) as the term is used generically is a means for updating one provider or organization about the care received elsewhere by patients. But as generally implemented, HIE is additive and occurring at the edges of the enterprise's and EHR system's view of the patient. As implemented by a number of initiatives in the U.S. in particular, HIE has been criticized as being essentially equivalent to an electronic fax [25]. The data are provided, but they must be examined, reconciled, and integrated into existing records by a more-or-less manual additive process if used at all.

## 33.1.1   Why Is Transformation an Issue Now?

Why is health care transformation a particularly urgent topic at this point in time? What are the disconnects between where we are and where we should be in terms of the IT environment to support health and health care, as the system transforms? The answer is that over the past decade or more, a number of disruptive forces have begun to take shape that radically alter the landscape. Most of these forces are being exerted around the world, although they may be taking different forms or manifesting with different priorities. The examples herein will largely focus on health and health care and the health IT systems of the U.S., partly because it has one of the most loosely coordinated (if not chaotic), locally (rather than globally) optimized, and least top-down governed health systems in the world, and is most in need of, yet resistant to, change.

An international perspective on this topic is provided by Fraser and Wyatt with respect to clinical decision support adoption [12]. The authors highlight some significant contrasts between a top-down approach to health IT in the United Kingdom and a more grass-roots, bottom-up approach in some developing nations, notably in sub-Saharan Africa. Fraser and Wyatt make the observation that the lack of legacy systems and infrastructure (and entrenched business interests) often can enable leapfrogging and rapid advance in the less developed settings.

An important question is whether health transformation will be the driver for health IT change or the reverse. In this book, this question of drivers for health transformation is dissected by O'Brien and Mattison (Chapter 12) and Silva and Ball (Chapter 27) This dialectic chicken-and-egg question does not have an either/or answer, and in fact, both answers are true. We couldn't imagine the disruptions in the publication industry, commerce, or media without the enabling technologies – change can't happen until it is technically possible. It is often not even proposed or on one's radar until the technological possibility creates new ways of seeing things and sparks innovative thinking.

But adoption also has to meet a need – business, socio/cultural, or political, so the technology imperative that existence will create its own need is not entirely true. EHR adoption is a case in point – it was not adopted broadly in the U.S. until the regulatory and incentive structure was in place to drive it.

**Table 33.1** The health care system is not set up to delivery optimal care and the health IT system supports this non-optimal delivery system

| Health care system | IT system |
| --- | --- |
| Siloized, fragmented | Practice- or enterprise-focused EHRs |
| Procedure-, action-, intervention-oriented | Support for office-specific optimization |
| Limited incentives for doing less, for prevention and wellness | Limited decision support, education, outreach |
| Not patient-centered | No lifetime record, limited use of patient data, limited patient control of use |

Considering this dialectic, it is helpful to examine first the nature of health care in the U.S. and the IT system (EHRs and clinical support information systems) that grew up to support it, as a contrast to what the disruptive changes now demand. Table 33.1 summarizes this legacy perspective. Health care has been delivered in silos and is fragmented. It has been procedure-, action-, and intervention-oriented, demand-based and largely compensated on a fee-for-service basis. There have been limited incentives for doing less rather than more, for carrying out prevention and wellness measures, or for expending effort to avoid care. Practices and organizations have been locally optimized, for efficiency and income maximization. From a global perspective, they are not particularly patient-centric but rather episode- or encounter- or organization/provider- centric. Sharing and exchange in this environment are considered additional tasks to do at the edges of the process, and only when considered necessary, not routinely.

It is not surprising therefore that the IT systems to match these delivery environments have also been provider- or enterprise- based, aimed at capturing (and billing for) transactions, and focused on optimizing local workflow and decision processes. There is no concept of a lifetime health record for a patient.

## 33.1.2 The Shift from a Health Care System to a Health System

The need for change is lately much on the minds of health care policy, business, and informatics and technology experts, and this health policy evolution is nicely summarized by Edmunds et al Chapter 8.

**The biggest overall change is an expanding perspective on health not just health care**. The 15-volume Institute of Medicine (IOM) Learning Health System Series over the past decade [27] reflects this evolving thinking. Obvious drivers are the growing age of the population, the increasing prevalence of chronic disease as the overall population gets older, and the increasing complexity of such patients as they have multiple diseases, treatments for them, complications of their diseases, and side effects of treatments. Without a fundamental shift in focus on better (and cooperative) management of the health of such patients, and different financial models for paying for and incentivizing optimal care (and prevention), costs will continue to rise and satisfaction and outcome will continue to be suboptimal, if not deteriorating further.

A concomitant shift in perspective is the recognition of the lifetime needs of the person, whether as a patient or not, for health maintenance and disease prevention, and early and proactive disease management, and for a system of healthcare that supports health as well as optimally manages episodes of disease. (See Grundy and Hodach (Chapter 15) for a focus on the care delivery models targeting these transformational goals.) Such a healthcare delivery system would necessarily require three main capabilities aimed at providing health and healthcare continuity across the spectrum of venues from home to provider office to hospital, intensive care, recovery, and all other processes and steps:

1. **Provider-centric care coordination**, especially across the transitions of care, including optimal decision processes and workflows and team communication.
2. **Patient-centric connected care**, in which patient mobile health, sensors, wearables, and other modes of self-management are highly integrated with provider-centric care processes, provide timely communication and data exchange, and enable early warning systems, education, and other support.
3. **Data analytics** to support the above, to provide research and quality measures, population management, predictive modeling, and direct patient decision support based on dashboards, feedback reports, retrieval of maximally similar cohorts, and other approaches.

The U.S. Office of the National Coordinator for Health IT (ONC) has released its draft 10-year interoperability roadmap [39]. The report's Appendix lists 56 driving use cases for increasing interoperability. I submit that the main categories of use case are the three kinds of capability listed above.

## 33.2   Eleven Disruptive Forces as Drivers for Health IT Transformation

Figure 33.1 highlights the disruptive forces that I believe capture the main dimensions of health and health care change now underway in our society. Collectively these point to the need for the above three kinds of capabilities. We shall return to this later.

This chapter is focused on the next decade, yet the seeds of many of the 11 areas or realms of disruption have already begun to take root over the past decade. Prior chapters in this book have touched on a number of them – McCallie's Chapter 1 traces CDS' fits and starts; Chapter 2 covers Sittig and colleague's definition of the "minimum" functional capabilities that clinicians have the right to expect in an EHR; and Ingram on the ambulatory EHR's rapid evolution in Chapter 3. And as the forward-looking chapters of Part IV describe, the new technologies, analytics, and developmental partnerships that are happening today are already bringing this

**11 new and coming disruptive transformations**
*changing the scope of what is required*

|  | Science | Technol. | Policy | Stds. | Soc./Cult. |
|---|---|---|---|---|---|
| 1. Precision medicine | X |  |  |  |  |
| 2. Biosensors |  | X |  |  |  |
| 3. Patient engagement |  |  |  |  | X |
| 4. Big data | X | X | X |  |  |
| 5. Pay for value |  |  | X |  | X |
| 6. Wellness & prevention |  |  | X |  | X |
| 7. Meaningful use |  |  | X | X |  |
| 8. Usability |  |  | X |  | X |
| 9. Rise of an app culture |  | X |  |  | X |
| 10. Interoperabiltity |  | X | X | X |  |
| 11. Augmented guidance |  | X |  | X | X |

**Fig. 33.1** Primary drivers for health system transformation and IT to support it

disruption into play (McCallie; Fackler; Sow; Hu et al.; and Dezarakon and Mehta in Chapters 28, 29, 30, 31, and 32 respectively). As we look back 10 years and forward to the next 10, it is likely that over this overall 20-year period, we will see more and more of this reality taking shape. Figure 33.1 indicates whether the driver or force is largely based on science, technology, policy, regulations and standards (which are of course, in some sense, policy-related), and business/organization, or social/cultural demands. There is some overlap among the 11 drivers, as indicated by the curly brackets to the left. The X's in the cells also indicate the multiple dimensions that often combine to manifest themselves as particular drivers.

The stakeholders for each of these drivers are somewhat different, although clearly overlapping. Care providers are most concerned with care efficiency, quality, and reimbursement. The patient/consumer is most concerned with personal health and communicating with his or her care provider. Public health, quality managers are concerned about population health and population management. Payers are concerned about individual patients, practice performance, and population-based process and outcomes data. Researchers are concerned with aggregate data for a diverse set of needs. The idealized structure for each of these purposes does not exist, and it is hard to see how one can get to it from the existing legacy systems, primordial personal health record initiatives, and patchworks of big data repositories.

In this section, we'll weave in the chapters in this book that are pertinent to our discussion, and outline some approaches that are being advocated, which could have the potential to converge on a unified model to meet the needs of these different categories of stakeholders. But again, as noted, while the science and technology goals are within reach, the timing will be greatly affected by leadership or lack thereof at the policy level, public/social support, and aligning incentives for coordinated effort. Several books have appeared recently about these trends [23, 44, 46]. We will briefly examine each of the 11 trends in terms of its implications for health IT system of the future, and then in the next section consider how they may come together over the next 10 years.

### 33.2.1   Precision Medicine

The terms *individualized* or *personalized* medicine are now referred to as *precision medicine*, in part due to recognition that we are not always truly getting down to the level of the "N of 1", where all patients are unique, although that remains the idealized goal. In the U.S., precision medicine has risen to the level of a Presidential initiative [36]. At heart, it is about harnessing the details of a person's innate biology (genomics), expression profile, phenomic characteristics, and environmental factors (together, constituting the other "omics"), to identify precise risks, disease states, and treatments. When one approaches these highly substratified cohorts, even if not the N of 1, the usual model of evidence-based medicine derived from population-based randomized clinical trials is no longer possible. One must be able to do highly specialized subcohort selection, analysis, and prediction, and must rely on increasingly large databases of gene variants and expression profiles such as the Million Veterans Biobank [15], NHGRI ENCODE project [10], national- or international- scale deep phenotyping initiatives [13], and eMERGE network/phenotype definitions [28].

IT implications include access to these databases, analytics, and prediction modeling. Clearly, it will be essential to create and maintain highly detailed clinical decision support resources, and actively use such resources, especially (and already occurring) in pharmacogenomics, and in selection of preventive measures based on risks. The importance of personal choice in such matters was dramatically demonstrated by the highly publicized "Angelina effect" of a well-known movie star having had prophylactic bilateral mastectomies because of BRCA1 positive gene mutations and having gone public about it [34].

### 33.2.2   Biosensors

We are seeing an explosion of fitness and other lifestyle monitoring tools, home health devices, and new and emerging technologies for breath analysis of peptides/metabolites, immunosignature analysis, lab-on-a-chip, and home instruments such as otoscopes and ophthalmoscopes. There is increased ability to do "lifelogging", as pursued by Quantified Self zealots [26], but which is becoming more mainstream, as apps provide continual situation awareness (in terms of our location, movement, environment, and social setting/friends/circles).

As individuals collecting such data (or perhaps in the future gaining access to it from third parties that are collecting it on us), we will increasingly need and want to have robust tools for dealing with and interacting with this potential mountain of data – tools for personal analytics, personal record banks and data management, integration with provider tools for notification and decision support, and motivational tools for adhering to lifestyle, health, and disease management regimens. We will come back to the personal record/data management issue in the next section.

### 33.2.3 Patient Engagement

Over the past decade or so, personal health records (PHRs) never really found a strong business case as stand-alone activities, and in fact, most health data access by individuals is managed through portals to enterprise health care systems. The latter are largely unidirectional, focusing only on episodes when the individuals are actually patients, and – even in these settings – with little opportunity to integrate data of the patient or his/her sensors, with EHR data or data from other care sites. The number of mHealth apps is growing rapidly, with some 40,000 identified as available through online app stores as of 2014 [35], although most are rarely used. Large IT companies like Microsoft, Google, Apple, and Samsung have all bet on the growth of wearables and sensors as driving this. Indeed the Consumer Electronics Show [4] each year has massive sections devoted to this area of innovation. Apple Inc. recently announced its HealthKit [9] as a platform for developing health apps and integrating sensors and other devices in a consistent framework. An intriguing announcement from Apple of an open ResearchKit platform [38] promises to enable thousands or even millions of smartphone users to sign up for clinical trials using devices that they are already carrying, creating an unprecedented opportunity for quickly generating large quantities of data for analysis. (See Chapter 22 by Zhu and Cahan for a look at the IBM vision for the "wearable revolution" and telehealth; as well as Chapter 13 by Watson for an example of how the digitization of care delivery has already redefined "point of care" to be geographically dispersed and wherever the patient is.) Patients are clearly having more opportunity for empowerment, and this is brilliantly reflected in Topol's new book, *The Patient Will See You Now* [45]. Topol points out that personal users (as patients or not) will be the primary force in driving change of health care to a health system and a lifetime continuous person-centric (patient-centric) activity.

Returning to the topic of personal health records, Yasnoff and colleagues have advocated a health record bank [48], a third-party resource that manages one's data. In Chapter 20 Yasnoff presents the need for a tool that can aggregate all records and patient data over the person's lifetime; and critiques prior efforts to provide such tools. Early business models for the health record bank concept relied on subsidies from advertisers and support to providers for their EHRs if compatible with and continually updating the health record bank data resource. However, I believe that collection and amassing of personal data from sensors, trackers, and other apps, will soon, if not already, be widely recognized as needing data management capabilities, and it will be clear that separate proprietary clouds (or storing the data locally) for all these sources are not feasible.

Therefore, it can be predicted that there will be an expanding effort to develop standards for interoperability, integration, and management of the data, and business models for providing these capabilities on a broad basis to the public. Concomitant with that will be the evolution of methods to integrate such data with providers as needed. An essential component, as addressed in a large part of the ONC draft 10-year vision [39] and the JASON report which influenced it [25], is the need for robust security and privacy protection, using role-based authentication and authorization controlled by the user (consumer or patient).

We will come back to this point later, but these future data management capabilities will clearly be one of the more impactful trends if and when it occurs, since it will change the primacy of data for health and healthcare from the enterprise-focused EHR to the patient-centric continuous (and greatly enhanced) lifetime record. EHRs will evolve to become views of and contributors to those data, combining them with applications that overlay health care organization/practice-specific business processes, business logic, and workflow processes and annotations thereof.

Other aspects of patient engagement involve greater access to knowledge, in the form of education and decision support, use of social media, and capabilities for shared decision making with the provider. The latter promises in the future to be a much more even rather than lopsided exchange, as has been the case to date, and tools to support it are needed.

## 33.2.4   Big Data

We have alluded to two major contributors to the growth of big data – namely precision medicine largely based on the growth of omics, and the predicted explosion in use of personal sensors and tracking devices. Let us consider several other contributors to big data: imaging data, natural language processing extraction from notes, and workflow/process tracking of care activities and outcomes. Lastly, various registries for tracking patients with specific conditions or treatments are being amassed across enterprises.

Big data efforts will require increased normalization and standardization of data elements. Major drivers include need for analytics to support care process characterization, outcome measurement, quality assessment and improvement, and risk or outcome prediction, for categories of patients – both for research, population management, and public health. Tracking of patterns can also provide information about changing underlying contributors to health, such as demographic, environmental, and exposure factors, and are needed for biosurveillance, epidemiology, health care resource estimation and projection, and for countless research investigations.

A major potential opportunity for big data analytics that is often overlooked is the ability to harness it for direct care. (Note that at times the data comparison cohort is quite local, and could really be referred to as "small data"). For direct care, the opportunities include use of dashboards and process monitoring tools at the enterprise, practice unit, or individual practitioner level, to identify patients needing attention, to identify areas for process improvement, and to provide individual decision support. An example of the latter is what can be called the "patients like mine" scenario, when there is no adequate knowledge-based decision support, e.g., in a complex patient with multiple co-morbidities. In this kind of situation, the responses of a cohort of maximally similar patients can shed light on the potential benefits of various treatments (e.g., drug A vs. drug B) these patients have had, or the risk/ likelihood of particular outcomes occurring (such as developing an infection, or short-term hospital readmission). This was done over 40 years ago in groundbreaking work in arthritis care beginning in the mid-1970s [14] and cardiac surgery [40] settings, and in other settings since then. But it has not been possible on a wide scale without a much broader effort to normalize and standardize EHR and other health data.

### 33.2.4.1    The Patient Identifier Challenge

A key consideration in achieving the benefits of analytics is how data sources will be assembled and made available. At the heart of this is the need for a reliable way of linking disparate sources of data on a per-patient basis and doing so over time for the patient's own benefit. Further, we need to enable aggregate research to occur as the norm when permission is given, rather than put up obstacles to deliberately prevent it.

This of course argues for the value of a single uniform patient identifier. Even without that, there are legitimate concerns about patient privacy and the dangers of breach. It could be argued that the disparate data sources and non-control over them by the patient are even more likely to be misused than if we had a system with a single identifier, but where access to data is highly coordinated and controlled by the patient, where role-based authentication and authorization is the norm, and where breaches are readily detected and appropriately penalized. Unfortunately, this is a hot-button political issue, and for years, debate has been stymied, not helped at all by the aforementioned breaches, and progress has been impeded by the well-intended HIPAA privacy rules that limit the ability to amass truly useful, updatable, aggregate databases of longitudinal patient data. However, there are signs that this question may yet be re-examined at the national level [30].

In the United States, the pursuit of the science and methodologies of big data analytics in biomedical science and health care is receiving focused attention by the National Institutes of Health and by the National Science Foundation, in several initiatives aimed at data management and curation, modeling, machine learning, and knowledge generation. This area of emphasis will hopefully continue to be a high priority, since it rightfully recognizes the needs for concerted effort.

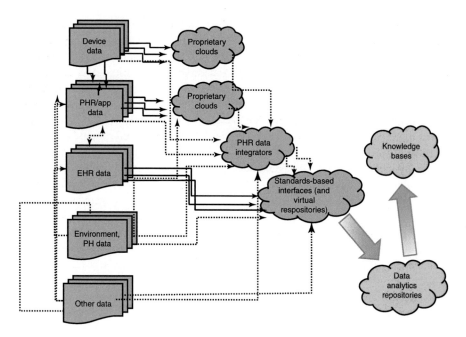

**Fig. 33.2** Data flow issues in considering sources of data, their progressive integration, normalization care processes, analytics, and knowledge generation. An important goal over the next decade is to focus on who the stakeholders are for each progressive step and how to align interests and incentives to yield greatest value along this pipeline

But major dimensions of the advances needed are in the policy and business spheres – around issues of security and privacy, as noted above, around access rights, around adoption of standards, and about aligning of interests to foster the construction of comprehensive data sets. It is clear that this will be a major area of attention in the coming decade. Consider the data flow issues depicted in Fig. 33.2, which demonstrates some of the multiple sources and transformations that need to occur to really get to robust uses of data for multiple purposes. As a society, we need to consider how to create the incentives for achieving these desired data flows and enabling appropriate access to the repositories. We must identify who the stakeholders are, who would operate the repositories, how the efforts would be sustained, and how access and appropriate use would be controlled.

### 33.2.5  Pay for Value

Value in health care is typically defined as quality/cost. That is a good metric for value of a particular service. But when one considers maximizing of health rather than achieving value in healthcare, the goal is to provide the appropriate service mix to maximize health at lowest overall cost. Reynolds and Jones (Chapter 14) and Yuen-Reed and

Mojsilović (Chapter 23) capture the new transformative changes that are driving reimbursement and patient choice changes that focus on paying for value and outcomes.

A major way to create incentives for holistic approaches to health (which includes both health maintenance and disease prevention, and early and aggressive management of healthcare to avoid or delay disease progression) is to reward the participants – the patients and the providers. If the reward system is aimed toward payment for episodes of care and the services received, then one can expect more services, highly optimized and efficiently delivered though they may be. If the reward system pays for keeping people well, or minimizing the effects of disease by early detection, engagement of patients, and active management, then one should presumably get higher overall value.

Reward systems also can be aimed at patients for active self-management and care compliance, such as reduced health care costs in terms of insurance, co-pays and deductibles. There are also strategies for aiming to maximize motivation and behavioral change through artificial challenges, gaming, and social network encouragement.

In the U.S., the Patient-Centered Medical Home (PCMH) model of care, with the primary care provider as the manager of the participation of the care system, and Accountable Care Organizations (ACOs), which use a capitated payment model for care of categories of patients with particular disease conditions and severities, are aimed at creating the dynamic to move to this mode of health/healthcare, with an emphasis on global optimization [22, 37]. However, saying that a transition to this model would be disruptive is an understatement. Hospitals, specialists, and high-technology services are especially at risk if systems that had previously been locally optimized to maximize their operational revenues and efficiencies are now part of a system that seeks to minimize their use for the purposes of global optimization. Also, services that have typically not been reimbursed to providers, such as preventive measures, patient education, email or telephone contact, and remote telecare, and thus tended to be avoided, become highly desirable to perform if the goal is overall optimization. Such approaches also require a high level of care coordination, team communication, patient engagement, and process and outcomes tracking across the entire spectrum of care. Incentives for savings need to be distributed across the participants. To do so optimally requires data on performance and outcomes at a level never previously available, and extending across the venues of care including self-care.

Informatics tools are needed also to enable the processes that facilitate these goals – e.g., to provide focused views on problems, tailored to the care setting, patient, and provider specialty, care pathway guidance and decision support, and a high degree of attention to the transitions of care.

## 33.2.6   Wellness and Prevention of Disease

Related to pay for value, the goal is to broaden the definition of our healthcare system to a "health system". This section is brief, not because it is unimportant but because it is already highlighted as a major overall driver in Sect. 33.1.2. The drive for wellness and prevention of disease means active involvement of the consumer/patient, but also more players, not just traditional care providers. Community-based services, public health, and other entities all have a stake in and bear on this broadened goal. So a challenge is how to engage and incorporate community-based entities, post-acute care providers and the consumer/patient into the ecosystem and information flow.

Also, as noted in the previous section, incentives need to be aimed at this goal of a broader "health system". Use of communication modes by providers that are typically not reimbursed per se – but that can lead to net benefit for the effort expended (such as email, phone, and remote telehealth consults). It definitely means active participation of the individual (which should be encouraged). It requires reward systems such as pay for value as well as incentives to the consumer/patient. And it needs active monitoring and decision support for early detection of deviations requiring attention, and thus active integration with the care system.

As already noted, this area is receiving a lot of attention due to lifestyle and mHealth apps, sensors, wearables, and approaches to begin to integrate them.

### 33.2.7   Meaningful Use

We use the term Meaningful Use as a proxy for a whole variety of top-down incentives and regulations fostering IT adoption. Besides financial and reimbursement models for care itself, government can play a key role in aligning interests by requiring certain levels of compliance in terms of the data, knowledge, and processes of care through IT systems – in order to be eligible for reimbursement, or by providing incentives and penalties (carrot and stick) for adoption of them. Recognizing that adoption of an EHR is not sufficient, the U.S. has defined the concept of Meaningful Use (MU) as a set of functionality that must be used [2, 29]. This set of requirements is being rolled out in a series of graduated levels of capability that must be attested to by health care organizations and providers. The expectations and requirements for MU are being elevated in stages roughly every 2 years, beginning in 2010. Required functionalities and performance include the use of computer-based provider order entry, clinical decision support, health information exchange, patient access to their records, quality monitoring, and public health reporting. The requirements for each of the various criteria start out being rather minimal, such as just demonstrating the presence of one clinical decision support (CDS) rule in Stage 1, to active use of several rules in subsequent stages.

MU has been a strong stimulus for standards adoption, and a lever for adoption of EHR functionality. At the same time, it has created a huge burden for both the EHR vendors and health care organizations and practices to ensure that they are installing and using systems that comply with escalating requirements. Because of the aggressive timetable, MU can perhaps be criticized as having the unintended consequence that it has brought about a hegemony of a few established legacy EHRs, because most other entities don't have the deep pockets to comply with all of these continually changing requirements and at the same time assure that current customers are also able to maintain compliance with current regulations. We will return to the consequences of this later.

### 33.2.8 Usability

As we gain more experience with the "science of implementation", it is increasingly clear that many systems have actually contributed to errors or inefficiencies or frustration, because they have been poorly matched to users' cognitive modes of reasoning, interactive preferences, and workflows. Many usability criteria have been developed, an example of which is the TURF project (Toward a unified framework) and framework of University of Texas Houston [49]. There have been many efforts to build better approaches to user interaction for managing of complex tasks, including problem-specific assembly of needed resources for an encounter, care pathway monitoring and dashboards, visualization tools for viewing trends, and tools for reconciliation of medications, problem lists, allergies, etc. Usability is the focus of Chapters 3 (Ingram) and 9 (Unertl et al).

Usability is an area where there needs to be continual research and innovation. As we shall discuss next, there is also a big opportunity for doing so through the development of apps for desktop or mobile use, if they can be interfaced with and interact with underlying EHR and other data sources.

### 33.2.9 Rise of an App Culture

The tremendous growth of "apps" (self-contained programs used to fulfill a particular purpose, for use on a mobile device such as a smartphone or tablet) and the sheer inventiveness of their design and use in many aspects of our society are testimony to the value of unleashing a platform such as the smartphone that enables this to occur. This has been true in media, finance, social networking, travel, and many other sectors. We noted earlier that although there are thousands of mobile health apps, only a small percentage are used frequently. Most of these are consumer- or patient- facing, and do not interact with the health care system per se, although apps for interacting with medical center patient portals are now appearing.

Health care organizations have sometimes needed to build apps in their own environments to meet various needs of their providers, not addressed by their EHRs per se. In this domain, we refer to apps not only as those on mobile devices but those on desktops. To provide needed functionality, these apps have needed to interact with their EHRs or pull data from secondary data sources such as their enterprise data warehouse, through various ad hoc approaches, and have created somewhat unique "bolt on" solutions. The difficulty of integration has been largely the consequence of the pervasiveness of the major EHR systems, which are legacy proprietary systems that are typically vertically integrated in terms of their data storage in proprietary formats, their tools for managing and editing knowledge and workflow processes, and their applications that use these resources. Communication with outside systems is typically done where necessary by HL7 messaging, and by production and consumption of documents such as those in C-CDA format for HIE [3].

There is some industry-wide movement toward supporting access to EHRs through FHIR (Fast Health Interoperability Resource) APIs – application programming interface – based on an initiative of HL7 that has begun to open up EHR systems to app developers, also discussed in Chapters 27 and 28 [11]. Notable among these are the SMART on FHIR apps that arose from an ONC-supported project to a group at Harvard [42] that enables a number of very well-designed apps to pull data from EHRs and to display lab result trends, analyses, or other useful information. But generally these are read-only, and more complex capabilities including two-way transactions, and orchestration of suites of apps are not able to be supported.

A number of external services are potentially available besides FHIR interfaces, to pull data from different sources, including those from mobile devices and sensors (such as Apple's HealthKit [9] or SamSung's SAMI platform [41]), to provide terminology services, to do authentication and authorization of users, to do master patient lookup, and for performing evaluation of CDS rules (such as OpenCDS [33]), but apps have not yet become easy to interface with EHRs or gained significant traction.

The Healthcare Services Platform Consortium (HSPC) is an organization led by health care organizations but with vendor participation, that seeks to push for more advanced adoption of capabilities for interoperability (see next section) to enable app development to flourish [24]. A main driver is the need to address the use cases of its member organizations not met by their EHRs such as those drivers we cited at the beginning of this chapter – care continuity, connected care, and the use of data analytics in care processes. Other organizations such as the Center for Medical Interoperability [5], the Argonaut Initiative [1], CommonWell [6], and Open Health Tools [31], have related missions. The U.S. Veterans Administration is working toward its next generation architecture, called Vista Evolution [7], which is based on a three-tiered model of an underlying EHR, middle-tier services, and apps on top of them. Conceptually, a model for app use in health care is depicted in Fig. 33.3.

A goal of this disruptive force and the drive for interoperability described in the next section is to enable and foster innovation, and the transition from a vertical, proprietary ecosystem, with interoperability only at the edges, to one in which solutions can be derived based on driving use cases and have the ability to interact with and build on the underlying resources – data, knowledge, and services.

### 33.2.10  Interoperability

The term "interoperability" can mean many things and be described at many levels, yet the term is often bandied about without defining what is meant. The simplest level (foundational interoperability) is the ability to exchange data among systems

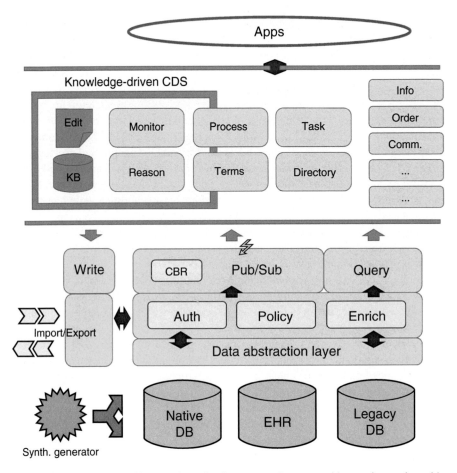

**Fig. 33.3** An example architecture for a development environment with apps integrating with underlying EHRs through middle-tier services (Based on AppWorks architecture [18])

in the form of messages, such as HL7 or HIE (health information exchange) Direct messages. We have already noted that the ability to provide apps to address needs in the healthcare environment not met by EHRs means that they must be able to interact with underlying EHRs and other data sources, to create useful summaries, analyses, or visualizations, and ideally to update the EHRs and submit actions to be performed (e.g., orders and notifications). If the underlying EHRs have similar interfaces, e.g., FHIR APIs, then the apps can have at least that level of interoperability. Data not only needs to be in similar format (structural interoperability) but coded via the same coding scheme (e.g., SNOMED) to achieve consistent meaning (semantic interoperability). Further, the information model needs to be consistent, in terms of the attributes that are associated with the data elements, such as date, specimen type, value type, and units of a laboratory test. Variants of this approach have been referred to as a Clinical Element Models [32] or as Archetypes [43].

To enhance the capabilities of EHRs or their subsystems, or of apps, a variety of services may be useful, invoked by APIs. Examples of typical services are those for access to data via the FHIR model, terminology, enterprise master patient index, record locator, authentication and role-based authorization, infobutton manager knowledge access [8], and clinical decision support. To the extent that these expect data in standard form and return results in similar form, they are interoperable and the applications and/or systems that depend on them are interoperable. Knowledge-based decision support services also need to have a consistent model for describing data elements on which they operate (e.g., a specific medication), and attributes of those data elements (e.g., dose, route of administration).

The ONC draft 10-year vision statement considers interoperability to be a very high priority [39], and attempts to define it. Important functional needs for interoperability relate to the exchange and reuse of data, the sharing of knowledge, and the ability of apps to operate in a variety of settings. An example of the ability to share knowledge spearheaded by ONC was the Health eDecisions (HeD) Initiative which was part of ONC's Standards and Interoperability Framework [21], which created a model-based formalism for representing decision rules, order sets, and documentation templates, and an editing tool for HeD artifacts [19].

It remains to be seen to what extent the three levels of interoperability we have identified above – for data, knowledge, and apps – actually come about. All of these require considerable cooperation among stakeholders, which depends on a compelling business case or "moral basis" for cooperating that does not yet exist. So it will be important for policy makers to consider how best to stimulate alignment of interests.

### 33.2.11   Augmented Guidance

Clinical decision support has had a tortured history, with much promise yet unfilled. Currently, EHRs typically use CDS either by explicitly invoking it or by having it triggered by user actions or background events like processing of a lab test with an above-threshold result. But this means laboriously considering and mapping all rules to the kinds of triggers and modes of interaction that will be most acceptable in particular settings. One size definitely does not fit all (See McCallie Chapter 1), and this need to tailor CDS with "setting-specific factors" has contributed to the multiple variations of similar rules, the time and effort needed to install and test them, and the difficulty in managing corpora of rules with subtle variations within an enterprise [16, 19].

Highly model-based representations of knowledge (such as the HeD editor described in the previous section) enable knowledge artifacts to be thoroughly tagged based on ontology classes and values used to characterize their parts, including descriptions of the settings and contexts in which they are to be used and the intended users. This is important in order to capture the setting-specific factors identified above as well as the problems, domains, settings, and classes of knowledge for maintenance of corpora of decision rule. Knowledge management is a significant challenge faced by large enterprises that must continually update their knowledge bases of hundreds or thousands of knowledge artifacts, where they typically have a number of variations and adaptions of such knowledge embedded in and running in operational settings in their various clinics, practices, and inpatient environments.

But such highly tagged knowledge resources also enable them to be retrieved easily as a function of context and situation. I use the term "augmented guidance" to refer to the ability to enhance all of our actions by situation- aware knowledge and advice. Situational awareness means a combination of context (who the user is, specialty orientation, level of expertise, location/setting, what devices or resources at hand or being used) and specific information about participants and their actions (patient information, including problems, status/degree of stress or urgency, immediate need, and options available).

Thus a possible mode of use, instead of specific triggering, is to always have knowledge that is pertinent to a given situation be available, much like the operation of a GPS (global positioning system), in which restaurant, service station, and ATM (automatic teller machine) nearest one's position on a roadway, or upcoming road hazards, are available and constantly updated as one moves or the situation changes. Infobuttons are a form of knowledge support that uses rather coarse determinations of context, like medication ordering or lab result viewing, but one can see an extension of this approach as ultimately providing highly tailored and pertinent advice. As more and more data about our setting and context can be automatically captured, the feasibility of this mode of CDS will greatly expand [17].

## 33.3 The Next Ten Years: A Projection

To summarize where we are and where we are going, the eleven disruptive factors we have considered above are all in place, and challenge the existing stovepipe EHR model. Some would advocate radical change, e.g., [47]. Yet there is no question that the health care "system" (or non-system) we have will evolve, and that these identified forces will be among the major ones that drive this evolution. But the next several years will be critical in shaping that, so that what results is a **more articulated, integrated health (not just health care) IT framework** for a **more articulated, integrated learning health system**. Weed and Weed's opening chapter for Section IV reviews the imperative for using technology to assist in all aspects of data gathering, decision making and care delivery in a framework that calls for structured documentation, CDS knowledge access, and analytics at point of care for the individual patient; as well as a call to fundamentally change the way we teach and prepare clinicians to practice in this digitized informatics world (Weed and Weed, Chapter 26).

Stakeholders need to take ownership of the future by responding to and helping to refine such proposed models as the 10-year vision of ONC, by forming interest groups and collaborative initiatives that will pursue aspects that are important to them and put resources into those activities. We see the critical factors being:

- The single uniform patient identifier. As highlighted earlier, this would be tremendously enabling, but depends on a concerted campaign and development of robust infrastructure to support the assurances that this would lead to reduced rather than heightened risk of misuse and breach.
- The person-controlled lifetime record. The trend is slow but building inexorably toward this, as we develop better ways to map, import, and synchronize information across venues and/or create virtualized versions of integrated records. When and if a person-controlled record becomes the primary repository against which all others are synchronized or into which they feed depend on whether a compelling business model can be found for creating significant enthusiasm for this among the consumer/patient public, and for the health care organizations and practices to update their data from these sources, by working with the EHR vendors to bring this about.
- Aligning of stakeholder interests around sharing of data. This challenge, as depicted in Fig. 33.2, of data as it moves along the various pipelines from local, proprietary, or device-specific, to more normalized, standardized data with both syntactic and semantic interoperability – will be primarily one of developing business cases for sharing. It is a given that this can only occur with appropriate and strong privacy protections
- The emergence of an app-based health information technology ecosystem. I believe that innovation will continue to be only incremental unless there is freedom to address problems beyond the scope of EHRs by unleashing cadres of informaticians, technologists, entrepreneurs, and investors in developing solutions for addressing the key problems of the transforming health system. We have shown in the previous section how disruptive those forces underlying the transformation are. Incremental change isn't going to address these substantial challenges. App-based ecosystems have begun to exert significant influence in almost every other sphere of society, and have wrought momentous – and largely beneficial – change. Health care is a hold out, but it can't withstand the inevitable and should not.

The above are all business and policy challenges more than technical challenges. In the U.S. we can consider the major drivers for these goals as: (1) the need for patient-centered continuous care management; (2) a focus on prevention, wellness, and active management of disease at early stages and with active patient engagement; and (3) the need for data analytics, to provide measures for assessing and providing feedback on outcome and performance, as a basis for value-based payment, for improved population health, and for many kinds of research. Thus efforts need to focus on how to align the various stakeholders to develop the business cases for longitudinal health records, care coordination, connected care, and cooperative development of the big data resources needed.

Various nations, economies, and cultures may have different priorities and mechanisms for fostering change. In the U.S. we can best foster this both at the individual or organization level and collectively. Individually/organizationally, the main power we have is through procurement language for future IT systems and components being purchased, insisting on interoperability at the various levels we have discussed. Collectively, the main means for fostering change is by creating large-scale and high-impact pilots and demonstrations that show the value that can be achieved, ideally through collaborations that show the power of replicating or sharing of achievements through interoperability; by engagement of key stakeholders in the standards development process; and by activism of prominent health care and health IT leadership to promote these goals at the policy, regulatory, and health care finance levels. We should not ignore the power of the consumer. Topol hits the mark [45] in his projection that the locus of care is on track to become the individual and his/her smartphone and connected devices – as the primary source of data, as the owner and person responsible for allocation of access rights to the data, and as the primary decision maker. This trend may be the most powerful of all.

## 33.4   Conclusion

The future will be quite different – but not all at once. The mantra going forward can be summed up by three words: *integration*, *interoperability*, and *innovation*. As various activities continue to advance through disparate developments and innovations of this field, there will be increasing emphasis on aligning these efforts, making them interoperable, and creating a more integrated ecosystem aimed at optimizing health. The ecosystem will not be new but rather will need to evolve from where we are now. Yet the shifts, e.g., in locus of control from provider to patient-centric, degree of integration of data from multiple sources, and the power of innovation, unleashed through apps and interoperable infrastructure, will be far-reaching – eventually – and the system that results will be quite different. Actually, I do think that 10 years may be a conservative estimate, because the trends are well underway. The future is ours to shape.

## References

1. Argo. HL7 launches joint argonaut project to advance FHIR. 2014. Available at: http://www.hl7.org/documentcenter/public_temp_8104FC82-1C23-BA17-0C7BF0F6526CE7DA/press-releases/HL7_PRESS_20141204.pdf. Accessed 21 Mar 2015.
2. Bendix J. Meaningful use 2: 2013's interoperability challenge. Connectivity barriers remain as physicians move from EHR implementation to data exchange, communication. Med Econ. 2013;90(18–19):24–7.
3. CCDA. Implementing Consolidated Clinical Document Architecture (C-CDA) for meaningful use stage 2. 2013. Available at: http://www.healthit.gov/sites/default/files/c-cda_and_meaningfulusecertification.pdf. Accessed 21 Mar 2015.
4. CEA. Future delivered: 2016 international CES. 2015. Available at: http://www.cesweb.org/. Accessed 21 Mar 2015.
5. CMI. Center for medical interoperability. 2015. Available at: http://medicalinteroperability.org/. Accessed 21 Mar 2015.

6. CommonWell. Why CommonWell Health Alliance: interoperability for the common good. 2014. Available at: http://www.commonwellalliance.org/. Accessed 21 Mar 2015.

7. Cullen T. VistA Evolution. Presentation to World Vista. 2014: worldvista.org/Conferences/conference_presentations/vcm28/VistA Evolution- Terry Cullen.pdf. Accessed 17 July 2015.

8. Del Fiol G, Huser V, Strasberg HR, Maviglia SM, Curtis C, Cimino JJ. Implementations of the HL7 Context-Aware Knowledge Retrieval ("Infobutton") Standard: challenges, strengths, limitations, and uptake. J Biomed Inform. 2012;45:726–35.

9. Developer. HealthKit. 2015. Available at: https://developer.apple.com/healthkit/. Accessed 21 Mar 2015.

10. ENCODE. The ENCODE project: ENCyclopedia of DNA elements. 2015. Available at: http://www.genome.gov/encode/. Accessed 21 Mar 2015.

11. FHIR. FHIR DSTU 1 (V0.0.82): welcome to FHIR. 2014. Available at: http://www.hl7.org/implement/standards/fhir/. Accessed 21 Mar 2015.

12. Fraser H, Wyatt J. International dimensions of clinical decision Support. In: Greenes RA, editor. Clinical decision support: the road to broad adoption. 2nd ed. New York: Elsevier; 2014. p. 241–67.

13. Frey LJ, Lenert L, Lopez-Campos G. EHR big data deep phenotyping: contribution of the IMIA genomic medicine working group. Yearb Med Inform. 2014;9:206–11.

14. Fries JF. The chronic disease data bank: first principles to future directions. J Med Philos. 1984;9:161–80.

15. Gaziano JM. Million veteran program. 2015. Available at: http://www.nih.gov/precisionmedicine/workshop-presentations/day-1/06-million-veteran.pdf. Accessed 21 Mar 2015.

16. Greenes R, Bloomrosen M, Brown-Connolly NE, Curtis C, Detmer DE, Enberg R, Fridsma D, Fry E, Goldstein MK, Haug P, Hulse N, Hongsermeier T, Maviglia S, Robbins CW, Shah H. The morningside initiative: collaborative development of a knowledge repository to accelerate adoption of clinical decision support. Open Med Inform J. 2010;4:278–90.

17. Greenes RA. Clinical decision support: the road to broad adoption. 2nd ed. New York: Elsevier; 2014.

18. Greenes RA, Boxwala A. AppWorks – an innovative design and delivery tool for interoperable health apps. 2015. Available at: https://sites.google.com/site/appworkshealth/home. Accessed 21 Mar 2015.

19. Greenes RA, Sottara D, Haug PJ. Authoring and editing of decision support knowledge. In: Zhang J, Walji M, editors. Better EHR: usability, workflow and cognitive support in electronic health records. Houston: University of Texas; 2014.

20. HealthIT. Health IT Quick Stats. Health IT Dashboard. 2015. Available at: http://dashboard.healthit.gov/quickstats/quickstats.php. Accessed 21 Mar 2015.

21. HeD. Health eDecisions homepage. 2014. Available at: http://wiki.siframework.org/Health+eDecisions+Homepage. Accessed 21 Mar 2015.

22. Helfgott AW. The patient-centered medical home and accountable care organizations: an overview. Curr Opin Obstet Gynecol. 2012;24:458–64.

23. Herzlinger R. Who killed health care? In: America's $2 trillion medical problem – and the consumer-driven cure. New York: McGraw-Hill; 2007.

24. HSPC. The healthcare services platform consortium. 2015. Available at: http://healthcaresoa.org/. Accessed 21 Mar 2015.

25. JASON. A robust health data infrastructure. AHRQ publication no. 14-0041-EF, 2015. 2014. Available at: http://healthit.gov/sites/default/files/ptp13-700hhs_white.pdf. Accessed 21 Mar 2015.

26. Krynsky M. Lefelogging/quantified self. 2015. Available at: http://lifestreamblog.com/lifelogging/. Accessed 21 Mar 2015.

27. LHS. Continuous improvement and innovation in health and health care. 2015. Available at: www.iom.edu/learninghealthsystem. Accessed 21 Mar 2015.

28. McCarty CA, Chisholm RL, Chute CG, Kullo IJ, Jarvik GP, Larson EB, Li R, Masys DR, Ritchie MD, Roden DM, Struewing JP, Wolf WA. The eMERGE Network: a consortium of

biorepositories linked to electronic medical records data for conducting genomic studies. BMC Med Genomics. 2011;4:13.

29. Murphy J. The journey to meaningful use of electronic health records. Nurs Econ. 2010;28:283–6.
30. NatPatID. National patient ID system: debate stoked. 2013. Available at: http://www.informationweek.com/administration-systems/national-patient-id-system-debate-stoked/d/d-id/1109314? Accessed 21 Mar 2015.
31. OHT. Improving the world's health and well-being by unleashing health IT innovation. 2015. Available at: http://www.commonwellalliance.org/. Accessed 21 Mar 2015.
32. Oniki TA, Coyle JF, Parker CG, Huff SM. Lessons learned in detailed clinical modeling at Intermountain Healthcare. J Am Med Inform Assoc. 2014;21:1076–81.
33. OpenCDS. Open Clinical Decision Support (OpenCDS) tools and resources. 2015. Available at: http://www.opencds.org/. Accessed 21 Mar 2015.
34. Park A, Kluger J. The Angelina effect. 2013. Available at: http://time.com/3450368/the-angelina-effect/. Accessed 21 Mar 2015.
35. Powell AC, Landman AB, Bates DW. In search of a few good apps. JAMA. 2014;311:1851–2.
36. PrecisMed. FACT SHEET: President Obama's precision medicine initiative. 2015. Available at: https://www.whitehouse.gov/the-press-office/2015/01/30/fact-sheet-president-obama-s-precision-medicine-initiative. Accessed 21 Mar 2015.
37. Reddy J, Kennedy K. From medical home to ACO: a physician group's journey. Healthc Financ Manage. 2013;67:38–42.
38. ResearchKit. Now everybody can do their part to advance medical research. 2015. Available at: https://www.apple.com/researchkit/. Accessed 21 Mar 2015.
39. Roadmap. Connecting health and care for the nation: a shared nationwide interoperability roadmap. 2015. Available at: http://www.healthit.gov/sites/default/files/nationwide-interoperability-roadmap-draft-version-1.0.pdf. Accessed 21 Mar 2015.
40. Rosati RA, McNeer JF, Starmer CF, Mittler BS, Morris Jr JJ, Wallace AG. A new information system for medical practice. Arch Intern Med. 1975;135:1017–24.
41. SAMI. SAMI: a data exchange platform that defines a new paradigm. 2015. Available at: https://developer.samsungsami.io/. Accessed 21 Mar 2015.
42. SMART. SMART: tech stack for health apps. 2015. Available at: http://docs.smarthealthit.org/. Accessed 21 Mar 2015.
43. Tapuria A, Kalra D, Kobayashi S. Contribution of clinical archetypes, and the challenges, towards Achieving Semantic Interoperability for EHRs. Healthc Inform Res. 2013;19:286–92.
44. Topol EJ. The creative destruction of medicine: how the digital revolution will create better health care. New York: Basic Books; 2013.
45. Topol EJ. The patient will see you now. New York: Basic Books; 2015.
46. Wachter R. The digital doctor: hope, hype, and harm at the dawn of medicine's computer age. New York: McGraw-Hill; 2015.
47. Wears RL. Health information technology and victory. Ann Emerg Med. 2015;65:143–5.
48. Yasnoff WA, Sweeney L, Shortliffe EH. Putting health IT on the path to success. JAMA. 2013;309:989–90.
49. Zhang J, Walji MF. TURF: toward a unified framework of EHR usability. J Biomed Inform. 2011;44:1056–67.

# Index

© Springer International Publishing Switzerland 2016                                601
C.A. Weaver et al. (eds.), *Healthcare Information Management Systems:*
*Cases, Strategies, and Solutions*, Health Informatics,
DOI 10.1007/978-3-319-20765-0